Principles of One Health for a better planet

Principles of One Health for a better planet

Edited by

Barbara Häsler,

Asta Tvarijonaviciute

and

Sara Savić

CABI

CABI is a trading name of CAB International

CABI
Nosworthy Way
Wallingford
Oxfordshire OX10 8DE
UK

Tel: +44 (0)1491 832111
E-mail: info@cabi.org
Website: www.cabi.org

CABI
200 Portland Street
Boston
MA 02114
USA

Tel: +1 (617)682-9015
E-mail: cabi-nao@cabi.org

A catalogue record for this book is available from the British Library, London, UK.

ISBN-13: 9781800622982 (hardback)
9781800622999 (ePDF)
9781800623002 (ePub)

DOI: 10.1079/9781800623002.0000

Commissioning Editor: Alexandra Lainsbury
Editorial Assistant: Emma McCann
Production Editor: Rosie Hayden

Typeset by Straive, Pondicherry, India
Printed and bound in the UK by Bell & Bain, Glasgow

Contents

Contributors

Alberto Muñoz-Prieto, Interdisciplinary Laboratory of Clinical Pathology, Interlab-UMU, Campus of Excellence Mare Nostrum, University of Murcia, Murcia, Spain and Internal Diseases Clinic, Faculty of Veterinary Medicine, University of Zagreb, Zagreb, Croatia.

Alexander Navas Panadero, Faculty of Agricultural Sciences, Universidad de La Salle, Bogotá, Colombia.

Ana Gloria Fonseca, NOVA Medical School, Campo Mártires da Pátria Lisbon, Portugal; Department of Medicine, Hospital Garcia de Orta, Almada, Portugal, Network for Ecohealth and One Health (NEOH).

Ana Maria Castro, Faculty of Agricultural Sciences, Universidad de La Salle, Bogota, Colombia.

Anaïs Léger, Federal Food Safety and Veterinary Office, Switzerland.

Angel M. Kennedy, Faculty of Health Sciences, Simon Fraser University, Burnaby, British Columbia, Canada.

Asta Tvarijonaviciute, Interdisciplinary Laboratory of Clinical Pathology, Interlab-UMU, Campus of Excellence Mare Nostrum, University of Murcia, Murcia, Spain and Network for Ecohealth and One Health (NEOH).

Barbara Häsler, Veterinary Epidemiology Economics and Public Health Group, Department of Pathobiology and Population Sciences, Royal Veterinary College, London, United Kingdom and Network for Ecohealth and One Health (NEOH).

Barry J. McMahon, UCD School of Agriculture & Food Science, University College Dublin, Dublin, Ireland and Network for Ecohealth and One Health (NEOH).

Brigitte Bagnol, Department of Infectious Disease and Global Health, Cummings School of Veterinary Medicine at Tufts University, Boston, USA and Network for Ecohealth and One Health (NEOH).

Caoimhe Doyle, UCD School of Agriculture & Food Science, University College Dublin, Dublin, Ireland.

Catharina B.M. Maassen, Centre for Infectious Disease Control (CIb), National Institute for Public Health and the Environment (RIVM), Bilthoven, The Netherlands and Network for Ecohealth and One Health (NEOH).

Christina Pettan-Brewer, School of Medicine and Center for One Health Research, School of Public Health, University of Washington, USA. UNEP Nature for Health (N4H) TAG, International Alliance against Health Risks and Wildlife Trade Steering Committee, CABI One Health Executive Editorial Member and Federal Schools of Minas Gerais (UFMG) and Parana (UFPR), *Faculdade Pontificia Catolica* (PUC), One Health Brasil (ABRASUNI) Brazil, OHLAIC/CYTED Latin America.

Claire Lajaunie, Inserm, LPED (IRD-Aix-Marseille Université), Marseille, France and Strathclyde Centre for Environmental Law & Governance, Strathclyde University, Glasgow, Scotland and Network for Ecohealth and One Health (NEOH).

Claire Martin, UCD School of Agriculture & Food Science, University College Dublin, Dublin, Ireland.

Craig Stephen, McEachran Institute, Nanoose Bay, British Columbia, Canada.

Cyril Caminade, Earth System Physics Department, The Abdus Salam International Center for Theoretical Physics, Trieste, Italy; Institute of Infection, Veterinary and Ecological Sciences, University of Liverpool, Liverpool, UK.

Dai Nakae, Department of Medical Sports, Faculty of Health Care and Medical Sports, Teikyo Heisei University, Chiba, Japan.

Daniela Figueroa, Carrera de Medicina Veterinaria, Facultad de Recursos Naturales y Medicina Veterinaria, Universidad Santo Tomás, Santiago, Chile and One Health Latin America, Ibero and The Caribbean Network (www.ohlaic.org).

Daniele de Meneghi, Department of Veterinary Sciences, University of Turin, Turin, Italy and Network for Ecohealth and One Health (NEOH).

Deborah J Thomson, One Health Lessons, Arlington, Virginia, USA and Network for Ecohealth and One Health (NEOH).

Diana Rosas Morales, Doctoral student of Social and Political Sciences at the University of Liège, Liège, Belgium.

Didier Wernli, Global Studies Institute, University of Geneva, Geneva, Switzerland and Network for Ecohealth and One Health (NEOH).

Dominic Travis, The Marine Mammal Center, Fort Cronkhite, Sausalito, USA.

Elena Boriani, EB consult, Hellebæk, Denmark and Network for Ecohealth and One Health (NEOH).

Gabrielle Laing, Unlimit Health, London, United Kingdom and Network for Ecohealth and One Health (NEOH).

Gillian Penn, Colorado School of Public Health University of Colorado, Denver, USA.

Glen Cousquer, University of Edinburgh, Edinburgh, Scotland, UK.

Grace Patterson, Department of Population Medicine, Ontario Veterinary College, University of Guelph, Guelph, Canada.

Hamisi Msagama, One Health Society, Dar es salaam, Tanzania and Network for Ecohealth and One Health (NEOH).

Hans Keune, Faculty of Medicine and Health Sciences, Department Family Medicine and Population Health, Chair Care and the Natural Environment, University of Antwerp, Antwerp, Belgium and Network for Ecohealth and One Health (NEOH).

Ilias Chantziaras, Faculty of Veterinary Medicine, Ghent University, Merelbeke, Belgium and Network for Ecohealth and One Health (NEOH).

Joana Pessoa, Technical University of Denmark, National Food Institute, Kongens Lyngby, Denmark.

John Berezowski, Centre for Epidemiology and Planetary Health, Scotland's Rural College (SRUC), Inverness, Scotland, UK and Network for Ecohealth and One Health (NEOH).

Julie Garnier, Odyssey Conservation Trust, Bakewell, UK and Network for Ecohealth and One Health (NEOH).

K. Marie McIntyre, Modelling, Evidence and Policy Group, School of Natural and Environmental Sciences, Newcastle University, Newcastle, United Kingdom and Network for Ecohealth and One Health (NEOH).

Kevin Queenan, Veterinary Epidemiology Economics and Public Health Group, Department of Pathobiology and Population Sciences, Royal Veterinary College, UK.

Laura Cristina Falzon, Institute of Infection, Veterinary and Ecological Sciences, University of Liverpool, Liverpool, UK and International Livestock Research Institute, Nairobi, Kenya.

Lorena Franco-Martínez, Interdisciplinary Laboratory of Clinical Pathology, Interlab-UMU, Campus of Excellence Mare Nostrum, University of Murcia, Murcia, Spain and Moorepark Animal and Grassland Research Center, Teagasc, Irish Agriculture and Food Development Authority, Cork, Ireland and Network for Ecohealth and One Health (NEOH).

Luís Pedro Carmo, Norwegian Veterinary Institute, Ås, Norway and Network for Ecohealth and One Health (NEOH).

Manuela Vilhena, Mediterranean Institute for Agriculture, Environment and Development & CHANGE (MED), Global Change and Sustainability Institute, Departament of Veterinary Medicine, University of Evora, Evora, Portugal and Network for Ecohealth and One Health (NEOH).

Margarida Simões, Veterinary Medicine Department, University of Évora and Comprehensive Health Research Centre, Portugal and One Health International Network and Network for Ecohealth and One Health (NEOH).

María Guerra-Zúñiga, Department of Public Health, School of Medicine, Universidad de Valparaiso, Valparaiso, Chile.

Martin Hitziger, Section of Epidemiology, Vetsuisse Faculty, University of Zurich, Zurich, Switzerland and Network for Ecohealth and One Health (NEOH).

Massimo Canali, Department of Agricultural and Food Sciences, University of Bologna, Bologna, Italy and Network for Ecohealth and One Health (NEOH).

Maurizio Aragrande, Department of Agricultural and Food Sciences, University of Bologna, Bologna, Italy and Network for Ecohealth and One Health (NEOH).

Maya K. Gislason, Faculty of Health Sciences, Simon Fraser University, Burnaby, British Columbia, Canada.

Natalia Cediel Becerra, Faculty of Agricultural Sciences, Universidad de La Salle, Bogota, Colombia and Network for Ecohealth and One Health (NEOH).

Nathaly Jimenez, Association Amazona, Putumayo, Colombia.

Neil Anderson, Royal (Dick) School of Veterinary Studies and the Roslin Institute, University of Edinburgh, Scotland, UK.

Nicolas Antoine-Moussiaux, Faculty of Veterinary Medicine and Faculty of Medicine, University of Liège, Liège, Belgium and Network for Ecohealth and One Health (NEOH).

Parntep Ratanakorn, Thailand National Wildlife Health Center, Faculty of Veterinary Science, Mahidol University, Nakhon Pathom, Thailand.

Patrícia Inácio, LEAF (Linking Landscape, Environment, Agriculture and Food Research Unit), ISA School of Agriculture, University of Lisbon and National Institute for Agrarian and Veterinary Research, IP, Portugal and Network for Ecohealth and One Health (NEOH).

Raffaella Campaner, Department of Philosophy, University of Bologna, Bologna, Italy.

Richard Kock (in retirement) Independent Scholar, Providence House, Green Hill Lane, Harrietsham, Kent, UK; Chief Editor on Research Directions One Health.

Roseanna Collins, UK Health Security Agency, London, UK.

Sara Savic, Scientific Veterinary Institute 'Novi Sad', Novi Sad, Serbia and Network for Ecohealth and One Health (NEOH).

Séverine Thys, ASTRE, University Montpellier, CIRAD, INRAE, Montpellier, France and Network for Ecohealth and One Health (NEOH).

Simon R. Rüegg, Section of Epidemiology, Vetsuisse Faculty, University of Zurich, Zurich, Switzerland and Network for Ecohealth and One Health (NEOH).

Sithar Dorjee, Khesar Gyalpo University of Medical Sciences of Bhutan, Thimphu, Bhutan.

Steve Unwin, Wildlife Health Australia, Canberra, Australia and School of Biosciences, University of Birmingham, Edgbaston, UK.

Thomas Jaenisch, Heidelberg Institute of Global Health (HIGH), Heidelberg University Hospital, Germany; Center for Global Health, Colorado School of Public Health, Aurora, USA and Network for Ecohealth and One Health (NEOH).

Tieble Traore, Emergency Preparedness and Response (EPR) Cluster, World Health Organization, Regional Office for Africa – Dakar Emergency Hub, Dakar, Senegal WHO Regional Office for Africa, Dakkar, Sénégal.

Tithipong Plangsangmas, Chulabhorn Royal Academy, Bangkok, Thailand.

Valentina Suprani, Department of Agricultural and Food Sciences, University of Bologna, Bologna, Italy.

Verónica Ormea, Faculty of Health Sciences, Universidad Peruana de Ciencias Aplicadas, Lima, Peru. Red One Health Latinoamerica, Ibero and The Caribbean Network (y El Caribe - OHLAIC)

Editors' Foreword

We have written this book thinking about our beautiful planet and what we can contribute to preserve it for present and future generations.

The world is facing an unprecedented set of challenges on a planet that is sustaining a huge number of people and domestic animals with rapidly dwindling wildlife populations and alarming reductions in biodiversity. Every day we hear stories about disease, violence, pollution, climate change, inequality, skewed power distribution, and lack of agency of the most affected, the most vulnerable and the most marginalized – including the populations that cannot speak for themselves and require human stewardship.

The challenges that we face are often interconnected and occur in complex systems where an action can have a multitude of effects – both intended and unintended. But too often still we try to fix complex problems in complex systems with simple solutions. The linear and siloed thinking that is so common nowadays is the result of increasing specialization and reward systems that incentivize silver bullet solutions with clear cause and effect messages. Combined with the technological progress that has allowed many of us to disconnect from nature, many people have grown to believe that there will be technical fixes to the most pressing problems. However, if we want to disentangle and address the multifaceted and integrated drivers of the problems we are seeing, we need to act and think differently.

We know that tinkering is not enough and business as usual has failed and continues to fail us. Many before us have said that we need to embrace holistic and interdisciplinary approaches that recognize the intricate web of interactions in our socio-ecological systems. But how do we break free from the many silos and structures that hold us back and impede the innovations, adaptations and changes that we need? One Health is one of the several approaches available that is supporting systemic solutions, collaborations, thinking and acting in interconnected ways, and seeing ourselves as integral parts of natural systems where each one has a role to play and consequently a responsibility. One Health can help us to break down silos, expand our minds, reach out to others and embrace the complexity, variable perspectives and uncertainty that comes with letting go of the safety of one's comfort zone. We are mindful of the fact that One Health is not a panacea, but we believe that it can help us achieve solutions for better health for all.

This book is about opening your mind to new possibilities that come with One Health. We have written it to facilitate the acquisition of competences that help you connect with others, learn together, question and critique, reflect, be emotional, and link up efforts systematically so that we can make progress. It is led by the Network for Ecohealth and One Health, NEOH (formerly the COST-funded Action Network for Evaluation of One Health), and created by many NEOH members, collaborators and friends.

Our entry-level book aims to contribute to your One Health literacy and to encourage you to look at problems in a different way, embracing the untapped potential stored in collaboration and thinking in systems. We have put it together as multi-author teams with diverse people who have varying skills, knowledge, experience and expertise. This not only allowed us to create a book for people who would like to learn more about One Health, but also gave us all an opportunity for reflection and our own learning. You find in this book a richness of different perspectives that we encourage you to explore even if it may feel uncomfortable at first. We hope that our book helps you to complement your existing skills and knowledge with new competences that unlock new pathways for you to do things differently and that it empowers you to facilitate collective action, foster resilience, and promote sustainable practices that benefit both present and future generations.

Barbara Häsler, Asta Tvarijonaviciute, Sara Savić

Quality Assurance

Here is an overview of the quality assurance process followed for this textbook:

1. Conceptual outline development: Initially, all editors and authors collaborated to create a conceptual outline tailored to the target audience, outlining objectives and predicted content.
2. Publisher review: The book proposal underwent a review by the publisher to assess its viability and alignment with market needs.
3. Feedback integration: Feedback from the publisher and any other initial reviews was incorporated, and the conceptual outline was refined accordingly.
4. Chapter alignment: Regular meetings were held among the editors and authors to ensure that individual chapters were cohesive, complementary, and aligned with the nine core competencies defined for the book.
5. Author teams, first draft and editorial review: Authors prepared the first draft of their chapters. Chapters benefited from multi-author inputs based on the authors' expertise and knowledge; an effort was made to be inclusive. The draft chapters underwent an in-depth editorial review conducted by at least two of the three editors. This step focused on content accuracy, consistency, adherence to the outlined objectives and chapter alignment.
6. Author revisions: Review comments were communicated to the authors, who made necessary revisions to adjust the content based on the editorial feedback.
7. External and internal review: The revised version was sent to external reviewers from the target audience to gather unbiased feedback. We made sure to select people from different fields, regions of the world, gender, and level of seniority. The external reviewers were asked to judge the following:

- Is the chapter accessible for an entry-level learner? If there are sections that appear not accessible, please mark them in the file/add a note.
- Does the flow work (is it logical)? If not, please point that out in the file.
- Is learning made easy? If not, what could be improved?
- Does it allow you to achieve learning on the competencies that have been ticked?
- Is the content comprehensive and accurate as far as you can judge given your current knowledge?

Additionally, at least one internal reviewer from the author group provided feedback. The internal reviewers were instructed to comment on the following:

- Is the content comprehensive, accessible and accurate?
- Does the chapter align with your own chapter and are the messages consistent?
- Are cross-references included correctly?
- Does the chapter explicitly facilitate learning of the competences that have been ticked at the beginning of the chapter?

Authors were encouraged to connect for these cross-chapter reviews to align messaging and facilitate exchange and learning. An additional editorial high-level check was performed concurrently at this stage, and further comments were provided as needed. For Chapter 1, a review was invited from a senior One Health expert to ensure accuracy of the content.

Chapters that ticked the competency 'social, cultural and gender equity and inclusiveness' were further reviewed by the gender group of the Network for Ecohealth and One Health to ensure consistency across the book.
8. Final version preparation: Authors incorporated the feedback from both internal and external reviewers (and editors where relevant) to prepare a final version of their chapters.
9. Final editorial check and submission: A final editorial check was conducted to ensure that revisions were done appropriately and final files were submitted to the publisher for editing and typesetting.
10. Proofreading: All chapters were subjected to careful proofreading by the chapter authors and the editors.

Artificial Intelligence (AI) use and statement

No generative AI was used in the writing of this book for the majority of the chapters, apart from Chapters 1, 10 and 13 where AI was used to suggest a few short paragraphs that were then reviewed and manually revised by the authors and for the creation of images in Chapter 16.

For the majority of chapters, AI-based tools like Microsoft Editor, Grammarly or Deeple were used in order to check grammar and spelling. Two chapters also made use of Google Translate to check certain sentences where the authors were unsure if they had captured the meaning as intended. The authors reviewed and revised all content as needed and take full responsibility for the content of their chapter.

The authors of Chapters 5, 8 and 12 expressively prohibit any entity from using their chapter for purposes of training AI technologies. The authors of the other chapters reserve all rights to license uses of this work for generative AI training.

Acknowledgements

We would never have been able to bring this book to the light of day, if it wasn't for the people believing in One Health and supporting it. Thus, we are most grateful to the very many lead authors and co-authors who provided their skill, expertise and enthusiasm to this book in-kind.

It was important for us to publish this book as an open resource to help facilitate wide access. This was made possible through the generous financial support provided by the Interlab-UMU Research Group at the University of Murcia for the publication fee and smaller contributions made by the Network for Ecohealth and One Health (NEOH) and the Royal Veterinary College for the cover and icon design. We thank Martin Dudek (Not a Binary World, https://notabinaryworld.com) for the beautiful designs of the cover and icons and Jeanne Peter (University of Zürich, Switzerland) for the skilful creation of the One Health implementation cycle figure.

We would also like to thank CABI who provided a discount for their open access as part of their commitment to One Health.

Moreover, we are greatly indebted to our external reviewers and contributors who agreed to support our book by sharing with us their skill, insights and time, and providing valuable feedback – at times within a very short time window! They were selected and approached to have a good geographic distribution and cover different backgrounds and expertise. The majority of them also represented the target audience.

- Kurt Arden (United Kingdom)
- Praise Adeyemo (Nigeria)
- David João Cordeiro Fernandes (Portugal)
- Evan Griffith (United States of America)
- Fairouz Larfaoui (Italy)
- Valeria Moreno Garcia (Colombia)
- Jessica Myers (United Kingdom)
- Helena Ngowi (Tanzania)
- Dirk Pfeiffer (Hong Kong SAR)
- Amira Preure (Switzerland)
- Eleanor Raj (United Kingdom)
- Stéphane de la Rocque (Switzerland)
- Evelyn Segredo (Uruguay)
- Sean Sum (Singapore)

We are also very grateful to all the chapter (lead) authors who engaged in cross-chapter review and provided useful comments and suggestions.

Lastly, we express our gratitude to everyone practicing and advancing One Health, providing inspiration and valuable examples in pursuit of more sustainability and a better planet.

Introduction

1 Why and How to Use This Book

Welcome to 'Principles of One Health for a Better Planet'!

We have designed this textbook as an entry-level resource for a diverse audience encompassing undergraduates, postgraduates and professionals who possess a foundational knowledge and understanding of relevant disciplines or fields such as public health, human health, animal health, environment health, medicine, and are interested in exploring the intersection of these disciplines with wider integrative aspects. Whether you are a researcher, clinician, practitioner or policy maker, this book provides an entry point to the holistic and interconnected world of One Health.

Understanding the complexity of One Health and its intersection with policy requires a thoughtful and accessible approach. We recognize that our readers bring diverse backgrounds, experiences and levels of expertise. Therefore, we aimed to make this book accessible to a wide and mixed audience who have tertiary education or equivalent experience or knowledge, but do not (yet) know much about One Health. With this book, we are aiming to give you an opportunity to gain essential competencies related to the principles, practices and ***policy*** dimensions of One Health so that you can complement your existing skills, values and knowledge.

To guide your learning, we have structured this book around nine key competencies elaborated in the Network for Ecohealth and One Health (whose members have led the creation of this book) and detailed in Laing *et al.* (2023). These competencies serve as a roadmap for your learning, ensuring that you develop essential skills for navigating the dynamic landscape of One Health.

In this book, we focus particularly on connective and underlying competencies that can be useful for any One Health initiative, e.g. surveillance, education, research or interventions targeted at any type of specific problem, such as infectious disease, pollution, biodiversity loss or antimicrobial resistance. They can complement or be complemented by technical skills in alignment with your professional needs (e.g. epidemiology, microbiology, sociology, computational or other skills). We offer a structured learning approach based on pedagogical principles to help you gain a One Health foundation upon which you can build in the future should you be motivated to continue your One Health journey.

We have pulled together the different chapters in multi-author teams to make use of the rich experience and expertise available in the One Health community. Because the book has been led by members of the Network for Ecohealth and One Health, which is mainly a European network with global links, we have a predominance of European authors with the corresponding cultural, societal and worldview influences. Wherever possible, however, we made a conscious effort to collaborate with colleagues from around the world to bring in broader perspectives, interpretations and examples. Because of the multitude of authors, you will find different writing styles in this book, but all chapters follow the same basic principles to guide your learning as explained below.

2 Core Competencies Covered

The foundational or core competencies covered in this book are shown in Fig. 1 (Laing *et al.*, 2023). You might learn about them now to see how the book is structured and make a note of how you understand them. Each competency is briefly described below based on the

DOI: 10.1079/9781800623002.0001

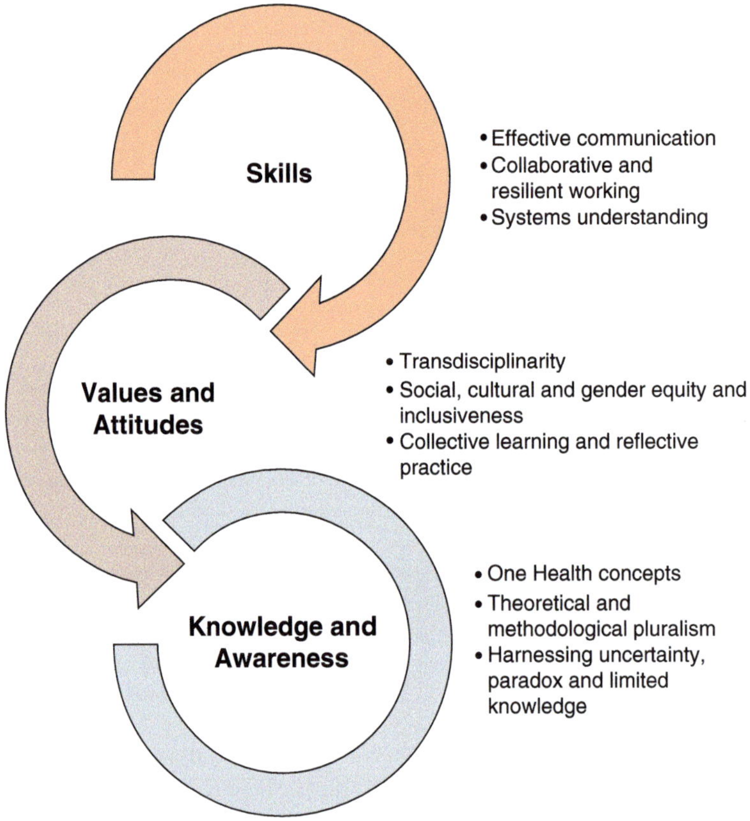

Fig. 1. Nine core competencies covered in this book grouped by skills, values and attitudes, and knowledge and awareness. From Laing *et al.* (2023), unchanged (CC4 BY 4.0 DEED; https://creativecommons.org/licenses/by/4.0/).

details provided in Laing *et al.* (2023). We appreciate that at this stage you may not yet grasp the full meaning of these competencies, but the content of the different chapters will cover these topics in depth. Later on, once you have engaged with the content of this book, it might be helpful to return to this chapter and see whether and how your understanding of the competencies might have evolved.

2.1 Effective communication

Effective communication is pivotal in One Health, where collaboration spans diverse ***sectors*** and societal groups. Different communication models exist that are helpful for One Health, including the transaction model that highlights that communicators are both senders and receivers, integrating social, relational and cultural contexts into dialogues. In One Health, this is crucial for seamless transdisciplinary collaboration, where co-generating and negotiating meaning is essential.

Communication barriers, including language, physical, emotional, cultural, interpersonal and gender barriers, are common in One Health. For instance, sectoral and disciplinary cultures create communication gaps, while gender and cultural differences shape power dynamics.

A One Health competent individual is acutely aware of these barriers and possesses skills such as public speaking, cultural and gender awareness, active listening, and media training. These skills are indispensable for overcoming communication challenges, fostering collaboration and effectively conveying complex One Health concepts. Effective communication is the linchpin for successful collaboration and the advancement of One Health in a globally interconnected and multidisciplinary landscape.

2.2 Collaborative and resilient working

Effective One Health practitioners demonstrate the ability to collaborate seamlessly with diverse partners, fostering a common understanding and shared goals. Treating others with courtesy, sensitivity and respect is paramount in navigating the innate diversity of approaches, people and perspectives in One Health.

The dynamic nature of One Health challenges demands rapid adaptation to new information, changing conditions and unexpected obstacles. Competence in conflict management and quick recovery is often essential. When working together, we ideally manage differences rather than eliminate or ignore them, allowing collaborators to choose forms of collaboration relevant to their needs. Establishing common goals and defined responsibilities enables network success in specific outcome-driven scenarios.

Resilient approaches to One Health challenges involve adaptive capacities and collaborative governance. Literature indicates that increased adaptive capacity, coupled with collaborative governance, enhances resilience to interlinked and multiscale changes. Emotional resilience is imperative when working across disciplines and sectors, and requires acknowledging and working through a range of emotions that might arise when differing perspectives are coming together and potentially clash. This includes negative feelings, emphasizing the ability to adapt under challenging circumstances and recover from adverse emotions.

2.3 Systems understanding

One Health competent persons comprehend the intricate interconnections between humans, animals, plants and ecosystems. They study these dynamic influences, managing boundaries across scales and identifying stakeholders within complex adaptive systems.

Approaching situations with systems thinking, it is possible to identify relevant elements, relationships and interactions. This involves recognizing patterns and conducting analyses across scales, allowing a nuanced understanding of problems as they emerge. One Health explicitly addresses the multiple interconnections between the health of all living beings within shared environments, viewing health as a dynamic property emerging from interactions within complex adaptive systems.

One Health competent individuals can uncover underlying structures and mechanisms by identifying temporal and spatial patterns in various contexts. They adapt to perpetual changes in complex systems by continuously shifting boundaries and perspectives, ensuring a comprehensive understanding of evolving issues. The systems thinking mindset extends to teams and projects, where embracing a dynamic approach is encouraged.

2.4 Transdisciplinarity

In transdisciplinarity we transcend disciplinary and sectoral confines to engage in seamless collaboration across diverse societal groups. This competency is rooted in the collective pursuit of solutions, emphasizing the synthesis of many forms of knowledge from different groups and transformative social engagement.

Multiple key characteristics of transdisciplinarity have been described that underscore the interplay between knowledge integration and social transformations. At its core, transdisciplinarity requires individuals to navigate the complex interplay of different perspectives, knowledge forms and problem conceptualizations as they are presented from different groups that are affected by a problem or interested in understanding or tackling it.

In essence, transdisciplinarity calls for a re-evaluation of the way we work, urging professionals to embrace collaborative efficiency over isolated achievement. It encourages a shift towards collective, holistic problem solving in pursuit of meaningful societal impact.

2.5 Social, cultural and gender equity and inclusiveness

Understanding and fostering equity and inclusiveness in multiple health contexts is another core competency in One Health. This involves acknowledging and incorporating considerations of gender, culture and the inherent interconnectedness between human, animal, plants and the environment.

Equity and inclusiveness, within the One Health framework, extend beyond human realms to encompass all living beings. An inclusive and biocentric perspective helps overcome barriers in the One Health space, such as a human-centred view contributing to ecological crises and gender and cultural discrimination leading to health disparities.

This competency challenges a human-centric perspective on nature and health, gender discrimination, cultural biases, societal homogeneity, and the reliance solely on technological solutions. It underscores the interconnectedness of social, environmental and health crises, and highlights the need for an inclusive approach rooted in justice, integrity and the recognition that humanity is an integral part of nature.

2.6 Collective learning and reflective practice

Demonstrating collective learning and reflective practice involves a commitment to continuous self-assessment, recognizing personal values, and maintaining a humble and active stance as a continual learner.

In One Health, reflective practices underscore the importance of incremental learning from each new experience. Lifelong learning is emphasized, acknowledging ambiguities and uncertainties that come up when dealing with complex problems. Some One Health projects have institutionalized self-reflective processes (e.g. as part of project evaluations) to drive changes in collective learning and practice. Even experiences that yield small learning opportunities can provoke incremental changes in behaviour and foster adaptability to different circumstances.

Reflective practice encompasses a detailed understanding of situations, emotional responses, critical review and future insights, and helps to have an improved awareness of how to integrate one's knowledge into One Health practices. The active acquisition of competencies by individuals is facilitated by a community ethos of self-reflection, promoting a culture of continual learning within the One Health community.

2.7 One Health concepts

A One Health competent individual possesses a deep understanding of various One Health theories, frameworks and methods. The concept of One Health has evolved from a mere mindset to a comprehensive approach, underpinned by diverse theories such as collaboration, communication, transdisciplinarity, collective learning and systems thinking. The continuous expansion of knowledge in this field reflects the dynamic nature of complex health problems and emerging perspectives.

As the definition of One Health has evolved, so has the body of literature, including economic considerations and evaluation methods relevant to issues occurring at the human–animal–plant–environment interface or in socio-ecological systems. A One Health practitioner equipped with knowledge of these evolving definitions, theories, frameworks and methods can navigate the diverse landscape of One Health activities. Informed choices grounded in nuanced understanding and evidence-based justifications become possible, aligning actions with the ever-expanding body of One Health knowledge.

2.8 Theoretical and methodological pluralism

The coexistence of diverse theories and methods requires practitioners to comprehend, apply and integrate knowledge, theories and ideas from diverse forms of knowledge. One Health, by its nature, draws from a multitude of disciplines and stakeholder perspectives, necessitating a nuanced understanding of ontology, epistemology and philosophical perspectives.

The competent One Health practitioner appreciates the fundamental elements of ontology, addressing what can be known; epistemology, exploring how knowledge is created; and the influence of philosophical perspectives on action choices. The understanding of relationships between truth, models, beliefs and the legitimacy of reasoning processes is crucial. This awareness allows for the moderation and collaboration across the plurality of theories and methods, fostering their coexistence.

In practice, One Health professionals adept in methodological and theoretical pluralism facilitate the synthesis of evidence from various sources. They navigate diverse epistemic and ontological standpoints, including local and indigenous knowledge, fostering a comprehensive system understanding.

2.9 Harnessing uncertainty, paradox and limited knowledge

Effectively managing the inherent complexity of One Health demands an understanding of the incomplete and uncertain knowledge base associated with these complex problems. One Health challenges, characterized by diverse stakeholder perspectives and interlinked complexities, extend beyond technical solutions, requiring adaptive mindsets and behaviours suited for complex systems.

One Health problems are usually inherently wicked (i.e. are difficult to define, have many stakeholders with varying interests, and lack a clear solution due to their ambiguous nature and evolving characteristics), existing within unique contexts and spanning diverse domains, making traditional technical solutions insufficient. Data limitations and time constraints further complicate decision making, necessitating a trade-off between timely action and an acceptable decision base for stakeholders. A One Health competent person navigates uncertainty and ambiguity and facilitates effective decision making.

A One Health competent individual further recognizes the incompleteness of knowledge and gains a meta-perspective on challenges, appreciating the potential for emerging solutions from diverse viewpoints while respecting that some positions may be incommensurable.

3 Where the Competencies are Covered

The One Health core competencies are addressed in different ways throughout the book, as you can see in Table 1. By re-visiting the core competencies multiple times in relation to diverse topics, you can deepen your learning. It also gives you the opportunity to engage with different perspectives on the same topic and reflect on differing interpretations.

The topics covered in the book are all contemporary topics as they relate to the current understanding of One Health and are essential to the advancement of One Health. While the chapters are structured primarily with the core competencies in mind, they go beyond that to look at relevant technical, social, policy, governance, economic and evaluation aspects with the view to facilitate the design, implementation and improvement of One Health. In each chapter, apart from the theoretical content, there are questions, thought-provoking activities and applied examples waiting for you to help you acquire the competencies in a practical way.

The introductory chapters trace the historical trajectory of One Health, Ecohealth and Planetary Health, setting the stage for an in-depth analysis. We then provide a comparative examination of One Health and Ecohealth in relation to other integrated approaches to health. The nuanced discussion provides insights into the unique strengths and contributions of these frameworks within the broader health landscape.

Inter- and transdisciplinarity in One Health takes centre stage in another section, highlighting the importance of collaborative approaches in addressing complex health challenges. Knowledge integration, both in the realms of science and decision support, emerges as a critical theme. A detailed exploration of a Data–Information–Knowledge–Wisdom framework offers a structured approach to solving intricate One Health problems, highlighting the need for a holistic perspective.

The practical aspects of One Health intervention and implementation, professional reflexivity, and reflective practice are carefully examined, providing valuable insights into the operationalization of One Health initiatives. Evaluation approaches for One Health initiatives, along with economic considerations, policy, governance and gender equality, are introduced and discussed.

The book expands its scope to encompass the intersections between One Health and Sustainable Development Goals, biodiversity conservation and ecosystem services. It further explores the social determinants of

Table 1. Overview of the nine core competencies and where they are addressed in the book.

Competency	Chapter number
1. Effective communication	6, 7, 10, 11, 14, 16
2. Collaborative and resilient working	1, 2, 3, 4, 7, 9, 10, 11, 14
3. Systems understanding	2, 4, 7, 8, 9, 10, 11, 12, 13, 15
4. Transdisciplinarity	1, 3, 4, 7, 8, 9, 10, 11, 15
5. Social, cultural and gender equity, and inclusiveness	1, 7, 8, 9, 10, 11, 14, 16
6. Collective learning and reflective practice	1, 2, 3, 4, 6, 7, 9, 11, 12, 14, 15, 16
7. One Health concepts	1, 2, 7, 11, 12, 13, 16
8. Theoretical and methodological pluralism	2, 3, 4, 11
9. Harnessing uncertainty, paradox and limited knowledge	4, 5, 6, 7, 11, 13, 14

health at the human–animal–ecosystem interface, acknowledging the interconnectedness of these elements.

Closing chapters delve into the concept of bringing 'One Health' home, emphasizing its relevance and applicability in local contexts. Overall, the book offers theoretical insights and practical guidance for addressing contemporary health challenges from a holistic perspective.

4 Navigating the Textbook

Our structured and modular approach enables you to study at your own pace and in the way that works best for you. Each chapter is crafted to build on the previous one, ensuring a gradual and cohesive exploration of One Health concepts and competencies. Despite the gradual increase in complexity and connectivity of topics, the chapters can also be studied individually depending on your interests and experience. At the beginning of each chapter, you will find the following information that will help you to navigate the content easily:

- Elevator pitch
- Book objectives to which the chapter relates
- One Health competencies covered
- Learning outcomes
- Summary

In each chapter, you also find the following icons to help you navigate the content and facilitate your learning:

Key term: Key terms are important words or phrases highlighted within the main text of the textbook, critical to understanding the main concepts and topics discussed in the chapters. They will be in dark blue and in CAPITALS, as well as being flagged using the key term icon, e.g. ONE HEALTH.

Glossary terms are words or phrases with definitions and explanations for these terms that are usually specialized terms that not everyone might understand and that are used regularly throughout the book. A glossary helps you understand the content better. These words will be dark blue and bold, e.g. **wellbeing**, and you will find them explained at the end of the book. A key term that is also in the glossary will be dark blue, bold and in CAPITALS, e.g. **HEALTH**.

Key concept: A key concept refers to an essential idea, theory or principle that is critical for understanding the broader topic. These concepts provide an important foundation for acquiring the core competencies and guide your learning throughout the book.

Activity: There are several learning questions, exercises and reflexive intermissions woven throughout the text to enhance understanding and application. For each activity, an example answer is usually provided to help you see how the activity could have been conducted. However, because there are very many possible ways of answering a question or conducting an activity, these example answers are just given as guidance. They serve to provide ideas and viewpoints that you may not have considered, and they allow you to reflect on your own answer. Besides the yellow icon, activities are also marked with a yellow background highlight.

Applied example: In each chapter, you will find case studies and examples that illustrate how theoretical knowledge is applied in practical, context-specific situations. At least the first paragraph of the applied example has a green background highlight.

To bridge theory with real-world application, we provide insights from practitioners, policy makers and researchers who have successfully navigated the challenges and opportunities within the One Health landscape. This contextualization helps you envision how the principles discussed in this textbook translate into action within diverse professional settings.

Our book invites you to explore, engage and contribute to the advancement of One Health. Whether you are taking your first steps into this interdisciplinary realm or are refining or expanding your existing knowledge, we hope that this book becomes a good companion in your One Health learning journey.

Reference

Laing, G., Duffy, E., Anderson, N., Antoine-Moussiaux, N., Aragrande, M. *et al.* (2023) Advancing one health: Updating core competencies. *CABI One Health* 2023, 1–13.

1 Introduction and Evolution of One Health, Ecohealth and Planetary Health

Sara Savić[1,2], Angel M. Kennedy[3], Hans Keune[2,4], Thomas Jaenisch[2,5], Gillian Penn[6], Barbara Häsler[2,7], Margarida Simões[2,8], Maya K. Gislason[3] and Christina Pettan-Brewer[9]

[1]Scientific Veterinary Institute 'Novi Sad', Novi Sad, Serbia; [2]Network for Ecohealth and One Health (NEOH); [3]Faculty of Health Sciences, Simon Fraser University, Burnaby, British Columbia, Canada; [4]Faculty of Medicine and Health Sciences, Department Family Medicine and Population Health, Chair Care and the Natural Environment, University of Antwerp, Antwerp, Belgium; [5]Heidelberg Institute of Global Health (HIGH), Heidelberg University Hospital, Germany; Center for Global Health, Colorado School of Public Health, Aurora, USA; [6]Colorado School of Public Health, University of Colorado, Denver, USA; [7]Veterinary Epidemiology Economics and Public Health Group, Department of Pathobiology and Population Sciences, Royal Veterinary College, London, UK; [8]Veterinary Medicine Department, University of Évora and Comprehensive Health Research Centre, Portugal and One Health International Network; [9]School of Medicine and Center for One Health Research, School of Public Health, University of Washington, USA, UNEP Nature for Health (N4H) TAG, International Alliance against Health Risks and Wildlife Trade Steering Committee, CABI One Health Executive Editorial Member and Federal Schools of Minas Gerais (UFMG) and Parana (UFPR), Faculdade Pontificia Catolica (PUC), One Health Brasil (ABRA-SUNI), Brazil, OHLAIC/CYTED Latin America

Contents

 Principles of One Health for a better planet (eds B. Häsler, A. Tvarijonaviciute and S. Savić)
DOI: 10.1079/9781800623002.0002

Chapter Overview

Elevator pitch

Health is not confined to individual beings, but encompasses the delicate balance of ecosystems, animals, humans and plants. This chapter helps you to understand the meaning of One Health. We also take you on a journey through time, tracing the roots of the One Health approach and looking at how it has evolved dynamically to tackle complex and interconnected issues of sustainability and balance, including health. We explain how One Health and Ecohealth are related and how they have changed over time, and where convergence points are where they deviate.

Book objectives the chapter relates to

- ☑ 1. Understand what One Health and Ecohealth mean
- ☑ 2. Think in a One Health and Ecohealth way
- ☐ 3. Apply One Health and Ecohealth in their professional and personal life
- ☐ 4. Know how to share One Health and Ecohealth knowledge
- ☐ 5. Integrate One Health and Ecohealth knowledge actively
- ☑ 6. Acquire or enhance core One Health competencies

One Health competencies covered

- ☐ 1. Effective communication
- ☑ 2. Collaborative and resilient working
- ☐ 3. Systems understanding
- ☑ 4. Transdisciplinarity
- ☑ 5. Social, cultural and gender equity and inclusiveness
- ☑ 6. Collective learning and reflective practice
- ☑ 7. One Health concepts
- ☐ 8. Theoretical and methodological pluralism
- ☐ 9. Harnessing uncertainty, paradox and limited knowledge

After having worked through this chapter, you will be able to understand what One Health and Ecohealth mean and how they have evolved over time.

Learning outcomes

1. Understand what One Health problems are and how the One Health approach can be useful to tackle them.
2. Comprehend the meaning of the terms One Health and Ecohealth, their similarities and differences.
3. Highlight the moments in history when the concepts of One Health and Ecohealth gained public recognition.
4. Evaluate critically how One Health and Ecohealth changed over time and what communities they are speaking to.

Summary

The realization that the health of people, animals and the environment are connected has been pivotal to human survival since time immemorial and is sustained in the present day by Indigenous Peoples around the world and communities whose health and wellbeing is directly connected to the natural world. Within modern science, however, it has only been in the last several decades that integrated approaches to health have gained formal recognition and begun to shape policy and practice domains around the world. In this chapter, you will explore the emergence and evolution of One Health and learn about and reflect on the contemporary understanding of One Health. We highlight the importance of participatory and transdisciplinary work rooted in systems thinking and the power of using these approaches to address global health challenges such as malnutrition, disease emergence or pandemics. The evolution of One Health within the context of the development of complementary and synergistic approaches such as Ecohealth and Planetary Health is presented. You will look at their similarities and differences and consider the contributions that the various orientations can make to strengthening health and wellbeing around the world. Because it is important to understand where we have been and what has led to where we are today, we also present a historical timeline of the development of One Health and Ecohealth and highlight key events that fostered sharing, collaboration and transdisciplinary work in service of addressing interconnected human, animal and ecosystem health challenges.

1.1 Health, Disease and One Health

The **One Health approach** recognizes that the health of humans, animals, plants and the environment[1] is closely linked and interdependent within the environments they share and shape across time and space (Adisasmito *et al.*, 2022; RSC, 2022).

While there are a variety of ONE HEALTH definitions, notions of **health** more broadly are also varied. For example, individualized notions of health generally refer to the overall **wellbeing** and harmonic functioning of an individual's (whether animal or human) physical, mental and behavioural states and the degree to which they can lead a fulfilling life within their species-specific context. Health goes beyond the absence of disease or illness and includes the presence of positive factors that contribute to quality of life, equity and wellbeing. Health in humans and non-human animals[2] (subsequently called animals in this book) can be conceptualized at the level of individuals or populations. However, definitions of intersubjective health, for example the relational production of health across human–animal interactions, is less often formally defined. Moreover, a definition of health for animals as an intrinsic state of being remains poorly defined. Furthermore, when extending the definition of health to the **ecosystem** the notion of individuality is de-centred and the functioning of the unit as a whole is foregrounded. For example, the health of the ecosystem can be defined as 'the extent to which the environment is able to function, maintain biological and chemical processes, and adapt to change or cope with the impacts of human activity' (FAO *et al.*, 2022).

To understand **HEALTH** and wellbeing, it is important also to understand the continuum of states of being that include **pathological states or disease**, which are terms used to describe a deviation from normal physiological functioning in an individual, leading to a disturbance in its health and wellbeing. Disease refers to a specific condition or disorder that adversely affects structure or function, resulting in recognizable signs, symptoms, and often a negative impact on the individual's overall wellbeing (Boorse, 2011). Diseases can manifest in various ways and are caused by a wide range of factors, including infectious agents (such as bacteria, viruses and parasites), genetic mutations, environmental factors, poor diets, and a combination of these factors. Some diseases are acute, have a sudden onset and a relatively short duration, while others are chronic, persisting over a longer period. The term disease is not commonly used to describe the health of ecosystems or **environment** in the same way it is used for individuals or populations. Ecological systems can, however, experience disruptions, imbalances and degradation that are analogous to diseases in living organisms. Significant disturbances that lead to a decline in the functioning of ecosystems and the environment and the communities they sustain include **biodiversity** loss, pollution, resource depletion and **climate** change (Dornelas, 2010).

There are differences in how different **disciplines** and practitioners conceptualize health and tackle disease or disturbances. Paradigmatically, the differences can be attributed to the historical and disciplinary perspectives that have shaped how to view health. For example, human health has traditionally been the primary focus due to the centrality of humans in society (except in Indigenous communities). Medical science and healthcare have evolved to prioritize human wellbeing, resulting in a robust framework for measuring and addressing human health issues. Similarly, veterinary medicine acknowledges that animals, like humans, have their own physiological, behavioural and health-related needs that require specialized knowledge and care. However, as our understanding of ecological systems and interdependencies has grown, an increasing need has emerged to address complex health challenges that transcend traditional boundaries, prompting the development of One Health and **Ecohealth** and other integrated approaches to health, which recognize the links between humans, animals and plants within the ecosystems.

A One Health problem is a multifaceted challenge that transcends the boundaries of the health of humans, animals, plants and the ecosystems. When it involves multiple species, complex interactions between humans, animals and the environment, shared determinants (including social factors), and interconnected systemic influences and necessitates collaborative, holistic solutions, then the use of a One Health approach is indicated. One Health problems include: **zoonotic diseases** (where **pathogens** are transmitted between animals and humans in both directions); antimicrobial and anti-parasitic resistance; food safety; vector-borne and neglected tropical diseases; climate change; pollution; biodiversity loss; food system crises; non-communicable diseases; and malnutrition. Finding optimum solutions for many of the most important health challenges facing humanity has proven to be difficult. Effective solutions to some of these challenges remain elusive for many reasons, including their complex or wicked nature, siloed approaches to addressing these problems, and our lack of a complete understanding of them. Integrated approaches to health offer concrete ways to advance thinking, practice and policy formation.

- **Complex problems** involve multiple interconnected causes, factors, variables, components and effects that cause their complex nature. These factors cannot be understood and analysed individually or linearly as they interact in nonlinear ways, making them difficult to predict or control. They require creativity, collaboration and critical systems thinking to solve them.
- **Wicked problems** are challenging because of their ill-defined (with no clear starting and ending point) and dynamic nature. They can have multiple possible solutions, yet, given their complexity, efforts to solve them tend to produce unintended consequences and **trade-offs** that vary across contexts (Waltner-Toews, 2017).

(One) Health problems can be expressed differently across different scales (e.g. individual, community, population, ecosystem and global scale), temporal dimensions (short, medium, long term; future generations), geographic boundaries (local, national, international), populations and **sectors** (biotic and aniotic environment, humans, animals), and perspectives (e.g. **ecocentric**, **anthropocentric**). It is these characteristics and the dynamic interconnections that make it difficult to understand them comprehensively.

Integrated approaches to health, like One Health or Ecohealth, constitute holistic approaches that consider the interconnected aspects of health including social, economic, environmental, biological and spiritual factors. They involve collaboration among diverse people, including Indigenous knowledge holders, medical professionals, veterinarians, ecologists and policy makers in collaboration with communities, to address complex health challenges. Some authors researching the history and development of One Health conclude that while 'there are movements towards the broader integration of different disciplinary conceptualizations of health, the associated complexity – biological, geophysical and social – remains a challenge' (Assmuth *et al.*, 2020). Yet, by recognizing the intricate relationships between humans, animals, plants and the environment, an integrated approach to health can emphasize the importance of understanding and mitigating the factors that contribute to health issues across multiple dimensions, ultimately leading to healthier populations, ecosystems and global **sustainability**. Integrating the needs, values and opinions of multiple disciplines, sectors and **stakeholders** can prove difficult owing to the complexity of their structures and dynamics, but the urgency and necessity to respond to many emerging and re-emerging health challenges underscores that it is imperative to invest in learning how to do this work well. A growing number of scholars and practitioners, therefore, are advocating for 'investing in a transdisciplinary approach that connects disciplines and communities engaged in coproduction, co-interpretation and co-utilization of knowledge' (see Chapter 3 for more information on **transdisciplinarity**). These authors propose the term 'transdisciplinary health' to signify the need for broad integration across fields and the study of dynamic interaction across research, practice and society as a whole on all scales that range from (and link) the local to global (Assmuth *et al.*, 2020).

Learning questions 1: Think of a One Health problem relevant to your context.

1. Why is it a One Health problem?
2. What kind of One Health problem is it?
3. For whom is it a problem?
4. Is this problem complex or wicked, and if so, in what ways?
5. Who needs to be involved in the attempt of solving it?
6. What are some possible solutions to the problem and how will you know once you have solved the problem?

Example answer: Below is an example answer from a Western Balkan country in Europe. Please note that your One Health problem may be very different depending on the context / your situation as such; please view this as an example from one particular context.

The One Health problem relates to increased spreading of vector-borne diseases in humans and animals in the region. This is due to two factors: (i) the number of vectors is rising in the region (ticks, mosquitoes, sand flies) due to change of climate conditions or, in other words, higher temperatures during summer and longer period of vector activity; (ii) people and animals (mostly pets) are often travelling from and to the region, and in that way increase the possibility of contact with pathogens in vectors. Some diseases are endemic for this region such as Lyme disease, dirofilariasis, West Nile, and some are emerging such as canine leishmaniasis, ehrlichiosis, anaplasmosis, babesiosis and tick-borne encephalitis. Most of these diseases are zoonotic and therefore can be found in humans and animals, but all of them are transmitted by a vector. That is why this is a One Health problem involving human health, animal health (domestic, pets and wildlife) and environment. However, this issue is not systematically investigated at the country or regional levels, but is left for single cases to be resolved, even though reported cases are found in both humans and animals. People and animals (mostly pets) travelling more and more contributes to the problem; this is linked to economic and transport development. When combined with the increasing vector presence, which cannot be resolved, this issue becomes a complex problem. The solution is neither simple nor easy and involves commitment of public health, animal health, environment control, preventive measures and public awareness. The problem would be considered under control if there were no outbreaks of the diseases either in humans or in animals and if preventive measures would be applied in humans and animals, with complete public awareness on how to behave in environments with persisting vectors.

In the next section, the meaning and evolution of One Health and Ecohealth will be introduced to you in more detail.

1.2 The Meaning of One Health

1.2.1 Contemporary understanding of One Health

One Health originated as a formal concept in the mid-1900s with the recognition of the interconnectedness of humans, plants, animals and the influence of the environment they live in, with the key being the importance of collaboration between sectors. It gradually gained attention in the health, science and ecological fields, and in the early 2000s expanded into a commonly used approach to address various interconnected health problems. The One Health approach is used in most health sectors around the world and has gained substantial momentum during the past decade. Ever evolving, it is now a commonly used noun and approach to tackling some of the world's most complex health problems at all levels of society and government, including the UN's **Sustainable Development Goals** (SDGs) (see Chapter 15).

One Health has been defined as an:

> integrated, unifying approach that aims to sustainably balance and optimise the health of people, animals and ecosystems. This recognises that the health of humans, domestic and wild animals, plants, and the wider environment (including ecosystems) are closely linked and interdependent. The approach mobilises multiple sectors, disciplines and communities at varying levels of society to work together to foster wellbeing and tackle threats to health and ecosystems, while addressing the collective need for clean water, energy and air, safe and nutritious food, taking action on climate change, and contributing to sustainable development.
>
> (Adisasmito *et al.*, 2022)

This definition, developed by the One Health High-Level Expert Panel (OHHLEP), was welcomed by the Quadripartite for One Health, i.e. the Food and Agriculture Organization of the United Nations (FAO), the United Nations Environment Programme (UNEP), the World Health Organization (WHO) and the World Organisation for Animal Health (WOAH) and used in their One Health Joint Plan of Action (OH JPA). The OH JPA expresses the joint commitment of the four organizations towards One Health and promotes the mainstreaming of One Health around six interconnected action tracks with objectives, activities and deliverables, namely: (i) enhancing One Health capacities to strengthen health systems; (ii) reducing the risks from emerging and re-emerging zoonotic epidemics and pandemics; (iii) controlling and eliminating zoonotic, neglected tropical and vector-borne diseases; (iv) strengthening the assessment, management and communication of food safety risks; (v) curbing the silent pandemic of antimicrobial resistance (AMR); and (vi) integrating the environment into One Health.

Another definition of One Health is that 'One Health is a collaborative, multisectoral, and transdisciplinary approach, working at local, regional, national, and global levels to achieve optimal health and wellbeing outcomes recognising the interconnections between people, animals, plants and their shared environment' (One Health Commission, 2022). Another one says that 'One Health is people interested in protecting human, animal and environmental health, coordinating, collaborating and communicating to achieve the best health outcomes for our planet' (CDC, 2022). One Health is also seen as a framework to understand the interconnectedness of development problems and to achieve transformative outcomes such as better food, improved ecological services and reduced disease risks (Habib *et al.*, 2022). However, the OHHLEP definition is the broadest and most all-encompassing so far and explicitly integrates the environment. It comes with a set of underlying principles:

1. Equity between sectors and disciplines;
2. Sociopolitical and multicultural parity (the doctrine that all people are equal and deserve equal rights and opportunities) and inclusion and engagement of communities and marginalized voices;
3. Socioecological equilibrium that seeks a harmonious balance between human–animal–environment interaction and acknowledging the importance of biodiversity, access to sufficient natural space and resources, and the intrinsic value of all living things within the ecosystem;
4. Stewardship and the responsibility of humans to change behaviour and adopt sustainable solutions that recognize the importance of animal welfare and the integrity of the whole ecosystem, thus securing the wellbeing of current and future generations; and
5. Transdisciplinarity and multisectoral collaboration, which includes all relevant disciplines, both modern and traditional forms of knowledge and a broad representative array of perspectives.

(Adisasmito *et al.*, 2022)

These five underlying principles form an important element of the One Health definition and summarize essential characteristics that One Health practitioners should strive for. Their application and the resulting effects would ideally form part of One Health monitoring and evaluation frameworks and activities (see Chapter 12 on **evaluation**).

Learning questions 2: Have a look at the underlying five principles of the One Health definition and note for each what they mean for One Health. Do you know what the different terms mean? What are potential implications of these principles for One Health?

Example answer:

1. Equity refers to the concept of fairness, justice and impartiality in the distribution of resources, opportunities and benefits within a society or community. It involves ensuring that everyone has an equal chance to succeed, regardless of their background, identity or circumstances. Equity goes beyond mere equality, recognizing that different individuals and groups may require different levels of support or accommodations to achieve truly equal outcomes (Hirschhorn *et al.*, 2021). Equity between disciplines or sectors refers to the fair and just treatment of different fields of study, professions or sectors within an organization, community or society. It involves ensuring that no discipline or sector is favoured or disadvantaged over others, and that resources, opportunities and recognition are distributed fairly and without bias. This is particularly challenging in One Health, because of the unequal resource availability. For example, the global health expenditures in 2020 were estimated at US$9 trillion (approximately 11 % of global GDP) (WHO, 2023), whereas the expenditures for biodiversity loss were about US$95 billion (OECD) and the animal health expenditures a fraction of that (TEEB, 2018; WHO, 2018, 2023). In comparison, while the human biomass is smaller than those of the other sectors, because of an entrenched existing imbalance in how the value of human and animal life is perceived, equity between sectors is hard to achieve. See also Chapter 8 on social determinants, Chapter 9 on **gender** and Chapter 15 on SDGs.

2. Socio-political and multicultural parity refers to achieving fairness, equality and representation in terms of social, political and cultural aspects within a diverse society. It encompasses creating a balance in power, influence and opportunities for individuals and groups from different backgrounds, ensuring that all voices are heard and valued in decision-making processes and societal structures. It includes giving a voice also to disadvantaged, disempowered and marginalized groups, which requires the establishment of participatory engagement processes, which is linked to transdisciplinarity (Chapter 3).

3. Socio-ecological equilibrium refers to a state of balanced and harmonious interaction between humans, animals and the environment within an ecosystem. This concept recognizes the intricate interdependencies and relationships that exist among these components and emphasizes the importance of maintaining this balance for the wellbeing of all living beings. It values biodiversity, equitable access to resources, and the intrinsic worth of all life forms and emphasizes sustainability, stewardship and a holistic perspective to ensure that interactions within the ecosystem are responsible, inclusive and supportive of long-term wellbeing. There are very wide and often diverging views on which living beings have intrinsic values and what the magnitude is of such value. Consequently, moving towards a common value understanding is a major challenge in One Health. See Chapters 10 and 11 for more information on **systems**.

4. Stewardship highlights the human responsibility to modify their behaviour and adopt sustainable practices that prioritize animal **welfare** and the overall health of the ecosystem. By doing so, this approach aims to ensure the wellbeing of both present and future generations, reflecting a commitment to preserving the environment and its inhabitants for the long term. See Chapter 7 on biodiversity and conservation and Chapter 13 on One Health economics (including **valuation**).

5. Transdisciplinarity (Chapter 3) refers to going beyond the boundaries of individual disciplines to address complex problems and challenges. It involves collaboration and integration of knowledge from multiple people, communities and sources of knowledge to gain a comprehensive understanding of a particular issue. It commonly spans multiple groups in society to have a holistic and synergistic collection of perspectives and knowledge that allows for a deeper exploration of problems that cannot be adequately addressed by a single discipline alone. Because of epistemic differences in knowledge this requires an awareness of and application of **knowledge integration** (see Chapter 4 on knowledge integration).

Ideally, One Health constitutes a local, national and global transdisciplinary and practical effort to elevate the health and long lasting of the environment, animals and humans through the principles above and by looking at ecological and other relationships (Coker *et al.*, 2011; Currier and Steele, 2011; Calistri *et al.*, 2012; Buse *et al.*, 2018; Trinh *et al.*, 2018). It calls on the collaboration of researchers, biologists, academics, veterinarians, ecologists, doctors, anthropologists, physicians, zoologists, demographers, agencies, governments and other professionals to promote health (including the health of nature) and sustainability and mitigate interconnected health risks (Day, 2011; Ruscio *et al.*, 2015; Destoumieux-Garzón *et al.*, 2018; Keune *et al.*, 2022). These collaborations can take place in different settings and multiple ways, e.g. disease control, research, policy, funding, community engagement and environmental health movements (Day, 2011; Kingsley and Taylor, 2017).

Because of the many connections between humans and domestic or wild animals and the similarities of the human and animal medical professions, One Health started with collaborations across the human and animal health sectors mainly around medically influenced topics like zoonoses, foodborne disease issues and antimicrobial resistance (AMR). These topics for many are still considered as the priorities of One Health and are the focus of many studies happening at the human–animal–environment interface. There has, however, been an effort in recent years to broaden the One Health concept to include not only central considerations of animal and human health, but also ecology, climate change, agriculture, biodiversity and other social determinants of health (Lerner and Berg, 2017). It has also expanded to include exploration into chronic non-infectious diseases, ecotoxicology and health in built environments (Destoumieux-Garzón *et al.*, 2018; Mackenzie and Jeggo, 2019). A subset of scholarship in the One Health field has further involved recommendations for holistic health interventions that are grounded in several bodies of knowledge, and do not solely rely on purely allopathic (conventional or Western medicine) assumptions (Kingsley and Taylor, 2017). Increasingly, the One Health approach challenges the 'reductionism of biomedical approaches by locating human and animal health within their wider ecological context' (Harrison *et al.*, 2019). To apply the One Health approach practically, researchers must be aware of the relationship between species, groups and ecosystems, as this will 'result in better science' (Lerner and Berg, 2015). As such, several scholars have noted an opportunity to work across the fields of One Health, Ecohealth and **Planetary Health**. The One Health approach has opportunities to work with Ecohealth and Planetary Health approaches, which when consolidated create increased collaborations by 'uniting and strengthening human, animal and environmental health, environmental management, natural resource management, and Indigenous local knowledge' (McFarlane *et al.*, 2019). The similarities and differences between these approaches are explored in Section 1.2.2.

Learning questions 3: One Health has been conceptualized visually in a variety of ways, changing as it has shifted and expanded over its lifespan. Have a look at Figures 1.1, 1.2, 1.3 and 1.4 provided below. They were all developed to depict One Health. How well do they convey the meaning of One Health? Do they resonate with you and why / why not?

Example answer: One Health is often pictured as three entities including: (i) human health, (ii) animal health and (iii) ecosystem, environment or plant health overlapping at the intersection (Figs 1.1 and 1.3). The use of the term environmental health can still be seen in many depictions even though it refers to an anthropocentric[3] concept, namely as the branch of public health 'concerned with studying and regulating factors in the environment that affect human health and disease and those with alleviating detrimental effects; often attributive; (also) the general condition of the natural environment' (FAO *et al.*, 2022). More recent illustrations use the term environment. As One Health has evolved, it has grown to take on a much larger focus incorporating all aspects of health, social, economic and ecological wellbeing including climate change issues, challenges with sustainable urbanization, human migration / climate refugees, and infectious diseases (novel and classic) of humans, animals and plants while recognizing the effect socio-economic status has on all of these factors (Day, 2011). The idea of balance in a **socio-ecological system** is depicted in the right-hand side of Fig. 1.3 where human health, animal health and environment health are embedded within the One Health realm, further highlighting the importance of interconnectedness and dependence. The illustration from Chidawanyika *et al.* (2023) puts the plant health separately from environment in the One Health circle with interconnections between animals, humans, plants and environment, thereby emphasizing

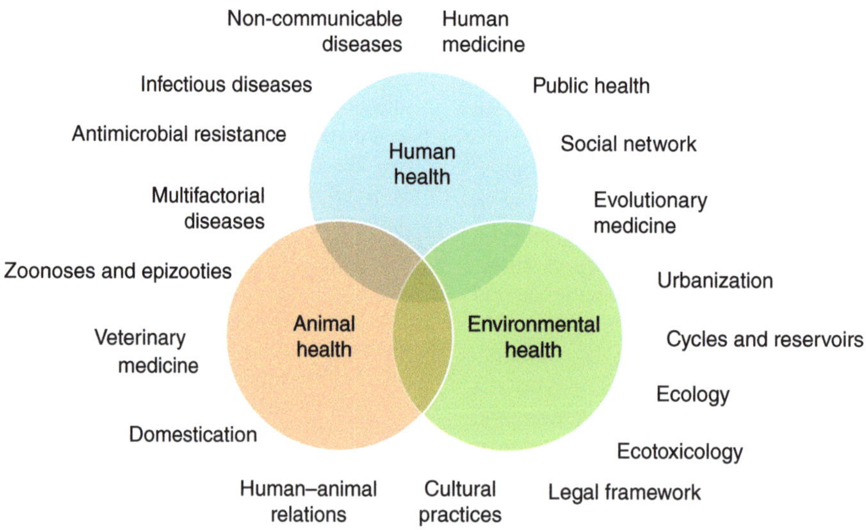

Fig. 1.1. A three-health Venn diagram of synergies and collaboration between animal, human and environmental health in the One Health approach. From Destoumieux-Garzón *et al.* (2018), unmodified (CC BY 4.0 DEED: https://creativecommons.org/licenses/by/4.0/).

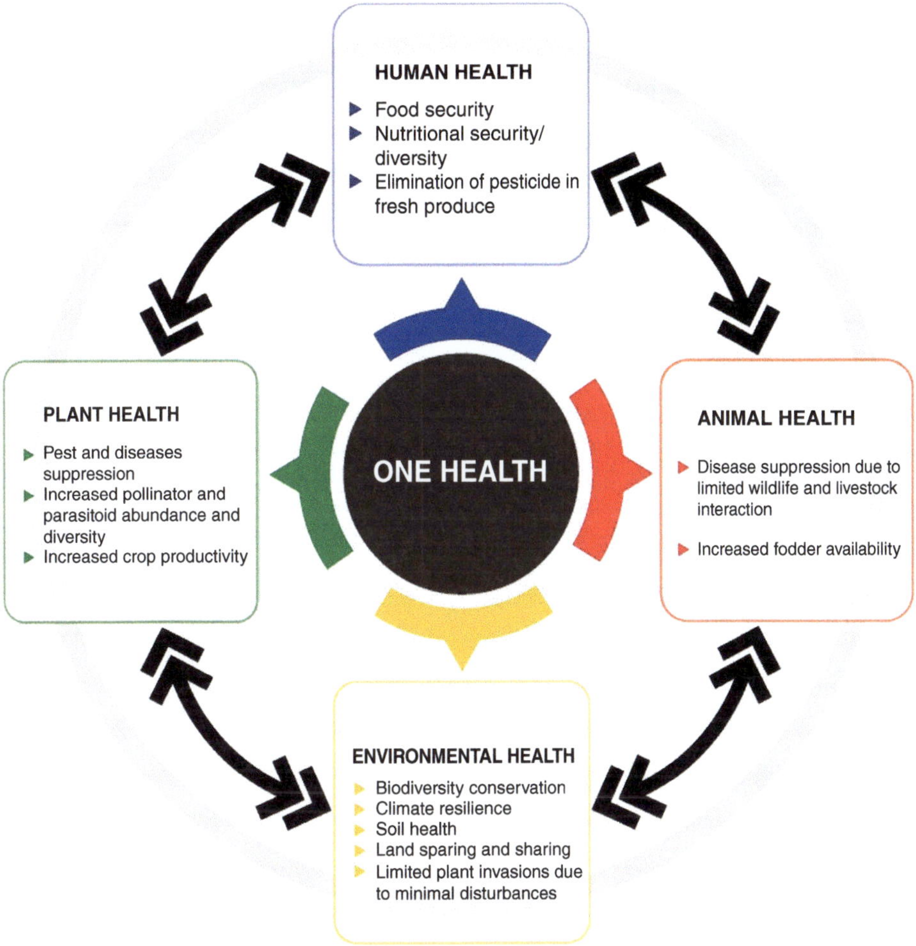

Fig. 1.2. Provisions of the sustainable vegetable integrated pushpull technology (VIPPT) in alignment with the One Health approach. From Chidawanyika *et al*. (2023), unmodified (CC BY 4.0 DEED: https://creativecommons.org/licenses/by/4.0/).

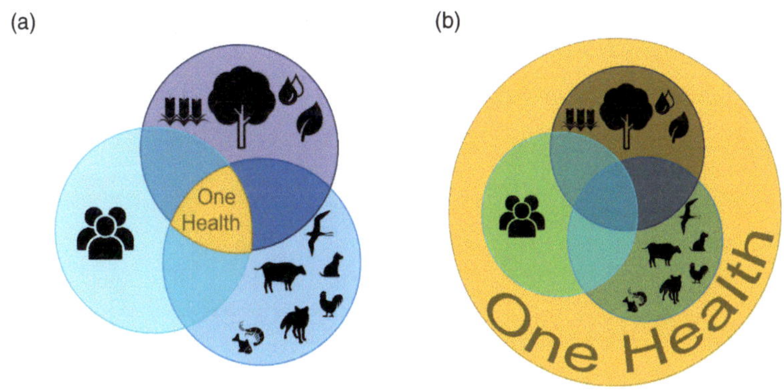

Fig. 1.3. Two streams of One Health that depict (a) a medically oriented stream focusing on the problems at the interfaces, and (b) a socio-ecological balance-oriented stream. From Laing *et al*. (2023), unmodified (CC BY 4.0 DEED: https://creativecommons.org/licenses/by/4.0/).

the importance of the plant health as an equal point within One Health (Fig. 1.2). The OHHLEP illustration in Fig. 1.4 has several of the common elements seen in the other figures, but also embeds working principles of communication, coordination, capacity building and collaboration as well as key principles around inclusivity, equity and access.

An awareness of the environment, animal and human health dimensions of One Health problems is not enough. One Health researchers and practitioners need to be able to recognize 'traps' or 'silos', to identify interconnections and interactions between the dimensions of the problems they work on, and they need specific skills to foster meaningful collaboration and co-production of knowledge between experts, institutions and stakeholders that represent differing paradigms. Global collaborations within the various human- and animal-related health and environmental science fields have led to strengthened relationships between fields, and a more elaborate approach for addressing critical needs (Calistri *et al.*, 2012; Lerner and Berg, 2015). This is particularly important when tackling global challenges that span multiple scales, including sectors (Calistri *et al.*, 2012). As explained by Hueffer *et al.* (2019), One Health's 'proactive, interdisciplinary, constructivist, and collaborative approach promise[s] earlier detection of risks and threats, as well as more effective responses, in part by engaging community level stakeholders in all stages of the process'. Moreover, One Health collaboration can enable the development of common understanding and values, the ability to recognize and deal with trade-offs, and the capacity to develop systems understanding and more sustainable solutions; more information on these topics is provided in Chapters 10–13 where we look at the One Health project life cycle.

Systems approaches are increasingly used to study One Health systems; you will find many examples and references throughout the book. Members of the Network for Evaluation of One Health proposed an integrative systems approach to evaluate One Health initiatives based on four elements that are: '(i) the definition of the initiative and its context; (ii) the description of the theory of change with an assessment of expected and unexpected outcomes; (iii) the process evaluation of operational and supporting infrastructures (the "One Health-ness"); and (iv) an assessment of the association(s) between the process evaluation and the outcomes produced' (Rüegg *et al.*, 2018a, b). Wernli *et al.* (2017) used a systems approach to propose a monitoring and evaluation framework to evaluate progress in the implementation of actions against AMR. Majowicz *et al.* (2018) used causal loop diagrams to map non-traditional stakeholders with whom to

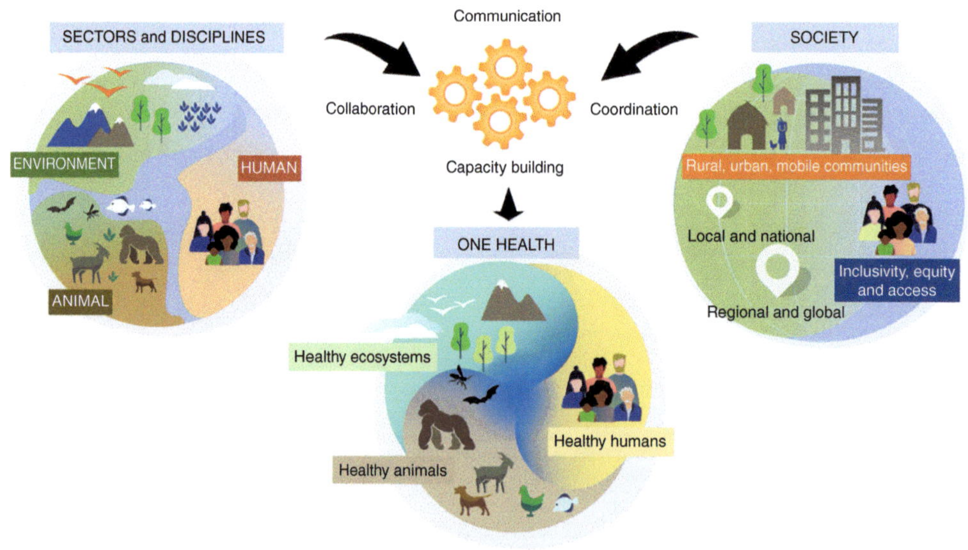

Fig. 1.4. Sectors, disciplines and society coming together in a process of communication, collaboration, coordination and capacity building to achieve healthy ecosystems, humans and animals through One Health. From Adisasmito *et al.* (2022), unmodified (CC0 1.0 DEED: https://creativecommons.org/publicdomain/zero/1.0/).

engage, when mitigating AMR in foodborne pathogens. A systems dynamic approach has been used to understand the relationship between various disciplines in the One Health context (Xie *et al.*, 2017). These examples underline the growing importance of systems thinking for One Health (see Chapter 10 for more information on systems approaches).

Wallace *et al.* (2015) extended the perspective of One Health to include the socio-economic perspective more clearly, in what they termed 'Structural One Health'. They criticized the earlier One Health concept for omitting to address fundamental structural political and economic causes underlying collapsing health ecologies highlighting different characteristics of different health approaches and interventions. Structural One Health involves analysing and addressing social, economic, environmental and political determinants of health that impact both human and animal populations. It recognizes that health outcomes are influenced not only by individual behaviours or biological factors but also by broader societal structures and systems. By addressing structural determinants such as poverty, inequality, environmental degradation and access to healthcare, Structural One Health aims to promote **health equity** and sustainable development while addressing complex health challenges at their roots (Wallace *et al.*, 2015).

1.2.2 Other integrated approaches to health

Although sometimes used as synonyms, the terms One Health, Ecohealth, Planetary Health, **One Welfare** and One Wellbeing represent different concepts linked to the same foundational values. There is some controversy around the similarities and differences of these terms; these aspects are explored in Chapter 2. While for some people these integrated approaches essentially have the same aims and work in a very similar way, others differentiate them based on their historical roots, disciplinary influences, and their **ANTHROPOCENTRIC** (humans at the centre of importance), **ZOOCENTRIC** (special focus on animals and their welfare, including ethics), **BIOCENTRIC** (values all living beings, including animals, and considers their intrinsic worth and rights; recognizes the importance of non-human life forms and ecosystems), or **ECOCENTRIC** (prioritizes the wellbeing of entire ecosystems and the environment as a whole) priorities.

The various integrated approaches to health do not necessarily result in identical definitions of nature and linkages with human health, nor in common framing of challenges and remedies, even if they share rather similar integrative and holistic new notions (Keune and Assmuth, 2018). One example concerns nature-related health effects: one community of experts mainly focuses on nature-related health benefits, and the other mainly on risks that the environment poses to health (Keune and Assmuth, 2018). This may result in different views for practice: either a plea for nature-based solutions as a path to a better future, or treating nature as an extreme danger to human health from which yet unknown threats could emerge and should be avoided. Mutsaers (2015) illustrates the biosecurity framing as 'intervene in the conditions of emergence of the future, before one may be besieged by nature's own act of emergence', out of which, next to development of vaccines, also ethically, culturally and practically harmful interventions may result, like preventative culling of wildlife and domestic animals. In line with One Health concepts such as those from OHHLEP, a balancing of perspectives is needed.

Because different integrated health approaches speak to different communities, which can facilitate successful collaboration and advancement of the field, we are looking here briefly at similarities and differences of One Health, Ecohealth and Planetary Health. For a more detailed description of the historical roots of these approaches, their convergence and divergence and epistemic difference, please refer to Chapter 2.

1.2.2.1 Ecohealth

Ecohealth, or eco (systems) approach to health, is a field based on the premise that human health and wellbeing are dependent on that of the environment (Lebel, 2003). The foundation of Ecohealth is primarily credited to the Canadian International Development Research Centre (IDRC), which supported transformative initiatives in human and ecosystem health with an early recognition that human health is inexorably linked to the environment.

The Ecohealth framework is described as an ecosystem research approach to human health, utilizing an integrated, applied and participatory action methodology (Charron, 2012). It offered a new perspective to managing health in the way ecologists approach problems by relating to natural and environmental resources and also integrating the many anthropogenic components: social, economic and cultural factors (Feola and Bazzani, 2001). This method of solving problems specifically involves those within the community (action–participatory). Six principles guide Ecohealth research, namely systems thinking, transdisciplinary research, participation, sustainability, gender and social equity, and knowledge to action (Charron, 2012). Ecohealth strives to promote the sustainable health of humans and animals through the acquisition of healthier ecosystems and by breaking down the compartmentalization of various policy agendas that are classically in place with an emphasis on integration (Charron, 2012). A basic tenet of Ecohealth is that human and animal health and wellbeing cannot be sustained in a resource depleted, contaminated and socially unstable planet (Lebel, 2003; Charron, 2012). Ecohealth practitioners, therefore, often engage in bottom-up activities that promote sustainable ecosystem health, foster social stability and promote the sustainable and equitable coexistence of humans, animals and the environment. Ecohealth tends to be informed by a constructivist epistemological position, whereby knowledge is considered to be socially constructed. Ecohealth typically recognizes that research is an exercise in knowledge creation (Charron, 2012; Vansteenkiste, 2014), and that researchers themselves are active participants in the generation of subjective 'truths' (Charron, 2012). In this view, knowledge and what is 'true' is considered flexible, temporal and contextually situated. Ecohealth's leaning towards ***CONSTRUCTIVISM*** (people actively create their own understanding and knowledge by building on their experiences and interactions with the world around them) is informed by its transdisciplinary nature, and in particular its tendency to draw not only on the natural sciences, but also on the humanities and social sciences with a goal of creating more just and sustainable solutions (Charron, 2012). More on this topic can be found in Chapter 2.

1.2.2.2 Planetary Health

Planetary Health is an emerging field that focuses on the intricate connections between the health of human populations, the health of ecosystems, and the health of the planet as a whole, all through an anthropocentric lens. While Planetary Health also emphasizes the importance of addressing global challenges such as climate change, loss of biodiversity and pollution in a comprehensive and collaborative manner, it highlights and addresses these issues in how they affect human health. This concept was initially mainstreamed in 2015 with a target audience of 'health professionals' and since has grown in popularity and notoriety with common mention in popular scientific publications. It calls for an integrated approach that considers social, political and economic factors, and acknowledges that solutions to these challenges must be found collectively across disciplines, sectors and nations. It is important to highlight the clear difference between the previous two approaches (One Health and Ecohealth) and Planetary Health: the first two wholly recognize and appreciate an intrinsic value in ecosystem and animal health, while Planetary Health places limited value on inherent values of other systems. Although some discussions in Planetary Health relate to animal health, it is only through their contribution to human health and disease, such as transmission of disease to humans and as commodities (Lerner and Berg, 2017). More on Planetary Health can be found in Chapter 2. The Commission on Planetary Health provided the original definition:

> the achievement of the highest attainable standard of health, wellbeing, and equity worldwide through judicious attention to the human systems – political, economic and social – that shape the future of humanity and the Earth's natural systems that define the safe environmental limits within which humanity can flourish. Put simply, planetary health is the health of human civilization and the state of the natural systems on which it depends.
>
> (Whitmee *et al.*, 2015)

1.2.2.3 Complementarity

The One Health approach is in a reciprocal relationship with Ecohealth. More specifically, One Health's economic analysis components and emphasis on animal health can enrich Ecohealth, and Ecohealth's focus on environmental degradation and over-development can be similarly emphasized by the One Health approach (Harrison *et al.*, 2019). While these two are similar, Ecohealth reminds us of the importance of place-based approaches to problem solving where a ground-up strategy is developed through an equity and sustainability lens. Planetary Health combines both top-down and bottom-up approaches, but has an underlying anthropocentric philosophy, while Ecohealth leans towards ecocentrism and One Health strives for cross-sectorial equity for the purpose of health. All three have experienced a common driver despite arising from different backgrounds and disciplines. One Health originated mainly from a medical perspective, drawn from similarities and common challenges, while Ecohealth was mainly oriented by ecology and conservation actions and Planetary Health driven by the desire to safeguard people and the planet. The creativity to address perceived threats and problems manifested in similar holistic approaches, with a different starting framework but aimed at generating integrated practices and participatory resolutions. They all appeal for paradigm shifts based on the complexity of problems that can only be tackled by multisectoral and collaborative efforts. All concepts and approaches are constantly evolving as their scope of activity and transdisciplinarity also broadens to address the constantly arising health and evolving sustainable issues.

With the environment, systems thinking and participatory aspects more commonly being integrated into One Health, there is an increasing convergence with other integrated approaches to health. None the less, the historical roots continue to influence the character of One Health. The remainder of the book focuses on One Health concepts and **core competencies.** Given the increasing convergence and the need to be equipped to tackle complex or wicked problems through collaboration, transdisciplinarity (for more details, see Chapter 3) and systems thinking, many of the competencies described in the book will also be directly relevant to other integrated approaches.

Learning questions 4: For the One Health problem that you described above in Learning question 1, reflect on the following:

1. What perspective did you use (ecocentric, anthropocentric, zoocentric, biocentric)?

2. What stakeholders (e.g. government officials, implementer, scientists) may be needed to tackle the problem?

3. What perspectives might they bring to the table?

Example answer: Below is an example answer provided from the same region from Learning question 1 in relation to the One Health problem already described previously. Please note that your experience might be different, as it is context-specific and personal.

The chosen perspective was anthropocentric and zoocentric owing to the fact that people and animals are actually in danger of getting sick. The anthropocentric component is probably stronger; an outbreak in humans that is usually seen as 'more important' or 'more visible' than when it occurs in animals. The main drivers of disease reduction are the concern about public health and the associated data that show the negative health impacts on people. Fortunately, activities conducted for reducing vector-borne diseases in humans imply preventive measures in animals, thereby benefiting the animals too. Considerations of costs are a crucial aspect of control. At the moment, all costs of possible preventive measures for animals are from the animal owner's budget. If those costs would be covered from the local government budget, a lot more animals would be likely to receive treatment. Also, if more biological measures were undertaken for vector control that would result in a long run with fewer vectors present. Stakeholders integral to addressing this One Health problem ideally encompass a diverse range of expertise: local government officials, healthcare professionals as well as animal health professionals, environmental scientists, entomologists, green space designers, media and citizens. For example, scientists advocate for an increase in public awareness, presenting the facts about pathogen presence and vector movement, while citizens have an important role in control of disease by reporting every contact with vectors or illness in animals. Collaboratively, these stakeholders navigate the intricate web of factors linking human health, animal wellbeing, environmental integrity and socio-economic considerations, forging comprehensive strategies to mitigate the One Health problem.

1.3 Connections and Synergies Between One Health and Ecohealth – Historical Evolution

Holistic health approaches have been used in practice across various cultures throughout history, e.g. by **Indigenous Peoples** around the world, as stewards of the diverse landscapes and ecosystems that make up this planet since time immemorial. Rooted in traditional knowledge, Indigenous Peoples have supported diverse ecosystems through reciprocal relationships, well before terms like One Health, Ecohealth and Planetary Health were coined. It was not, however, officially or publicly recognized as an approach until recent history. The anthropocentric point of view, with the main principle of human existence has dominated other cultures which were in harmony with nature, but they had less economic power. We have included a historical timeline in the following pages of this chapter to highlight important points in One Health and Ecohealth evolution.

One early record of the principle of One Health is from the Fourteen Rock Edicts, which were tall pillars or large stones placed near roads throughout India around 300 BC (see Point of Interest; Fig. 1.5). Historically, insights of interconnection and health are found in Western philosophy and the development of allopathic medicine and public health. Yet, over the centuries, these holistic insights have been replaced by atomized notions of the body and specialisms focused on discrete systems. This approach has lost touch with the notion of interrelated health that can be found in the original writings of the Greek physician Hippocrates (460–367 BC). In his work 'On Air, Waters and Places, ('Aere, Aquis et Locis'), he identified and described the interdependence of public health with the environment and how all forms of illness had natural causes (Francis Adams, 1849; Miller, 1962). This innovative work appeared during a time when most people attributed diseases to the wrath of gods and superstitions. After that, Aristotle (384–322 BC) introduced the concept of comparative medicine to studies of various epizootic diseases of humans and other animal species, maintaining an integrity with the ecosystem written in a series of books. Later, this material was translated and published in Zurich (1551–1558) and in 1587 became an encyclopaedic 'An Inventory of Renaissance Zoology' by Swiss physician, naturalist, bibliographer and philologist Conrad Gessner (1516–1565). Gessner was a medical doctor and professor at the Carolinum in Zurich, the precursor of the University of Zurich. Nearly 2000 years later, Giovanni Maria Lancisi (1654–1720), an Italian physician, veterinarian and a pioneer epidemiologist, initiated epidemiological strategies to control and prevent diseases such as quarantines, drainage of swamps and vector protection through management for prevention of rinderpest and human malaria. In 1712, Claude Bourgelat, the founder of the first veterinary school of medicine in Lyon, France, established in Europe the interaction between

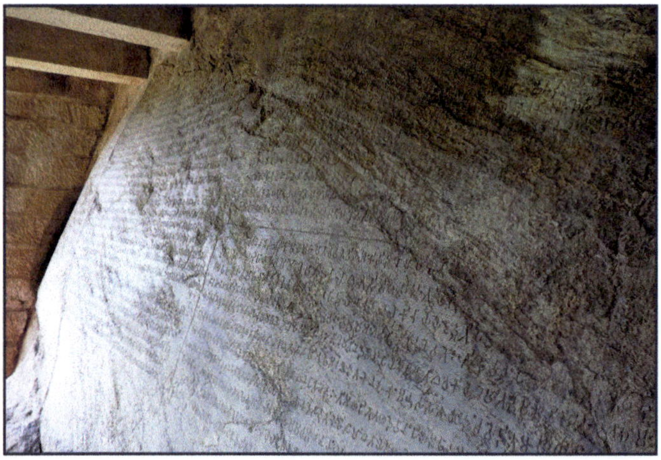

Fig. 1.5. Point of Interest: the Rock Edicts of Ashoka. The Fourteen Rock Edicts are large stones or tall pillars with regulations placed near roads from the reign of King Ashoka (ca 304–232 BC) in India. They provided messages as reminders to the people of how they should adhere to certain principles: '...everywhere has Beloved-of-the-Gods, King Piyadasi, made provision for two types of medical treatment – medical treatment for humans and medical treatment for animals. Wherever medical herbs suitable for humans or animals are not available, I have had them imported and grown. Wherever medical roots or fruits, I have had them imported and grown. Along roads I have had wells dug and trees planted for the benefit of humans and animals' (Dhammika, 1993). From Ankur Panchbudhe (on flickr.com), unmodified (CC BY 2.0 DEED, https://creativecommons.org/licenses/by/2.0/).

animal and human health and subsequently known as public health. In the 19th century, the pathologist Rudolf Virchow, MD (1855) studied *Trichinella spiralis* in swine and recognized the similarities with the disease in people; he coined the term zoonosis and later William Osler, MD (1870) declared his interests in connections between human and veterinary medicine.

In 1947, James H. Steele founded the Veterinary Public Health Division at the Centre for Disease Control. He recognized the connection between health in animals and public health. The Veterinary Public Health Division was particularly important during that time as public health was dealing with zoonotic diseases such as rabies, brucellosis, salmonellosis, Q fever, bovine tuberculosis and leptospirosis. This was the entry door for veterinary medicine into public health.

In the 1960s, Calvin Schwabe, a Doctor of Veterinary Medicine, founded the Department of Epidemiology and Preventive Medicine in the Veterinary School at UC Davis (1966), the first department like this ever in a veterinary school. In 1964, he promoted the collaboration of medical and veterinary workers against zoonotic diseases and used the term 'One Medicine' for the first time, emphasizing a need for collaboration between human and veterinary medicine (Schwabe, 1964).

Ecofeminism developed as a branch of feminism and political ecology. From the concept of gender, the relationships between humans and the natural world were analysed. The term was coined in 1974 by the French writer Françoise d'Eaubonne in her book *Le Féminisme ou la Mort*. Ecofeminism presents a feminist perspective of Green politics calling for an egalitarian, collaborative society in which there is not one dominant group.

In 1992, the International Development Research Centre (IDRC) launched its Health, Society and Environment Program, which explored how environmental factors influence health and brought together specialists from different fields. The IDRC of Canada was very influential in the Ecohealth world at that time.

In 1996, the IDRC created the Ecosystem Approaches to Human Health Program that was eventually shortened and is now known as Ecohealth (2001) and supported Jean Lebel in publishing the first textbook on ecosystem approaches to health in 2003. In the same year, it hosted the International Forum on Ecosystem Approaches to Human Health in Montreal, Canada.

In 2004, the *EcoHealth* journal was launched. Also in 2004, the influential 12 'Manhattan Principles of One Health' were published by the Wildlife Conservation

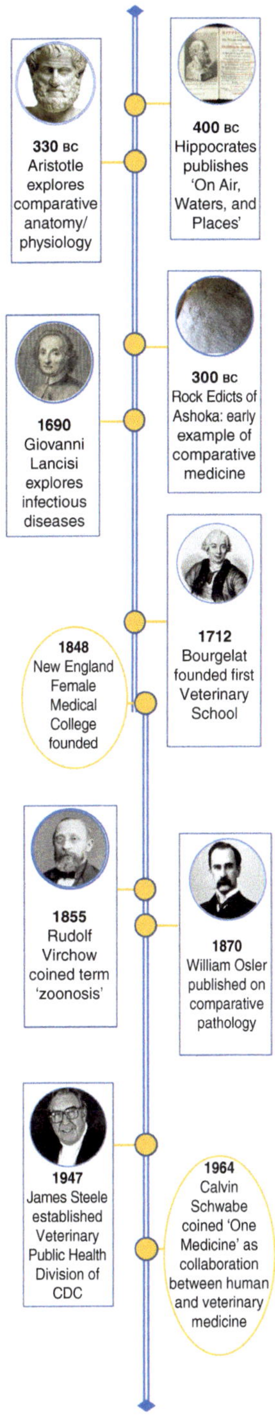

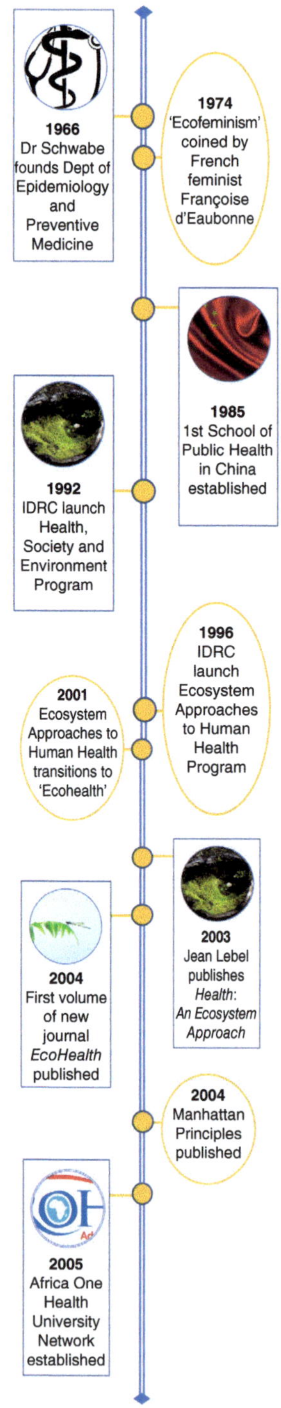

Society. At a symposium entitled Building Interdisciplinary Bridges to Health in a 'Globalized World', several human and animal health experts came together and discussed human, domestic animal and wildlife diseases. As a result, 12 priorities were set on how to fight the threats to human and animal health, and they were named the 'Manhattan Principles'. This point in history is most frequently considered as a moment when the basis of the 'One Health, One World' concept was formed. The Manhattan Principles also formed the basis for the later Berlin Principles on One Health, bridging global health and conservation (Gruetzmacher *et al.*, 2021). The Berlin Principles were created in 2019 because much had changed on the planet during the previous 15 years.

The International Association for Ecology and Health (IAEH) was formed in 2006 and hosted a series of biennial conferences, such as in the USA in 2006, Mexico in 2008, the UK in 2010, China in 2012, Canada in 2014, Australia in 2016, Colombia in 2018 and South Africa in 2022.

In 2006, limited, non-sustained, person-to-person-to-person (3rd generation) spread of highly pathogenic avian influenza AI(H5N1) virus occurred. Some researchers think that this was the moment when a large part of the scientific community started to embrace One Health. In 2007, the International Ministerial Conference on Avian and Pandemic Influenza was held in New Delhi, India. A total of 111 countries participated and were encouraged to embrace One Health by way of establishing connections between human and veterinary health systems for pandemic preparedness in order to keep the public safe. In the same year the American Medical Association and the American Veterinary Medical Association called for collaboration between the human and veterinary medical communities.

The year 2007 brought with it the official introduction of One Health to Brazil, where the first One Health Symposium was held. The 'One World, One Health' conference was held with the Wildlife Conservation Society (WCS) and EcoHealth Alliance. The main focus points revolved around the downstream effect of environmental destruction on human health through wildlife's ability to act as reservoirs and sentinels of disease.

The 2008 International Ministerial Conference on Avian and Pandemic Influenza in Sharm el-Sheikh, Egypt hosted 120 countries that endorsed a new strategy for fighting avian influenza and other infectious diseases in areas where animals, humans and ecosystems meet. The strategy was named Contributing to One World, One Health™: A Strategic Framework for Reducing Risks of Infectious Diseases at the Animal–Human–Ecosystems Interface. In 2008, the Canadian Community of Practice in Ecosystem Approaches to Health (CoPEH Canada) was created, including the formation of workshops and an Ecohealth field school. The IDRC later supported the development of an Ecohealth field-building Leadership Initiative in South-east Asia designed to strengthen the field through training, evidence-building and linking researchers. The Southern African Center for Infectious Disease Surveillance (SACIDS) was founded in January 2008 as a regional disease surveillance hub. It was then transformed in 2018 by the Council of Sokoine University of Agriculture (SUA) into the SACIDS Foundation for One Health, operating as a university research and training institute with the South African National Institute for Communicable Diseases and other member institutions across Africa (SACIDS: http://www.sacids.org/).

In 2009, the United States Agency for International Development (USAID) launched the Emerging Pandemic Threats Program for preventing the emergence of diseases of animal origin which could threaten human health. The Emerging Pandemic Threats Program aimed to improve US public health by addressing inadequacies through building national and local One Health capacities for early disease detection, laboratory-based disease diagnosis, rapid disease response and containment, and risk reduction.

In 2010, the 'Outcome and Impact Assessment of the Global Response to the Avian Influenza Crisis' was published by the Publications Office of the European Union (EU): 'The European Union has already taken new initiatives under the One Health umbrella and will continue to do so in the coming years', meaning that the One Health concept was to be applied into practical policies and strategies. In the same year, the United Nations and the World Bank released the 'Fifth Global Progress Report on Animal and Pandemic Influenza', where adopting the One Health approach was highlighted to keep developing pandemic preparedness and building on One Health response to emerging diseases and threats. Also in 2010, there was a meeting between the Center for Disease Control (CDC), World Organisation for Animal Health (OIE, now designated as WOAH), the Food and Agriculture Organization of the United Nations (FAO) and the World Health

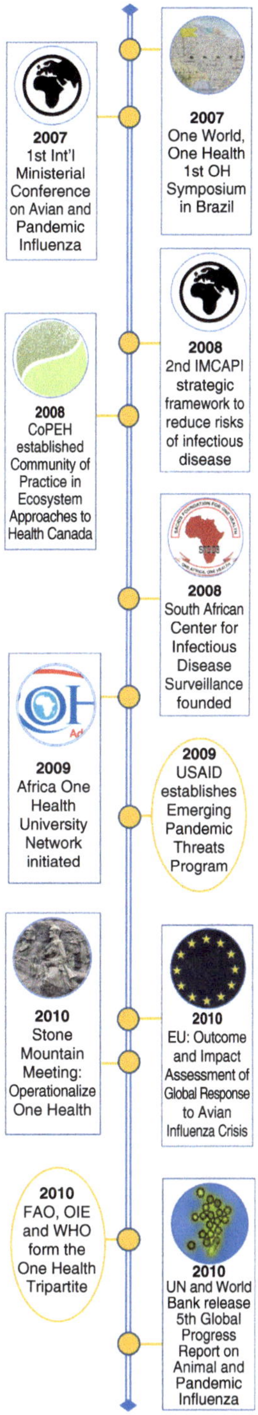

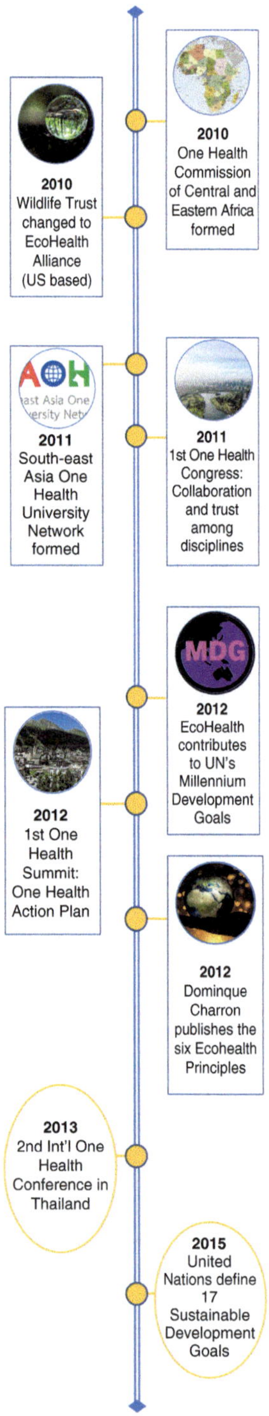

Organization (WHO) called the 'Stone Mountain Meeting', where seven key activities to advance the One Health concept were identified in a document named 'Operationalizing "One Health": A Policy Perspective – Taking Stock and Shaping an Implementation Roadmap'. Finally, in 2010, a Tripartite Concept Note was published by OIE, FAO and WHO together, proposing international collaboration, sharing responsibilities and coordinating global activities to address health risks. In 2010, the International Ministerial Conference on Avian and Pandemic Influenza in Hanoi, Vietnam was held where 71 countries participated in adopting the Hanoi Declaration. The Hanoi Declaration recommended the broad implementation of One Health.

The Africa One Health University Network (AFROHUN) came from the Leadership Initiative of Public Health in East Africa (LIPHEA) and the Health Alliance, both spearheaded by Makere University School of Public Health (MakSPH) in Uganda, in collaboration with Muhimbili University of Health and Allied Sciences (MUHAS) School of Public Health in Tanzania, established in 2005 with support from USAID. The formation of One Health of Central and East Africa (OHCEA) was inaugurated in October of 2010 from LIPHEA and many schools of public health and faculties of veterinary medicine in Democratic Republic of Congo, Ethiopia, Kenya, Rwanda, Tanzania and Uganda. The focus was initially on disaster preparedness and response. Ultimately, the One Health Workforce was strengthened in Africa under the umbrella of USAID. The initial geographic focus was East and Central Africa; however, the network continues to expand, embracing West African universities in Senegal and beyond (AFROHUN: https://afrohun.org/).

Also in 2010, the organization Wildlife Trust changed its name to EcoHealth Alliance. In the following year, 2011, the South-east Asia One Health University Network (SEAOHUN) was established, working to expand the One Health workforce capacity across 92 universities in eight South-east Asian countries (usaid.gov). The first international One Health congress in Melbourne, Australia was held in 2011 with 650 attendees from 60 countries promoting the One Health approach. At this congress it was agreed that, in addition to human, animal and environmental health, for the One Health approach it is important to include disciplines such as economics, social behaviour and food safety.

The year 2012 marked the first One Health Summit in Davos, Switzerland where the One Health concept was presented through the Davos One Health Action Plan, considering ways to improve public health through multisectoral and multi-stakeholder cooperation. In the same year, Dominique Charron published the six overarching guiding principles for Ecohealth. Later that year, the Kunming Position Statement was released, identifying Ecohealth's contributions to the Millennium Development Goals.

In 2013, the second One Health Congress was held with 1000 attendees from 70 countries, probably being the biggest One Health congress of all.

In September 2015, at the UN Sustainable Development Summit, the 2030 Agenda for Sustainable Development, with 17 Sustainable Development Goals (SDGs) at its core, was adopted. These 17 SDGs were the starting point for many 'equities'. The 2030 Agenda for Sustainable Development, adopted by all United Nations Member States, provides a shared blueprint for peace and prosperity for people and the planet, now and into the future (https://sdgs.un.org/2030agenda).

As the first centre for One Health in China, the One Health Center of Excellence for Research and Training at Sun Yat-Sen University held international symposia in 2014 and 2019. These meetings laid the foundation for implementing the One Health concept and strategy in China. The Sino-Italian Food Safety Dialogue, held in Beijing in 2016, brought the One Health concept to bear on food safety issues. In February 2017, the Liaocheng City of Shandong Province held the academic conference 'One World, One Health', where experts expressed their positive response to promoting the One Health concept to address the challenges of infectious disease (Li *et al.*, 2022).

In 2016, a joint International One Health Congress and Biennial Conference of the International Association for Ecology and Health took place in Australia.

In 2018, the International Association for Ecology and Health transformed into Ecohealth International, then the following year, in 2019, the Network for Ecohealth and One Health (NEOH) became EcoHealth International's European Chapter. Within NEOH, several working groups started to grow, namely: Promoting Transdisciplinarity in Health Sciences, Communication and Collaboration, Learning Organization, Theoretical Dimension of One Health and Ecohealth, and Education in One Health and Ecohealth.

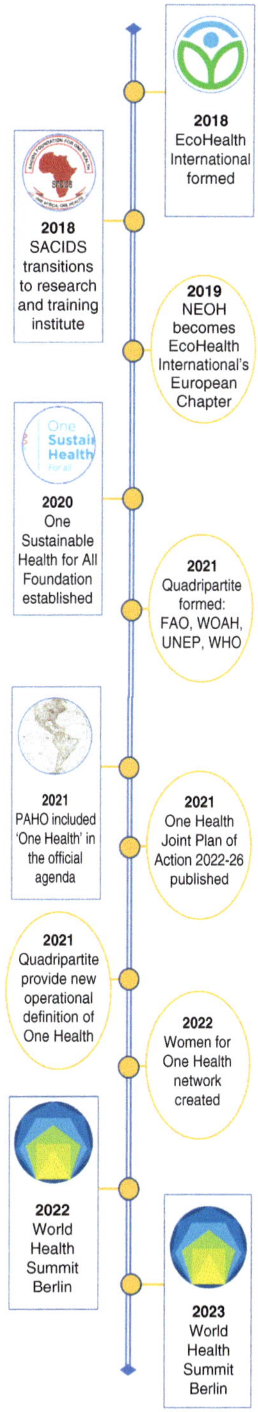

The One Sustainable Health forum was launched in July 2021 in Lyon, bringing together European and global professional and civil society organizations working on a holistic approach to health, taking into account human, animal and environmental health. The One Sustainable Health for All Foundation was created on 1 September 2020 in Lyon, France, as a response to the COVID-19 pandemic, with the objective to increase dialogue and innovative projects between public and private partners in favour of a holistic approach to health. It brings several new dimensions: (i) sustainability; (ii) for all (diversity / inclusiveness / gender); and (iii) by all (in a participatory way and without speaking in the name of others, deciding for others).

In 2021, the Quadripartite for One Health (FAO, UNEP, WHO, WOAH) promote the newly formed operational definition of One Health from their advisory panel, the One Health High-Level Expert Panel (OHHLEP). This is followed in 2022 by the publication of the Quadripartite's One Health Joint Plan of Action.

In 2022, a network, Women for One Health, was founded. The network represents parity across gender and other historically marginalized groups, to create a more equitable and inclusive scientific and One Health community. The Women for One Health network is promoting the importance of diversity and equity.

In 2022 and 2023, the World Health Summit (WHS) was held in Berlin bringing together leaders, health professionals, ministries and stakeholders for important public policy discussions and governance decisions for the future of One Health, Ecohealth and Planetary Health. A pre-workshop, 'Breaking Barriers: Advancing the One Health Agenda with a Focus on Environment', preceded the 2023 WHS organized by the German Federal Ministry for Economic Cooperation and Development (BMZ), the German Federal Ministry for the Environment, Nature Conservation, Nuclear Safety and Consumer Protection (BMUV), the Quadripartite Collaboration on One Health, the Wildlife Conservation Society (WCS), the Sector Initiative One Health of the German Society for International Cooperation (GIZ), and the International Alliance against Health Risks in Wildlife Trade. It brought together decision makers, scientists and implementers taking action related to the environmental pillar of the One Health approach to push the agenda towards action and important collaborative decisions for the future of One Health, Ecohealth and Planetary Health (https://oneworldonehealth.wcs.org/EVENTS/Breaking-Barriers.aspx).

There is still one part of One Health that is being underrepresented, namely plant health. The first and possibly most obvious link between human/animal health and plant health is the use of plants as food. Unhealthy plants as crops or vegetables directly influence dietary needs of humans and animals and can lead to food insecurity and different diseases as a consequence of malnutrition. Apart from serving as food, plants also serve as habitats and contribute to biodiversity, nutrient cycles and ecosystem services. Plants contribute to environmental sustainability by stabilizing soils, preventing erosion, sequestering carbon dioxide and improving air quality. For example, forests as 'lungs of the planet', once unhealthy or taken down, will not be able to clear the air adequately. Plants provide medicinal compounds and dietary nutrients, and contribute to traditional medicine practices. Overall, the wider recognition of plant health as an integral component of One Health is growing, but still modest; further attention needs to be attributed to plant health to realize fully the interconnectedness and holistic nature of the One Health approach.

Learning questions 5: Try to identify One Health / Ecohealth activities that were celebrated in your country or region, such as One Health Day, One Health/Ecohealth Conferences, Associations, or similar.
Example answer: If you were not able to think of something, or you do not know where to find information, you may want to look at websites from government, universities and non-government organizations. Or you might look at the One Health commission website (https://www.onehealthcommission.org) where many One Health activities are listed; it also includes a map of who is who in One Health. On this website, you can also search the events by country or by region.

1.4 Conclusions

1. Integrated health approaches have ancient origins in various cultures, but the naming of this formal recognition of interconnectedness between the health of people, animals and the environment is a relatively recent development. From early historical records to modern initiatives such as One Health and Ecohealth, the journey of recognizing and addressing the interdependence of living beings and ecosystems has led to collaborative efforts and interdisciplinary approaches to tackle shared health challenges.

2. The One Health approach recognizes the interconnectedness of human, animal, plant and environment health. It emphasizes collaborative, holistic solutions to complex health challenges that transcend traditional boundaries, involving diverse disciplines and sectors to promote healthier populations, ecosystems and global sustainability. The evolution described in this chapter shows that it is highly adaptable to new global challenges and applicable across settings and complex issues.

3. The term originated in the mid-1900s and has gained substantial momentum during the past decade, rising to widespread international recognition as an approach for addressing complex global health challenges with specific expertise in the study of zoonotic diseases, many of which are driving the emergence of global pandemics. It aims to balance and optimize sustainably the health of people, animals and ecosystems through interdisciplinary collaboration, societal engagement and principles such as equity, stewardship and transdisciplinarity. One Health is evolving to include broader considerations such as climate change, sustainability and social justice.

4. One Health, Ecohealth and Planetary Health are integrated approaches to health that share a foundation but have different emphases. While they all promote holistic and transdisciplinary thinking to address health challenges, they differ in their perspectives on anthropocentrism, zoocentrism, biocentrism and ecocentrism. They are similar in that they highlight the interconnectedness of human, animal and environmental health, and emphasize collaboration across disciplines and sectors to find sustainable solutions to complex global challenges.

Notes

[1] 'The natural world or physical surroundings in general, either as a whole or within a particular geographical area' FAO *et al.*, 2022).

[2] 'Human animals' is a term used to emphasize the biological and physiological aspects of human beings within the context of the broader animal kingdom. It highlights the fact that humans are a species of animals, sharing many biological characteristics and evolutionary history with other animals while also possessing unique cognitive, cultural and technological attributes. By using the terms 'human and non-human animals', the anthropocentric status of humans is questioned and a sense of humility and connection with the rest of the natural world promoted, recognizing that our existence and behaviours are deeply rooted in nature.

[3] In an anthropocentric viewpoint, human needs, desires and interests are often prioritized over the wellbeing and rights of other species or the natural world. This approach can lead to human-centred decision making, where the impact on humans is the central concern, sometimes at the expense of environmental sustainability or the rights of animals.

References

Adams, F. (1849) *The Genuine Works of Hippocrates, translated from the Greek with a Preliminary Discourse and Annotations by Francis Adams, LL.D.* Sydenham Society, London.

Adisasmito, W.B., Almuhairi, S., Behravesh, C.B., Bilivogui, P., Bukachi, S.A. *et al.* (2022) One Health: A new definition for a sustainable and healthy future. *PLoS Pathogens* 18(6), e1010537. DOI: 10.1371/journal.ppat.1010537.

Assmuth, T., Chen, X., Degeling, C., Haahtela, T., Irvine, K.N. *et al.* (2020) Integrative concepts and practices of health in transdisciplinary social ecology. *Socio-Ecological Practice Research* 2, 71–90. DOI: 10.1007/s42532-019-00038-y.

Boorse, C. (2011) Concepts of health and disease. In: Fred, G. (ed.) *Handbook of the Philosophy of Science, Vol. 16.* Philosophy of Medicine, North-Holland, pp. 13–64. DOI: 10.1016/B978-0-444-51787-6.50002-7. ISSN: 18789846, ISBN: 9780444517876.

Buse, C.G., Oestreicher, J.S., Ellis, N.R., Patrick, R., Brisbois, B. *et al.* (2018) Public health guide to field developments linking ecosystems, environments and health in the Anthropocene. *Journal of Epidemiology and Community Health* 72(5), 420–425.

Calistri, P., Iannetti, S.L., Danzetta, M., Narcisi, V., Cito, F. *et al.* (2012) The components of 'one world–one health' approach. *Transboundary and Emerging Diseases* 60, 4–13.

CDC (2022) About One Health. Available at: https://www.cdc.gov/onehealth/basics/index.html (accessed 15 July 2024).

Charron, D.F. (2012) In: Charron, D. (ed.) *Ecohealth Research in Practice. Insight and Innovation in International Development, Vol. 1.* Springer, New York. DOI: 10.1007/978-1-4614-0517-7_22.

Chidawanyika, F., Muriithi, B., Niassy, S., Ouya, F.O., Pittchar, J.O. *et al.* (2023) Sustainable intensification of vegetable production using the cereal 'push-pull technology': Benefits and one health implications. *Environmental Sustainability* 6, 25–34. DOI: 10.1007/s42398-023-00260-1.

Coker, R., Rushton, J., Mounier-Jack, S., Karimuribo, E., Lutumba, P. *et al.* (2011) Towards a conceptual framework to support one-health research for policy on emerging zoonoses. *The Lancet Infectious Diseases* 11(4), 326–331.

Currier, R.W. and Steele, J.H. (2011) One Health – One medicine: Unifying human and animal medicine within an evolutionary paradigm. *Annals of the New York Academy of Sciences* 1230(1), 4.

Day, M.J. (2011) One health: The importance of companion animal vector-borne diseases. *Parasites & Vectors* 4(1), 1–6.

Destoumieux-Garzón, D., Mavingui, P., Boetsch, G., Boissier, J., Darriet, F. *et al.* (2018) The one health concept: 10 years old and a long road ahead. *Frontiers in Veterinary Science* 5, 14.

Dhammika, V.S. (1993) *The Edicts of King Asoka: An English Rendering.* Buddhist Publication Society, Kandy, Sri Lanka. Available at: https://bps.lk/olib/wh/wh386_Dhammika_Edicts-of-King-Asoka.pdf (accessed 15 July 2024).

Dornelas, M. (2010) Disturbance and change in biodiversity. *Philosophical Transactions of the Royal Society of London. Series B, Biological Sciences* 365(1558), 3719–3727. DOI: 10.1098/rstb.2010.0295.

Feola, G. and Bazzani, R. (eds) (2001) *Challenges and Strategies for Implementing the Ecosystem Approach to Human Health in Developing Countries: Reflections from Regional Consultations.* International Development Research Centre and United Nations Environment Programme, Uruguay.

Food and Agriculture Organization of the United Nations, World Organisation for Animal Health, World Health Organization and United Nations Environment Programme (2022) One Health Joint Plan of Action (2022–2026): Working Together for the Health of Humans, Animals, Plants and the Environment. Rome.

Gruetzmacher, K., Karesh, W.B., Amuasi, J.H., Arshad, A., Farlow, A. *et al.* (2021) The Berlin principles on one health – Bridging global health and conservation. *Science of the Total Environment* 764, 142919. DOI: 10.1016/j.scitotenv.2020.142919.

Habib, N., Parry, J., Elfving, R. and Dunn B. (2022) Practical Actions to Operationalize the One Health Approach in the Asian Development Bank, ADB East Asia Working Paper Series No. 50/May. DOI: 10.22617/WPS220202-2.

Harrison, S., Kivuti-Bitok, L., Macmillan, A. and Priest, P. (2019) EcoHealth and One Health: A theory-focused review in response to calls for convergence. *Environment International* 132, 105058.

Hirschhorn, L.R., Magge, H. and Kiflie A. (2021) Aiming beyond equality to reach equity: The promise and challenge of quality improvement. *BMJ* 374, n939. DOI: 10.1136/bmj.n939.

Hueffer, K., Ehrlander, M., Etz, K. and Reynolds, A. (2019) One health in the circumpolar North. *International Journal of Circumpolar Health* 78(1), 1607502.

Keune, H. and Assmuth, T. (2018) Framing complexity in environmental and human health. In: *Oxford Research Encyclopedia of Environmental Science.* Oxford University Press, Oxford, pp. 1–35. DOI: 10.1093/ACREFORE/9780199389414.013.350. ISBN: 978-0-19-938941-4.

Keune, H., Payyappallimana, U., Morand, S. and Rüegg, S. (2022) One Health and biodiversity. In: Visseren-Hamakers, I. and Kok, M. (eds) *Transforming Biodiversity Governance.* Cambridge University Press, Cambridge, pp. 93–114.

Kingsley, P. and Taylor, E.M. (2017) One Health: Competing perspectives in an emerging field. *Parasitology* 144(1), 7–14.

Laing, G., Duffy, E., Anderson, N., Antoine-Moussiaux, N., Aragrande, M. *et al.* (2023) Advancing One Health: Updated core competencies. *CABI One Health* 2023: 1–13. DOI: 10.1079/cabionehealth.2023.0002.

Lebel, J. (2003) Health: An Ecosystem Approach. International Development Research Centre, Ottawa, Canada. ISBN: 1-55250-012-8.

Lerner, H. and Berg, C. (2015) The concept of health in One Health and some practical implications for research and education: What is One Health? *Infection Ecology & Epidemiology* 5(1), 25300.

Lerner, H. and Berg, C. (2017) A comparison of three holistic approaches to health: One Health, eco health, and planetary health. *Frontiers in Veterinary Science* 4, 163. DOI: 10.3389/fvets.2017.00163.

Li, Q., Guo, C., Hu, H. and Lu, J. (2022) Towards One Health: Reflections and practices on the different fields of One Health in China. *Biosafety and Health* 4(1) 23–29. DOI: 10.1016/j.bsheal.2021.12.004.

Mackenzie, J.S. and Jeggo, M. (2019) The One Health approach – why is it so important? *Tropical Medicine and Infectious Disease* 4, 88. DOI: 10.3390/tropicalmed4020088.

Majowicz, S.E., Parmley, E.J., Carson, C. and Pintar K. (2018) Identifying non-traditional stakeholders with whom to engage, when mitigating antimicrobial resistance in foodborne pathogens (Canada). *BMC Research Notes* 11, 170. DOI: 10.1186/s13104-018-3279-8.

McFarlane, R.A., Horwitz, P., Arabena, K., Capon, A., Jenkins, A. *et al.* (2019) Ecosystem services for human health in Oceania. *Ecosystem Services* 39(C), 100976.

Miller, G. (1962) 'Airs, waters, and places' in history. *Journal of the History of Medicine and Allied Sciences* 17, 129–140.

Mutsaers, I. (2015) One-health approach as counter-measure against 'autoimmune' responses in biosecurity. *Social Science & Medicine* 129, 123–130. DOI: 10.1016/j.socscimed.2014.09.042.

One Health Commission (2022) What is One Health? Available at: https://www.onehealthcommission.org/en/why_one_health/what_is_one_health/ (accessed 15 July 2024).

RSC (2022) Strengthening a One Health approach to emerging zoonoses. Available at: https://rsc-src.ca/sites/default/files/OH % 20PB_EN.pdf (accessed 15 July 2024).

Rüegg, S.R., Häsler, B. and Zinsstag, J. (2018a) *Integrated Approaches to Health, A Handbook for the Evaluation of One Health.* DOI: 10.3920/978-90-8686-875-9. eISBN: 978-90-8686-875-9, ISBN: 978-90-8686-324-2.

Rüegg, S.R., Nielsen, L.R., Buttigieg, S.C., Santa, M., Aragrande, M. *et al.* (2018b) Systems approach to evaluate One Health initiatives. *Frontiers in Veterinary Science* 5. DOI: 10.3389/fvets.2018.00023.

Ruscio, B.A., Brubaker, M., Glasser, J., Hueston, W. and Hennessy, T.W. (2015) One Health – A strategy for resilience in a changing arctic. *International Journal of Circumpolar Health* 74(1), 27913.

Schwabe, C.W. (1964) *Veterinary Medicine and Human Health.* Published 1984 by Williams & Wilkins. ISBN: 0683075942, ISBN13: 9780683075946.

TEEB (2018) The Economics of Ecosystems and Biodiversity (for National and International Policy Makers). Available at: https://www.teebweb.org/wp-content/uploads/Study%20and%20Reports/Reports/National%20and%20International%20Policy%20Making/TEEB%20for%20National%20Policy%20Makers%20report/TEEB%20for%20National.pdf (accessed 15 July 2024).

Trinh, P., Zaneveld, J.R., Safranek, S. and Rabinowitz, P.M. (2018) One health relationships between human, animal, and environmental microbiomes: A mini-review. *Frontiers in Public Health* 6, 235.

Vansteenkiste, J. (2014) Considering the ecohealth approach: Shaping Haitian women's participation in urban agricultural projects. *Development in Practice* 24(1), 18–29. DOI: 10.1080/09614524.2014.867307.

Wallace, R.G., Bergmann, L., Kock, R., Gilbert, M., Hogerwerf, L., Wallace, R. and Holmberg, M. (2015) The dawn of Structural One Health: A new science tracking disease emergence along circuits of capital. *Social Science & Medicine* 129, 68–77. DOI: 10.1016/j.socscimed.2014.09.047. ISSN: 0277-9536.

Waltner-Toews, D. (2017) Zoonoses, One Health and complexity: Wicked problems and constructive conflict. *Philosophical Transactions of the Royal Society of London. Series B, Biological Sciences* 372(1725), 20160171. DOI: 10.1098/rstb.2016.0171.

Wernli, D., Jørgensen, P.S., Harbarth, S., Carroll, S.P., Laxminarayan, R., Levrat, N. *et al.* (2017) Antimicrobial resistance: The complex challenge of measurement to inform policy and the public. *PLoS Medicine* 14(8), e1002378. DOI: 10.1371/journal.pmed.1002378.

Whitmee, S., Haines, A., Beyrer, C., Boltz, F., Capon, A.G. *et al.* (2015) Safeguarding human health in the Anthropocene epoch: Report of The Rockefeller Foundation-Lancet Commission on planetary health. *Lancet* 386(10007), 1973–2028. DOI: 10.1016/S0140-6736(15)60901-1. Erratum in *Lancet* 2015 Nov 14; 386(10007), 1944.

WHO (2018) WHO Report by Director General (A71/10). Available at: https://apps.who.int/gb/ebwha/pdf_files/WHA71/A71_10-en.pdf (accessed 15 July 2024).

WHO (2023) Nature, Biodiversity and Health. Available at: https://www.who.int/europe/news-room/fact-sheets/item/nature--biodiversity-and-health (accessed 15 July 2024).

Xie, T., Liu, W., Anderson, B.D., Liu, X. and Gray, G.C. (2017) A system dynamics approach to understanding the One Health concept. *PLoS ONE* 12(9), e0184430. DOI: 10.1371/journal.pone.0184430.

2 Comparing One Health and Ecohealth with Other Integrated Approaches to Health

Gillian Penn[1], Christina Pettan-Brewer[2], Neil Anderson[3], Margarida Simões[4,7], Hans Keune[5,7] and Thomas Jaenisch[6,7]

[1]Colorado School of Public Health, University of Colorado, Denver, USA; [2]School of Medicine and Center for One Health Research, School of Public Health, University of Washington, USA, UNEP Nature for Health (N4H) TAG, International Alliance against Health Risks and Wildlife Trade Steering Committee, CABI One Health Executive Editorial Member and Federal Schools of Minas Gerais (UFMG) and Parana (UFPR), Faculdade Pontificia Catolica (PUC), One Health Brasil (ABRA-SUNI), Brazil, OHLAIC/CYTED Latin America; [3]Royal (Dick) School of Veterinary Studies and the Roslin Institute, University of Edinburgh, Scotland, UK; [4]Veterinary Medicine Department, University of Évora and Comprehensive Health Research Centre, Portugal, and One Health International Network; [5]Faculty of Medicine and Health Sciences, Department Family Medicine and Population Health, Chair Care and the Natural Environment, University of Antwerp, Antwerp, Belgium; [6]Heidelberg Institute of Global Health (HIGH), Heidelberg University Hospital, Germany and Center for Global Health, Colorado School of Public Health, Aurora, USA; [7]Network for Ecohealth and One Health (NEOH)

Contents

DOI: 10.1079/9781800623002.0003

Chapter Overview

Elevator pitch

One Health and Ecohealth have diverse origins and with this, varied ways of relating to other similar integrated approaches to health. This chapter is dedicated to the many integrated approaches closely related to One Health and Ecohealth, while also recognizing the contribution and origination of integrated approaches from Indigenous cultures across the world. By understanding how these similar concepts revolve around and relate to One Health or Ecohealth, we hope to help the reader orient themselves and maximize opportunities to address health imbalances in all facets of our world: humans, animals, plants and our ecological settings. The effects of synergy between various integrated approaches have the potential to be greater than the sum of different, non-articulated interventions.

Book objectives the chapter relates to

☑ 1. Understand what One Health and Ecohealth mean
☑ 2. Think in a One Health and Ecohealth way
☐ 3. Apply One Health and Ecohealth in their professional and personal life
☐ 4. Know how to share One Health and Ecohealth knowledge
☐ 5. Integrate One Health and Ecohealth knowledge actively
☐ 6. Acquire or enhance core One Health competencies

One Health competencies covered

☐ 1. Effective communication
☑ 2. Collaborative and resilient working
☑ 3. Systems understanding
☐ 4. Transdisciplinarity
☐ 5. Social, cultural and gender equity and inclusiveness
☑ 6. Collective learning and reflective practice
☑ 7. One Health concepts
☑ 8. Theoretical and methodological pluralism
☐ 9. Harnessing uncertainty, paradox and limited knowledge

Learning outcomes

1. Describe the context in which different integrated approaches to health originated.
2. Analyse the differences and the synergies between these concepts and One Health or Ecohealth.
3. Evaluate calls for convergence in scholarship and joined action.

Summary

This chapter is an overview of several of the various integrated approaches to health, namely One Health, Ecohealth, Planetary Health, Conservation Medicine, Environmental Health, One Welfare, Comparative Medicine and One Ocean Health. A description is provided of the historical roots of each of these science-based approaches, while considering the convergence and divergence of each to the others. This chapter also highlights the importance of contributions from Indigenous Peoples and traditional knowledge that have influenced these more recent concepts. In this chapter you will learn about many of the different ways we approach health and comparatively dive into the discussion on differences and similarities to each of the approaches. You will then have the opportunity to consider arguments for or against calls for convergence. Complementary to Chapter 1, there is a more expansive timeline provided throughout the text highlighting various important dates, people and events in each of the respective histories. Throughout this chapter we aim for you to become more familiar with the use of a systems-thinking approach across a transdisciplinary and cross-sectoral playing field, by comparing the many integrated health approaches. We highlight the importance of effective communication, cooperation amongst all sectors through the collective learning process and reflective practice that are fundamental to One Health and Ecohealth.

2.1 The Many Integrated Approaches to Health

A number of **integrated approaches to health** have been developed, each originating from different epistemological (the perspective through which **knowledge** and its acquisition are understood) or academic traditions. These integrated approaches conceptualize the connectedness of the **environment**, human, plant (photosynthetic organisms) and animal health. While the multitude of approaches can lead to confusion among practitioners and academics, these approaches also represent the rich history of efforts within and across scientific **disciplines** to address the complex interactions between the health of humans, animals, plants and their environment (FAO *et al.*, 2022).

The ever-evolving scope of **One Health** and **Ecohealth** poses a challenge in providing a single, clear definition of the concept. In this chapter, we focus on natural science-based integrated approaches to health as we discuss the concepts listed later in the chapter (see Table 2.1). While we recognize the importance of fields such as social sciences, economics and political ecology (which are crucial to some of the integrated approaches to health), these are not discussed in their own right in this chapter, as we focused on highlighting the need for holistic contributions to solve complex health issues. The same applies to concepts such as International Health, Geographical Health or Global Health, which are not included because of their focus on human health. We also did not include more methodologically oriented approaches like disease ecology.

We do recognize, however, the contribution of Indigenous, traditional and cultural influences to the understanding of the interconnectedness of life on Earth and to the integrated approaches to health (Box 2.1). For example, from an Australian Aboriginal perspective, 'One Health is highly […] applicable within indigenous communities as it adopts a holistic approach and is in line with indigenous cultural beliefs […] of health' (Riley *et al.*, 2021). An Indigenous approach often utilizes a 'whole-society' lens, involves community engagement, is inclusive, utilizes partnerships, and acknowledges the importance of cultural knowledge (Riley *et al.*, 2021). While we have chosen to focus on conventional academic approaches, we encourage the exploration into some of the Indigenous resources for more information on cultural approaches to health, such as the traditional knowledge of and practices by the Suquamish people and Māori (see: https://suquamish.nsn.us/; https://www.thelancet.com/journals/lancet/article/PIIS0140-6736(22)01596-3/fulltext, respectively).

Box 2.1. Significance of Traditional Healthcare

Traditional healthcare, while viewed with scepticism through a Western medicine lens, is commonly preferred over Western medicine in many parts of the world. In recognition by the international community of the rights of Indigenous Peoples' cultural beliefs in 2007, 143 member states adopted the United Nations Declaration on the Rights of Indigenous Peoples (UNDRIP), which is an internationally agreed upon set of principles acknowledging the human right to culturally determined traditional medicines, thereby allowing people to maintain their health practices (United Nations, 2008).

What follows is a non-exhaustive review of integrated approaches to health with an exploration through their synergies as well as the differences compared to One Health and Ecohealth. For orientation purposes, we present a timeline of the history of integrated approaches to health in this chapter (in the margins of some pages in this chapter with points in the text). Prior to our discussion of conventional academic approaches, we felt it important to discuss briefly the contributions of Indigenous or traditional cultures, highlighting regional examples of Indigenous, traditional connections to the land, animals, plants, Spirit and Mother Earth. While this does not cover the full breadth or depth of these concepts and cultures, we hope to provide these examples in a respectful and meaningful way to show that these belief systems hold the very essence of our more recent understanding of integrated approaches to health.

Finally, this chapter concludes with a discussion around calls for convergence between some of the approaches listed, given their inherent synergies and partially overlapping agendas. While we cover the history of integrated approaches closely related to One Health and Ecohealth, a more thorough description of the history of One Health and Ecohealth itself can be found in Chapter 1.

2.2 Contributions of Traditional and Indigenous Knowledge to Integrated Approaches to Health

The discussion of concepts around integrated approaches to health would not be complete without the recognition of the significance of Indigenous and traditional belief systems that hold the very essence of the more classic One Health approach. A commonly understood tenet of many ancient, **Indigenous and traditional belief systems** is that the health of the environment is inherently linked and inseparable from the physical and spiritual health of humans, animals and plants (QingWen *et al.*, 2010; Kimmerer, 2015; Pettan-Brewer *et al.*, 2021; Riley *et al.*, 2021; Pettan-Brewer *et al.*, 2024).

Task: Consider the key concept, 'A commonly understood tenet of many ancient, Indigenous and traditional belief systems is that the health of the environment is inherently linked and inseparable from the physical and spiritual health of humans, animals and plants'. As you read through this chapter, consider how this idea is related to, or differs from, the various approaches to health discussed. Additionally, consider how the traditional Indigenous knowledge has provided a foundation to the integrated approaches to health.

Example answer: Indigenous communities often use a holistic approach to health, including the spiritual dimension of each individual and community with Nature. These practices are the basis for modern integrated approaches, contrasting with the reductionist interventions performed in Western medical specialization.

There are many examples repeated across time and place that showcase the importance of the interconnectedness of the land, the environment, plants, animals and the people that share these values and resources. While **Indigenous Peoples** make up only 6% of the world's population, they live within and protect areas that hold up to 80% of the world's **biodiversity** according to the World Bank (Worldbank.org, 2022). More information on the importance of Indigenous Peoples' stewardship can be found in Chapter 7.

2.2.1 North America

Native American, First Nations, Inuit and Métis cultural beliefs are as varied as the tribes themselves. There are over 600 Tribal Nations in Canada and the USA (Government of Canada, 2023), each with their own Creation stories. We share, with gratitude, some of the stories with consideration of the connectedness to the holistic principal concepts of One Health and Ecohealth and to exemplify how they have been applied well before these terms became popularized. Robin Wall Kimmerer shares the traditional Potawatomi creation story in her book *Braiding Sweetgrass* (Kimmerer, 2015). She describes how Skywoman fell to the water-covered Earth and the animals worked together for her survival, including the geese who flew up to catch her. Turtle who offered his back for her to rest. Muskrat who gave his life diving deep into the water to collect a handful of mud from which the land grew. Skywoman shared the seeds and fruits of many plants from the Tree of Life, thereby feeding and nourishing all of the creatures. Kimmerer impresses that the beauty of this story is what was created from the collaboration of the animals and Skywoman's gratitude toward them.

Animals play an important role in many Tribal Nations; great respect is held for all living things, including animals. The Tlingit (phonetically 'klin-kit') People of Alaska carry a beautiful story as to the origin of the aurora borealis. The Tlingit people believe that each life we live on the Earth holds a lesson for our Spirit to learn from and that we continue to have many lives to learn the necessary lessons. The final lesson on Earth, the last lesson in a living body, is experienced in the body of a sacred animal. At the close of this final transition on Earth, the Animal Spirit is released to the heavens; the aurora borealis is the display of the Animal Spirits playing in the sky (Watermolen, 2022).

2.2.2 South America

Animals and plants have also influenced human history in an adaptive and interdependent human–animal relationship in South America (Vergara,

2018). Although the use of animals in conventional medicine has been comparatively recent, a **meta-analysis** (a statistical technique used in research to combine and analyse **data** from multiple independent studies on a particular topic) of historical and archaeological evidence indicated that animals have been used in traditional medicine in South America since ancient times, similar to other Indigenous cultures (Montenegro and Stephens, 2006). This was considered a 'faunal drugstore'. Animals, mostly wild species, were seen as healing instruments and considered sacred in native rituals and ceremonies (Alves and Souto, 2011). Plants have also been used for both human and animal care in South America (Alves *et al.*, 2010), demonstrating the environmental health **impact** on One Health. In contrast, animals have historically threatened human health prior to European arrivals, such as the Yanomami indigenous communities of Northern Brazil, which have been faced with high burdens of **zoonotic disease** from soil-, water- and food-borne zoonoses, including larvae of the native sand flea, which causes severe disability of hands and feet (Ehrenberg and Ault, 2005).

2.2.3 Asia

Classic Eastern belief systems hold animals in high prestige, including the belief in the cyclical embodiment of all living beings or reincarnation. Many incorporate a doctrine of nonviolence, which is extended to animals. Buddhism holds that killing animals is karmically equivalent to killing humans, therefore animal welfare is placed in high importance to everyday life. The Islamic religion teaches that unnecessary use or careless entertainment from animals is to disobey Allah's will (Szucs *et al.*, 2012). As of the time of writing, in parts of Asia, specifically India, it remains controversial to euthanize animals, making disease management and population control challenging, particularly with zoonotic diseases such as rabies and leishmaniasis (Srinivasan *et al.*, 2020).

Learning question: Consider the example above. What is your own country's approach to disease management or population control regarding animals (domestic, production or wild animals)?

Example answer: In Brazil, domestic animals are vaccinated against rabies as part of a national plan of vigilance and control. According to the World Health Organization (WHO), Food and Agriculture Organization of the United Nations (FAO) and World Organisation for Animal Health (WOAH):

> Mass dog vaccination is a proven, cost-effective way to save human lives by stopping transmission of rabies at its source. (...) dogs are responsible for 99% of human cases. (...) real-world experience shows that sustained vaccination coverage of 70% of dog populations is sufficient to stop transmission of the disease between dogs, and from dogs to humans.
>
> WHO *et al.* (2018)

Through the One Health approach, vaccinating feral dogs can contribute to the decrease of rabies in wildlife.

2.2.4 Africa

African Traditional Religion (ATR) and African Traditional Medicine (ATM) are the traditional beliefs, convictions and heritage handed down from generation to generation by African people. It is the 'cumulative knowledge and practices among Africans used in the diagnosis, prevention and elimination of physical, mental or social imbalance and the restoration of health and weakness' (Ajima and Ubana, 2018). Medicines, in many traditional therapies and specifically African traditional medicines, refer to healing agents such as plants, but also ritual or spiritual practices and objects (Ajima and Ubana, 2018). African traditional belief systems posit that we as humans should strive to maintain a harmonious relationship with all forces in the entire world, which is seen as a flowing, connected unit where all entities contribute to the relationship including spirits, plants, animals, the elements, humans and the dead (Ajima and Ubana, 2018).

Task: Identify the One Health core competencies discussed in the Introduction Chapter and throughout the text that are exemplified by Indigenous and traditional teachings / knowledge.

Example answer: Indigenous communities use practical skills of systems understanding based on their values and attitudes, applying collective learning and reflective practice.

2.3 Emergence of the Different Integrated Approaches to Health

2.3.1 Environmental Health

The origin of the concept or science of **Environmental Health** is less defined than many of the other concepts around One Health. The ambiguity arises, in part, as there was not a single entity that popularized the concept throughout history; the understanding of the role of the environment in health and disease was a gradual, evolving process (Gochfeld and Goldstein, 1999). The concept was formalized across Europe in the early 1800s with the discovery of the causal relationship of poor living conditions and dirty water to disease in humans. Similarly in the USA, Environmental Health Science arose from a branch of Sanitary Science in the late 1800s and was adapted by various universities across the USA to a variety of studies (University of Michigan, 2021).

The US Center for Disease Control (CDC) established the Center for Environmental Health in the 1980s and the concept of Environmental Health was eventually adopted and popularized by the World Health Organization (WHO) in the early 1990s. The study of Environmental Health has held an anthropocentric public health policy focus and has become an umbrella term for many related sciences including environmental toxicology, ecotoxicology, industrial hygiene, occupational health studies, etc. Environmental Health studies work to identify and evaluate environmental sources of hazardous agents and explore ways to limit exposures to such toxic environmental agents in water, soil, food and air that may affect human health (NEHA, 2013).

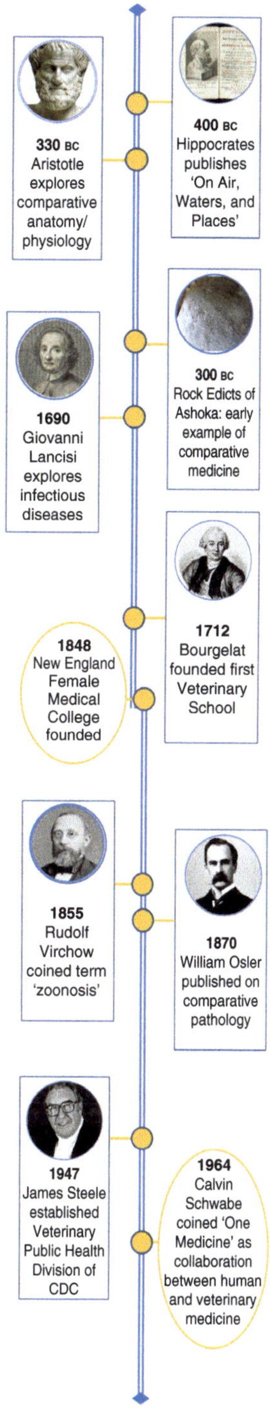

2.3.2 One Medicine Leading to One Health

The **One Medicine** concept has significant overlap with One Health as the originating concepts arose and evolved throughout history, at times in parallel and at others tangentially. Contemporarily, One Medicine was conceptualized in part by the recognition that animals share similar physiology to humans, while sharing the same environment. There are various references across pre-industrial history noting the link between human and animal health (Woods, 2017; King, 2021). The Industrial Revolution in Europe brought with it a number of scientific and medical advances, many guided by animal dissection, anatomical exploration and animal experimentation.

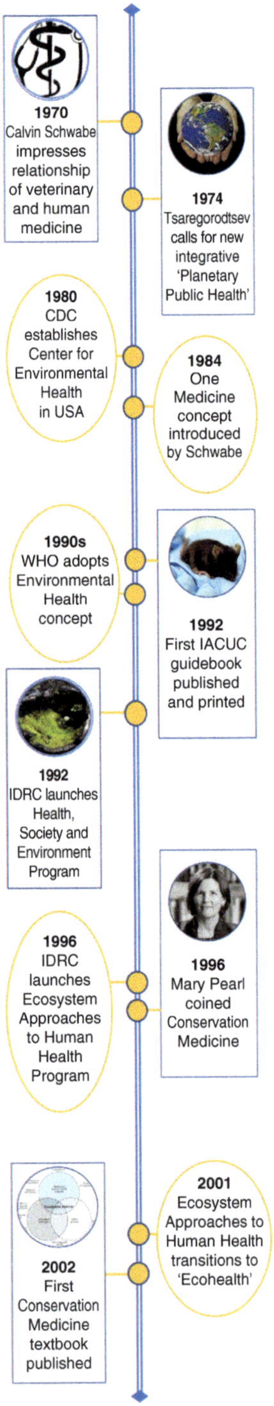

The German physician and pathologist Rudolf Virchow (1821–1902) is credited with the origination of the One Medicine concept in the 1800s with the recognition and investigation of transmissible disease between animals and humans, thereby familiarizing the term 'zoonosis' (Gyles, 2016) in the Global West. The concept was supported in 1870 with William Osler's publication on Comparative Pathology (Gyles, 2016). Continuing to recognize the importance of the study of animal health and disease transmission in relation to human health, James Steele was successful in the establishment of the Veterinary Public Health Division of the CDC in 1947 (Gyles, 2016). It was not until Calvin Schwabe at UC Davis popularized the term One Medicine, however, and spearheaded the integrative collaboration between veterinarians and human medical doctors in the 1960s that the term became part of common vernacular in the field (Gyles, 2016). Dr Schwabe revolutionized the One Medicine field, highlighting how veterinary medicine is directly related to human health and establishing the first Department of Veterinary Epidemiology in the USA at UC Davis (Zinsstag *et al.*, 2011). Interestingly, much of Schwabe's influence on the Global West understanding of One Health came from his time spent in Africa working with native Dinka pastoralist people (Zinsstag *et al.*, 2011). The terms and ideas around One Medicine have gradually evolved since origination, progressing and continuing toward a more comprehensive and holistic approach that commonly sits within the concept of One Health.

These leaders in One Health exemplify the core competencies of One Health through their spearheading of ideas incorporating collective learning and reflective practice, understanding of the inherent interconnectedness between humans, plants, animals and **ecosystems**, transcendence of disciplinary and sectoral confines engaging diverse groups through a collaborative, systems-thinking approach with effective communication (Laing *et al.*, 2023). In 2004 following outbreaks of Ebola Hemorrhagic Fever, SARS, Mpox and West Nile Virus, the 'One World, One Health' conference was held with a focus on the emergence and resurgence of infectious disease, pollution, habitat degradation, biodiversity loss and global **climate** change. Here, the 12 Manhattan Principles were envisioned as recommendations to establish a comprehensive approach to preventing infectious diseases and maintaining ecosystem integrity (Cook *et al.*, 2004).

Of note, many oncological advances in human chemotherapeutics and radiation methodologies were gained in part due to the collaboration and overlap between veterinary and human medicine (see Section 2.3.4 on Comparative Medicine below).

2.3.3 Conservation Medicine

Conservation Medicine first emerged as a concept in the 1990s in response to the growing health concerns associated with environmental degradation and biodiversity loss (Pokras *et al.*, 1999; Tabor, 2002; Daszak *et al.*, 2004; Jakob-Hoff and Warren, 2012). The term was first used in 1994 and has been attributed to Mary Pearl. The first textbook (*Conservation Medicine: Ecological Health in Practice*) was published in 2002 (Aguirre, 2002) as an output from a multidisciplinary conference in 1999 in Florida, USA. A Symposium on Conservation Medicine was launched in June 2000 at the annual meeting of the Society for Conservation Biology. The Center for Conservation Medicine was established as a collaboration between Tufts University School of Veterinary Medicine and the Wildlife Trust, later designated Ecohealth Alliance, while the Harvard Medical School Center for Health and Global Environment expanded to become the Consortium for Conservation Medicine in 2000. At the time, conservation practitioners recognized that the health of all species was an important factor limiting the success of conservation and development programs. Conservation Biology had been widely adopted by ecologists and conservation practitioners since the 1970s to develop strategies to address declines in wildlife species and the loss of biodiversity. Conservation Biology was heavily influenced by Rachel Carson's *Silent Spring* in 1962, a transformative call to attention towards the interconnected relationship of humans and the natural environment, including animals and plants (Carson, 1962, republished 2022). However, the scope of Conservation Biology was considered too narrow to address some of the complex health challenges related to conservation, which required a more integrated and holistic approach, focusing on the health sciences (Tabor *et al.*, 2001).

The emergence of Conservation Medicine was influenced by conservation biology, veterinary science and human medicine (Meffe, 1999). Joint meetings and conferences were held between conservation biologists and veterinary, medical and public health fields, framing biodiversity conservation firmly within the context of global health (e.g. the AHEAD meetings

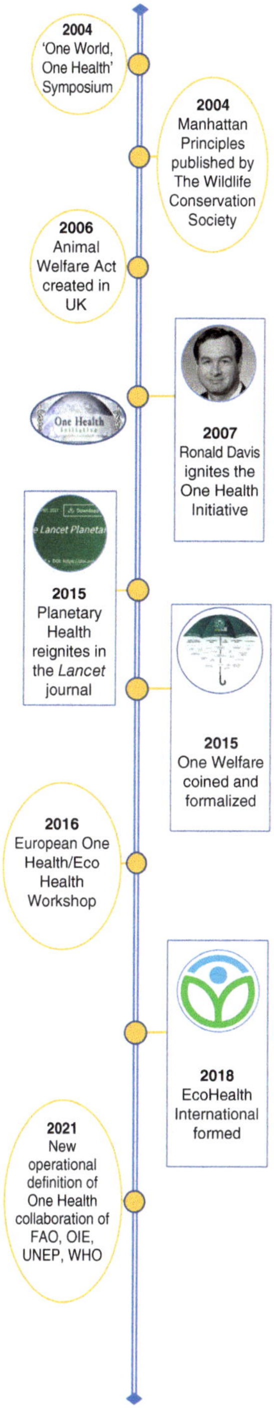

sponsored by the Wildlife Conservation Society and Cornell University since 2004). An important belief underpinning the newly emergent field was that conservation of biodiversity, and of functional healthy ecosystems, was necessary for the health of human and animal populations. It has many similarities in this regard to Ecohealth and has been described as the pursuit of ecological health, or ecological health in practice (Aguirre, 2002). It forms part of an intellectual trend beyond the species-specific approach to focus instead on ecosystems.

The approach has developed substantially since its origins. In its most holistic form, its scope may be as broad as that of One Health, including both the natural sciences and the social sciences. Similar to One Health, it focuses on the interactions between humans, animals and the ecosystems that they inhabit (Tabor, 2002; Deem, 2015); however, it has primarily been promoted by the veterinary profession and those working in the field of wildlife health. For example, it has been popular amongst zoo veterinarians and has been promoted by the American Association of Zoo Veterinarians. Inclusion of the term 'medicine' within the name has had the unfortunate effect of reinforcing the misguided belief that this field should be the domain of veterinarians, rather than a truly holistic and integrated approach to health.

This limited scope is not reflected in the most commonly cited definitions. Reflecting the more holistic view of Conservation Medicine, Aguirre (2002) states that 'conservation medicine examines the interactions between pathogens and disease and their linkages with the synergies that occur between species and ecosystems'. Deem (2015) considers it to be 'a transdisciplinary approach to study the relationships among the health states of humans, animals, and ecosystems to ensure the conservation of all, including *Homo sapiens*'. Defined this way, there is little difference from One Health apart from the emphasis on ensuring the conservation of all. Conservation Medicine therefore fosters an interdisciplinary, or ideally a transdisciplinary, approach and has a similar philosophy and epistemological basis to One Health. Indeed, it may be described as the application of One Health to the conservation of biodiversity.

2.3.4 Comparative Medicine

The discipline of **Comparative Medicine** is an interdisciplinary and translational approach to biomedical research benefiting animal and human medicine, commonly correlating with animal models of disease (Macy and Horvath, 2017). In other words, it relates to and leverages biological similarities and differences among species, including humans, to gain a better understanding of the mechanism of human and animal disease for treatment, drug discovery and vaccine production. It has also been defined as a study of similarities and unique differences between human and veterinary medicine, including the critical role veterinarians play in understanding animal diseases as spontaneous and natural models for human diseases. It, thus, improves human health, including neglected and emerging zoonotic diseases (zooanthroponosis, or reverse zoonosis, refers to diseases transmitted from humans to non-human animals; anthropozoonosis refers to diseases transmitted from animals to humans). For example, the COVID-19 pandemic has highlighted the utmost importance of veterinarians in One Health, Global Health and Population Health for the prevention and control of pandemics (as in the latest paper by Bernstein *et al.*, 2022). Comparative Medicine has been instrumental in moving forward the concept of One Health and promoting some of the most important medical advances in the 21st century. In addition, the Institutional Animal Care and Use Committees (IACUC) have played major roles in facilitating and ensuring humane animal welfare and reproducible laboratory results in studies involving research animals. The 19th-century German physician Rudolf Ludwig Carl Virchow, widely known as the 'Father of Modern Pathology' and the founder of the science of veterinary pathology, wrote: 'Between animal and human and medicine, there is no dividing line – nor should there be. The object is different, but the experience obtained constitutes the basis of all medicine.'

The recognition of highly identical biological mechanisms shared among the animal kingdom (humans included) was the basis for the continuity of this crossover discipline and forwarded translation studies ever since. Sadly, the comparative efforts maintained an anthropocentric vision with results mainly benefiting humans. More recently, translation research has been applied with a special attention on naturally occurring diseases in animals that are almost completely identical to human diseases. This allows an acceleration of knowledge gaining that would be much harder to obtain via inducing these conditions in a lab setting, fully representing the common vision of shared problems and shared solutions (Macy and Horvath, 2017). This comparative trend to use 'naturally occurring/spontaneous' animal models has gained traction only fairly recently (2010 onwards) with the legal settings in place to attend 'Replacement, Reduction and Refinement – the Three Rs' (Tannenbaum and Bennett, 2015).

Historically, Comparative Medicine can be traced back to 1927 when Sir Bradley presented the arguments for the parallel practices of human and veterinary medicine. A renewed interest began in the 1960s with Gordon Theilens' groundbreaking research in veterinary oncology and viral oncology advancing oncological treatments and opening new doors in other fields of health sciences by unravelling mechanisms and providing solutions based on translational medicine research. Interestingly, Comparative Medicine recognizes and serves as the basis for the study of similarities and differences, which was also used as a favourable argument for animal experimentation. In an attempt to promote a more ethical use of animals, Russel and Burch edited what is known as the 3Rs (Replacement, Reduction, Refinement) guiding principles, while also promoting efforts to find alternatives to animal use for education purposes and testing (Cozigou *et al.*, 2015). This acknowledgement that animals are sentient beings laid the groundwork for other approaches that include **welfare** as an intricate part of the health status, see section 2.3.7.

2.3.5 Ecohealth

The foundation for the Ecohealth concept was laid in the early 1990s using the term 'Ecosystem health' (Mageau *et al.*, 1995; Rapport *et al.*, 1998), which was also the name of a journal that was issued from 1997 to 2001 and then discontinued (Rapport *et al.*, 1999). In 1992, the International Development Research Centre (IDRC) in Canada launched its Health, Society and Environment Program, which explored how environmental factors influence health. In 1996, the IDRC created the Ecosystem Approaches to Human Health Program, and later in 2003 coined the term 'Ecohealth'. Shortly after, the IDRC hosted the International Forum on Ecosystem Approaches to Human Health in Montreal, Quebec, Canada, and in 2004 the new *EcoHealth* journal was launched. This journal was associated with the International Association for Ecology and Health (IAEH). The IAEH was formed in 2006 and hosted a series of biennial conferences, such as in the USA in 2006, Mexico in 2008, the UK in 2010, China in 2012, Canada in 2014, Australia in 2016, Colombia in 2018 and South Africa in 2022. The IAEH parted from the journal in 2016 and *EcoHealth* was henceforth managed by the Ecohealth Alliance (https://www.Ecohealthalliance.org). In 2016, a joint International One Health Congress and Biennial Conference on the International Association on Ecology and Health took place in Australia. In 2018, the IAEH transformed into Ecohealth International. In 2019, the Network for Ecohealth and One Health (NEOH) became Ecohealth International's European Chapter.

In 2008, the Canadian Community of Practice in Ecosystem Approaches to Health (CoPEH Canada) was created, including the formation of workshops and an Ecohealth field school. The IDRC later supported the development of an Ecohealth field-building Leadership Initiative in South-east Asia designed to strengthen the field through training, evidence-building and linking researchers. In 2012, Dominique Charron published the six overarching guiding principles (systems thinking, transdisciplinary research, participation, sustainability, gender and social equity, and finally, knowledge-to-action) for Ecohealth (Charron, 2012). Later that year, the Kunming Position Statement was released, identifying Ecohealth contributions to the Millennium Development Goals. In 2017, the Tackling Infections to Benefit Africa (TIBA) Initiative was funded to work in transdisciplinary ways to reduce the threat of infectious diseases in Africa through health policy and system interventions.

Common themes in Ecohealth and One Health include a systems approach to health and holistic understanding of the linkages between human and animal health. Ecohealth emphasizes the intertwined connections between health and sustainable development, which have recently also gained momentum in One Health. The One Health movement has achieved a considerable footprint in the areas of zoonotic disease control and emergence, including very recently during the COVID-19 pandemic (WHO, 2021). A key assumption of Ecohealth is that humans can only survive in healthy, diverse ecosystems. Ecohealth with its focus on Ecosystems is situated at an 'intermediate level' of complexity compared to One Health on one side and **Planetary Health** on the other side.

2.3.6 Planetary Health

The concept of Planetary Health was popularized in 2014 and 2015 to a wider audience after being published in the *Lancet* (Horton *et al.*, 2014; Whitmee *et al.*, 2015). It is closely linked to prior global concerted efforts assessing the status of global environmental / climate change like the Brundtland Commission ('Our Common Future', 1987, United Nations; https://sustainabledevelopment.un.org/content/documents/5987our-common-future.pdf), the Millennium Ecosystem Assessment (https://www.millenniumassessment.org/en/index.html) and the reports of the International Panel on Climate Change (IPCC) (https://www.ipcc.ch/). The term 'Planetary Health' was introduced previously, as early as the 1970s–1980s (Prescott and Logan, 2019). Currently, the movement mostly follows an anthropocentric approach, but also includes the more abstract concepts of 'Planetary Boundaries', which put the focus on the maintenance of key biophysical functions necessary for human health and growth (Rockstroem *et al.*, 2009).

For Planetary Health, human **health** and **wellbeing** depends on the wellbeing of the Earth, attending to its living and non-living systems, for long-term sustainability and balance (Lerner and Berg, 2017; Hill-Cawthorne, 2019). Contrastingly, Rabinowitz *et al.* (2018) defend that One Health embraces both Ecohealth and Planetary Health concepts. For many researchers and practitioners, the dividing line between One Health and Ecohealth is that One Health does not include a health definition on the systems level, even if the importance of the systems approach to health is stressed for scientific inquiry and practice.

The proponents of the Planetary Health movement state that while a global improvement in human health was achieved over the last century, the natural systems of the Earth have deteriorated, which will have implications for human health in the future. Planetary Health now is being supported by the Lancet Planetary Health Commission and the Rockefeller Foundation. The secretariat of the Planetary Health Alliance is located at Harvard University, USA (https://www.planetaryhealthalliance.org/). Ferretto *et al.* (2022) discuss the operationalization of Planetary Boundaries taking into account Doughnut economics (see Chapter 13 for more information on different schools of economic thought), and point out that global-level policies require local-scale implementations in order to have meaningful impact and preserve the social components of each country/region.

2.3.7 One Welfare

Animal rights and animal welfare are commonly overlapping. In sum, sentient animals have similar moral rights and worth as humans, and should be allowed to live free from human exploitation while welfare is based on the relationship between humans and animals, relying on the five freedoms, namely: freedom from hunger and thirst, discomfort, pain, injury or disease, freedom to express normal behaviour, and freedom from fear and distress. Laws were published almost 200 years ago in the United Kingdom, with animal welfare legislators passing the Act to Prevent the Cruel and Improper Treatment of Cattle in 1822 based on the acknowledgement that animals are sentient beings (not commodities), making the UK the first nation to regulate animal rights and welfare. Soon, this prompted the first animal welfare charity named the Society for the Prevention of Cruelty to Animals (SPCA), which later had royal patronage (1837) and since 1840 has been called the RSPCA. Still in the UK, Pease's Act of 1835 extended the prohibition of cruelty towards dogs and other domestic animals, and other activities envisioned as cruel to animals, while appealing for better standards and handling in slaughterhouses. The Protection of Animals Act, the first animal protection law, was approved in 1911, leading on to the more recent Animal Welfare Act (2006).

Many countries do not recognize animals as sentient beings, so offer no protection for their welfare, while other countries are making great strides to support empathic and respectful animal handling. According to the World Organisation for Animal Health (WOAH), animal welfare is 'the physical and mental state of an animal in relation to the conditions in which it lives and dies'. Still, WOAH emphasizes animal welfare practices in Asia, the Far East and Oceania, by the regional animal welfare strategy (https://rr-asia.woah.org/en/projects/animal-welfare/, accessed 13 March 2024). WOAH also identified two major tools to overcome welfare issues as being education and training in animal welfare through active professional awareness and community engagement. All animal–human interactions should assess animal welfare, considering necessities (nutrition, environment and possibility to behave as in a natural setting) along with the physical and mental health status, according to the 5 Domains Model. In line with this call for action, several international organizations, e.g. Veterinarians Without Borders International and Brooke Organization (Action for Working Horses and Donkeys), and others, advocate for animal welfare, voicing concerns for laboratory animal conditions and improving standards for trade and transport conditions for animals (Tarazona *et al.*, 2019; UN Conventions on Animal Health Protection, https://www.globalanimallaw.org/gal/projects/uncahp.html).

More recently, in 2015, a group of veterinarians came together and coined the **One Welfare** concept defending the 'interconnection between animal welfare, human wellbeing and their physical and social environment' (Pinillos *et al.*, 2016; Bourque, 2017). This initiative promotes the awareness of the consequences of human activities with animals (direct and indirect use), which have profound impacts on the environment, law making, commerce and finance development, and ultimately conditioning humans' and animals' health. For this, the One Welfare framework champions a One Health approach with the appeal for multisectoral-approach collaborations to attain health for all and to help prevent zoonotic disease emergence, while defending equity stewardship and compassionate professional practices both for animal welfare and human wellbeing (Fawcett *et al.*, 2018; Pinillos, 2021). Overall, One Welfare based its conceptual approach on the One Health vision and practices along with other initiatives that contribute to One Health evolution (Radeski *et al.*, 2018).

Notably, the initial protective laws for the respect of animal welfare also helped set the tone for later protection laws for children (1880) and women in the UK, and throughout the world. These achievements can be related to the definition for human health, 'A state of complete physical, mental and social well-being and not merely the absence of disease or infirmity', inscribed in the Constitution of WHO in 1948. Health in an integrated approach means basically the same for humans, animals and the environment they inhabit.

2.3.8 One Water, Oceans Health and One Health

Oceans cover more than 70% of our planet and represent over 95% of the biosphere. Hence there is an urgent need to develop the underlying One Health concept and approaches of global sustainability, based on an understanding of the fundamental interactions between oceans and health. This requires a new research and education paradigm that embraces aquatic ecosystems' complexity, which integrates the physical, biological and social sciences, and uses an integrated natural systems approach (https://www.cabidigitallibrary.org/journal/cabioh/special-issues/beyond-one-ocean-health; https://oceanandsociety.org/en/projects/b1oh-beyond-one-ocean-health).

> Marine and coastal habitats cover a diverse spectrum (...) such as coral reefs, mangrove forests, seagrass beds and estuaries, (...) open ocean, hydrothermal vents, seamounts and soft sediments on the ocean floor. (CBD)

One Ocean, One Health has been previously described and published in the first edition of *EcoHealth* (Wilcox and Aguirre, 2004). The authors discuss the paradigm, applying the concept of health to ecosystems,

Box 2.2.

For many decades, a well-known correlation between marine ecosystem distress caused by nutrient loading and potential contributions of anthropogenic global climate change is associated with the frequency and intensity of harmful algal blooms (HABs) and their associated toxicity for marine mammals and humans. Indeed, the horror movie *The Birds* by Alfred Hitchcock (1963) reflects a real event that happened in Monterey, California in 1963 and an example of domoic acid toxicity and algal blooming. Pseudo-nitzschia is a marine planktonic diatom genus that accounts for 4.4% of pennate diatoms found worldwide. Some species are capable of producing harmful blooms and toxicity that affects humans and animals. Many populations of marine animals, marine birds and sea turtles are exposed to pollutants from water and agricultural runoff, human sewage, including pathogens of terrestrial origin best described as pathogen pollution, antimicrobial-resistant (AMR) genes and microplastics. Thus, marine mammals and birds can serve as sentinel species for environmental and human health, reflecting their ecosystems.

addressing the links between oceans, wildlife, plants and human health. In addition, the authors discuss the economic and social value that provides the importance of subsistence, health and equity for more than 200 million people and animals.

A Beyond One Ocean Health Action (B1OH) Initiative based in Kiel, Germany is led by collaborative partnerships and supported by the Ocean Decade and a Special One Oceans Health Edition (https://www.cabidigital-library.org/journal/cabioh/special-issues/beyond-one-ocean-health) is available at CABI One Health Journal. Thus, the **Beyond One Ocean Health** perspective includes issues related to: health and disease in the ocean, ocean-mediated human disease, ocean-related prevention, healing including physical and spiritual wellbeing concepts, the morality and justice of interventions with environmental health **outcomes**, and understanding and living within planetary limits (https://oceandecade.org/actions/beyond-one-ocean-health/).

Finally, we must '**Go Blue**' and be concerned that the current biodiversity loss, ocean pollution and anthropogenic threats will cause planetary health distress if we continue to ignore sustainability and health of the oceans.

Crossword puzzle. Using your newly gained knowledge, see if you can solve the crossword puzzle below.

Learning question: Using the examples provided in Table 2.1, discuss the following questions:

- How unique is each approach? Is the suitability in different scenarios the answer to opt for one instead of another?
- What are the difficulties with these different approaches that are all similar, but yet quite different?
- What does it mean for working together in practice in the same setting?

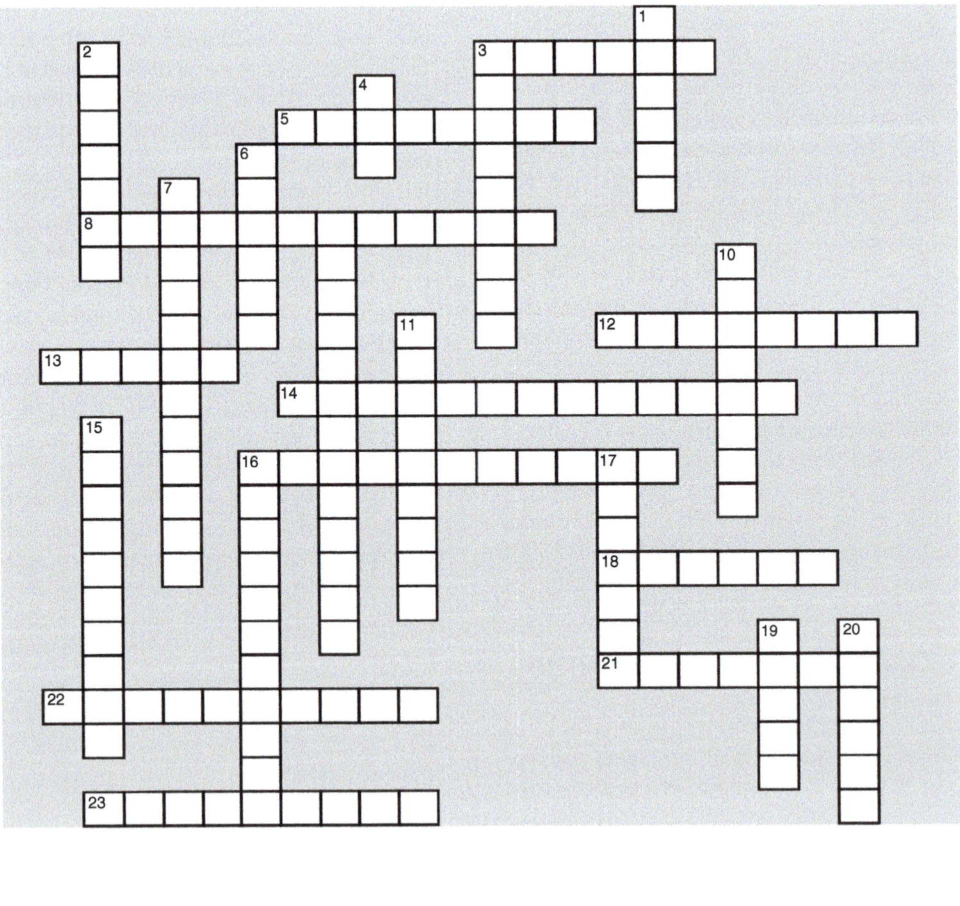

	Across		Down
3	These 'medicines' are also ritual and spiritual objects in many African traditional therapies	1	Veterinarian and pioneer who worked to establish the Veterinary Public Health Division of the CDC in 1947
5	Environmental Health originally came about as the study of ______________ sciences	2	A leader in the One Medicine movement who established the first department of veterinary epidemiology in the US
8	Conservation Medicine arose due to health concerns associated with environmental degradation and __________ loss	3	This health concept is often prioritized by physicians taking an anthropocentric approach to human and environmental health
12	In the 1700s Darwin discussed infectious diseases of humans and animals in his book called ________________	4	___________ Medicine concept, shares similarities with One Health in that animals are physiologically similar to humans and share the same environment
13	Leading biologist (last name) who spear headed the Conservation Medicine movement	6	The Tlingit people of Alaska believe the aurora borealis is the display of the sacred ___________ Spirits playing in the sky
14	One Health conceptualizes the __________________ between animal, plant, environment and human health	7	_____________ Medicine is a health concept that is influenced by conservation biology, veterinary science and human medicine, focusing on the interactions between humans, animals and their environment
16	This health concept, __________________ Medicine, leverages biological similarities and differences among species in health and pathology, including an important focus on zoonotic diseases	9	This health concept discussion includes a focus on toxin exposure
18	Woman author (last name) who helped set the stage for the environmental movement in the US in the 1960s and 1970s	10	Researcher (last name), veterinarian and public health professional who focuses on zoonoses and is active in the One Health and Ecohealth fields
21	The initial protective laws for animal _______________ helped set the tone for children and women protection laws later in history	11	These 12 'Principles' arose at the 'One World, One Health' Conference as recommendations to establish a more holistic approach to prevent infectious disease and maintain ecosystem integrity
22	Practically, ____________________ cultural beliefs preceded many of the same concepts currently embodied within the One Health paradigm	15	The third 'R' of the 3Rs, a principle referencing animal experimentation to find alternatives to animal testing, to find ways to limit the number of animals and adopt methods to alleviate stress
23	Systems-thinking approach that includes the principles of transdisciplinarity, participation, sustainability, equity and knowledge-to-action	16	A call for the synergism between the varied and integrated approaches to health around One Health
		17	Early notable physician who recognized and published on investigation of transmissible disease between animals and humans
		19	Acronym for the committee that ensures humane animal welfare and reproducible laboratory results in studies using research animals
		20	The One ________________ concept is one that integrates unifying approaches to sustainably balance the health of humans, animals and ecosystems through multidisciplinary involvement

Table 2.1. Integrated approaches to health in the context of their academic origin.

Concept	Historical origin and notable dates	Stakeholders / target audience	Key concepts and tenets	Journals (J), conferences (C), societies (S)
Environmental health	Initiated from the Sanitary Sciences[a] 1800s	Ecologists, biologists, public health professionals, students of the natural sciences	Anthropocentric approach of how the environment affects human health	J: *Environmental Health Perspectives*; *Healthy People 2030*; *BMC Journal of Environmental Health*, *International Journal of Environmental Research* and *Public Health* C: WHO Annual Ministerial Conference on Environmental Health, Global Summit on Environmental Health S: US National Environmental Health Association (NEHA), National Institute of Environmental Health Sciences (NIEHS), International Federation of Environmental Health
One Medicine (precursor to traditional One Health)	Virchow and Osler (1800s) embraced One Medicine and coined the term zoonosis. Schwabe in 1964 revived the concept[b] and Zinsstag (2000s) implemented practices for pastoralists in developing countries[c]	Medical professionals (human and animal), microbiologists, geneticists, medical researchers	Collaboration between human and veterinary medical professionals	J: *Emerging Topics in Life Sciences*, *Journal of Veterinary Medical Education*, Veterinary Medicine and Medical Journals C: Zoobiquity Symposiums and Conferences, One Medicine Day Seminar S[d]: Zoobiquity (books) and Humanimal Trust (HUB)
One Health	Modern One Health History[e]. While the term 'One Health' arose in the early 2000s, the concept has been around for hundreds of years. The use of the term arose largely in response to infectious disease (SARS, MERS, Ebola) as a transition from One Medicine through the lens of the broader Ecosystem approach to health	Human, animal, plant and environmental health professionals, public health professionals, politicians/ governmental officials and communities, anthropologists, journalists	Collaboration between every sector to promote cross-sectoral and transdisciplinary changes to improve health of humans, animals and ecosystems. Central tenet revolves around the inter connectedness of all systems where an impact or alteration in one system affects all other systems. Incorporates components of food safety, antimicrobial resistance, and environmental contamination	J: *One Health*, *One Health Outlook*, *Infection Ecology* and *Epidemiology*, *Lancet*, *Frontiers*, *CABI* C: World One Health Congress, WVA/WMA Global Conference on One Health, yearly One Health Symposiums (international) S: One Health Commission; Network of Ecohealth and One Health (NEOH); One Health Initiative, Health in Harmony, International Alliance against Health Risks in Wildlife Trade; continental One Health networks; Nature4Health

Continued

Table 2.1. Continued.

Concept	Historical origin and notable dates	Stakeholders / target audience	Key concepts and tenets	Journals (J), conferences (C), societies (S)
Conservation Medicine	Emerged in the 1990s out of a recognition of the importance of health in conservation problems	Veterinarians and other wildlife health professionals, biologists	The central principle of Conservation Medicine is that the health of animals and humans is connected with the ecosystems in which they live. This fosters an interdisciplinary or transdisciplinary approach	J: No dedicated journal – however, *EcoHealth* has promoted itself as a Conservation Medicine journal C: Annual Wildlife Disease Association Conference S: No global society exists, although Ecohealth International focuses on common areas; regional societies exist including the Asian Society for Conservation Medicine Conferences and Societies[f]
Comparative Medicine	The legacy for this approach includes Hippocrates, Aristotle, Virchow, Steele and many more	Medical professionals (human and animal), biomedical, biosciences and translational researchers	'Inclusive crossover discipline'. Understanding of shared / similar physiological and pathological processes (humans and other animals). Fundamentals for medical and translational research (anthropogenic)	J: *Comparative Medicine*[g], *Clinical and Translational Medicine*, *Journal of Translational Medicine*, *Current Research in Translational Medicine*, SAGE journals, *European Journal of Medical Research* C: Combivet, AALAS, Zoo and Wildlife Health Conferences S: The Royal Society of Medicine (UK), Centre for Comparative Medicine (SE, ES), Einstein Center 3R (DE), The 3Rs Collaborative (US, UK)
Ecohealth	The underlying Ecosystems approach to health[h] was established in part by the French Canadian-based International Development Research Centre (IDRC) in the 1990s	Biologists, ecologists, conservationists	The central tenet of Ecohealth is the premise that human and animal health and wellbeing are dependent on that of the environment and cannot be sustained in a resource-depleted, contaminated and socially unstable planet. Ecohealth recognizes the importance of inclusivity, gender and social equity and contributions of holistic and Indigenous views	J: *Ecosystem Health*; *EcoHealth* C: Ecohealth International Biennial Conference series S: Ecohealth International; Ecohealth Alliance; Network of Ecohealth and One Health (NEOH)

Continued

Table 2.1. Continued.

Concept	Historical origin and notable dates	Stakeholders / target audience	Key concepts and tenets	Journals (J), conferences (C), societies (S)
Planetary Health	Concept was first introduced in the 1970s–1980s. Repopularized and publicized in 2015 by the Lancet Commission and the Rockefeller Foundation	(Human) medical professionals	Anthropomorphized view of the impact of and interconnectedness of humans with the Earth at all levels	J: *Lancet Planetary Health* (Lancet Commission on Planetary Health); *Panorama*[i] C: Annual Planetary Health Conference S: Planetary Health Alliance
One Welfare	This approach emerged in 2015 to promote the links between animal welfare and human wellbeing	Animal welfare scientists and veterinarians / veterinary nurses	One Welfare serves to highlight the interconnections between animal welfare, human wellbeing and the environment. It fosters interdisciplinary collaboration to improve human and animal welfare internationally	J: *Animal Welfare*[j] C: Variety of conferences related to animal welfare, One Welfare World Conference; UFAW S: One Welfare[k]
Beyond One Ocean Health (B1OH)	The Ocean Decade integrates and recognizes the impacts of environmental change on the health of ecosystems and organisms, with an emphasis on the ocean domain	Oceanographers, economists, science and health professionals, modelling engineers, fisheries and oceanography, coastal and river communities	Oceans Health or Beyond One Ocean Health highlights transdisciplinary actions emphasizing aquatic ecosystems and all interconnected integrated systems and health through sustainable development. It links a healthy ocean with health and equity	J: *One Earth, Environmental Justice, EcoHealth, Planetary Health* and *One Health* C: The Ocean Decade Conferences, International Ocean Health Symposium on Emerging Marine Diseases, Regulating Functions and Governance S: Ocean Decade, ECOHA, Oceans Health Associations and Institutions

[a] https://sphweb.bumc.bu.edu/otlt/mph-modules/ph/publichealthhistory/publichealthhistory7.html
[b] Schwabe (1964)
[c] Zinsstag *et al.* (2011)
[d] https://www.zoobiquity.com/ and https://www.humanimalhub.org.uk/
[e] Pettan-Brewer *et al.* (2024)
[f] http://www.ascminfo.org/ and https://www.eazwv.org/events/EventDetails.aspx?id=1002188
[g] https://www.scimagojr.com/journalsearch.php?q=21383&tip=sid
[h] https://www.cbd.int/ecosystem/ and https://www.unep.org/unepmap/what-we-do/ecosystem-approach
[i] https://www.panoramaglobal.org/
[j] https://www.scijournal.org/impact-factor-of-anim-welfare.shtml
[k] https://www.onewelfareworld.org/

- What does it mean for funding potential vs funding struggles?
- What does it mean for solving problems jointly?
- How can we make connections across these different approaches and communities?

Example answer: 'What does it mean for funding potential vs funding struggles?': Planetary Health has substantial funding since its origin because it is focused on human health (anthropocentric). In contrast, One Health initiatives have encountered unsustainable funding as the investment return is not so evident for human health (human–animal–plant–environment based), disregarding the long-term gains of this integrated approach.

Learning question: Consider the various integrated health concepts and approaches above. What two stand out to you the most (perhaps the one you most agree with and the one you most disagree with)?

List the pros and cons for each, then create a visual representation of the relationships between considering how each would approach a multisectoral challenge such as increasing incidence of infectious disease in human health related to climate change (consider pandemics, disease transmission, natural disasters), public health and disaster preparedness, or human/animal migrations.

Example answer: See the Venn diagram in Fig. 2.1. The pros and cons of each domain are shown through the One Health lens.

2.4 Future Perspectives and Calls for Convergence

The synergies and partially overlapping agendas between some of the integrated approaches for health have led to **calls for convergence**, for example, in the case of **Ecohealth and One Health**, which we will concentrate on from this point. In this case, the proponents of the convergence share a broad notion of One Health, which is sometimes distinguished from a more focused tradition in One Health (of which both are coexisting) (Stephens and Karesh, 2014; Harrison *et al.*, 2019; Laing *et al.*, 2023). Areas supporting this convergence have been identified as the research around zoonotic disease and emergence, as well as pandemic threats

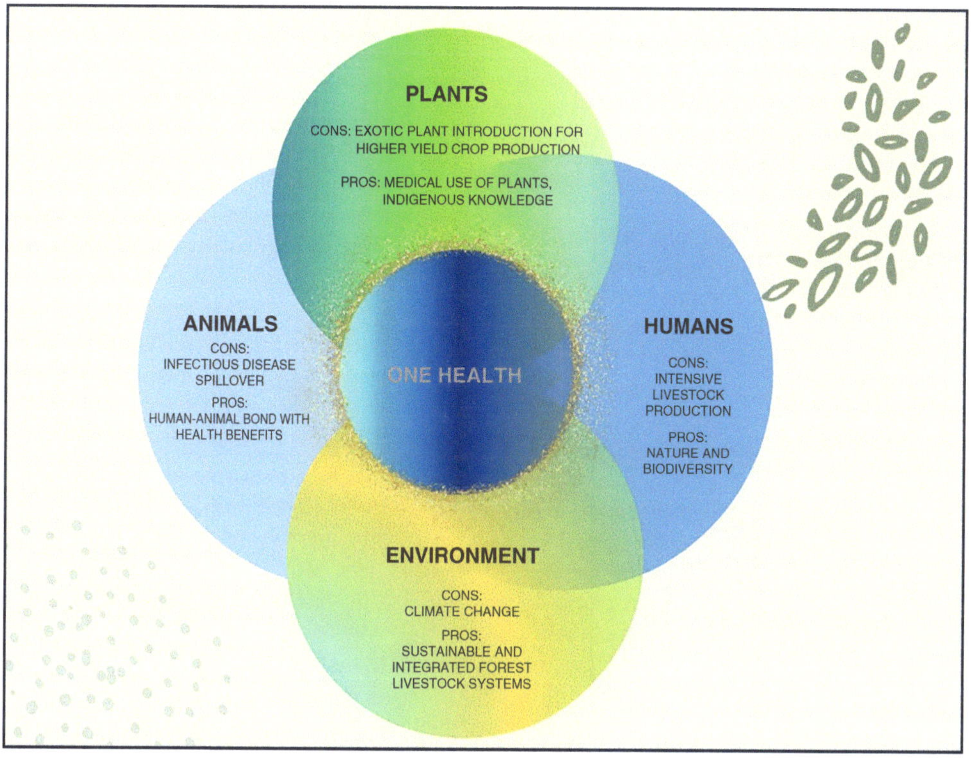

Fig. 2.1. Venn diagram showing the pros and cons relating to plants, animals, humans and environment viewed through the One Health lens.

(Zinsstag, 2012). According to Zinsstag *et al.* (2022), both approaches can benefit from each other's strengths and complementary perspectives. Practical synergies would include joint conferences, integrated health education, curricula development, shared training opportunities, research partnerships and transdisciplinary community involvement as efforts to boost transformative change (Zinsstag *et al.*, 2022).

However, the question is whether the different epistemological heritage as well as the academic disciplines standing behind one versus the other approach can easily be united or reconciled. Some of the epistemological differences between One Health and Ecohealth are related to **ontology** (understanding the categories and relationships that exist within a knowledge domain) and environmental ethics, referring to bearers of health, integrity and value. Thus, taking Ecohealth and One Health as examples, the differences between different integrated approaches to health are related to the background histories and epistemologies and might preclude a full convergence; nevertheless, convergence of practice might be achievable in many cases (Harrison *et al.*, 2019).

The future relies on strengthening the practical initiatives that have previously faced unforeseen challenges, forging non-competitive alliances, operating with transparent communication, trust and **inclusiveness.**

In order to achieve wellbeing for humans, animals and supporting ecosystems, integrated concepts need to be fostered by policy makers and put into practice by societies.

Task: Consider the integrated health approaches described above and the common problem of urban sprawl into natural places. Consider the impact on nature of the urban expansion, increased stress on the environment, encroachment of humans into animal spaces, disease transmission, reduced environmental resources and pollution and how this impacts climate change. Choose two of the above approaches and describe how each would address this problem, listing priorities, possible solutions and challenges faced for each. Finally, indicate the major differences (at least one or two) between these two approaches in addressing this dilemma.

Example answer:

- Extreme weather events related to climate change:
- Planetary Health lens – human deaths, human communities' displacement, increased risk of human diseases (anthropogenic vision)
- Ecohealth lens – Terrestrial environmental destruction, aquatic habitat disruption, animals, humans and plants die off

2.5 Conclusions

This chapter's learning points offer practical applications to better understand and implement integrated approaches to health, especially One Health and Ecohealth. The historical background, individual description of each health perspective and comparative analysis were presented to address complex health challenges at the interfaces of human–animal–plant–environment.

- Emphasize the importance of multisectoral collaboration involving various disciplines such as human health, veterinary medicine, agriculture, environmental sciences and social sciences attending the concepts evolution and key players.
- Encourage breaking down silos between different sectors to achieve a more integrated approach to health management, especially considering the traditional Indigenous knowledge and practices.
- Promote global awareness of health-related integrated approaches, especially among students, through initiatives like One Health Day (and promoting active interplay with associations, foundations, etc.).
- Highlight the need for identifying and prioritizing research gaps as, for example, in zoonoses, emerging infectious diseases, antimicrobial resistance and other multifaceted issues, by shared evidence and knowledge.
- Stress the significance of international collaboration, education and coordination using available technology for controlling outbreaks effectively, promoting a preparedness mindset towards a health continuum of ecosystems, plants, animals and humans.
- Advocate for policy integration across sectors to overcome challenges related to disease control and prevention programmes, from bottom-up and top-to-bottom strategies, and mostly involving community approach to decision making.

References

Aguirre, A.A. (2002) *Conservation Medicine: Ecological Health in Practice*. Oxford University Press, Oxford, UK. ISBN: 9780195150933.

Ajima, O.G. and Ubana, E.U. (2018) The concept of health and wholeness in traditional African religion and social medicine. *Arts and Social Sciences Journal* 9, 4. DOI: 10.4172/2151-6200.1000388.

Alves, R.N., Barboza, R.R.D. and Souto, W.D.M.S. (2010) *Plants Used in Animal Health Care in South and Latin America: An Overview*. Available at: https://www.taylorfrancis.com/chapters/mono/10.1201/EBK1420045604-15/plants-used-animalhealth-care-southand-latin-america-david-katerere-dibungi-luseba?context=ubx&refId=7e4e76c7-0179-4e7d-9a43-0e0f43d38ac1 (accessed 19 July 2024).

Alves, R.R. and Souto, W.M. (2011) Ethnozoology in Brazil: Current status and perspectives. *Journal of Ethnobiology and Ethnomedicine* 7, 22. DOI: 10.1186/1746-4269-7-22.

Bernstein, A.S., Ando, A.W., Loch-Temzelides, T., Vale, M.M., Li, B.V. *et al.* (2022) The costs and benefits of primary prevention of zoonotic pandemics. *Science Advances* 8(5), eabl4183. DOI: 10.1126/sciadv.abl4183.

Bourque, T. (2017) One welfare. *The Canadian Veterinary Journal = La Revue Vétérinaire Canadienne* 58(3), 217–218.

Carson, R. (2002) [1st. Pub. Houghton Mifflin, 1962]. *Silent Spring*. Mariner Books. ISBN: 978-0-618-24906-0. *Silent Spring* initially appeared serialized in three parts in the June 16, June 23 and June 30, 1962, issues of *The New Yorker* magazine.

Charron, D. (ed.) (2012) *Ecohealth Research in Practice: Innovative Applications of an Ecosystem Approach to Health*. Springer, Cham, Switzerland.

Convention on Biological Diversity (CBD), https://www.cbd.int/

Cook, R., Karesh, W.B. and Osofsky, S.A. (2004) *The Manhattan Principles*. Wildlife Conservation Society, Bronx, New York, USA. Available at: https://oneworldonehealth.wcs.org/About-Us/Mission/The-Manhattan-Principles.aspx (accessed 19 July 2024).

Cozigou, G., Crozier, J., Hendriksen, C., Manou, I., Ramirez-Hernandez, T. and Weissenhorn, R. (2015) The European Partnership for Alternative Approaches to Animal Testing (EPAA): Promoting alternative methods in Europe and beyond. *Journal of the American Association for Laboratory Animal Science: JAALAS* 54(2), 209–213.

Daszak, P., Tabor, G.M., Kilpatrick, A.M., Epstein, J. and Plowright, R. (2004) Conservation medicine and a new agenda for emerging diseases. *Annals of the New York Academy of Sciences* 1026, 1–11.

Deem, S.L. (2015) Chapter 73 – Conservation medicine to One Health: The role of zoologic veterinarians. In: Miller, R.E. and Fowler, M.E. (eds) *Fowler's Zoo and Wild Animal Medicine*, Vol. 8. W.B. Saunders, St. Louis.

Ehrenberg, J.P. and Ault, S.K. (2005) Neglected diseases of neglected populations: Thinking to reshape the determinants of health in Latin America and the Caribbean. *BMC Public Health* 5, 119. DOI: 10.1186/1471-2458-5-119.

FAO, UNEP, WHO and WOAH. (2022) *One Health Joint Plan of Action (2022–2026). Working Together for the Health of Humans, Animals, Plants and the Environment*. FAO, UNEP, WHO, WOAH, Rome. DOI: 10.4060/CC2289EN.

Fawcett, A., Mullan, S. and McGreevy, P. (2018) Application of Fraser's 'practical' ethic in veterinary practice, and its compatibility with a 'One Welfare' framework. *Animals: An Open Access Journal from MDPI* 8(7), 109. DOI: 10.3390/ANI8070109.

Ferretto, A., Matthews, R., Brooker, R. and Smith, P. (2022) Planetary Boundaries and the Doughnut frameworks: A review of their local operability. *Anthropocene* 39, 100347. DOI: 10.1016/j.ancene.2022.100347.

Gochfeld, M. and Goldstein, B.D. (1999) Lessons in environmental health in the twentieth century. *Annual Review of Public Health* 20(1) 35–53. DOI: 10.1146/ANNUREV.PUBLHEALTH.20.1.35.

Government of Canada. (2023) *Indigenous Peoples and Communities*. Available at: https://www.rcaanc-cirnac.gc.ca/eng/1100100013785/1529102490303 (accessed 19 July 2024).

Gyles, C. (2016) One medicine, one health, one world. *The Canadian Veterinary Journal = La Revue Vétérinaire Canadienne* 57(4), 345–346.

Harrison, S., Kivuti-Bitok, L., Macmillan, A. and Priest P. (2019) Ecohealth and One Health: A theory-focused review in response to calls for convergence. *Environment International* 132, 105058. DOI: 10.1016/j.envint.2019.105058.

Hill-Cawthorne, G. (2019) *One Health/Ecohealth/Planetary Health and Their Evolution*. DOI: 10.2307/j.ctvggx2kn.6.

Horton, R., Beaglehole, R., Bonita, R., Raeburn, J., McKee, M. and Wall, S. (2014) From public to planetary health: A manifesto. *Lancet* 383, 847. DOI: 10.1016/S0140-6736(14)60409-8.

Jakob-Hoff, R. and Warren, K.S. (2012) Chapter 3: Conservation medicine for zoo veterinarians. In: Miller, R.E. and Fowler, M. (eds) *Fowler's Zoo and Wild Animal Medicine*. W.B. Saunders, Saint Louis.

Kimmerer, R.W. (2015) *Braiding Sweetgrass*. Milkweed Editions, Minneapolis, MN.

King, T.A. (2021) The One Medicine concept: Its emergence from history as a systematic approach to re-integrate human and veterinary medicine. *Emerging Topics in Life Sciences* 5(5), 643–654. DOI: 10.1042/ETLS20200353.

Laing, G., Duffy, E., Anderson, N., Antoine-Moussiaux, N., Aragrande, M. *et al.* (2023) Advancing One Health: Updated core competencies. *CABI One Health* 2023: 1–13. DOI: 10.1079/cabionehealth.2023.0002.

Lerner, H. and Berg, C. (2017) A comparison of three holistic approaches to health: One Health, ecohealth, and planetary health. *Frontiers in Veterinary Science* 4, 163. DOI: 10.3389/FVETS.2017.00163.

Macy, J. and Horvath, T.L. (2017) Comparative medicine: An inclusive crossover discipline. *Yale Journal of Biology and Medicine* 90(3), 493–498.

Mageau, M.T., Costanza, R. and Ulanowicz, R.E. (1995) The development and initial testing of a quantitative assessment of ecosystem health. *Ecosystem Health* 1, 201–213.

Meffe, G.K. (1999) Conservation medicine. *Conservation Biology* 13, 953–954.

Montenegro, R.A. and Stephens, C. (2006) Indigenous health in Latin America and the Caribbean. *Lancet* 367, 1859–1869. DOI: 10.1016/S0140-6736(06)68808-9.

National Environmental Health Association (NEHA) (2013) New perspectives on environmental health: The approval of new definitions. *NEHA NEWS* Available at: https://www.neha.org/Images/resources/NEHA_Adopted_EH_Definition_July_2013.pdf (accessed 19 July 2024).

Pettan-Brewer, C., Martins, A.F., de Abreu, D.P.B., Brandão, A.P.D., Barbosa, D.S. *et al.* (2021) From the approach to the concept: One Health in Latin America – experiences and perspectives in Brazil, Chile, and Colombia. *Frontiers in Public Health* 9, 687110.

Pettan-Brewer, C., Penn, G., Biondo, A.W., Jaenisch, N., Grutzmacher, K. and Kahn, L.H. (2024) Who coined the term 'One Health'? Cooperation amid the siloization. *One Health* 18, 100678. DOI: 10.1016/j.onehlt.2024.100678.

Pinillos, R.G. (2021) One welfare impacts of COVID-19: A summary of key highlights within the one welfare framework. *Applied Animal Behaviour Science* 236, 105262. DOI: 10.1016/j.applanim.2021.105262.

Pinillos, R.G., Appleby, M.C., Manteca, X., Scott-Park, F., Smith, C. and Velarde, A. (2016) One Welfare: A platform for improving human and animal welfare. *Veterinary Record* 179(16), 412–413. DOI: 10.1136/vr.i5470.

Pokras, M., Tabor, G., Pearl, M., Sherman, D. and Epstein, P. (1999) Conservation medicine: An emerging field. In: *Nature and Human Society: The Quest for a Sustainable World.* National Academy Press, Washington, DC, pp. 551–556.

Prescott, S.L. and Logan, A.C. (2019) Planetary health: From the wellspring of holistic medicine to personal and public health imperative. *Explore* 15(2), 98–106. DOI: 10.1016/j.explore.2018.09.002.

QingWen, S., Huo, C.-H., Wang, Y.-F., Li, L. and Zhang, M. (2010) Study on natural medicinal chemistry and new drug development. *Chinese Traditional and Herbal Drugs* 41(10), 1583–1589.

Rabinowitz, P.M., Pappaioanou, M., Bardosh, K.L. and Conti, L. (2018) A planetary vision for one health. *BMJ Global Health* 3(5), e001137. DOI: 10.1136/bmjgh-2018-001137.

Radeski, M., O'Shea, H., De Meneghi, D. and Ilieski, V. (2018) Positioning animal welfare in the one health concept through evaluation of an Animal Welfare Center in Skopje, Macedonia. *Frontiers in Veterinary Science* 4, 238. DOI: 10.3389/fvets.2017.00238.

Rapport, D.J., Constanza, R., Epstein, P.R., Gaudet, C. and Levins, R. (1998) *Ecosystem Health.* Blackwell Science, Malden, MA.

Rapport, D.J., Böhm, G., Buckingham, D., Cairns Jr., J., Costanza, R. *et al.* (1999) Ecosystem Health: The concept, the ISEH, and the important tasks ahead. *Ecosystem Health* 5(2).

Riley, T., Anderson, N., Lovett, R., Meredith, A., Cumming, B. and Thandrayen, J. (2021) One Health in Indigenous Communities: A Critical Review of the Evidence. *International Journal of Environmental Research and Public Health.* Available at: https://pdfs.semanticscholar.org/9d16/22b54a13e22159da1d67af04a70d5d7632c1.pdf?_ga=2.166723710.1106852886.1669765631-1335074918.1669671428 (accessed 19 July 2024).

Rockstroem, J., Steffen, W., Noone, K., Persson, A., Chapin, F.S. 3rd *et al.* (2009) A safe operating space for humanity. *Nature* 461, 472–475.

Schwabe, W. (1964) *Veterinary Medicine and Human Health.* Williams & Wilkins, Baltimore, Maryland.

Srinivasan, K., Kurz, T., Ramp, D. and Pearson, C. (2020) *Remaking One Health: Decolonial Approaches to Street Dogs and Rabies Prevention in India.* Available at: https://wellcome.org/grant-funding/people-and-projects/grants-awarded/remaking-one-health-decolonial-approaches-street (accessed 19 July 2024).

Stephens, C. and Karesh W.B. (2014) Introduction: Is One Health delivering results? *Revue Scientifique et Technique (International Office of Epizootics)* 33(2), 375–379.

Szucs, E., Geers, R., Jezierski, T., Sossidou, E.N. and Broom, D.M. (2012) Animal welfare in different human cultures, traditions and religious faiths. *Asian-Australasian Journal of Animal Sciences.* DOI: 10.5713/ajas.2012.r.02. Available at: https://www.ncbi.nlm.nih.gov/pmc/articles/PMC4093044/pdf/ajas-25-11-1499-1.pdf (accessed 19 July 2024).

Tabor, G.M. (2002) Defining conservation medicine. In: Aguirre, A.A., Ostfeld, R.S., Tabor, G.M., House, C. and Pearl, M.C. (eds) *Conservation Medicine: Ecological Health in Practice.* Oxford University Press, Cary, New York.

Tabor, G.M., Ostfeld, R.S., Poss, M., Dobson, A.P. and Aguirre, A. (2001) Conservation biology and the health sciences: research priorities of conservation medicine. In: M.E. Soule and G.H. Orians (eds). *Conservation Biology: Research Priorities for the Next Decade*, 155–74. Island Press, Washington, DC. http://www.caryinstitute.org/reprints/Tabor_et_al_2001_p155-174_in_Soule_and_Orians_Conservation_Biology.pdf.

Tannenbaum, J. and Bennett, B.T. (2015) Russell and Burch's 3Rs then and now: The need for clarity in definition and purpose. *Journal of the American Association of Laboratory Animal Science* 54(2), 120–132.

Tarazona, A.M., Ceballos, M.C. and Broom, D.M. (2019) Human relationships with domestic and other animals:

One Health, One Welfare, One Biology. *Animals* 10(1), 43. DOI: 10.3390/ani10010043.

United Nations. (2008) *United Nations Declaration on the Rights of Indigenous Peoples.* Available at: https://www.un.org/esa/socdev/unpfii/documents/DRIPS_en.pdf (accessed 19 July 2024).

University of Michigan (2021) *History of Environmental Health Sciences.* Available at: https://sph.umich.edu/ehs/history.html (accessed 19 July 2024).

Vergara, G. (2018) Animals in Latin American history. In: *Oxford Research Encyclopedia of Latin American History.* Oxford University Press, New York. DOI: 10.1093/acrefore/9780199366439.013.436.

Watermolen, S. (2022) *Tlingit Nation Member.* Personal communication.

Whitmee, S. *et al.* (2015) Safeguarding human health in the Anthropocene epoch: Report of The Rockefeller Foundation-Lancet Commission on planetary health. *Lancet* 386, 1973–2028.

WHO (2021) Available at: https://www.who.int/health-topics/one-health#tab=tab_1 (accessed 13 March 2024).

WHO, FAO and OIE (2018) Zero by 30: The global strategic plan to end human deaths from dog-mediated rabies by 2030. Available at: https://iris.who.int/bitstream/handle/10665/272756/9789241513838-eng.pdf?sequence=1 (accessed 17 July 2024).

Wilcox, B.A. and Aguirre, A.A. (2004) One ocean, One Health. *Ecohealth* 1, 211–212. DOI: 10.1007/s10393-004-0122-6.

Woods, A. (2017) From one medicine to two: The evolving relationship between human and veterinary medicine in England, 1791–1835. *Bulletin of the History of Medicine* 91(3), 494–523. DOI: 10.1353/bhm.2017.0058.

WorldBank.org. (2022) *Indigenous Peoples.* Available at: https://www.worldbank.org/en/topic/indigenouspeoples (accessed 17 July 2024).

Zinsstag, J. (2012) Convergence of ecohealth and One Health. *Ecohealth* 9(4), 371–373. DOI: 10.1007/s10393-013-0812-z.

Zinsstag, J., Schelling, E., Waltner-Toews, D. and Tanner, M. (2011) From 'one medicine' to 'one health' and systemic approaches to health and well-being. *Preventive Veterinary Medicine* 101(3–4), 148–156. DOI: 10.1016/j.prevetmed.2010.07.003.

Zinsstag, J., Hediger, K., Osman, Y.M., Abukhattab, S., Crump, L. *et al.* (2022) The promotion and development of One Health at Swiss TPH and its greater potential. *Diseases* 10(3), 65. DOI: 10.3390/diseases10030065.

3 Inter- and Transdisciplinarity in One Health

Nicolas Antoine-Moussiaux[1,2], Luís Pedro Carmo[2,3], Anaïs Léger[4] and Margarida Simões[2,5]

[1]*Faculty of Veterinary Medicine and Faculty of Medicine, University of Liège, Liège, Belgium;* [2]*Network for Ecohealth and One Health (NEOH);* [3]*Norwegian Veterinary Institute, Ås, Norway;* [4]*Federal Food Safety and Veterinary Office, Switzerland;* [5]*Veterinary Medicine Department, University of Évora and Comprehensive Health Research Centre, Portugal and One Health International Network*

Contents

DOI: 10.1079/9781800623002.0004

Chapter Overview

Elevator pitch

Understanding and solving complex health issues requires multiple perspectives and complementary knowledge. Collaborative approaches, such as multi-, inter- or transdisciplinarity, can help us gather and make the best of that diverse knowledge. Far from being a magic bullet, collaborative approaches entail major challenges for science and society as a whole. A deep understanding of the challenges and potential of the diverse collaborative modes is needed in order to mobilize these strategically and harvest their benefits.

Book objectives the chapter relates to

☐ 1. Understand what One Health and Ecohealth mean
☑ 2. Think in a One Health and Ecohealth way
☑ 3. Apply One Health and Ecohealth in their professional and personal life
☐ 4. Know how to share One Health and Ecohealth knowledge
☑ 5. Integrate One Health and Ecohealth knowledge actively
☑ 6. Acquire or enhance core One Health competencies

One Health competencies covered

☐ 1. Effective communication
☑ 2. Collaborative and resilient working
☐ 3. Systems understanding
☑ 4. Transdisciplinarity
☐ 5. Social, cultural and gender equity and inclusiveness
☑ 6. Collective learning and reflective practice
☐ 7. One Health concepts
☑ 8. Theoretical and methodological pluralism
☐ 9. Harnessing uncertainty, paradox and limited knowledge

After having worked through this chapter, you will be able to reflect critically on the need for and constraints of collaborative approaches, identify disciplines and stakeholders to include and propose a plan to mobilize inter- and transdisciplinarity in a given context, including categories of methods to facilitate the process.

Learning outcomes

1. Discuss the meaning of multi-, inter- and transdisciplinarity.
2. Recognize these collaborative approaches as critical components of One Health activities.
3. Identify the benefits, challenges and limits of the different collaborative approaches according to the context and goals.
4. Identify categories of methods, including creativity methods, to be further explored in your other learning.

Summary

Working in multi-, inter- and transdisciplinarity means that more than one scientific discipline and possibly other knowledgeable actors collaborate to tackle complex real-life problems. These collaborative approaches are at the centre of One Health operationalization. This chapter first discusses these distinct collaborative approaches and their respective contribution to One Health. Based on the proposed definition, you learn about barriers and conditions to their implementation. The divides and specificities of disciplines will be presented, considering their diversity as the resource to be harnessed. You will then look at how inter- and transdisciplinarity can be considered as creative processes for collective problem solving, and how these approaches can be implemented in practice.

3.1 Introduction: One Health, the Challenge of Approaching Wholeness

One Health, **Ecohealth** and **Planetary Health**, beyond their differences (see Chapters 1 and 2), all embrace the concept that the **health** of humans, animals, plants and, as a whole, the **ecosystems** they share and constitute, are tightly intertwined. In that understanding and for the sake of simplifying the expression, this chapter will refer to 'One Health' in this broader acknowledgement. As you will further discover in the chapters dedicated to **systems thinking** (Chapter 10) and **knowledge integration** (Chapter 4), this wholeness has been approached in manifold ways by a variety of sciences, practices, traditions and spiritualities. Among these approaches, a significant part of modern science has taken a reductionist turn (see Chapter 4 on knowledge integration), cutting this complexity down into manageable pieces and producing the basis of a substantial segment of current education programmes worldwide. Across the globe, professionals are most often trained in a defined set of sciences and practices, with the prospect of taking charge of one of these pieces: forest management, fisheries, urban planning, veterinary medicine, human medicine, and so on. As will be further outlined in this chapter, these segments of **knowledge** and practices are called **disciplines**, the term here referring indiscriminately to scientific branches (e.g. sociology, epidemiology), humanities or professions. Yet, through its subdivision in disciplines, science and science-based professions have lost the sense of the wholeness that is needed to embrace the One Health concept. Also, by the dominant position that it has taken in many societies across the globe and in international spheres, science has regrettably set aside many other forms of knowledge (see Chapter 4 on knowledge integration).

Hence, to address appropriately the complexity of the intermingled health of life forms, multiple 'disciplines' must be involved, as the knowledge required to frame the problem and investigate and implement solutions cannot lie in a single branch of science or a single profession. The One Health approach leads us to raise questions pertaining to many domains of application, hence, to mobilize many disciplines but also to acknowledge, do justice to and leverage other forms of knowledge. Also, well beyond a simple re-branding of current dominant approaches, One Health must be a complex re-braiding of a diversity of threads of knowledge to produce a colourful and supple fabric. Indeed, as proposed in this chapter, One Health is not 'just' a matter of efficient collaborations but about vivid and fruitful co-creation. This chapter proposes an introduction to these forms of collaboration and creativity, proposing a first set of conceptual landmarks to start your journey across disciplines and beyond.

Throughout your reading, please keep in mind that the authors of this chapter, although they have evolved in very distinct ways away from their initial training, are all anchored in a mix of life and social sciences, leaving out of reach a wealth of considerations that you will be able to discover by reading authors from other disciplinary origins across sciences, arts and humanities. Also, as a joint production, the chapter does not aim at exploring the diversity of thoughts within the team of authors. Rather it proposes a common basis to pave your first steps towards wider and more diverse explorations.

3.2 Multi-, Inter- and Transdisciplinary Work in One Health

One Health dialogues must include a wide spectrum of disciplines and professions, involving or based on life science, social science and humanities, as well as technology, mathematics and engineering. These various disciplines or, better said, the collaborators representing them will bring complementary knowledge and a multitude of perspectives, which enrich our understanding of these complex problems. Therefore, as outlined in the introduction, knowledge sharing and articulation among multiple disciplines, **sectors** and groups in society are at the core of integrated approaches to health (as seen in Chapter 1). Hence, the terms **multi-**, **inter-** and **transdisciplinarity** are often associated with the work conducted using the One Health approach. None the less, these represent distinct modalities of collaboration and should not be used interchangeably.

In the realm of health, Choi and Pak (2006) reviewed the definitions of the three terms according to multiple sources. The results showed that the terms are ambiguously defined, which these authors consider to be a cause of confusion and misinterpretations. While the ambiguity of terms may in fact be appreciated for the freedom of interpretation and creativity that it allows, at this step of your learning, it seems wise to start from a first set of beacons, under the form of definitions that you will be later able to re-consider and critique. Indeed, for the sake of clarity, we will propose here a brief summary of our current understanding of each type of collaboration. Be aware, nevertheless, that the literature may contain many nuances in the interpretation of these terms, showing that the debate is vivid and that our experience of collaborations between disciplines is still evolving.

MULTIDISCIPLINARITY refers to collaborations that use knowledge and practices from different disciplines but stay within the boundaries of each field. Hence, multidisciplinary collaboration represents merely an addition of different disciplines. Courses at university level are often built in a multidisciplinary fashion: students from health-related areas need to study different disciplines (e.g. microbiology, pathology, parasitology) to complete their course. Due to the lack of integration of the knowledge of different disciplines, this can be considered the least collaborative of the approaches here described. Therefore, multidisciplinarity may not be considered an 'integrative' approach.

INTERDISCIPLINARITY requires an intersection of knowledge between two or more disciplines to tackle a common problem. This goes beyond the additive nature of multidisciplinary collaborations because it requires an integration of knowledge from the disciplines involved (for further insight on knowledge integration, see Chapter 4). This means that, in interdisciplinary works, collaborating disciplines hold direct interactions and mutual adaptation of their questions, methods and tools. They are learning from each other and producing approaches and knowledge that would not be reachable by each discipline on its own or by simply adding to each other. During the COVID-19 pandemic, many countries created task forces to control the disease. These task forces included virologists, epidemiologists and clinicians, among others. Actors in such task forces often collaborated in an interdisciplinary fashion to advise authorities about the control measures to be taken. This happened through direct dialogues between the representatives of the various disciplines involved. Such task forces, however, often failed to integrate other types of disciplines, notably across social sciences and humanities or environmental sciences. Therefore, let us note here that reaching the degree of co-learning between disciplines that interdisciplinarity is conveying does not reveal anything about the diversity of the disciplines involved.

TRANSDISCIPLINARITY often refers to the realm of scientific research, hence to trandisciplinary research (see, for example, Scholz and Steiner, 2015). This then means that the knowledge production efforts involve knowledgeable actors across society, beyond scientific disciplines. Hence, there is an integration of knowledge from scientific and other sources. This transdisciplinary research is focused on solving problems within society, involving the needed **stakeholders** and leveraging the diversity of their knowledge (experiential, traditional, and so on). The scientific realm investigates a given problem while society needs to handle that problem (or a societal group, not necessarily the society as a whole) (Pohl *et al.*, 2017). Along the steps of the transdisciplinary collaboration (framing the problem, analysing the problem and exploring the impact of potential solutions – more detail on this can be found in the One Health implementation cycle, Chapter 10), there is an involvement from both the scientific and the societal actors. Let us use the example of sustainable food systems in the 21st century. Such a complex topic cannot be solved by science on its own. Even if multiple scientific disciplines collaborate to develop technical solutions and a fine understanding of social and economic stakes, their applicability might be limited if critical actors, such as the food industry and the consumers, are not engaged throughout the process. To provide sustainable options, societal actors need to perceive the current system as a problem and be involved in the scientific exploration of solutions.

As illustrated in the definition of transdisciplinarity, these three forms of collaboration are often evoked in the particular context of research, with the term 'disciplines' then covering 'scientific disciplines'. This dominant use can be seen as still influencing the writing of this chapter. However, these terms also apply to the collaboration between different professions, different institutions, and different sectors of activity. In this case, it may be proposed to apply the term 'transdisciplinarity' to cases where the boundary to be crossed is the one delimiting not only science from society, but more generally professional actors (e.g. medical doctor, nurse, social worker, veterinarian, epidemiologist, agronomist) from other knowledge holders who are not commonly considered legitimate to influence the professional decision of the former (e.g. pet holders for veterinary decision making, a patient group for therapeutic strategy, citizen groups for the control of an epidemic). Transdisciplinarity has been a particularly successful and debated term, with some authors pointing more recently to it as being a 'way of living' (Rigolot, 2020), significantly opening the box and creating a space that you will be able to inhabit through your evolving practice.

These three modalities can be seen as a collaboration continuum, where multidisciplinarity requires the least intense collaboration and transdisciplinarity entails the most engagement from various scientific disciplines and societal actors. Between those extremes, interdisciplinarity covers a wide range of collaborative efforts, depending on the number of disciplines, their diversity and the depth of integration that is meant. In perspective, this does not mean that there is an approach that is per se better or has more worth than the others. Much can be achieved by scientific disciplines in isolation, taking advantage of specialization and sharp expertise on well-delimited topics.

The choice of the collaborative modality should be made based upon the problem to be solved. As a matter of fact, not all health problems require a collaborative approach. Social change for health purposes will eventually require wide transdisciplinary collaborations, but these changes will also be fuelled by knowledge produced by disciplines in isolation. Moreover, one given societal problem requiring transdisciplinary approaches will in fact be tackled in different phases. Each of these may require distinct depths of collaboration, with multi-, inter- and transdisciplinary stages (Hurni and Wiesmann, 2004). Thus, there is a dynamic of collaboration, with each form of collaboration holding distinct roles in problem solving. In other words, there is no point in demeaning shallower forms of collaborations or in idealizing deeper ones. The quest will be one of a flexible and adapted course to one or the other form to address challenges in a feasible way.

Interdisciplinarity and transdisciplinarity represent fields of knowledge and practices in their own right, being developed and reflected upon in a plurality of communities of practice, around various concerns and challenges, well beyond integrated approaches to health (see Chapter 6 on reflexivity and Chapter 10 on communities of practice). Therefore, interdisciplinary and transdisciplinary efforts made in the pursuit of One Health implementation are a particular case of application of these fields, and remain mostly a work in progress, not to say a promise. For instance, in the case of antimicrobial resistance, which is addressed by many One Health endeavours, it is widely accepted by professionals across medical and veterinary sectors that social sciences can help understand practices and habits of farmers, veterinarians, patients and medical doctors that impact antimicrobial consumption. This in turn can help generate more adequate measures to curb the use of antimicrobials and protect the efficacy of these drugs for use in animals and humans, consequently also lowering their impact on the **environment**. Some may even be well aware that social sciences and humanities more fundamentally provide critical analyses of the current ways of living, thinking and doing, which can be leveraged to re-think more fundamentally ourselves and our societies (see Chapter 6 on reflexivity), including obviously the healthcare and the food system that are home to this overuse and misuse of antibiotics. It is also widely understood that environmental sciences will shed light on how antimicrobial resistance affects ecosystems and how it spreads and persists in a diversity of conditions, and eventually how it will respond or not to interventions we aim at. Yet, despite their obvious relevance, social and environmental sciences are often poorly represented in One Health endeavours.

This is to highlight the difficulty of translating these principles into practice and the efforts that remain to be done. Indeed, establishing collaborations across disciplines comes with considerable challenges that will be addressed in this chapter. Before entering into the more systematic discussion of these challenges, let us first stress that a main difficulty in this regard will be that any collaboration is, at the end of the day, a matter of learning and unlearning, a matter of deep reflection and reflexivity (see Chapter 6). This constant effort to deepen our understanding of the world and critically view what we do and how we think, beyond our 'common understanding' and 'good practices' (Antoine-Moussiaux and Leyens, 2023), remaining open to contradictions, emanating from our collaborators or from reality, is difficult. Nevertheless, if we are to create bright futures, we do not have another option.

Task: Consider a One Health problem of your choice (e.g. control and prevention of a defined zoonosis, non-communicable disease, antimicrobial resistance, food safety and security in a defined socio-economic context). For the sake of this exercise, let us focus on addressing the problem you identified using the most integrative collaboration approach we discussed in this chapter: transdisciplinary collaborations. You can also complete this activity by addressing the identified problem using a less integrative collaborative approach.

1. Describe the One Health problem you aim to address: type of health matter, context (geographic, social, economic, etc.), stakeholders, i.e. people impacting or impacted by the health issue and its control (e.g. health professionals, patients, economic actors, authorities), type of action you would focus on.
2. Identify which scientific disciplines should be engaged in your initiative and explain their relevance to your project. Start with the wide categories of disciplines: life sciences (including biomedical and environmental sciences), engineering and technologies, social sciences and humanities. Then explore each of these categories and be as precise as you can about the disciplines that should be involved. What kind of study/action would each discipline be requested to conduct?
3. Describe which societal actors should also be engaged in your study or initiative and explain their relevance to your project. Be explicit about your expectations: Do you need them to define the questions or actions with you? Do you need them to share their knowledge and produce new knowledge together with scientists?
4. Consider the potential negative and positive consequences of your intervention for the different stakeholders. Who would have something to gain or to lose if an intervention is put in place? Try to think of coping strategies to face the negative consequences.

Reflect on the advantages and disadvantages of your collaborative approach to address the One Health problem under analysis, when compared to other collaborative options (or no collaboration at all).

Once you have concluded this exercise, have a look at the example answers provided below and compare them with your answers. Think about how they differ and what may be the reasons for this difference.

Example answers: Caveat – This example is written in a short and simplified way, from a restricted perspective, for the sake of clarity. Please keep in mind that integrated approaches to health will always call its practitioners to bring up complexity onboard by gathering distinct and even divergent perspectives. This brief and illustrative example cannot be interpreted as a valid analysis. For the same reasons, the proposals are not criticized here for their feasibility.

- **One Health problem description:**
  Let us consider antimicrobial resistance in a rural area of a low-income country.

  The context may be characterized grossly by a high rate of poverty and low literacy of population with great disparities between small commercial centres and more remote communities. Overall, transport and communication infrastructures are weak. The local authorities lack means of action but are well-rooted in the communities with community-based workers being active across the territory. On average, the access to healthcare services is very low and a high prevalence of self-medication exists, the drugs being purchased in informal markets. Main health concerns in the region relate to maternal health, with a high rate of child mortality tied to poor hygiene, poor vaccination coverage, food and water insecurity and high prevalence of diarrhoeal and respiratory diseases. People live mainly from agriculture, and livestock mainly consist of a few backyard or free-ranging animals (chickens, pigs, goats). Some commercial broiler and layer production is developing near the commercial centre.

  The stakeholders include patients, practitioners in health centres, community-based workers, local authorities, animal smallholders, poultry producers, drug sellers on the informal markets, established pharmacies and traditional healers.

  Potential topics of focus are the monitoring of resistance, the development of alternative treatments, the control of antimicrobial use, and so on. Let us choose for the rest of the example the case of the delivery of antibiotics in informal markets.

- **Scientific domains and disciplines to be included:**

  When considering this part, you will observe it is probably easier to imagine roles for different categories of sciences for different types of actions. Hence, for antimicrobial resistance, life science would find an obvious role in the surveillance of resistance, technologies in the development of alternative treatments, social science in the study of consumption and health-seeking behaviour. However, let us try to focus on one single type of action to increase the ability of these specialists to interact around the same topic and learn together. In our case, focusing on informal markets of antibiotics in low-income countries would call for **life sciences** to characterize the diseases that led buyers to seek antibiotics in informal markets for human use and animal use, to characterize the environmental impact of that supply chain and its waste production; **technologies** would develop capacities for the rapid testing of the quality of antibiotics or communication technologies would increase the access to health expertise despite remoteness; **social science** would study the organization of these informal markets for antibiotics to understand consumer behaviours.

  For the sake of brevity, we will develop only one scientific area here. Let us focus on the study of informal markets by social science and humanities. This can include a **value chain analyst** to study the product flows, values, profits and interests of different actors, a **behavioural economist** to study the willingness of consumers to pay for better quality products, a **health anthropologist** to study the representation of health products in general, and antibiotics in particular, among sellers and buyers, a **sociologist** to study social networks of cooperation and influence among sellers, a second sociologist to characterize the types of consumers buying antibiotics in such markets and their motives not to go through formal markets, a **philosopher** to reflect on ethical issues, such as the right to access health products and social justice matters in controlling informal markets of antibiotics for human and for animal use.

- **Societal actors:**

  Patients and artists can help in designing effective communication materials. School teachers can help in designing sessions to explain the issue to children. Traditional healers can help in identifying alternative treatments that have better accessibility for people. Local authorities can contribute their knowledge of the context and legal or administrative constraints. It is important here to go beyond the mobilization of stakeholders as mere implementers and to really include them as contributors to problem analysis or solution design.

- **Consequences for stakeholders:**

  Drug sellers in informal markets would lose from this regulation. It would be wise in this case to think about a way to compensate for this loss by the development of other business opportunities respecting the sound use of antibiotics. Maybe some would be ready to specialize in drug delivery and find an economic role in collaboration with pharmacists, to increase the access of people to quality products, respecting good conditions of conservation and distribution, as well as waste management. What new scientific questions would this raise?

  An improvement of the drug supply chain and better access to healthcare will have a cost. Who would bear that cost? Is it possible to develop local health insurance schemes? What new scientific questions would this raise?

  Lowering the use of antibiotics for poultry producers will have consequences on their profitability and will increase the technicality of production, requesting higher biosecurity standards, better use of vaccination and ensuring sources of good quality inputs (day-old chicks, feed). What new scientific questions would this raise?

- **Advantages and disadvantages of collaboration:**

  The collaboration will need time to be implemented and will generate some complexity in the coordination of the interventions of experts in the field. However, this might also generate some logistic advantages, by collecting, for example, the needed situational diagnostic information in one single survey. If all these specialists focus on the same topic, we can expect them to learn from each other and generate new ideas, refine their scientific questions and increase the overall relevance of the study and the ensuing action.

The involvement of stakeholders will also require a lot of time, at first to generate the needed trust between them and scientists, and then to develop a mutual understanding that would allow them to produce new knowledge and solutions together. The advantage will be that the study will produce more adapted solutions, with several stakeholders already being fully convinced of their interest.

Reflexive intermission: You have read the caveat and then the proposed example. What would you think could be other ways to frame the same example from a different perspective? What would you deem not feasible? Would you be able to imagine alternatives to compensate for what you deemed not realistic?

3.3 Institutional Barriers to Collaboration Between Disciplines and Between Sectors

The challenges of putting One Health into practice are more than many. A significant number of those challenges are directly due to the difficulty of fostering the needed collaborations between disciplines and between sectors. Hereafter, the term 'sector' will be used as an encompassing term to refer to the set of agencies, institutions, professions and actors operating throughout society around one domain of concern. Possibly, the practical division of the concern may define 'sub-sectors'. For example, we may consider human health as a sector, which may encompass a sub-sector of healthcare and one of health promotion. Another sector would be agriculture, which includes crop production and livestock. The latter can be proposed as two 'sub-sectors'. The preservation of ecosystems would be another sector. Other examples of sectors are the bio-pharmaceutical sector, the industry sector, the energy sector, the education sector, and so on. Let us note that people from one given discipline (e.g. mathematical modelling) can be active in different sectors (e.g. one in agriculture, the other in health). A collaboration between them would be intersectoral but not interdisciplinary.

Let us first consider some of the barriers and constraints that are embedded in our current modes of organization (Table 3.1). Indeed, across the globe, administrations, research institutions and private companies commonly work in a highly segmented fashion. Sectors of activity are separated and work in parallel; likewise, governance is based on a clear distribution of roles and competencies. This mode of organization is often mentioned as working in 'silos' (e.g. faculties in universities, departments in ministries or agencies), stressing the lack of communication and collabor-

Table 3.1. Examples of barriers to collaborations, with some solutions and values or competencies that are key to their success.

Categories	Examples	Potential solutions	Key value or competency needed for success	References
Political	Territorial sovereignty	Transboundary and multi-country projects	Transparency, leadership	Pettan-Brewer *et al.* (2021); Caron *et al.* (2022)
Economic	Competition for funding	Cost–benefit analysis to prove the value added of collaboration	Equity	Häsler *et al.* (2013)
Scientific	Ignorance about other disciplines	Joint training in One Health programmes	Inclusivity, knowledge sharing	Sidikou *et al.* (2022)
Institutional	Lack of established procedures for data sharing	Inter-institutional agreement	Engagement, transparency	See Tripartite and Quadripartite agreements
Ethical	Data ownership	Clear and enforceable agreements on data sharing	Effective communication, responsibility	Capps (2022)

ation between sectors once the work has been distributed. This siloed organization of work is based on historical development and has successfully dealt with specific problems. For example, within an academic context, we can highlight how the division of a university in faculties or colleges can help each of those address more specifically the needs of their curriculum and students. The needs of a student in engineering are distinct from the needs of a veterinary student. It seems wise to allow each faculty to manage their needs separately to provide suitable services to their students, developing and managing their specific infrastructures. This will lead each faculty to develop ways of working that will be distinct from others. Across society, it is easy to imagine the benefits obtained in the last two centuries from the specialization of medicine at large. Considering the development on the one side of a diverse set of medical specialities and on the other side of bio-pharmaceutical industry, we can understand that this allowed the development of an array of high-quality healthcare services. In the first line of healthcare, the recognition and development of nursing as a speciality and profession on its own, with duly standardized curricula and the emergence of very active nursing science, helped improve the services rendered to society but obviously created a distinction between nurses and other professions around the care of people. Specialization in livestock production, e.g. in milk production, has generated considerable gains in productivity, improving the availability and quality of milk products worldwide. Through that specialization, dairy production has gradually distanced itself from other agricultural activities, turning a former peasant system integrating crops and livestock into well-separated activities, sometimes just connected through feed markets. Hence, specialization and division of labour appear almost an inherent feature of human activity once it involves large groups. By tackling issues in a siloed way, however, solutions of one sector will generate new problems outside of the sector, which we call 'externalities'. For example, intensive livestock production and large-scale bio-pharmaceutical production both generate important environmental issues (see Chapter 7 for information on **biodiversity** and food production). It is important to note in this critical domain of One Health, touching on deep and pressing concerns of justice and **sustainability**, that these accounts of the process of specialization are meant as didactic illustrations, leaving aside the otherwise crucial questions of the merit of the goals pursued or of means employed.

Based on jurisdictional divides, each sector has developed distinct practices and modes of working that might not be compatible with one another. Hence, this reinforces a sector's individuality and autonomy. In this context, collaborations are often perceived by a sector as a threat to its sovereignty (Jerolmack, 2013). This may be exemplified in the case of the outbreak investigation of a **zoonotic disease**. Indeed, veterinarians will obviously be in charge of managing animal cases, and they will treat, cull or sample animals according to the state of the art of veterinary science, reporting information to their hierarchy. In the same way, medical doctors will handle patients independently, with due confidentiality. This segmented way of working, each following their own procedures, will not be prone to the sharing of information that would be needed to correctly assess the situation and react accordingly.

Nowadays, the acknowledgement of the interconnectedness and interdependence of many issues, as in the case of One Health, unveiled the fragilities and incapability of these single vertical structures to properly address and solve the multidimensional, complex problems (Destoumieux-Garzón *et al.*, 2018). Therefore, across the world, efforts are underway to build interministerial and intersectoral bridges around One Health, at national and decentralized levels, through permanent commissions (as the National One Health Coordination Mechanisms, also termed 'One Health platforms') or other kinds of agreements (e.g. fusion of scientific institutes or public administrations). However, as a matter of fact, the integrative thinking and interdisciplinary and inter-agency collaborations of One Health often remain trapped in the unique views of each 'organizational silo' and face the difficulty of bridging the articulation with other 'organizational cultures' (Jerolmack, 2013).

Alongside the institutional barriers, the distinct habits of each profession (e.g. ways of communicating, kinds of hierarchical relationships) also contribute to the lack of common understanding, in turn leading to non-sharing practices (e.g. of **data**), many times aggravated by context barriers (e.g. territorial borders), which have long been contributing to the missed opportunities for One Health integrative efforts (Kayunze *et al.*, 2014). Therefore, effective partnerships are often impeded by lack of communication, mistrust and conflicts of ego, entrenched in 'silo' bureaucracies and hierarchy. Coupled with insufficient coordination, these culminate in disarticulation and flawed integration between organizations or sectors (Uchtmann *et al.*, 2015).

Mirroring the segmentation of professional realms, the segmentation of academic disciplines also further cultivates this differentiation and transfers them to the next generation. This segmentation in training and education appears necessary to reach relevant levels of specialization and standardization of practices and competencies (to be sure that diplomas are well certifying the set of expected competencies from a practitioner). Moreover, this segmentation coincides with a hierarchical differentiation between professions (e.g. nursing and medical sciences). Each sector's set of priorities, necessarily aligned to its domain of knowledge and expertise, contributes to the disparities in working relationships (Humboldt-Dachroeden, 2021). Finally, this institutional segmentation within higher education and research produced deeper divides between people, in their mode of thinking and in conceiving the world, its issues and our knowledge itself. The next section will consider those divides in the modes of thinking.

Naturally, as this book illustrates, much effort is devoted in several domains to produce the interdisciplinary curricula that would respond to complexity of world problems: classical or more recent examples can be highlighted here as land planning, public health, environmental management or food systems. Because those problems are all interconnected, however, each of those already integrated curricula will have to establish bridges with the others to build One Health capacities. Since knowledge grows together with its segmentation and since integration efforts must always concentrate on defined problems, interdisciplinarity seems a never-ending effort, always searching for the missing collaboration, with people having the knowledge and abilities we are missing but also distinct ways of thinking and working.

Task: Imagine you are part of a One Health team with secured funding for the next three years. The One Health research project adopts a community-based approach and aims to study a waterborne zoonotic disease that afflicts wildlife, domestic mammals and humans.

1. List the various disciplines and stakeholders that you expect to be involved, and ascribe responsibilities to each of them.

2. Anticipate the barriers to collaboration that you will be confronted with, considering interacting stakeholders.

3. How would you term the competency that we have to foster to overcome your examples of expected barriers to collaboration?

4. Develop working rules that would help in avoiding each of these difficulties.

Once you have concluded this exercise, have a look at the possible answers provided below and compare them with your answers. Reflect on how they differ and what may be the reasons for this difference.

Example answers:

1. We may propose to include in your team an infectiologist, an epidemiologist, a socio-anthropologist, a biologist specialized in aquatic ecosystems, a livestock specialist, an economist and a land planner. Among stakeholders, you may consider hunters, birdwatchers, conservationists, farmers, local veterinarians, public health professionals and healthcare professionals. Regarding their respective responsibilities, among scientists, the socio-anthropologist could characterize the relationship between distinct social categories and the ecosystem (representation of wildlife, perception of the zoonotic risk, cultural role of hunting, etc.). Among stakeholders, one example could be to ascribe a role to birdwatchers in the reporting of mortalities in wild birds or other unusual observations.

2. Let us consider as an example the expected barriers to collaboration between the biologist of aquatic ecosystems and the socio-anthropologist. The latter might have a clear view of human stakes at the community level and be sensitized to poverty issues or the importance of cultural habits that drive poaching behaviours. The former may not have that understanding, being personally more sensitized to the uniqueness of the biotope and the need to protect it from any human-origin disturbance. They will not agree in the way the issue may be expressed. The socio-anthropologist will be used to long stays in the field to interview people and live with them, whereas the biologist will rather consider short interventions to take samples and set up monitoring tools. The socio-anthropologist may not directly understand the relevance of the list of figures and graphs that the biologist will produce to describe the ecosystem dynamic. The biologist may not perceive the general scientific relevance of an in-depth case study where the socio-anthropologist would detail the people's motives, history, gender relations or familial organization.

3. Both the socio-anthropologist and the biologist will have to gain literacy in the other's methodologies and focus of interest. Fundamental competencies will be humility and open-mindedness, but also a basis in epistemology (see below). Both will require systems thinking to learn the value of connecting their information, respective pieces of understanding and (maybe contradictory) perspectives (see Chapter 4 on knowledge integration to read more on the topic).

4. In our example, rules could be to hold regular meetings to update the other on progress in the understanding of the situation. Such a meeting could rigorously set the same time for each partner to speak, to make sure that each holds an equitable place in the collaboration.

3.4 Divides in the Modes of Thinking

The deepest barriers to collaboration are embedded in the cores of disciplines or professions, i.e. in the way each discipline thinks and conceives of the world (Antoine-Moussiaux *et al.*, 2019). This section will consider two levels of this divide: first considering the different ways in which disciplines tackle complex problems, and then the way each discipline thinks about knowledge itself.

3.4.1 Disciplines and disciplinarity, an evolving set of fuzzy (sub)divisions

Above, we considered implicitly the term 'discipline' as commonly shared and understood; however, its meaning is not so obvious. Let us sum up here the elements already shared about disciplines in an attempt to circumscribe the term. Each discipline will have a distinct focus that defines it. To tackle that subject of concern, a discipline includes a set of methodologies and tools. Disciplines are organized around key concepts (see Box 3.1 for further discussion on the role of concepts in inter- and transdisciplinarity) and key theories, as well as founding authors or even heroes. The members of a discipline thus share a history and most often sharing this will entail that they share values, and a common representation of what science is or must be, or what a good practice is or must be. To hand over this legacy between generations, a discipline is created by the establishment of a curriculum, a standardized training that makes sure that every member of the discipline holds that common basis of concepts, theories, tools, authors, heroes and values (sometimes very explicitly, as exemplified by the Hippocratic Oath). An important heterogeneity in the size and nature of disciplines emerges from the diversity of nature and degrees of precision of topics of concern. Indeed, a discipline can be organized around a very broad and fundamental topic, such as biology studies life, chemistry the molecular interactions, or physics the principles governing energy and matter. Other disciplines will organize around a practical problem, such as medicine, urban planning or climatology, merging elements from several fundamental disciplines. The focus of interest may be very precise, making the discipline very specialized, resulting most often from a specialization from a discipline of origin. This means that the reality covered by the term discipline may vary greatly and evolve through time, through a continuous process of differentiation and merging around topics of concern.

Even more tricky will be to circumscribe the term disciplinarity, the meaning of which has also been held implicit in the above. In fact, we did not use the term 'disciplinarity' on its own but always with a prefix (multi-, inter- and trans-), on which the first section focused its definitional effort. Let us now spend some time on the term of disciplinarity. From the way it has been mobilized in the above, we can propose disciplinarity to be the way that people will work within and across disciplines. Indeed, given the evolving reality of scientific enquiry and professional practices, it may not be easy for anyone to state the discipline to which they belong or the discipline they practise. Translating this difficulty, quite often, scientists will merge terms to describe the discipline they practise: immuno-pathologist, socio-anthropologist, socio-economist or eco-infectiologist. Disciplinarity may thus be considered as the tendency of anyone to consider her or his own practice as embodied (or not) in the limits circumscribed by the established curricula we mentioned earlier. This points to the individual abilities and mindset that inter- and transdisciplinarity call for (Max-Neef, 2005; Darbellay,

2015), what other authors – playing with words – will call 'indiscipline' (Pasquier and Schreiber, 2007; Wolton, 2013). Disciplinarity appears as a field of tension between the societal need to frame and format professional practices (including science) and the need for individuals or communities to evolve, using the available degrees of freedom (or creating them).

As we already mentioned, each discipline will have a distinct focus, and this will translate to distinct ways of approaching a given health concern. For example, biology will study living beings and processes that sustain their development and how they interact in ecosystems, sociology will study the way that humans interact in societies, while epidemiology will study the distribution of health events in space and time and the drivers of that distribution. If we are facing a potential zoonotic risk, the biologist might focus on the ability of the **pathogen** to jump from one species to another and the genetic mechanisms allowing for those jumps; the sociologist will highlight how our way of living is creating special risks for certain categories of people (e.g. women, children, farmers); and the epidemiologist will work on mathematical models of disease spread to predict the risk and inform policy makers. Certainly – and that is the very interest of collaborative approaches – all these contributions are interrelated, and those professionals would learn from collaborating directly. Indeed, each actor generates information and questions for the others. However, one cannot learn everything and one needs to be anchored in one or a small subset of disciplines, with varied degrees of specialization. Also, it may prove unrealistic to expect to have a complete view of the rapidly changing landscape of scientific disciplines and professions. Therefore, each will have only a partial understanding of what the others study and can bring, if not false beliefs about what others do. In particular, the challenge for life scientists to understand and engage in fruitful collaborations with social scientists has been experienced and commented in the context of One Health research, calling for mutual learning and understanding (Barnett *et al.*, 2020).

To this diversity of contributions by discipline, one must add a diversity within disciplines. Indeed, we

Box 3.1. Nomadic concept

The chapter has mentioned the importance of concepts in the constitution of disciplines, their identity and the way they view and analyse the world. Therefore, the diversity of understanding of concepts between disciplines may be a barrier to collaboration. Yet, concepts can also be bridges between disciplines and their diversity can be a rich source of ideas. This box explores how concepts play a manifold role in inter- and transdisciplinary collaborations, as developed by Antoine-Moussiaux and Leyens (2023).

Working in One Health, one will often face the issue of terms not being understood in the same way by different disciplines. A classical and important example of this is the term 'resilience', but widely used terms are just as diversely understood, though central to our actions: justice, poverty, development, nature, environment. The method of nomadic concepts aims at taking advantage of the diversity of understanding to foster critical and creative thinking. Those concepts are called 'nomadic' or 'travelling' because they have been subsequently used and appropriated by different disciplines. During that travel, they gained an array of distinct understandings and modes of implementation. Taking the example of resilience, it emerged in physics as a property of matter, to gain later uses in psychology, ecology and risk management. Organizing a workshop with different users of the term will first generate a better awareness of that diversity, and of the limits of action derived from an ill-defined term. Later in the process, the confrontation between viewpoints will help the group coin a common understanding of the term and establish together the practical steps that should be followed to act in accordance with that way to conceive the issue or the goal. Creativity may also be fostered by making a concept travel, hence by trying to transpose the terms of one discipline into another to allow cross-fertilization. In this sense, technical terms from one discipline (as was the case for resilience coming from physics) can first appear as a metaphoric use in the other discipline, holding some fuzziness in its practicality but raising interest and curiosity. If the new term proves relevant, going through mutual learning between disciplines, this use may gradually gain precision about its frame of application and limits, as well as practical consequences in the discipline adopting it.

For a detailed explanation of a workshop based on the idea of nomadic concepts, see Rossini (2020).

mentioned here above widely defined disciplines. However, biologists can work from the level of the pathogen to that of the ecosystem. Social scientists may hold very diverse stances in their analysis of society, sometimes holding conflicting views and analyses (Moon and Blackman, 2014). Epidemiologists may be specialized in the design of a diversity of models, mobilizing distinct streams of data, and being more or less acquainted with the use of qualitative or participatory approaches... and resulting in distinct predictions or appreciation of risks. Within each of these 'sub-disciplines', individual scientists tend to focus on particular topics, of which they become specialists. Hence, there is a tendency towards fragmentation of expertise that goes hand in hand with the need for specialization of scientists. Specialization, however, is itself manifold. One can be a specialist of a context (e.g. health in slums in low-income countries), wherein a set of intertwined problems arise. Another may be a specialist of an infectious agent, which may infect a range of hosts in a diversity of ecosystems and contexts. Yet another will be a specialist of a methodology that can be applied to a wide range of problems and in diverse contexts (e.g. network analysis that can be applied to epidemiology, study of innovation, social or economic organization, mindmaps and learning). Hence, we understand that, specializing around different objects, each scientist and practitioner will show some degree of specialization together with some generalist skills that will allow the application of this speciality in diverse ways.

Despite this fortunate plasticity, quite understandably, scientists or practitioners focusing on a defined problem (e.g. one working on the surveillance of chemical risks to health linked to water contamination) will tend to ascribe to their topic of interest a considerable importance. By knowing all the details and ramifications of one topic and by ignoring other dimensions of the same complex problem, one will naturally hold a biased appreciation of the importance of that topic within the complete picture. In that complete picture, each scientist or other professional will tend to see their part bigger than it may be in reality. This will eventually result in an underestimation of the importance ascribed to other dimensions of the same problem. Hence, as a general observation, each professional will have a distinct focus of interest within the range of their discipline, leading them to ignore or downplay the importance of realities outside of that focus (Assmuth and Hilden, 2008). Holding only partial or even false ideas of what other disciplines can bring can hamper the establishment of needed collaboration. Interestingly, we may note the particular role that specialists in contexts or in methods can play to bridge 'problem-centred' approaches (Antoine-Moussiaux, 2018).

3.4.2 Epistemologies: distinct relations to knowledge and to the world

Let us now consider the diversity in the ways of thinking about knowledge itself. Different disciplines hold unique views on science and on what constitutes valuable work. These divergent conceptions of knowledge are referred to as the 'epistemological' divides between disciplines. **EPISTEMOLOGY** is the branch of philosophy that tackles questions around knowledge, its nature, origin and limits. Among other topics, epistemology will be concerned by the criteria of validity of knowledge. This means that different disciplines will have divergent criteria to judge the validity of statements or practices. Hence, the proponents of one given discipline might consider what other disciplines produce as being of lesser scientific value because it rests on a distinct epistemological criterion (Albert *et al.*, 2008). To start with a caricatural situation, a natural scientist who works on the statistical analysis of quantitative data collected on a random sample of thousands of people may not easily perceive the scientific value of an approach based on the interpretation of the discourse of a handful of purposefully selected stakeholders (see Box 3.2 for further comments on the divide between 'quantitative' and 'qualitative' methods). For example, an epidemiologist may follow the issue of obesity in a population and be interested in estimating as precisely as possible its prevalence and the correlation with defined risk factors. That scientist will base the assessment of quality of the information provided on the sampling size and method and the sophistication of the statistical models in order to produce objective figures about what influences or causes obesity. Let us consider now a sociologist who would work on a small set of in-depth interviews about the personal history of persons suffering with obesity, in order to understand the social determinants and consequences of obesity and the potential for public preventative action. Our imagined epidemiologist may consider that this interpretative work lacks scientific value and does not produce generalizable knowledge, being too particular to the few interviewees (Flyvbjerg, 2006). Conversely, the social scientist might miss the meaning that is conveyed by the figures produced by the statistical analysis, considering that the figures miss the depth of how the problem of obesity unfolds in people's life. This social scientist would maybe consider the statistical work as lacking conceptual grounding and missing the question of causation of obesity. To keep our example caricatural, both scientists will eventually consider that the knowledge produced by the other fails at producing valuable evidence and understanding of the reality of the disease in society. This stereotyped example is just here to illustrate that the scientific rigour and the notion of quality of the scientific work diverge between disciplines. These epistemological divides are major barriers to inter- and transdisciplinary collaborations.

Everybody wants to do quality work. Hence, if one underestimates the quality of what another does, then effective collaborations are hindered.

Box 3.2. Quantitative, qualitative and mixed methods

The example described comments on the difficulties that different disciplines may encounter in understanding each other. Many discussions about these difficulties in interdisciplinary collaborations in science revolve around an opposition between the so-called 'quantitative' and 'qualitative' methods. As a matter of fact, many One Health studies will combine these two types of studies, sometimes in the same protocol, then termed as 'mixed methods'. However, those terms (quantitative, qualitative, mixed) have to be handled with caution, often being imprecise and misunderstood. A first confusion appears when applying those terms to variables or to methods. Regarding variables, the difference is quite straightforward: those that are measured and expressed in numbers are quantitative (e.g. body weight), those that are qualified through words to distinguish between categories are qualitative (e.g. coat colour). But if you count the frequency of coat colours in a cow population, you are mobilizing a quantitative approach to a qualitative variable. Hence, we need to be explicit about what we are doing. Methods that are typically referred to as 'quantitative' in public health are population studies, aiming at establishing the distribution of some variable in a population based on samples. The main concern of validity will then be the 'representativeness' of the sample, i.e. whether or not the values calculated on the sample may be considered as good approximations of those values at the level of the whole population. But one can also mobilize measured values to investigate and characterize a case study, without any claim for representativeness and no will to infer on population values. This then rather pertains to a qualitative approach despite the mobilization of quantitative variables. However, very often, the term 'qualitative' will be used to indicate methods based on a textual analysis of themes occurring in the discourse of interviewees. The quality of the data in such studies will not be tied to its representativeness, but rather to its relevance and how exemplary the situation may be of recurrent situations. The trustworthiness of those data will be tied to a constant rigour to identify possible bias and cross-check all that can be cross-checked (a process known as 'triangulation'). Those qualitative methods often discard any use of quantified measures to qualify a particular case/person. However, psychometric tests exist that allow the 'measurement' of, *inter alia*, people's perceptions, emotional states or degree of agreement with opinions. Those might be used within both quantitative and qualitative approaches. You can observe here that those notions are intermingled and would deserve a richer vocabulary than 'qualitative' or 'quantitative'. Finally, while the joint use of different methods can be easily termed 'mixed', again a more precise description of your methods will be needed if you want to avoid misunderstandings about your work. Therefore, without pursuing any further here the disentanglement of these different terms, this box should raise awareness of the importance for One Health practitioners to keep a critical eye on the rigour of their approaches, with precise notions of what in these approaches may limit data validity and applicability to draw practical conclusions and formulate policies.

Our explanations focused on the cases of scientists. Nevertheless, all these comments apply equally to professional contexts, each profession being trained in a defined set of scientific disciplines. Therefore, both the biased perspective on the relative importance of topics within complex problems and the lack of mutual understanding or appreciation apply to health practitioners, such as veterinarians, medical doctors, nurses, social workers or pharmacists. The more the diversity of professions involved in the collaboration increases, the more these internal barriers will inhibit fruitful partnerships. Yet, One Health approaches naturally call for the involvement of a diversity of professions well beyond the health sector. Let us be clear: these misunderstandings do not totally preclude collaboration; rather, they will keep the collaboration at the level of multidisciplinarity, failing to develop a direct co-learning between partners and keeping them working in parallel.

To become an effective One Health collaborator, it is necessary for a person to make the time and effort to learn about, and from, other disciplines and professions. Naturally, the goal is not to become a specialist in all these disciplines. Rather, one will aim at gaining just enough knowledge to understand others and be able to develop collaborations. This means that we have to understand at the very least what others can bring, what their areas of interest are and their overall way of working.

Task:

1. Consider the following four domains of knowledge: (i) life science, (ii) social science, (iii) humanities, (iv) technology, engineering and mathematics, and provide for each three names of (sub-)disciplines that are relevant to obesity. Try to elaborate on the kind of contribution they may bring.
2. Taking the case of rabies, try to formulate questions you think that a statistician, a sociologist and a philosopher would formulate about the management of that disease.
3. Taking the case of antimicrobial resistance, try to formulate questions you imagine that a veterinarian practitioner, a nurse and a policy maker would formulate about its management.
Once you have concluded this exercise, have a look at the possible answers provided below and compare them with your answers. Think about how they differ and what may be the reasons for this difference.

Example answers:

1. Life science: medical doctors and nutritionists to care for individual cases, epidemiologists to follow the evolution of the problem, its drivers and co-morbidities, agriculturalists to analyse the orientation of current food production, zootechnicians and veterinarians to work on animal nutrition, lowering fat content of animal products and influencing the fatty acid ratios, and so on. **Social science**: anthropologists to investigate the representation of food, nutrition for people and how it evolves in particular social categories that are more prone to obesity, sociologists to investigate the social drivers and consequences of obesity and how this problem can be shared by people and their pets, value chain economists to analyse the orientation of food systems towards more healthy food, behavioural economists to study the consumers, habits, and so on. **Humanities**: philosophers to raise ethical questions around social exclusion or stigmatization of obese persons and the extent to which obesity has to be considered as a disease, media analysts to explore the place of bodyweight in cinematographic productions and television series, historians to analyse how obesity emerged as a public problem through the last century, and so on. **Technology and engineering**: bio-engineers and food technologists to develop transformation and conservation methods to improve the shelf-life of fresh fruits and vegetables, data analysts to explore how big data and natural language analysis can help track food habits, their drivers and detect emerging tendencies.
2. Statistician: Can Bayesian methods generate more accurate estimations of prevalence of rabies? **Sociologist**: What are the social drivers of dog vaccination? **Philosopher**: Can a level of risk of rabies be considered acceptable?
3. Veterinarian practitioner: What alternatives can I use to lower my prescriptions of antibiotics? **Nurse**: How can I improve my practice to avoid hospital-acquired infections? **Policy maker**: What antibiotics should we forbid the use of in veterinary practice?

3.5 Implementation of Inter- and Transdisciplinarity as a Creative Process

We have proposed that the realization of inter- and transdisciplinarity entails the need for all contributors to engage in a process of mutual and shared learning. Facing complex issues and ever evolving challenges, this learning process must also be a creative one. Inter- and transdisciplinarity indeed appear as a way to mix knowledge, line looks very cramped with little space between words; please improve spacing world issues. Indeed, researchers describe our time as a 'transitional time', where issues are identified as radically new and increasingly complex (e.g. global warming). Also called 'interregnum', this expression stresses the need for new approaches and new skills for today's and tomorrow's professionals (Montuori and Donnelly, 2016). These 21st-century skills are communication, collaboration, critical thinking and creativity (Reilly, 2010). Inter- and transdisciplinarity are a way to foster the latter skill of creativity, especially needed to face the lack of ready-made answers. Hence, collaborations between disciplines centrally call for methods to foster creativity. This last section of the chapter explores inter- and transdisciplinarity as a source and soil for creativity, discussing its social and individual parts and the need for specific spaces and methods.

First, creativity insists on its social nature. Along with this view, **creative thinking** does not appear as a point-in-time event. Rather it is a process needing interactions between people in a defined context. Being recognized as a social process, creativity then requires stimulation by social interactions hosted by a favourable environment (Johnston, 2008; DeHaan, 2009; Hugill and Smith, 2013; Klein, 2017). Inter- and transdisciplinarity have been recognized as an enhancing environment, where these interactions are facilitated and opportunities for novelty are always present. To be successful, collaborative initiatives have to offer flexibility and dynamism, developing core qualities such as centrality of communication, curiosity, commitment, critical awareness and connectedness, fostering creativity (Hall and O'Rourke, 2014). Also, inter- and transdisciplinarity must create spaces of perceived freedom, allowing individuals to voice views not normally expected in their prescribed roles. Environmental factors thus seem crucial to enhance and sustain these creative processes. The pressure of time, money or other resources needed can, however, force people to settle with the 'first or easiest' answer to their problem, preventing the longer process of maturation, ideation and exchange that creativity is calling for. The provision of an enhancing environment has to be critically considered, in ways that have to adapt to circumstances and to the actors involved, addressing the diverse dimensions of the identified problem. The thinking about inter- and transdisciplinary spaces is still relatively new. Therefore, their evolution and adaptation often require participants to be supported by experienced facilitators and always to share their respective experiences to foster valuable context for creativity (Pineo *et al.*, 2021).

Design theory to renew research on antimicrobial resistance in animal health: Antimicrobial resistance (AMR) is a highly complex issue that requires innovative solutions. Therefore, current AMR research should expand the boundaries of knowledge, ways of conducting research and transcending disciplines. It should include many types of actors, researchers and stakeholders to foster innovative approaches. To this end, Vourc'h *et al.* (2018) created a research network (R2A2, Réseau Recherche Antibiotiques Animal) focused on antimicrobial use and microbes' resistance to antimicrobials in animals. The objectives were the development of cross-disciplinary thinking and to enhance the emergence of atypical research projects. According to the network evaluation, it was a successful approach to raise important applied questions to fight against AMR and to build cross-disciplinary research projects. This evaluation also identified key factors behind the success of the network. First, it adopted the concept–knowledge (C–K) design theory from the start, which is a theory that seeks to understand the reasonings according to which innovation occurs. It models that pathway as a diagram and helps explore new innovative design paths. Developing such a diagram at the onset of the network allowed the participants to keep an overview, connecting and understanding the diversity of subjects across workgroups. The diagram was constantly updated, revealing that 'a more cross-disciplinary approach was emerging, which essentially resulted from the adoption of an alternative mode of partitioning'. The C–K diagram is one important tool, recognized to enhance cross-disciplinary thinking, and already has many successful adaptations. Among others, it helps integrate the point of view of individual interests and collective interest. Finally, adaptability and flexibility of the network were two essential components for the evolution and completion of the project. Among several examples, they changed the frequency of the meetings over time, the number of participants was fluid (open registration in the network), and the network format was adapted to diverse profiles and backgrounds. The network adapted over time to respond to the participants' needs.

Second, creativity is understood and studied as an individual skill. As such, it has long been perceived as a fuzzy and uncontrollable process or aptitude. However, more and more studies show that it can be encouraged and enhanced in individuals. Individual factors that have been identified as enabling creativity are personality, motivation/individual attraction, knowledge and capacity for problem definition. Traits of personality that would be more prone to creativity are cognitive flexibility, personal experience and feelings, resources for new insights and synthesis. Contextual factors are also pinpointed by this thread of research, such as work conditions and incubation process (Gilhooly, 2016). Interestingly, creativity might not be linked to the time spent working in a field (Mumford *et al.*, 2010). Moreover, adapted training enhances the individual aptitude for creativity and educators developed tools to teach and trigger creativity. Among these tools, one is known as 'broadening the problem' (Ness, 2011), i.e. including other aspects and disciplines into a case study, which directly points to the benefits of inter- and transdisciplinarity in problem solving.

Finally, many tools are now available to apply a creative approach to diverse issues (e.g. design theory, TRIZ method, role plays). Many researchers are using them on a daily basis to improve their creativity and problem-solving skills, with diverse practices developing in distinct disciplines. Thanks to inter- and transdisciplinarity, these tools and approaches can further be shared between disciplines. Creativity has to be understood as emerging from trainable individual qualities, group-working abilities and enhancing contexts. The open sharing of knowledge and ideas is its very substance.

Learning questions:

1. From your experience, how would you describe the process and triggers for creativity? Where do you think new ideas come from?
2. What tools have you already used to create and generate ideas? What kind of expression medium would you be more open to and why: open discussions, structured questions and answers, free drawing, structured diagramming, role play, song writing?
3. If you were to address a One Health problem, in which domain could you see a more creative approach to be implemented? Please describe your targeted One Health problem and the creative approach you can imagine.

For this exercise, we leave it up to your own experience and reflection. No example answer is provided. To further explore the domain of creativity, you might start by reading the literature to which this section refers.

3.6 Conclusions

Far from being a magic bullet, collaboration between disciplines entails major challenges for science and society as a whole. The One Health concept places these collaborations at the very heart of their definition in order to tackle the most pressing health challenges of our times. Therefore, the deep understanding of barriers to such collaborations is essential to every One Health practitioner, who will not be above those constraints but will have, on the contrary, to engage in a perpetual effort to overcome them and harvest the benefits from crossing intellectual, philosophical and practical barriers. Because inter- and transdisciplinarity aim at producing new solutions to old problems by looking at them with fresh eyes and a renewed understanding, their practical implementation must be conceived as a creative effort, one where all professionals involved will get inspired by and learn from other disciplines, to constantly reflect critically on their own practices.

Additional activity: If you are interested in another activity to deepen your learning and think about the practical applications of inter- and transdisciplinarity, you can work through the exercise provided below.

Conceptual map and interdisciplinary contributions

Develop a conceptual map, either on paper or using mind-mapping software (Cmap tool, Institute for Human-Machine Cognition, allows you to create and freely arrange elements and named links), illustrating the main interactions between human activities, domestic animals, ecosystems and the spread of H5N1 Highly Pathogenic Avian Influenza (HPAI).

- Identify key elements for human activities, veterinary services, health systems, domestic animals and ecosystems, and create boxes labelled with their names.
- Establish links gradually between these boxes, labelled with active verbs.

Based on this map, imagine and outline the contributions of different disciplines to solving the issue. Focus on disciplines such as epidemiology, veterinary medicine, environmental science and public health. Consider the specific perspectives each discipline brings and potential blind spots. Identify which discipline could offer insights to address these blind spots.

- Create boxes labelled with these disciplines.
- Create links between the disciplines and the problem's elements, labelled with their type of contribution. If needed, add intermediate boxes in order to keep links labelled only with active verbs.

For at least two disciplines, formulate research questions that would contribute to understanding and managing HPAI. For example, in epidemiology, you might ask about disease spread patterns, and in veterinary medicine, you might explore effective vaccination strategies for domestic poultry.

Role play scenario

Imagine a dialogue between different actors involved in addressing HPAI. Assume roles such as epidemiologist, veterinarian, environmental scientist, etc. Think individually about the priorities and actions each role would propose within the complexity of the issue. Consider both a conflictual scenario and one that generates consensus.

Nomadic concept

Choose a concept that appears relevant to you to manage HPAI (you may choose from the following examples: resilience, vulnerability, responsibility, precaution). Write down your own definition, being as precise as possible. Look for reference papers exploring the chosen concept (if possible, choose papers in different disciplines). Note any differences in interpretations within your own definitions. Ask colleagues about their spontaneous understanding of the concept.

Based on your personal definition and insights from literature exploration, work towards a common definition of the chosen concept in the context of HPAI. Consider the various elements raised by different perspectives and aim to synthesize a definition that encapsulates interdisciplinary insights.

New perspective? Own action within interdisciplinary partnerships

Did the preceding exercises inspire some new perspectives on HPAI management? Did you identify relevant partnerships that you had not considered before?

Choose an action that your discipline may be responsible for within a project aimed at managing HPAI. Draw a theory of change for that action (linking the actions to their direct outputs, the outcomes that the latter will enable and finally the broader impact these outcomes would contribute to). Identify blind spots in your study and propose improvements that could involve researchers from different disciplines. If possible, reflect on these points with researchers from other relevant disciplines to explore shared interests and potential collaborative work.

Brief comments to guide your resolution of the exercise

While building your conceptual map, please consider the following elements (not specific to HPAI):

- *Human Activities*: Includes various activities that bring humans into contact with domestic animals and ecosystems. May involve agriculture, animal husbandry, hunting and healthcare practices.

- *Transmission Routes*: Represents pathways through which zoonotic pathogens can be transmitted from animals to humans. Routes may include direct contact, consumption of contaminated food or water, and vectors.
- *Domestic Animals*: Encompasses animals kept by humans, such as livestock and pets. Consider the diversity of livestock-keeping systems: different systems may show unique roles in epidemiology. Consider the potential role of these animals and their products as reservoirs/vehicles for zoonotic pathogens.
- *Interactions and Exposures*: Signifies the various ways in which humans come into contact with domestic animals and potential sources of zoonotic pathogens. In the case of production animals, think of the whole value chain. Also think of other uses of domestic animals.
- *Ecosystems*: Involves the natural environment where wild fauna and vectors reside. Acknowledges the role of ecosystems in the maintenance and transmission of zoonotic diseases.

Here is a list of key stakeholders and their roles in implementing the One Health approach, potential incapacities and challenges. Use this list to confront with your map and exercise.

- Public Health Agencies
  - Role: Monitor and respond to human cases of zoonotic diseases.
  - Contribution: Provide expertise in epidemiology, disease surveillance and public health interventions.
  - Blind spots / limits: Focus limited to the human health aspects and sometimes insufficient collaboration with other disciplines.
- Veterinary Services
  - Role: Monitor and manage health in domestic animals, including early detection and control of zoonotic diseases.
  - Contribution: Conduct surveillance, implement preventive measures and collaborate with public health agencies.
  - Blind spots / limits: Focus limited to animal health aspects and sometimes insufficient collaboration with other disciplines.
- Environmental Agencies
  - Role: Monitor and assess the health of ecosystems, wildlife and vectors.
  - Contribution: Contribute to understanding the environmental factors influencing zoonotic disease transmission.
  - Blind spots / limits: Limited focus on clinical aspects of diseases and their direct impact on human and animal health. May not prioritize the immediate health concerns of domestic animals and human populations.
- Agricultural and Food Safety Authorities
  - Role: Oversee food production systems and safety.
  - Contribution: Implement measures to reduce the risk of zoonotic transmission through the food chain.
  - Blind spots / limits: May not fully consider ecological and social factors influencing disease emergence.
- Research Institutions and Academia
  - Role: Conduct research on zoonotic pathogens, transmission dynamics and innovative solutions.
  - Contribution: Generate scientific knowledge, educate professionals and contribute to evidence-based policy making.
  - Blind spots / limits: Scientific actors may disregard non-academic knowledge.
- Human and Animal Health Professionals
  - Role: Diagnose, treat and prevent zoonotic diseases in both humans and animals.
  - Contribution: Provide healthcare services, conduct surveillance and educate communities.
  - Blind spots / limits: A clinical work functions on a case-by-case basis and may miss the overall picture. The health systems may be biased toward curative interventions while neglecting prevention and health determinants.

- Pharmaceutical Industry
  - Role: Develop vaccines, treatments and other health devices.
  - Contribution: Support the development of tools to prevent and control zoonotic diseases.
  - Blind spots / limits: If technical innovation generates a potential, this does not translate into impacts if the social, political, economic and cultural context is not enabling that change.
- International Organizations (e.g., WHO, FAO, WOAH)
  - Role: Facilitate global collaboration and set international standards.
  - Contribution: Provide guidance, support capacity building and coordinate responses to zoonotic outbreaks.
  - Blind spots / limits: Normative approaches have to mind the gap of inequity due to the diverse abilities of actors to follow recommendations and norms. General recommendations may not be suited to some specific local conditions. Working at the international level involves many diplomatic sensitivities and pressures.
- Policy Makers and Government Agencies
  - Role: Develop and implement policies to address zoonotic risks.
  - Contribution: Enact and enforce regulations, allocate resources and support intersectoral collaboration.
  - Blind spots / limits: Challenges in translating policies into practical actions and ensuring compliance. Subject to local political and economic pressures.
- Community and Indigenous Groups
  - Role: Participate in surveillance, share local knowledge and implement preventive measures.
  - Contribution: Act as key partners in community-based interventions and awareness campaigns.
  - Blind spots / limits: Limited expertise in clinical aspects of diseases and ecological factors.
- Media and Communication Specialists
  - Role: Disseminate information, raise awareness and promote behaviour change.
  - Contribution: Communicate scientific findings to the public, facilitating understanding and cooperation.
  - Blind spots / limits: Communication focuses here on the diffusion of information. Yet, listening to the reactions of people, their beliefs and knowledge is a key aspect of successful management.

References

Albert, M., Laberge, S., Hodges, B.D., Regehr, G. and Lingard, L. (2008) Biomedical scientists' perception of the social sciences in health research. *Social Science & Medicine* 66, 2520–2531.

Antoine-Moussiaux, N. (2018) The bridging role of socio-economic reasoning in 'One Health'. *Bulletin of Royal Academy for Overseas Science* 64(1), 39–60. DOI: 10.5281/zenodo.3980725.

Antoine-Moussiaux, N. and Leyens, S. (2023) Harnessing concepts for sustainability: A pledge for a practice. *Sustainability Science* 18, 1–11. DOI: 10.1007/s11625-023-01375-4.

Antoine-Moussiaux, N., Janssens de Bisthoven, L., Leyens, S., Assmuth, T., Keune, H. *et al.* (2019) The good, the bad and the ugly: Framing debates on nature in a one health community. *Sustainability Science* 14(6), 1729–1738. DOI: 10.1007/s11625-019-00674-z.

Assmuth, T. and Hilden, M. (2008) The significance of information frameworks in integrated risk assessment and management. *Environmental Science & Policy* 11, 71–86.

Barnett, T., Pfeiffer, D.U., Hoque, M.A., Giasuddin, M., Florag, M.S. *et al.* (2020) Practising co-production and interdisciplinarity: Challenges and implications for one health research. *Preventive Veterinary Medicine* 177, 104949.

Capps, B. (2022) One health ethics. *Bioethics* 36(4), 348–355. DOI: 10.1111/bioe.12984.

Caron, A., Mugabe, P., Bourgeois, R., Delay, E., Bitu, F. *et al.* (2022) Social-ecological system health in transfrontier conservation areas to promote the coexistence between people and nature. *One Health Cases*. CABI, Wallingford, UK. DOI: 10.1079/onehealthcases.2022.0005.

Choi, B.C.K. and Pak, A.W.P. (2006) Multidisciplinarity, interdisciplinarity and transdisciplinarity in health research, services, education and policy: 1. Definitions, objectives, and evidence of effectiveness. *Clinical and Investigative Medicine* 29, 351–364.

Darbellay, F. (2015) The gift of interdisciplinarity: Towards an ability to think across disciplines. *International Journal for Talent Development and Creativity* 3(2), 201–211.

DeHaan, R.L. (2009) Teaching creativity and inventive problem solving in science. *CBE – Life Sciences Education* 8(3), 172–181.

Destoumieux-Garzón, D., Mavingui, P., Boetsch, G., Boissier, J., Darriet, F. *et al.* (2018) The One Health concept: 10 years old and a long road ahead. *Frontiers in Veterinary Science* 5, 14. DOI: 10.3389/fvets.2018.00014.

Flyvbjerg, B. (2006) Five misunderstandings about case-study research. *Qualitative Inquiry* 12(2), 219–245.

Gilhooly, K.J. (2016) Incubation and intuition in creative problem solving. *Frontiers in Psychology* 7, 1076.

Hall, T.E. and O'Rourke, M. (2014) Responding to communication challenges in transdisciplinary sustainability science. In: Huutoniemi, K. and Tapio, P. (eds) *Transdisciplinary Sustainability Studies: A Heuristic Approach*. Routledge, London, pp. 119–139.

Häsler, B., Gilbert, W., Jones, B.A., Pfeiffer, D.U., Rushton, J. and Otte, M.J. (2013) The economic value of One Health in relation to the mitigation of zoonotic disease risks. *Current Topics in Microbiology and Immunology* 365, 127–151. DOI: 10.1007/82_2012_239.

Hugill, A. and Smith, S. (2013) Digital creativity and TD at postgraduate level: The design and implementation of a TD masters programme and its implications for creative practices. *Digital Creativity* 24(3), 191–207. DOI: 10.1080/14626268.2013.827099.

Humboldt-Dachroeden, S. (2021) One Health practices across key agencies in Sweden: Uncovering barriers to cooperation, communication and coordination. *Scandinavian Journal of Public Health* 51, 535–541. DOI: 10.1177/14034948211024483.

Hurni, H. and Wiesmann, U. (2004) Towards transdisciplinarity in sustainability-oriented research for development. In: Hurni, H., Wiesmann, U. and Schertenleib, R. (eds) *Research for Mitigating Syndromes of Global Change. A Transdisciplinary Appraisal of Selected Regions of the World to Prepare Development-Oriented Research Partnerships. Perspectives of the Swiss National Centre of Competence in Research (NCCR) North-South, University of Berne*, Vol. 1. Geographica Bernensia, Berne, pp 31–41.

Jerolmack, C. (2013) Who's worried about turkeys? How 'organisational silos' impede zoonotic disease surveillance. *Sociology of Health & Illness* 35, 200–212. DOI: 10.1111/j.1467-9566.2012.01501.x.

Johnston, R.R. (2008) Of connection and community: Transdisciplinarity and the arts. In: *Transdisciplinarity: Theory and Practice 1*. Hampton Press, New York, pp. 223–236.

Kayunze, K.A., Kiwara, A., Lyamuya, E., Kambarage, D.M., Rushton, J. *et al.* (2014) Practice of One Health approaches: Bridges and barriers in Tanzania. *Onderstepoort Journal of Veterinary Research* 81(2), E1–8. DOI: 10.4102/ojvr.v81i2.733.

Klein, J.T. (2017) Creativity, design, and transdisciplinarity. In: *Creativity, Design Thinking and Interdisciplinarity*. Springer, Singapore, pp. 53–68.

Max-Neef, M.A. (2005) Foundations of transdisciplinarity. *Ecological Economics*, 53, 5–16.

Montuori, A. and Donnelly, G. (2016) The creativity of culture and the culture of creativity research: The promise of integrative transdisciplinarity. In: *The Palgrave Handbook of Creativity and Culture Research*. Palgrave Macmillan, London, pp. 743–765.

Moon, K. and Blackman, D. (2014) A guide to understanding social science research for natural scientists. *Conservation Biology* 28(5), 1167–1177.

Mumford, M.D., Antes, A.L., Caughron, J.J., Connelly, S. and Beeler, C. (2010) Cross-field differences in creative problem-solving skills: A comparison of health, biological, and social sciences. *Creativity Research Journal* 22(1), 14–26.

Ness, R.B. (2011) Commentary: Teaching creativity and innovative thinking in medicine and the health sciences. *Academic Medicine* 86(10), 1201–1203.

Pasquier, R. and Schreiber, D. (2007) De l'interdiscipline à l'indiscipline. Et retour? *Labyrinthe* 27(2), 91–108. DOI: 10.4000/labyrinthe.1983.

Pettan-Brewer, C., Martins, A.F., de Abreu, D.P.B., Brandão, A.P.D., Barbosa, D.S. *et al.* (2021) From the approach to the concept: One Health in Latin America – experiences and perspectives in Brazil, Chile, and Colombia. *Frontiers in Public Health* 9, 687110. DOI: 10.3389/fpubh.2021.687110.

Pineo, H., Turnbull, E.R., Davies, M., Rowson, M., Hayward, A.C., Hart G. and Aldridge, R.W. (2021) A new transdisciplinary research model to investigate and improve the health of the public. *Health Promotion International* 36(2), 481–492.

Pohl, C., Krütli, P. and Stauffacher, M. (2017) Ten reflective steps for rendering research societally relevant. *GAIA-Ecological Perspectives for Science and Society* 26(1), 43–51. DOI: 10.14512/gaia.26.1.10.

Reilly, E.T. (2010) The four C's: Executives say the 21st century requires more skilled workers. *Mworld* 9(2), 47.

Rigolot, C. (2020) Transdisciplinarity as a discipline and a way of being: Complementarities and creative tensions. *Humanities and Social Sciences Communications* 7, 100. DOI: 10.1057/s41599-020-00598-5.

Rossini, M. (2020) Nomadic concepts. Td-net toolbox profile (13). In: *Swiss Academies of Arts and Sciences: td-net Toolbox for Co-producing Knowledge*. Available at: www.transdisciplinarity.ch/toolbox. DOI: 10.5281/zenodo.3717144.

Scholz, R.W. and Steiner, G. (2015) The real type and ideal type of transdisciplinary processes: Part II – what constraints and obstacles do we meet in practice? *Sustainability Science* 10(4), 653–671.

Sidikou, D.I., Irabor, T.J., Bonfoh, B. *et al.* (2022) Teaching and learning for change: Analysis of a post-graduate One Health program. *Sustainability Science* 17, 65–80. DOI: 10.1007/s11625-021-01053-3.

Uchtmann, N., Herrmann, J.A., Hahn, E.C. 3rd and Beasley, V.R. (2015) Barriers to, efforts in, and optimization of integrated One Health surveillance: A review and synthesis. *EcoHealth* 12(2), 368–384. DOI: 10.1007/s10393-015-1022-7.

Vourc'h, G., Brun, J., Ducrot, C., Cosson, J.F., Le Masson, P. and Weil, B. (2018) Using design theory to foster innovative cross-disciplinary research: Lessons learned from a research network focused on antimicrobial use and animal microbes' resistance to antimicrobials. *Veterinary and Animal Science* 6, 12–20.

Wolton, D. (2013) Conclusion. Pour un manifeste de l'indiscipline. *Hermès, La Revue* 67, 210–222. DOI: 10.4267/2042/51919.

4 Knowledge Integration in One Health: Science and Decision Support

Martin Hitziger[1,2], Nicolas Antoine-Moussiaux[2,3], Diana Rosas Morales[4] and Didier Wernli[2,5]

[1]Section of Epidemiology, Vetsuisse Faculty, University of Zurich, Zurich, Switzerland; [2]Network for Ecohealth and One Health (NEOH); [3]Faculty of Veterinary Medicine and Faculty of Medicine, University of Liège, Liège, Belgium; [4]Doctoral student of Social and Political Sciences at the University of Liège, Liège, Belgium; [5]Global Studies Institute, University of Geneva, Geneva, Switzerland

Contents

 Principles of One Health for a better planet (eds B. Häsler, A. Tvarijonaviciute and S. Savić)
DOI: 10.1079/9781800623002.0005

Chapter Overview

Elevator pitch

Knowledge integration is key for tackling systemic challenges at the interface of science and society. Many tools and approaches have been developed in different disciplines to enable knowledge integration across stakeholder groups or societal actors. However, its roots in interdisciplinary thinking may be unfamiliar to many One Health learners. Its multidisciplinary origin also creates challenges for those who aim to learn about the field and to apply it. The chapter therefore introduces the field and relevant resources that may help you to acquire skills for using knowledge integration approaches in science and society.

Book objectives the chapter relates to

☐ 1. Understand what One Health and Ecohealth mean
☑ 2. Think in a One Health and Ecohealth way
☑ 3. Apply One Health and Ecohealth in their professional and personal life
☑ 4. Know how to share One Health and Ecohealth knowledge
☑ 5. Integrate One Health and Ecohealth knowledge actively
☑ 6. Acquire or enhance core One Health competencies

One Health competencies covered

☐ 1. Effective communication
☑ 2. Collaborative and resilient working
☑ 3. Systems understanding
☑ 4. Transdisciplinarity
☐ 5. Social, cultural and gender equity and inclusiveness
☑ 6. Collective learning and reflective practice
☐ 7. One Health concepts
☑ 8. Theoretical and methodological pluralism
☑ 9. Harnessing uncertainty, paradox and limited knowledge

Learning outcomes

1. Understand the concepts **knowledge**, **knowledge systems** and **knowledge integration** from a social science point of view.
2. Identify potential benefits and challenges of knowledge integration in systemic problems faced by science and society.
3. Understand basic characteristics of selected exemplary approaches to facilitate knowledge integration.
4. Recognize basic characteristics of applied examples of knowledge integration in published literature.
5. Be aware of relevant bodies of literature and educational opportunities for learning to apply key knowledge integration approaches in systems science and decision support.

Summary

This chapter starts in the first section (Section 4.1) with a diagnosis: it identifies the integration of knowledge as a challenge that is at the core of all One Health initiatives, and that can be more complex to address than it may seem at first. In the second section (Section 4.2) you will learn about key terms and concepts that will help you to understand knowledge integration in One Health initiatives and beyond, with a focus on knowledge systems and boundary management. This section will also enable you to familiarize yourself more deeply with applied knowledge integration methods and approaches, if you so wish. To enrich your understanding of knowledge integration, we will also look from another relevant angle to introduce concepts and applications relevant to knowledge integration, as they have been developed in systems thinking. The third section (Section 4.3) will revisit some of these concepts from the perspective of decision science to deepen and extend your understanding of links between knowledge integration and decision making. One of the challenges with knowledge integration is, as you will realize, that it itself has a multidisciplinary background – some relevant concepts are similar and overlapping as they developed in different disciplines. We are therefore providing relevant definitions where appropriate and are carefully linking key terms throughout the various sections. Overall, this chapter will help you to increase your understanding of the need to integrate information, data, techniques, tools, perspectives, concepts and theories from different bodies of specialized knowledge to advance fundamental understanding and to address One Health problems of which the solutions are beyond the scope of any single discipline or area of practice.

4.1 One Health as a Dialogue Between Multiple Forms of Knowledge

It is difficult to carry out a One Health approach in practice, because responsibilities are usually organized along sectoral lines, many **actors** are used to unisectoral and disciplinary work in their daily tasks, and their regular routines may be inclined towards such work styles. During the time of Descartes and Newton in the 17th century, reductionism started to dominate modern science (Elkana, 2012; Van Riel and Van Gulick, 2018).

METHODOLOGICAL REDUCTIONISM can be defined as the strategy of 'dividing a phenomenon into its constituent parts and studying them separately in the expectation that knowledge produced by narrow specialties can be readily combined into the understanding of the phenomenon as a whole' (Newell, 2004). Reductionism has produced much of what we know about the world and will continue to contribute to the scientific endeavour. It is also a root cause of the specialization of most educational and professional paths that create different perspectives on reality (Kuhn, 2012).

Yet, knowledge about finely subdivided phenomena produced by different actors with distinct perspectives on reality does rarely combine easily to a shared and overarching understanding of the whole. As it turned out, this reductionist idea encountered challenges when studying deeply interconnected biological, ecological and social systems that are at the core of One Health. The tendency to try to resolve such problems with unisectoral, disciplinary and reductionist approaches can undermine the impact of One Health initiatives (Wernli and Darbellay, 2016; Léger *et al.*, 2018). The beginning of the 21st century has been associated with an increasing awareness that the challenges we face require collaboration across **disciplines** (Wernli and Darbellay, 2016). As Capra and Luisi noted, 'at the forefront of contemporary science, we no longer see the universe as a machine composed of elementary building blocks. We have discovered that the material world, ultimately, is a network of inseparable patterns of relationships; that the planet as a whole is a living, self-regulating system' (Capra and Luisi, 2014). This systems paradigm contends that a holistic approach is needed to understand the world around us and to solve complex health problems (see also Chapters 1 and 3).

The relevance of meaningful cooperation for successful One Health implementation is well captured by Buttigieg and colleagues in the article entitled *Brucellosis Control in Malta and Serbia: A One Health Evaluation* (Buttigieg *et al.*, 2018). The case study in Malta reconstructs one century of Brucellosis control policies. Various uncoordinated and failed measures and setbacks led to the recognition that cooperation between disciplines and **sectors** was needed. The implemented measures ranged from relatively isolated initial actions such as processing of milk through pasteurization (introduced prior to the Second World War) to a more sectoral approach adopted in the 1980s. It was only upon the adoption of a One Health approach in the mid-1990s, however, that Brucellosis eradication was successfully achieved and maintained. Enforcement of existing and newly implemented legislation was crucial to this success and required collaboration by all **stakeholders** involved including public health, veterinary health, policy makers and legislators, as well as farmers and consumers' representatives. The next section of this chapter will enable you to better understand and address these aspects of One Health.

4.2 Integrating Knowledge

4.2.1 Knowledge integration and One Health

Let us try to understand the concept of knowledge integration, which is of such importance that it has been proposed as one of eight key challenges to public health in the 21st century (Khoury *et al.*, 2013).

KNOWLEDGE INTEGRATION has been defined as 'the cognitive process of critically evaluating insights and creating common ground among divergent perspectives to construct a more comprehensive understanding. The understanding is the product or result of the integrative process' (Repko, 2011). Knowledge integration is about building shared and meaningful syntheses between different disciplines, sectors, traditions or cultures, which usually have their own mental models, theories and methodology. Building shared and meaningful syntheses needs to be based on a recognition and explanation of the relevant differences between these models (Jahn *et al.*, 2012; Körner *et al.*, 2016). Rather than seeking consensus, knowledge integration has been likened to the weaving of multiple perspectives into a common vision or a search for coherence and correspondence (Wickson *et al.*, 2006; Klein, 2008). That means the key intention of knowledge integration is to understand the commonalities, differences and relationships between the knowledge and views of reality of different disciplines or perspectives. In simple terms, knowledge integration means to understand each other – in a conscious, reflective and profound way. It includes understanding how an actor perceives a situation and how – in that actor's view – this situation developed in the past and might further develop in the future. It also includes how this perception of the situation influences what that actor intends to achieve and why they hope to achieve these goals in certain ways.

These aspects are captured in three specialist terms (Pohl and Hirsch Hadorn, 2007):

- **SYSTEMS, OR DESCRIPTIVE, KNOWLEDGE** relates to perspectives on factual processes.
- **TARGET, OR NORMATIVE, KNOWLEDGE** relates to objectives and interests.
- **TRANSFORMATION, OR PRESCRIPTIVE, KNOWLEDGE** relates to the transformation of the current version of a system towards a more desired version.

Hitziger *et al.* (2018) describe how the implementation of One Health initiatives can benefit from integrating each of these dimensions of knowledge of various actors into each stage of projects or policies (Fig. 4.1):

1. Integrating systems knowledge at the **evaluation** stage of a project or **policy** can transform individual observations into narratives of how situations emerge and might unfold in the future.
2. Integrating target knowledge at the agenda-setting, policy formulation and decision-making stage can resolve **trade-offs** between participants of a One Health initiative, and can determine common vision and direction.
3. Integrating transformation knowledge at the implementation stage can strengthen networks for collective action.

See also Chapter 3, which covers **multi-, inter-** and **trans-disciplinarity**, and Chapter 10 for more information on the One Health project life cycle and knowledge integration in relation to the cycle and stakeholder engagement.

Have a look at the learning questions below and try to formulate your own answer. Subsequently consider the example answers to check whether they provide an additional perspective that complements your own answers. Also make sure to work through Chapter 6, which will build your understanding of **reflexivity** and **reflective practice** in knowledge integration, and offers you practical exercises to train your capacity for focused reflection as an important One Health competency.

Learning questions:

1. Identify an example from your own experience in which the collaboration of experts from different sectors was required. These could include professional jobs and projects, course work, internships, volunteering work or campaigns.
2. In this personal experience, can you identify these examples of knowledge integration?
  (i) Understanding aspects in which your own knowledge corresponds to someone else's knowledge, even if the two perspectives may be expressed differently.
  (ii) Accepting new pieces of knowledge into your own perspective by understanding what it adds to your previous knowledge.
  (iii) Understanding an aspect of someone else's knowledge without accepting it as an additional aspect of your own knowledge, but recognizing how the two perspectives differ.
  (iv) Recognizing the internal logic of someone else's knowledge by understanding how their systems, target and transformation knowledge cohere and understanding **why** their perspective differs from yours.
3. If you experienced knowledge integration, what effects did this have on the collaboration?

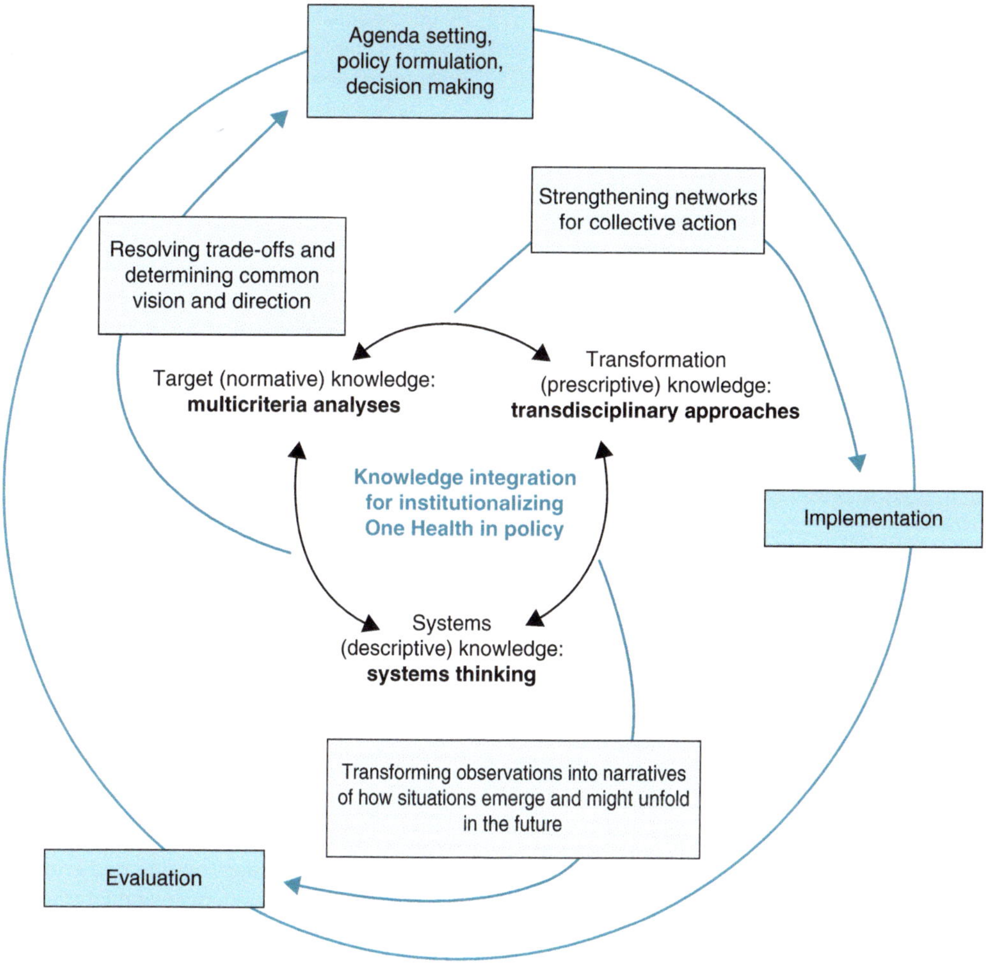

Fig. 4.1. Uses of knowledge integration in One Health. The outer and inner circles indicate the stages within each round of policy development and the approaches for integrating target, transformation and systems knowledge respectively. The text on the arrows summarizes the main benefits of knowledge integration for each stage of policy development. Figure from Hitziger *et al.* (2018), unmodified (CC BY 3.0 IGO DEED: https://creativecommons.org/licenses/by/3.0/igo/).

If you did not experience knowledge integration, what were the likely reasons for that?

4. Can you identify an example from your own experience in which knowledge integration was insufficient or unsuccessful, and can you identify how this obstacle hampered the overall success of the collaboration?

Example answers and reflection triggers:

1. If you cannot come up with an example from your professional context, think of discussions with fellow students, the last time you had some professional craftsman at your house for repairs, or when talking to your parents about their professional context. If you cannot immediately think of answers to these questions, we suggest you undertake an experimental approach and invite one person of your social context with expressly different views and opinions than yours to discuss a controversial topic in a thoughtful, in-depth manner, and answer these questions afterwards.

2. Alternatively, imagine a hypothetical discussion between a medical doctor, a political analyst, an activist from a local non-governmental organization (NGO) and an environmental scientist discussing a Cholera outbreak. Understanding the epidemiological incidence of Cholera, contributing environmental and societal factors, including those that enable, foster, delay or prevent effective responses, are part of systems knowledge. Characteristics of a human–environment system that would be desirable and probably stop the outbreak would be target knowledge. Designing surveillance and control interventions, or other forms of responses to the outbreak, would be transformation knowledge.

3. See **1** and **2**.

4. If you cannot identify an example from your own experience, think about a major conflict in the news. Why would you presume knowledge integration does not happen in this situation? Think about matters such as social contacts as opportunities for knowledge integration, emotional obstacles, language barriers, cultural barriers, diverging economic or political interests, the influence of social and political context on decision makers, as well as narrow-mindedness, ignorance and path-dependency (i.e. once a particular path or course of action is chosen, it can become increasingly difficult to deviate from that path). All of these may be reasons why knowledge integration was insufficient or unsuccessful.

4.2.2 Knowledge and knowledge systems in medicine and beyond

After the previous section, you may wonder how it arises that all sorts of matters are called 'knowledge'. Should matters as different as 'objective evidence' and personal experiences (systems knowledge), subjective aspirations, institutional goals and societal values (target knowledge), legal, practical, or interpersonal strategies and tactics related to achieving such objectives (transformation knowledge) – even beliefs that a scientist or expert practitioner may consider outright 'wrong' – all be treated as 'the same' and respected as simply 'another perspective'? This may be particularly challenging if you were trained in a discipline that is strongly anchored in the belief that knowledge is revealed from an objective and quantifiable (measurable) observation of the world and that there are hierarchies of the strength of evidence. In that case you may be more used to thinking from a stance that is sometimes called 'objectivist' or 'realist'. Even from such a stance, however, there remain a lot of matters that can – practically and pragmatically – not be unquestionably determined by unambiguous facts. A very incomplete list of such matters includes those of excessive scale or complexity, those that have not yet been sufficiently analysed by scientists or experts, those ruled by unpredictable dynamics that may seem 'chaotic' (Erdi, 2008), those dominated by uncertainty, and those influenced by human decisions that are never entirely rational, and may depend on feelings, personal experience, social context, institutional interests or cultural background. Moreover, from the perspective of science-policy initiatives or societal decision making at large, you will rarely come across any situation in which you can decide important matters just by yourself. To build coalitions and consensus towards joint action, you will need to build a shared perspective (sometimes called framing; Shiffman and Shawar, 2022), even if you are 'right' – and that includes dealing effectively with divergent perceptions and goals. As you may have realized, the situations touched upon above include any situation that would be considered a One Health matter. It is therefore appropriate and useful, in a One Health context, to start with the assumption of actors having partial but complementary knowledge, and decisions to also entail important subjective components. Such a stance is more inclined towards constructivism than to objectivism.

On the one hand, **CONSTRUCTIVISM** is a learning theory that states people actively create their own understanding and knowledge by building on their experiences and interactions with the world around them in a cognitive or social process that starts from subjective thoughts, perceptions and individual pieces of evidence. **OBJECTIVISM**, on the other hand, emphasizes the existence of objective reality and holds that knowledge and values are based on factual observation.

For Fredrik Barth (2002), knowledge is what a person employs to interpret and act on the world. Under this caption he includes feelings (attitudes) as well as information, embodied skills as well as verbal taxonomies and concepts: all the ways of understanding that we use to make up our experienced, grasped reality. Crucially, he also includes emotional judgements and cognitive inferences based on whatever criteria of truthfulness that we may embrace – above all, what others whom we trust tell us they believe. Thus, a person's stock of knowledge structures that person's understanding of the world and purposive ways of coping in it, including the knowledge that is employed to form preferences and objectives. That form of knowledge varies greatly between individuals, even those closely related, of similar age, or of common cultural, educational and professional backgrounds.

Reflective intermission: Before you continue reading, you may want to pause a moment. Think about the last instance in which you, somewhat defiantly, insisted to someone that you **knew** something. What role did feelings play in this knowledge? What is a fact for you? Where do you get knowledge from and why? Also, make sure not to miss Chapter 5, which provides you with a detailed understanding of the differentiations, interrelations and relevance of **data**, **information**, **knowledge** and **wisdom** (DIKW hierarchy) in One Health.

We learn much of our knowledge from others - including our preferences and our criteria for judging truthfulness that we have learned to use. Though it is experience-based, most knowledge thus is not private in an individual sense but is constructed within the social context, the 'traditions of knowledge' in which each of us partakes. According to Barth, such traditions are characterized by shared corpora of substantive assertions and ideas about the world, shared communicative media, and shared institutional knowledge transmission processes. In the context of One Health, where a transdisciplinary approach (Chapter 3) is often seen as the best way forward to tackle complex problems holistically and sustainably, a lot of distinctive knowledge traditions may come together, e.g. academic disciplines (medicine, public health, veterinary or environmental sciences), major institutions, or cultural or ethnic groups and networks.

Such traditions are embedded within **KNOWLEDGE SYSTEMS** – networks of linked actors, organizations and objects that facilitate communication and translation across perspectives and between actors, therefore linking knowledge and know-how with action (McCullough and Matson, 2011). The applied example below on biomedicine will deepen your understanding of knowledge and knowledge systems by analysing and comparing medical traditions of different cultures as part of those cultures' respective health systems – which in turn are knowledge systems as described in the present paragraph.

Biomedicine in the light of other health-related knowledge systems – acknowledging biomedicine as one of many medical systems:
Western health systems, with medical, pharmaceutical, financial, educational and **governance** institutions, as well as their scientific approach to health, have come to dominate, politically and legally, many competing health-related knowledge systems globally. Many people recognize biomedicine as **the** medicine, rather than as one version of the larger human concept of medicine as an interpretive and interventive social process.

This applied example will allude to some boundaries between these systems, using the example of Quechua medicine in the southern Peruvian Andes from the personal experience of one of the authors. Addressing other belief systems as a means for interpreting biomedicine, rather than the more usual converse approach, Thorne (1993) adopts a critical stance toward the assumptions, beliefs and behaviours underlying the Western biomedical tradition and provides an unusual angle from which to evaluate critically the way we think and behave. Through this converse perspective, we highlight some common misunderstandings and some commonalities between these knowledge traditions.

The meaning of health in Quechua societies

In the Quechua societies of the southern Andes, the notion of health, or *allin hampi*, refers to **wellbeing**, the absence of illness, and the maintenance of good relations with their **environment**. The healthy man (*qhali runa*) is the one exempt from pain and preoccupations. The categories *ñakary* (collective suffering) and *llaki* (grief, sadness, usually referring to the individual level) refer to experiences of discomfort (Pedersen *et al.*, 2010). Social relations involve humans, animals and supernatural entities such as the Apus, protective spirits of the community that live in the mountains. In Quechua mythology, humans and animals come from the same place (Rozas Álvarez, 2022), reflected in close interaction between humans, sacred spirits and the world (Flores Ochoa, 1974). Human beings have *animu*, an active force in movement that drives every being to its own realization (Lanata, 2007). When the *animu* is separated from the body, certain diseases occur. They may also be caused by another person, calling upon the *layqa*, the sorcerer who specializes in invoking the spirits that have the power to do harm. His counterpart is the *altomisayoq*, able to communicate directly with the sacred spirits of the mountains. He can thus re-establish the health balance compromised by illness (Lanata, 2007) of the person or social group.

According to Quechua traditional practices, after giving birth, women should maintain a salt-free diet for at least one month. The extended family (usually grandmothers and aunts), and sometimes the husband, prepare special foods, such as guinea pig broth. Another common practice is the *waltado*, which consists of wrapping the woman's torso to the hips, to recompose the body affected by the pressure exerted during childbirth. Newborn babies are also *waltado* to help fuse their bones, ensuring healthy and strong growth.

Yet, the provision of healthcare by the Peruvian state focuses on combatting the diseases conceptualized by biomedicine, excluding those specific to the Quechua system. These practices are considered as 'beliefs' or 'ancestral customs', as opposed to objective knowledge based on physical evidence or laboratory results (Good, 1994). A nurse's job is to instruct mothers in the care of newborns based on biomedical, not Quechua, practices. The Quechua medical system coexists with biomedicine, but the clash between knowledge systems remains unresolved. Depending on the symptoms, the illness and the economic conditions, families will resort to one or the other.

Contrasting key concepts in biomedicine and other medical systems

Thorne argues that biomedicine sees itself as based on mind–body dualism, science-based inquiries, and relatively rigorously established chains of causal factors, and that biomedicine tends to relegate loosely observed correlations, supernatural and spiritual elements in knowledge to the domains of superstition, religion and philosophy. The distinction is reflected in the terminological difference of objectively evidenced 'disease' and subjectively experienced 'illness'. Yet, Thorne identifies beliefs that go beyond immediate explanations and treatment of specific symptoms in the health systems of all cultures, including the wider public health knowledge system in the West. Examples are to interpret illness and disease as consequences of misbehaviour (e.g. failure to do sport during childhood, long-standing bad habits or diet, symptoms of Karma), of body–mind interactions (somatic consequences of psychological conditions, punishment of gods, or teachings from deceased elders).

Thorne analyses three key concepts of health-related knowledge systems: (1) the nature of health; (2) the nature of disease; and (3) the nature of healing and healers. You might realize that these three concepts by Thorne roughly relate to three forms of knowledge described in Section 4.2.1: (i) target knowledge; (ii) systems knowledge; and (iii) transformation knowledge.

1. Thorne points out that one of the most universal aspects of health is its links with social context. The Western term 'quality of life' might most closely approximate 'health' for most of the world's people. In line with a One Health perspective, 'health' can in most cultures not be understood without considering community, environment and spirit world. The more narrowly defined biomedical knowledge system, as analysed by Thorne, is unique in conceptualizing health as a physical attribute of the individual. Thus, the mind–body problem in biomedicine is merely an artefact of the biomedical approach to health. Yet, he observes how we, as a Western society, abuse our physical selves in search of psychosocial wellbeing, pay for expert medical advice we have no intention of following, and express considerable anxiety about the extent to which crime, environmental destruction and social injustice influence the 'health' of nations.

2. In contrast to most non-Western traditions, biomedicine interprets and treats illness largely in terms of single pathogens and specific etiologies. It often categorizes the wider interpretative approach of most non-Western traditions as 'religion', even though the role of faith in healing was always acknowledged in Western tradition. While all healing traditions have diagnostic procedures, Thorne asserts that contrary to biomedicine, such diagnostic processes in non-Western knowledge systems are more concerned with underlying causes, rather than specific pathological processes. Yet, the search for single pathogens and specific etiologies may be of limited value for the treatment of complex, chronic, non-infectious syndromes, and the larger questions of why specific individuals react to specific germs in the way they do has attracted considerable scientific controversy. In the opinion of some, as Thorne argues, the more particular biomedical approach has precluded serious consideration of the general conditions under which illness does and does not occur.

3. Thorne observes how many non-Western traditions emphasize preventive therapies or require the participation of the entire community in rectifying the cause of illness. In contrast, one frequent accusation against biomedicine is that it returns the patient to the same circumstances that caused their illness in the first place. Additionally, biomedicine is highly intolerant of the viability of shamanic healing because it cannot generally be scientifically tested. Yet, Thorne asserts that shamans explain natural phenomena, guard against dangerous behaviour, distinguish good from evil and channel aggression, and that these techniques perform their healing function most evidently in the preventive mode at the community level – in some ways similar to various kinds of religious or profane Western community workers.

Learning questions:

1. Referring to Barth, please identify all forms of knowledge that you employed to interpret and act in two specific moments of your professional career:

(i) When you were challenged with a factual or scientific problem (such as diagnosing a pathology or understanding an environmental problem that was at that moment not well known to you); and

(ii) When you were challenged with a social problem relating to your professional work (such as diagnosing a fearful and confused patient with limited skills in your usual professional language or being confronted with local stakeholders who feel threatened by environmental protection activities).

2. From your own experience, what would you consider key substantive assertions, communicative media, social organization and validity criteria of a health-related knowledge system that you are familiar with?

3. Can you identify any differences between two knowledge systems that you are familiar with?

Example answers and reflection triggers:

1. While answering this question, you may find it useful to consider what you were intending to achieve in situations (i) and (ii) (target knowledge). Make sure to consider all forms of knowledge in your answer, including feelings (attitudes), information, embodied skills, verbal taxonomies/classifications and theoretical concepts or assumptions. Lastly, you may want to consider whether your way of using your knowledge was likely to lead to your intended goals (transformation knowledge).

2. If you are struggling with this question, please re-read the applied example and focus on the presented information on Quechua healing and biomedicine. Which differences can you identify between them in terms of their ontological/metaphysical assumptions, their way of communicating knowledge, the social organization underpinning their medical traditions and health systems, and their ways of assessing the effectiveness of healing interventions?

3. See **2.**

4.2.3 Integrating knowledge across knowledge systems

Knowledge integration can and does occur naturally in many instances in which people communicate. It is the means to make interpersonal discussions, academic argumentations and practical collaborations in One Health fruitful, as described in Chapters 3, 10 and 11. Yet, the integration of knowledge between the actors from different knowledge systems can be hampered by boundaries that prevent meaningful communication and translation. In the case of One Health, such boundaries may prevent communication between researchers and decision makers, between representatives of different disciplines such as human medicine and veterinary medicine, or between actors who pertain to different societal sectors (e.g. experts, legislators/regulators, business stakeholders, local communities). Such boundaries can occur for multiple reasons. In some cases, they root in differing ontologies and epistemologies – such as different norms and expectations as to what constitutes reliable evidence, convincing arguments and appropriate characterization of uncertainty. Yet, many such boundaries are social or cultural in nature, and are constituted by differing technical jargons or styles of expression, notions of procedural fairness, or economic and behavioural differences in perceived status, influence and power (Cash *et al.*, 2003; Clark *et al.*, 2016).

The central idea or ultimate intention of collaborating across such boundaries (also called 'boundary work') is to manage tensions between different viewpoints and to enable creation of knowledge that all relevant knowledge systems consider **salient** (relevant to their needs), **credible** (adequate in its evidence and arguments) and **legitimate** (respectful of their values and beliefs, unbiased in its conduct, and fair in its treatment of opposing views and interests). Since these three attributes are tightly coupled and their perception may differ between knowledge systems, efforts to enhance any one for a particular knowledge system could incur costs to other attributes, or to their perception by other knowledge systems (Cash *et al.*, 2003; Clark *et al.*, 2016). For example, a common observation in science-policy initiatives revolves around some actors highlighting certain matters because they perceive these as relevant and problematic (salient), while other actors question the credibility of the highlighted matter on factual grounds and prefer to address issues and aim for solutions which they consider to be supported by more robust evidence. Yet others may question the appropriateness (legitimacy) of certain proposed solutions due to a perceived lack of fairness or cultural appropriateness. Successful boundary work needs to reconcile such views to create common ground for joint action.

Cash *et al.* (2003) propose that in its quest to mobilize knowledge that is seen by all actors as salient, credible and legitimate, boundary work fulfils three functions. First, it facilitates active, iterative and inclusive communication between knowledge systems. Yet, communication does not ensure that participants in the resulting conversation understand each other. Second, effective boundary work facilitates information flow by translation when, as is often the case, actors are divided by jargon, language, experiences and presumptions about what constitutes persuasive arguments. Yet, the trade-offs among salience, credibility and legitimacy are fundamental. Conflicts among efforts to attain them cannot always, or even often, be resolved merely by improving understanding. This is why mobilizing knowledge for One Health often requires active mediation of those conflicts. See Chapter 10 for more information on conflict resolution.

Similarly, but using a different terminology, Clark *et al.* (2016) suggest that successful boundary work is characterized by meaningful **PARTICIPATION** in agenda setting and knowledge production by stakeholders from all sides of the boundary; governance arrangements that assure **ACCOUNTABILITY** of the resulting boundary work to relevant stakeholders; and by the production of **BOUNDARY OBJECTS**.

The concept of boundary objects may be unfamiliar to you, but is crucial, and we will therefore explain it further and also provide an example. The term was initially developed by Star and Griesemer (1989) and is defined as collaborative products such as reports, models, maps or standards that are both adaptable to different viewpoints and robust enough to maintain identity across them. In simple terms, boundary objects are 'something' that all actors in a One Health initiative share access to, that they can 'experience and grasp with their own senses', and that they can relate to based on their own perspective. Crucially, the immediacy and intersubjectivity of the boundary object allows them to visually or otherwise explain or demonstrate their own perspective to others in a relatively hands-on manner.

There could be no clearer illustration of a boundary institution using a model as boundary object to link science and policy than the one given by Cash and colleagues on the management of acid rain (Cash *et al.*, 2003). They report that, during the early 1980s, countries used their own experts to bolster their negotiating position or to question the expertise of others. No widely accepted scientific assessment of the problem existed and no political agreement on action could be reached. Subsequently, 'a modeling effort linked researchers from various disciplines (producing a more credible model of acid deposition and impacts) with the multinational delegates negotiating emission reduction protocols (producing information more salient to the policy debate). The [...] model became a boundary object that facilitated discussion among parties with multiple interests regarding differences in perspective, methodology, preferences, values, and desired outcomes. The iterated process of its construction, revision, and application created communication between model producers and model users that assured its information outputs were salient to negotiators, credible to scientists of all nations, and legitimate in not favoring the interests of any particular country.'

Manifold methods and approaches can serve to strengthen the creation of knowledge that actors across the full spectrum of participants of One Health initiatives perceive as salient, credible and legitimate. Bergmann *et al.*

(2010) distinguish and describe seven aspects of collaborative initiatives that can foster knowledge integration: (i) integrative organization of the research process; (ii) conceptual clarification and framing; (iii) integrative research questions and hypotheses; (iv) interdisciplinary or transdisciplinary research methods; (v) integrative assessment procedures; (vi) abstract modelling; and (vii) boundary objects.

Reflective intermission: You may pause a minute and re-read the above example of a science-policy process relating to acid rain (environment health). Which of these seven aspects can you identify in the quoted example? We also encourage you to work through Chapter 10 and to familiarize yourself with systems thinking that will improve your ability to use several of the above-mentioned approaches.

The next applied example introduces a case study in which the concepts that define boundary work are applied to bridging the boundaries between the knowledge systems of traditional Indigenous medicine and Western biomedicine in the particularly challenging intercultural context of a society that is divided by historical, cultural, ethno-linguistic and socio-economic boundaries. The next section will give you an exemplary familiarity with one particularly relevant tradition of knowledge that is at the forefront of enabling knowledge integration: the role of systems thinking and participative modelling in creating common understanding of a situation and enabling joint action. As a side remark, readers might want to note some of the considerations relating to boundary work are as well explored in Chapter 9, which essentially describes the relevance of bridging boundaries between genders.

Boundary work to support communication, translation and mediation between traditional and Western medicine: a case study in Guatemala based on Hitziger *et al.* (2017):

The case study was developed in 2014–2015 in collaboration with two Indigenous councils of Mayan elders and the national cancer hospital (INCAN) as a follow-up to previous collaborative efforts. It was implemented because health services to Indigenous populations of Guatemala are hampered by barriers between Western and Indigenous population groups and between their respective health systems. Study objectives were to develop and test a boundary mechanism to facilitate intercultural collaboration, reflection and mutual learning between Mayan healing practitioners and biomedical doctors, despite considerable differences in how these medical conditions are described and treated in their respective medical systems.

The boundary mechanism (Fig. 4.2) consisted of:

1. Exchange workshops to discuss and clarify Mayan and biomedical concepts relating to health and disease, and to strengthen trust between participants.

2. Bridge persons and Institutions from Western academic institutions and Indigenous councils of elders, representing reputed organizations that are accountable within their respective societal systems, to coordinate the study and to support intercultural process.

3. Joint diagnoses and follow-up of Indigenous patients suffering from chronic non-infectious diseases. They serve as palpable subjects to whom practitioners from both medical systems can relate in the terms of their own knowledge and paradigm (termed 'boundary subjects').

Since Indigenous and biomedical practitioners would diagnose each patient in accordance with their own knowledge, and since insights from case studies of patients who they could directly observe were considered tangible and credible, practitioners perceived the study as salient, legitimate and credible. Using the case studies of ~35 patients, this boundary mechanism enabled interaction and coordination between individual biomedical and traditional practitioners and an initiation of medical partnerships – spaces for communication and coordinated interaction that were connected to the realms of the two health systems in which information could be translated from one system to another and conflicts could be mediated. In the context of Guatemala, ongoing work intends to build on these efforts to facilitate mutual learning between medical knowledge systems and to improve public health services to Indigenous populations with limited access to biomedical health services (Hitziger, 2016).

Learning questions:

Can you identify a One Health example from your own experience in which specific methods or approaches were used to systematically integrate knowledge across knowledge systems? Can you identify how this One Health example:

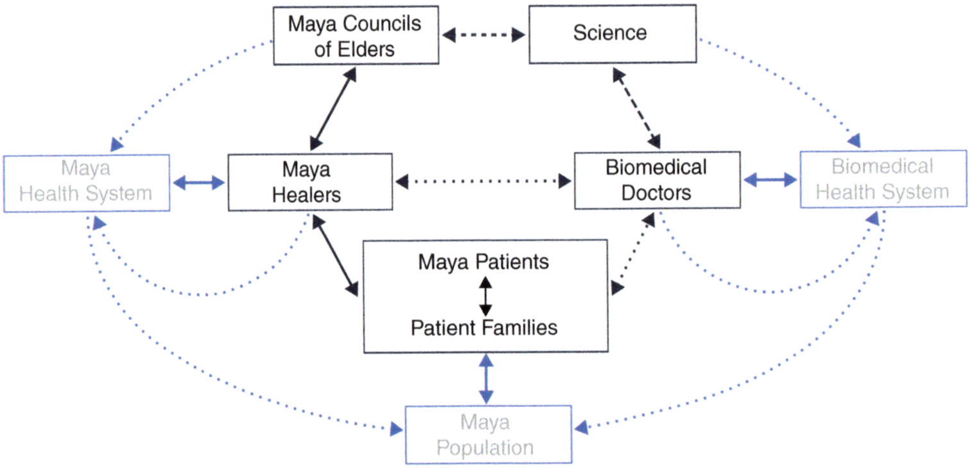

Fig. 4.2. Diagram with actors and relations involved in the case study. Left side: Mayan knowledge system. Right side: Biomedical knowledge system. Top: study coordination and facilitation. Centre: Medical systems. Bottom: Maya society. Black: Main actors and relations directly involved in the study. Grey: Contextual actors and relations influencing main actors. Solid arrows: relations that pre-date the project. Dashed arrows: Relations established during a previous project. Black dotted arrows: relations established by the research design. Grey dotted arrows: Potential future indirect impacts of the study outcomes. Figure from Hitziger *et al.* (2017), unmodified (CC BY 4.0 DEED: https://creativecommons.org/licenses/by/4.0/).

1. Implemented the three characteristics of boundary work elaborated by Clark *et al.*?
2. Implemented the three functions of boundary work proposed by Cash *et al.*?
3. Achieved the ultimate intention to foster the production of knowledge that is perceived as salient, credible and legitimate?

Example answers and reflection triggers:

If you cannot identify a One Health example from your own experience, please re-read the applied example case study in Guatemala. The following answers provide some additional leads on how authors would have answered this question for this applied example.

1. Participation ensured by involving practitioners from both health systems in exchange workshops, interviews, joint diagnoses and validation of fieldwork results. Accountability ensured by project implementation through institutions that constitute participants' professional authorities (councils of elders for healers, biomedical institutions for doctors). Though not objects in any literal sense, joint diagnoses of patients fulfil a boundary function as joint diagnoses constitute opportunities to relate knowledge and healing approaches to palpable exemplifications that are accessible of practitioners from each tradition, in terms of their own knowledge and experience.

2. Communication through facilitated workshops, iterative interactions, field researchers and co-ordinators as trusted bridge persons, and by ensuring practitioners feel their expertise is valued and relevant for the project. Translation provided in a literal sense (interpretation provided in workshops and fieldwork), as well as an overarching sense through involvement of bridge persons from both traditions, who are open to, and have become capable of, expressing knowledge in culturally appropriate ways. Mediation enabled through involvement of respected key authorities of both traditions, and through repeated negotiation of project objectives, methods and progress (including validation and interpretation of outcomes).

3. Knowledge perceived as salient as it relates to matters that are at the core of practitioners' professional focus. Knowledge perceived as credible as the project gave practitioners opportunity to build some trust with their counterparts, and relate to some of their counterparts' knowledge in experiential and palpable ways. Outcomes perceived as legitimate as they were achieved with involvement of respected authorities, resulted from a research process that was received to be fair to both traditions, and validated by practitioners from both sides.

4.2.4 Systems thinking and systems science – an approach and a toolbox for knowledge integration

SYSTEMS SCIENCE analyses the interactions of multiple interconnected system elements. Some methods deriving from systems science also form the basis for group modelling exercises, which is why interest has grown to use this tool for knowledge integration in One Health.

A 'system' in the most general sense is a set of three essential components: **parts** (which are generally the only component that can be directly observed); **interconnections** (that represent the (causal) relationships among the parts and determine how they interact); and **behaviour** (Banathy, 1997; Meadows, 2008); more information on this can be found in Chapter 10. System parts are related among themselves in a way that differs from the relationships they have with other elements in the surrounding environment. This difference is what we consider a boundary that defines the system (Mobus and Kalton, 2014). It may be helpful to reflect on the previous uses of the terms 'boundary' and 'knowledge system': In the context of systems science, societal boundaries differentiate 'systems' of societal actors (the system 'parts'), with common patterns of communication and interaction (the system 'interconnections'). These common patterns give rise to coordinated behaviour and a tradition of knowledge.

The concept of **complex adaptive systems** (CAS) refers to the limits of scientific reductionism that you are already familiar with from Section 4.1: the whole is more than the sum of the parts in the sense that, given the properties of the parts and their interactions, it is not trivial to infer the properties of the whole (Simon, 1962). CAS are built up from subunits, the interactions of which result in collective behaviour that feeds back into individual parts and determines the system's emergent dynamics (Simon, 1962; Brachthäuser, 2011; Mobus and Kalton, 2014). CAS are defined as 'large networks of components with no central control and simple rules of operation, which give rise to complex collective behavior, sophisticated information processing, and adaptation via learning or evolution' (Mitchell, 2009). Cells, living organisms, **ecosystems** and social organizations – including One Health systems and knowledge systems as defined earlier – are all examples of CAS.

Decision making and acting in CAS is fraught by obstacles. One such obstacle is **unintended consequences**, where side effects of action dominate over the intended outcomes (Merton, 1936) – we can never do merely one thing (Hardin, 1963). This means that any One Health action has implications that go beyond the intended goal. A second property is that CAS tend to be self-stabilizing. We observe this resistance to change from chemistry to ecosystems to policies (Scheffer, 2009). Policy resistance describes the tendency for an intervention to be defeated by the system's response to the intervention (Sterman, 2012). It arises because we do not understand the full range of feedback created by our decisions, including the responses of other actors and the ways in which experience shapes our goals (Sterman, 2006). Hence, the pervasive idea that One Health systems can and should be controlled is often an 'illusion of control' (Helbing, 2012).

CAS are difficult to control but can still be manageable – not by imposing structures but by creating the transactional rules needed to allow the system to find a state of stable organization. Acting in CAS entails identifying leverage points or 'levers', where a small shift in one thing can produce big changes in everything (Meadows, 2008). The power of an intervention comes from how it creates change within the system. Efforts targeted at government policy can have limited effectiveness if they are aimed at changing only relatively weak leverage points (Carey and Crammond, 2015). In other words, 'policy is designed to play a supporting role in an evolving structure – it is not designed to control the system' (Colander and Kupers, 2014). This approach stresses the relevance of alternative approaches to regulatory governance, including goals setting and establishment of common principles (Young, 2017). Finally, an important idea in the management of CAS is that the response to a problem should be commensurate with its complexity (Ashby, 1956). This means that a simple problem can be addressed by simple means, while a problem of increasing complexity requires more complex solutions. For the American anthropologist Joseph A. Tainter, the problem is that 'as systems develop more parts, and more complex interactions among these parts, the potential for problems, conflicts, and incongruities develops disproportionately' (Tainter, 1988).

Systems science provides a perspective on systems structure and systems behaviour that allows us to conceptualize One Health problems as emerging from interactions between parts and actors. It is similar to the previously introduced term 'systems knowledge', as it relates to factual circumstances and processes, including constellations of actors with differing perspectives and behaviours. Systems science also offers a toolbox of methods, and we encourage you to explore it elsewhere (e.g. see Sterman, 2000). As you are probably now able to see, systems science provides a powerful approach for knowledge integration across fields and disciplines. In terms of the model for One Health knowledge integration proposed by Hitziger *et al.* (2018) (Section 4.1 and Fig. 4.1), its tools, in particular when applied participatively as described in the applied example below on group model building, foster the integration of systems knowledge by transforming participants' observations into joint narratives about how situations emerge and how they might unfold in the future. They foster the integration of target knowledge by determining common vision and direction, which derives from the joint evaluation of the impact of potential scenarios of change. Importantly, the process of group model building can also be instrumental in strengthening trust between participants. By building trust between participating actors, and by creating a shared understanding of the situation and possible solutions, such an exercise furthermore integrates transformation knowledge and strengthens networks for collective action. The subsequent section will revisit some of the concepts introduced earlier to deepen and extend your understanding how knowledge integration can support robust decision making.

Group model building for knowledge integration:

Group model building uses rigorous computational tools in participatory settings aimed at integrating knowledge from across knowledge systems. Black and Andersen (Black and Andersen, 2012; Black, 2013) demonstrate how group model building, using a system dynamics tool, can act as a boundary object to facilitate the construction of shared meaning and of solutions among multiple stakeholders. Group modelling brings a selection of relevant experts and stakeholders together, in order to jointly develop an analytical model that describes a situation or a perceived problem. This model is intended to become a shared representation of the views, understandings and meanings perceived by the group. All participants share their views and understandings of the situation, and of subjective solutions to jointly develop and modify this model under the guidance of an expert facilitator. Knowledge is integrated by jointly assessing how these views link to, differ from or contribute to the overall model that is being constructed. Since all participants can suggest modifications, this boundary object is adaptable to their views, while retaining a shared identity that can be seen by all. Due to the possibility of 'running' the system dynamics model, all knowledge integrated into it contributes to visualizing scenarios of potential system changes, and their impact on the overall system. This is how the model enables the joint assessment of proposed solutions. Writing from the perspective of experienced workshop facilitators, their articles give precise and practical insights on best practice and common challenges of participative group modelling exercises.

Black and Andersen (Black and Andersen, 2012; Black, 2013) propose that participatively constructed system dynamic models are more likely to result in integrated knowledge that fosters collective action, if the models:

(i) are concrete, tangible two-dimensional or three-dimensional shared representations such as diagrams, sketches, prototype models or maps – they can include text but, by experience, the text is sparse;

(ii) portray dependencies and relationships among participants' objectives, expertise, decisions and actions;

(iii) can be modified by input from every participant – the facilitator needs to ensure a process that respectfully redistributes power away from existing institutional or social hierarchies, and allows perspectives to be considered on their merit rather than seniority or prestige, building trust between participants where possible, or enable anonymous sharing of perspectives, if necessary; and

(iv) are constructed iteratively and allow revision of earlier perspectives and contributions.

Learning questions:

1. Consider a system that you are familiar with and identify:

- **(i)** The elements of a complex adaptive system – its parts and interconnections.
- **(ii)** Examples of feedback between elements and of system behaviour (learning / adaptation).
- **(iii)** Examples of unintended consequences of an action taken by one of its actors.

2. Referring to the applied example on group model building, can you identify how participative modelling serves to:

- **(i)** Facilitate knowledge that all actors perceive as credible, salient and legitimate?
- **(ii)** Foster communication, translation and mediation?

3. Can you think of limitations of participative systems modelling for knowledge integration, or of situations in which such an approach might not work?

Example answers and reflection triggers:

1. For this example answer, let us allude to antibiotics use and management, as a commonly highlighted One Health issue.

- **(i)** When considering the parts of the system, pay attention to actors: human antibiotics consumers (e.g. patients), other users (e.g. farmers), producers (industry), other stakeholders (research institutions, regulatory bodies), other system parts such as antibiotics, animals, farms, wastewater treatment plants, environmental systems exposed to antibiotics. Consider material interconnections (stocks and flows, e.g. of antibiotics and their biochemical transformations), as well as information flows representing causal processes, information exchange between actors, and decisions. Note that by defining parts and interconnections that you include in your considerations, you are implicitly defining the scope of the system you are analysing. Can you sketch your system graphically?
- **(ii)** When considering feedback loops and adaptation, consider biological factors (such as reduced effectiveness of immune system responses, bacterial evolution towards antibiotics resistance) as well as human learning.
- **(iii)** Unintended consequences are one manifestation of complexity. They often exceed the system boundaries as implicitly or explicitly defined in the scope of your system analysis. Consider, for example, biological and evolutionary consequences in freshwater ecosystems exposed to antibiotic inflows.

2. If you are unsure about answering this question, please refer to the example answer in Section 4.2.3. Where do you see similarities of relevance to knowledge integration between the methodologies described in the applied example on the case study in Guatemala and that on group model building? Which of the elements of relevance to knowledge integration listed in the example answer in Section 4.2.3 seem to similarly apply to the applied example on group model building? Where do you see differences in the manner these two approaches foster knowledge integration?

3. If you are hesitating about limitations of group model building, consider hypothetical applications. Do you think group model building could be done without professional facilitators – or why not? Would it serve to design delivery of emergency interventions? Could it serve to discuss health impacts of poverty with illiterate communities? With stakeholder groups that represent divergent factions in violent conflicts or contexts of organized crime? Please use such trigger questions to list preconditions for the successful application of group model building in One Health contexts. Based on the list, try to summarize in one sentence when group model building actually is a promising approach.

4.3 Knowledge and Decision Making

4.3.1 Knowledge and decision making: the falsely blatant link

At first sight, you may think that the role of knowledge in decision-making appears obvious, especially once you do – for a moment – step away from the concept of knowledge as introduced in Section 4.2.2. From a 'natural science' understanding of knowledge as fact-based, objective information, you might assume that a decision that stems from a more complete knowledge of reality will better fit the needs of a situation. This understanding is reflected widely in concepts relating to decision making. It is often seen as common sense: knowledge is used to make right decisions, meaning that these decisions are in accordance with what we know. The more knowledge feeds into a decision, the better that decision will be, as it decreases what we do not know. For example, as a One Health practitioner, you might think that based on the diagnosis of a condition, you will decide the adequate treatment. Once you have more information on the history, the current state and context of the patient, you will be able to refine the treatment. This concept is also the foundation of evidence-based policy making, which originates in evidence-based medicine. It echoes the classical economic models depicting the decision maker (the famous *Homo oeconomicus*) as perfectly informed and rational, i.e. choosing the optimal solution in a truly mathematical sense. It also underpins models used to calculate the value of information: an additional piece of information will improve the decision by lowering the uncertainty; hence additional information will hold some value because it ascertains the decision (Yokota and Thompson, 2004).

Along that view, knowledge integration would improve decisions in an 'obvious' and 'natural' way and provide an additional rationale for using participatory methods in One Health as described in Section 4.2, and for democratic decision-making processes in societies at large. In fact, however, the link between knowledge and decision making in complex situations is far from obvious and One Health issues are never as simple as 'posing a diagnosis to recommend an adequate treatment'. One Health issues extend their ramifications across all levels of our lives: from the molecular to the global scale, going through local, national, regional and international levels. Their very nature is that they present a wide diversity of aspects, across the health of humans, animals, plants and ecosystems, across cultures, societies and economies, and across geographical levels of action. The 'simplistic' viewpoint thus forgets many complexities of real life that are at the core of the One Health concept, and issues at stake in One Health require us to consider a more complex perspective on decision making (please use any of the following key terms for your own research into the extensively available literature):

- Human decision makers show an imperfect ability to process information and are subject to cognitive limits, being simply unable to embrace manifold aspects of an issue when making a decision (Simon, 1959).
- Humans are subject to cognitive biases and perceive and handle situations with systematic inaccuracies or distortions, due to physiological traits, cognitive and mental habits, tricks, and rule-of-thumb-solutions (called 'heuristics') (Kahneman and Tversky, 1979). Examples of such cognitive biases are the tendency to downplay the probability of highly frequent events and the mirroring tendency to overweigh the probability of rare events. In One Health initiatives, an additional bias is the tendency to ignore or downplay the importance of what is outside the range of one's own expertise (Assmuth and Hilden, 2008).
- Human decision makers are emotional beings embedded in social interactions (Simon, 1959). They are not purely calculating consequences of options to choose the best. People are reacting, sometimes emotionally or intuitively, to a set of diverse stakes, either stakes for them personally or for the group. Stakes may also conflict with each other, the best solution for the individual not being the same as the best solution for the group or for different groups. Most often, stakes pose the question of how commons are collectively managed.

Reflective intermission:
Based on what you just read, you may wonder whether, when making decisions, we ignore more than we know, and are less independent than we believe? This feeling could be your first step towards becoming a more considerate decision maker!

Take some time to think about one or two of your recent decisions and whether you can now, upon reflection, identify aspects that you did not consider at the time of making this decision.

Also try to identify how your social context influenced your decision. Who or what else did exert influence on how you decided back then – not by their or its conscious actions, but simply through your own implicit and maybe even unconscious consideration or emotional attachment?

Reverting to a more complex 'social science' concept of knowledge as introduced in Section 4.2.2, the collective influence of cognitive limits, biases, heuristics and emotional factors on decision making is known as 'bounded rationality', a term that was coined by Simon (1957).

Being limited in their ability to address complex problems, humans then tend to opt for solutions that are '**satisficing**' rather than optimal (the term being a mix of 'satisfying' and 'sufficing'). As a result of the bounded rationality, much individual decision making will depend on its context – no knowledge can be considered as independent from its conditions of production (place, time, promotor) (Haraway, 1988). Moreover, no individual decision maker is socially independent (Antoine-Moussiaux, 2018): a farmer has a family, suppliers, lenders or may adhere to a cooperative; a minister has a cabinet, colleagues and voters – dependencies that imply risks and social consequences for those affected by decisions, as well as for decision makers themselves. One Health is often tied to a notion of socially contentious issues, where decision makers seem to bear particular responsibility. For example, in the face of an outbreak, would we stop economic activities to avoid any possible spillover? Such factual uncertainties can thus result in acutely felt psychological insecurity and be compounded by insecurity stemming from uncertainty about any social consequences of choices. The awareness of such uncertainties and complexities, of our ignorance and doubts, might even increase when presented with partial information that appears conflicting or contradictory (Assmuth and Hilden, 2008; Antoine-Moussiaux *et al.*, 2019), as is frequently the case in knowledge integration processes.

One lesson to learn from these explanations of the nature of decision making in One Health is that, in the siloed organizations that the One Health approach intends to connect, knowledge integration might also need to influence the very functioning of organizations or societies (i.e. knowledge systems) in which the One Health initiative is embedded. Another lesson is that knowledge integration will not distill an idealized decision process that eradicates cognitive limitations of the human being, factual uncertainties, or subjective and social aspects of decision making. Yet, broad consultations in knowledge integration processes can help to partially address factual uncertainty by reducing what we do not know, and will hopefully correct some of each other's biases and provide a more balanced, comprehensive, complete and complex understanding of a situation (credibility of information and salience of the addressed problems). At least as importantly, knowledge integration can render the positions of decision makers less subject to ulterior attacks or controversy. Communication, translation and mediation will build trust between partners and strengthen One Health initiatives by widening the coalition of actors who take ownership and collaborate towards common objectives (legitimacy of proposed ways forward). Indeed, if well done, knowledge integration provides scientifically robust information by shedding light on the limits of knowledge and enables societally robust decision making by instilling widely shared confidence in choices!

Learning question: Can you think of a decision or a situation in which the wealth of information did not help you decide? Can you identify reasons why the wealth of information was not helping your choice?

Example answer and reflection triggers:

If unsure about answering this question, try an experiment and make your next choice with full information. For example: Where and what to eat next. Start with listing all relevant criteria that ought to determine your decision, including from the One Health realms of human health, animal health and environmental health. Then proceed to identify what you need to know to make this choice with full information on all relevant criteria. Would you survive without food until you have compiled and comprehensively assessed all this information? If you are inclined to ensure your survival by making this decision under uncertainty – with incomplete information – and using bounded rationality only, what heuristics do you choose to use to simplify your decision? What role are your emotions and instincts playing in this decision?

4.3.2 Knowledge and decisions: matters of process

We have at various points in earlier sections casually mentioned 'knowledge integration processes' (also see Chapter 11 on the process to define One Health interventions). We will now explore this procedural aspect of knowledge integration. It stands opposite to the illusion of a decision that would occur at a given point in time, in an isolated manner. Instead, it rather resembles evolving strategies. Remember what you learnt about the contextualized nature of decision making: Any choice is taken within the context and organizational framework defined by earlier choices and will in turn set the context and organizational precedent for future decision making. For example, imagine a decision on rabies control: funding for the vaccination of dogs and wildlife reservoirs, dog population control and human post-exposure treatment will also depend on past decisions to invest in other vaccination services, in political decentralization, community empowerment and organization, or in surveillance in humans, domestic and wild animals. Conversely, it will be tied to decisions to be made now or later in urban planning, veterinary services, healthcare deployment, wildlife conservation or other zoonoses control.

Knowledge integration will not only shape a singular decision but will indeed shape the knowledge that we subsequently produce and the way we understand and frame future problems. The knowledge and its further evolution appear part of the same learning process. In this view, knowledge integration shapes the decision by shaping the way we formulate the issue and by shaping social interactions around that issue. In our rabies example, the integration of the knowledge from animal health, human health, environment or from communities and local governance would gradually shape the perceived problem that causes rabies to persist in a species population, and would direct surveillance and control efforts towards those aspects of the situation that are perceived as problematic. This role stresses the importance of a problem's structuring and framing in its solving (Antoine-Moussiaux *et al.*, 2019), evoking the claim that solving complex issues is less about 'getting the problem right' than 'getting the right problem' (note how this paragraph illustrates the concept of salience introduced earlier).

That shaping role of knowledge also holds long-lasting consequences for the way we organize ourselves. As already pinpointed, to influence decisions, the integration of knowledge may need to influence the societies, knowledge systems or organizations that frame these decisions. In fact, organizations or societies, i.e. the way people live and work together, are a result of knowledge that can be subject to integration. Indeed, theories on organizational learning consider knowledge as being translated into modes of functioning: our processes, routines, guidelines as well as tools or products (Argote and Miron-Spektor, 2011). Together, these types of knowledge shape how decisions are made, and integrating different knowledge systems can help organizations evolve into more flexible and effective entities. This process is often referred to as becoming a 'boundary organization', as proposed by Cash *et al.* (2003). This transformation appears as central to the implementation of One Health: the gradual bridging of boundaries between actors, sectors, disciplines and cultures, through a constant effort of each party towards knowledge integration.

Learning questions: Consider the final sentence of this section. Would you consider the 'gradual bridging of boundaries between actors, sectors, disciplines and cultures, through a constant effort of each party towards knowledge integration' as entirely desirable?

Example answers and reflection triggers: If you are unsure about this learning question, consider taking a hypothetical approach similar to the example answer to question 3 in Section 4.2.4. Imagine this sentence, in its literal sense, were to entirely come true. What would be disadvantages? Similarly, compare this extreme hypothetical vision of converging towards complete knowledge integration to your understanding of biological and cultural evolution: do you consider the scenario painted in the final sentence to be likely? Is such a scenario aligned with the nature of humans, societies and ecosystems? If it were to become real, what would be missing in such a world?

4.4 Conclusions

Knowledge integration, as presented in this chapter, is based on understanding knowledge as everything that a person employs to interpret and act on the world. Rather than seeking consensus, knowledge integration is being likened to weaving multiple perspectives into a common vision, or as a search for coherence and correspondence. Where knowledge is systematically integrated through networks of linked actors, organizations and objects that facilitate communication, translation and mediation, such an integration process can contribute to bridge existing traditions of knowledge and form new knowledge systems that support science and decision making. We hope that after working through this chapter, its applied examples and activities, we were able to convince you that this proposal has something very meaningful to offer to One Health and that you have become curious. We recommend you go back to the activities in this chapter and in Chapter 6 on professional reflexivity and reflective practice, to read additional sources and to understand some knowledge integration methods that we alluded to in depth.

Yet, the beauty of knowledge integration is that it goes beyond merely a different analytical skill and that it is more than just an additional set of methods. You can use it, improve your proficiency, and benefit from its application even away from your lab and desk, in your everyday life! Improve your listening, test your empathy. Change perspectives, through reflection or activities. Dare to venture into conversations or experiences with people with whom you happen to disagree in fundamental ways. Where you do not understand, ask questions or observe, rather than discontinue your engagement. Leave your comfort zone to see whether you might want to expand it. There is no need to take just any argument or suggestion, but there is a benefit from not discarding them all without consideration. Over time, you will realize that knowledge integration will broaden and enrich your experiences, sharpen your judgement, improve your professional track record as a One Health practitioner, deepen your wisdom, and become a habit and a character trait. Enjoy the journey!

References

Antoine-Moussiaux, N. (2018) The bridging role of socio-economic reasoning in 'One Health'. *Bulletin des Séances - Mededelingen der Zittingen* 64(1), 39–60.

Antoine-Moussiaux, N., de Bisthoven, L.J., Leyens, S., Assmuth, T., Keune, K. *et al.* (2019) The good, the bad and the ugly: Framing debates on nature in a one health community. *Sustainability Science* 14(6), 1729–1738.

Argote, L. and Miron-Spektor, E. (2011) Organizational learning: From experience to knowledge. *Organization Science* 22(5), 1123–1137.

Ashby, W.R. (1956) *An Introduction to Cybernetics*, Vol. 2. Chapman & Hall, London.

Assmuth, T. and Hilden, M. (2008) The significance of information frameworks in integrated risk assessment and management. *Environmental Science & Policy* 11, 71–86.

Banathy, B. (1997) Systems Inquiry [Internet]. Available at: https://web3.isss.org/primer2/bela3.html (accessed 23 July 2024).

Barth, F. (2002) An anthropology of knowledge. *Current Anthropology* 43(1), 1–18.

Bergmann, M., Jahn, T., Knobloch, T., Krohn, W., Pohl, C. and Schramm, E. (2010) *Methods for Transdisciplinary Research: A Primer for Practice*. Campus, Frankfurt am Main, Germany.

Black, L.J. (2013) When visuals are boundary objects in system dynamics work. *System Dynamics Review* 29(2), 70–86.

Black, L.J. and Andersen, D.F. (2012) Using visual representations as boundary objects to resolve conflict in collaborative model-building approaches. *Systems Research and Behavioral Science* 29(2), 194–208.

Brachthäuser, C. (2011) Explaining global governance: A complexity perspective. *Cambridge Review of International Affairs* 24(2), 221–244.

Buttigieg, S.C., Savić, S., Cauchi, D., Lautier, E., Canali, M. and Aragrande, M. (2018) Brucellosis control in Malta and Serbia: A One Health evaluation. *Frontiers in Veterinary Science* 5, 1–15.

Capra, F. and Luisi, P.L. (2014) *The Systems View of Life: A Unifying Vision*. Kindle edn. Cambridge University Press, Cambridge, UK.

Carey, G. and Crammond, B. (2015) Systems change for the social determinants of health. *BMC Public Health* 15, 662.

Cash, D.W., Clark, W.C., Alcock, F., Dickson, N.M., Eckley, N. *et al.* (2003) Knowledge systems for sustainable development. *Proceedings of the National Academy of Sciences of the United States of America* 100(14), 8086–8091.

Clark, W.C., Tomich, T.P., van Noordwijk, M., Catacutan, D., Guston, D. *et al.* (2016) Boundary work for sustainable development: Natural resource management at the Consultative Group on International Agricultural Research (CGIAR). *Proceedings of the National Academy of Sciences of the United States of America* 113(17), 4615–4622.

Colander, D.C. and Kupers, R. (2014) *Complexity and the Art of Public Policy: Solving Society's Problems from the Bottom Up*. Kindle edn. Princeton University Press, Princeton, New Jersey.

Elkana, Y. (2012) The university of the 21st century: An aspect of globalization. In: Renn, J. (ed.) *The Globalization of Knowledge in History*, Vol. 1. Max Planck Institute for the History of Science, Germany.

Erdi, P. (2008) *Complexity Explained*. Springer Verlag, Berlin, Heidelberg.

Flores Ochoa, J.A. (1974) Enqa, Enqaychu illa y Khuya Rumi: Aspectos mágico-religiosos entre pastores. *Journal de la Société des Américanistes* 63, 245–262.

Good, B. (1994) *Medicine, Rationality and Experience: An Anthropological Perspective*. Cambridge University Press, Cambridge, UK.

Haraway, D. (1988) Situated knowledges: The science question in feminism and the privilege of partial perspective. *Feminist Studies* 14(3), 575–599.

Hardin, G. (1963) The cybernetics of competition: A biologist's view of society. *Perspectives in Biology and Medicine* 7(1), 58–84.

Helbing, D. (2012) *Systemic Risks in Society and Economics in Social Self-Organization*. Springer, Heidelberg, Germany, pp. 261–284.

Hitziger, M. (2016) *Mayan Phytotherapy in Guatemala: A Transdisciplinary Study for Ethnographic Documentation and Local Empowerment*. ETH Zurich, Switzerland.

Hitziger, M., Berger Gonzalez, M., Gharzouzi, E., Ochaíta Santizo, D., Solis Miranda, R. *et al.* (2017) Patient-centered boundary mechanisms to foster intercultural partnerships in health care: A case study in Guatemala. *Journal of Ethnobiology and Ethnomedicine* 13, 44.

Hitziger, M., Esposito, R., Canali, M., Aragrande, M., Häsler, B. and Rüegg, S.R.R. (2018) Knowledge integration in One Health policy formulation, implementation and evaluation. *Bulletin of the World Health Organization* 96(3), 211–218.

Jahn, T., Bergmann, M. and Keil, F. (2012) Transdisciplinarity: Between mainstreaming and marginalization. *Ecological Economics* 79, 1–10.

Kahneman, D. and Tversky, A. (1979) Prospect theory: An analysis of decision under risk. *Econometrica* 47, 263–291.

Khoury, M.J., Lam, T.K., Ioannidis, J.P.A., Hartge, P., Spitz, M.R. *et al.* (2013) Transforming epidemiology for 21st century medicine and public health. *Cancer Epidemiology, Biomarkers & Prevention* 22(4), 508–516.

Klein, J.T. (2008) Evaluation of interdisciplinary and transdisciplinary research. A literature review. *American Journal of Preventive Medicine* 35(2 SUPPL.), 116–123.

Körner, M., Lippenberger, C., Becker, S., Reichler, L., Müller, C. and Zimmermann, L. (2016) Knowledge integration, teamwork and performance in health care. *Journal of Health Organization and Management* 30(2), 227–243.

Kuhn, T. (2012) *The Structure of Scientific Revolutions: 50th Anniversary Edition* (4th edn). University of Chicago Press, Chicago, Illinois.

Lanata, R. (2007) *Ladrones de Sombra: El Universo Religioso de los Pastores del Ausangate (Andes Surperuanos).* Institut Français d'études Andines, France.

Léger, A., Stärk, K.D.C., Rushton, J. and Nielsen, L.R. (2018) A One Health evaluation of the University of Copenhagen Research Centre for control of antibiotic resistance. *Frontiers in Veterinary Science* 5(August), 1–14.

McCullough, E.B. and Matson, P.A. (2011) Evolution of the knowledge system for agricultural development in the Yaqui Valley, Sonora, Mexico. *Proceedings of the National Academy of Sciences of the United States of America* 113(17), 4609–4614.

Meadows, D.H. (2008) *Thinking in Systems – A Primer.* Wright, D. (ed.) Chelsea Green Publishing Co., London.

Merton, R.K. (1936) The unanticipated consequences of purposive social action. *American Sociological Review* 1(6), 894–904.

Mitchell, M. (2009) What is complexity? In: *Complexity: A Guided Tour.* Oxford University Press, Oxford, UK.

Mobus, G.E. and Kalton, C.M. (2014) *Principles of Systems Science.* Kindle edn. Springer, New York.

Newell, W. (2004) Complexity and interdisciplinarity. In: *Encyclopedia of Life Support Systems.* EOLSS Publishers, Paris.

Pedersen, D., Kienzler, H. and Gamarra, J. (2010) Llaki and ñakary: Idioms of distress and suffering among the highland Quechua in the Peruvian Andes. *Culture, Medicine, and Psychiatry* 43(2), 279–300.

Pohl, C. and Hirsch Hadorn, G. (2007) *Principles for Designing Transdisciplinary Research.* Oekom Verlag, Munich, Germany.

Repko, A.F. (2011) *Interdisciplinary Research: Process and Theory* (2nd edn). SAGE Publications, Los Angeles, California.

Rozas Álvarez, W. (2022) El mito y el ritual andino. In: Yagi, Y. (ed.) *Etnografía Andina: Recorrido y Valoración Cultural.* SENRI Ethnological Studies, Osaka, Japan.

Scheffer, M. (2009) *Critical Transitions in Nature and Society.* Princeton University Press, Princeton, New Jersey.

Shiffman, J. and Shawar, Y. (2022) Framing and the formation of global health priorities. *Lancet* 399(10339), 1977–1990.

Simon, H.A. (1957) *Models of Man, Social and Rational: Mathematical Essays on Rational Human Behavior in a Social Setting.* John Wiley and Sons, New York.

Simon, H. (1959) Theories of decision-making in economics and behavioral science. *American Economic Review* 49(3), 253–283.

Simon, H.A. (1962) The architecture of complexity. *Proceedings of the American Philosophical Society* 106(6), 467–482.

Star, S. and Griesemer, J.R. (1989) Institutional ecology 'translations' and boundary objects: Amateurs and professionals in Berkeley's Museum of Vertebrate Zoology. *Social Studies of Science* 19, 387–420.

Sterman, J.D. (2000) *Business Dynamics: Systems Thinking and Modeling for a Complex World,* Vol. 19. Irwin/McGraw-Hill, Boston, Massachusetts.

Sterman, J. (2006) Learning from evidence in a complex world. *American Journal of Public Health* 96(3), 505–514.

Sterman, J.D. (2012) Sustaining sustainability: Creating a systems science in a fragmented academy and polarized world. In: *Sustainability Science.* Springer, Cham, Switzerland, pp. 21–58.

Tainter, J.A. (1988) *The Collapse of Complex Societies.* Kindle edn. Cambridge University Press, Cambridge, UK.

Thorne, S. (1993) Health belief systems in perspective. *Journal of Advanced Nursing* 18, 1931–1941.

Van Riel, R. and Van Gulick, R. (2018) Scientific reduction. In: *The Stanford Encyclopedia of Philosophy.* Department of Philosophy, Stanford University, California.

Wernli, D. and Darbellay, F. (2016) *Interdisciplinarity and the 21st Century University.* League of European Research Universities, Brussels.

Wickson, F., Carew, A.L. and Russell, A.W. (2006) Transdisciplinary research: Characteristics, quandaries and quality. *Futures* 38(9), 1046–1059.

Yokota, F. and Thompson, K. (2004) Value of information literature analysis: A review of applications in health risk management. *Medical Decision Making* 24, 287–298.

Young, O.R. (2017) Beyond regulation: Innovative strategies for governing large complex systems. *Sustainability* 9(6), 938.

5 A Data–Information–Knowledge–Wisdom Framework for Solving Complex One Health Problems

John Berezowski[1,2], Luís Pedro Carmo[2,3], Craig Stephen[4] and Laura Cristina Falzon[5]

[1]*Centre for Epidemiology and Planetary Health, Scotland's Rural College (SRUC), Inverness, Scotland, UK;* [2]*Network for Ecohealth and One Health (NEOH);* [3]*Norwegian Veterinary Institute, Ås, Norway;* [4]*McEachran Institute, Nanoose Bay, British Columbia, Canada;* [5]*Institute of Infection, Veterinary and Ecological Sciences, University of Liverpool, Liverpool, UK and International Livestock Research Institute, Nairobi, Kenya*

Contents

 Principles of One Health for a better planet (eds B. Häsler, A. Tvarijonaviciute and S. Savić)
DOI: 10.1079/9781800623002.0006

Chapter Overview

Elevator pitch

The goal of One Health is to address health challenges with solutions that benefit people, animals and the environment. Health challenges can be very complex and difficult to fully understand. Creating good solutions requires decision-making processes that are well informed with data, information, knowledge and wisdom (DIKW) from a wide variety of sources. In some cases, scientific information and knowledge may be insufficient to fully inform the decision-making process. Community members are an often overlooked source of additional DIKW that is not found in scientific domains, and engaging them may more fully inform decision-making processes. We use the DIKW framework to describe and understand some of the varied inputs into One Health decision-making processes and provide three case studies for illustrating some of these inputs.

Book objectives the chapter relates to

☑ 1. Understand what One Health and Ecohealth mean
☑ 2. Think in a One Health and Ecohealth way
☑ 3. Apply One Health and Ecohealth in their professional and personal life
☑ 4. Know how to share One Health and Ecohealth knowledge
☑ 5. Integrate One Health and Ecohealth knowledge actively
☑ 6. Acquire or enhance core One Health competencies

Main One Health competencies covered

☐ 1. Effective communication
☐ 2. Collaborative and resilient working
☐ 3. Systems understanding
☐ 4. Transdisciplinarity
☐ 5. Social, cultural and gender equity and inclusiveness
☐ 6. Collective learning and reflective practice
☐ 7. One Health concepts
☐ 8. Theoretical and methodological pluralism
☑ 9. Harnessing uncertainty, paradox and limited knowledge

After having worked through this chapter, you will be able to apply the DIKW hierarchy to the design and operationalization of One Health projects and programmes.

Learning outcomes

1. Learn the definitions of data, information, knowledge and wisdom and how they are related.
2. Understand how DIKW is used in One Health decision making.
3. Understand where DIKW comes from and the importance of engaging people with diverse backgrounds in the decision-making process.

Summary

In this chapter, you first get to know the data, information, knowledge, wisdom (DIKW) hierarchy, and its relevance to decision making in One Health programmes and activities. Focusing on each tier (data, information, knowledge, wisdom), you then get to see practical examples of each from the literature or our own field experience, specifically, the different kinds of data that can be collected, both tangible and intangible, and the various data collection methods employed. Next, you get to learn about different ways to generate information from these data, and how this information can then be incorporated into knowledge. Finally, you will learn about different types of wisdom that may come into play when making decisions. Throughout the chapter, there is a focus on how all these tiers are, or could be, connected to streamline the process while ensuring that all perspectives are represented. At the end of the chapter, we discuss how this hierarchy can be operationalized within all One Health activities and programmes.

5.1 Introduction

Making good decisions about how to respond to health challenges requires timely, fit-for-purpose information, knowledge and wisdom. These, however, are often insufficient, constraining our decision making so that some of our responses to health challenges fail or even cause additional, unexpected harm. **One Health** is an approach that aims to help people make better decisions by providing additional information, knowledge and wisdom through a collaborative process and integration mechanisms (see also Chapter 3 on **transdisciplinarity**, Chapter 4 on **knowledge integration** and Chapter 10 on **stakeholder** engagement). Good One Health decisions are those that maximize health benefits for people, animals, plants and the **environment**, given the resources available, **governance** structures and other constraints. In Chapters 3 and 4 you learn about the value of multi-, inter- and transdisciplinary approaches as well as barriers and challenges to their successful use (Chapter 3) and the meaning and importance of knowledge integration (Chapter 4). In Chapter 11 you gain further insights into effective communication in the One Health project life cycle. These chapters highlight that including people with different backgrounds, experiences, knowledge and wisdom brings additional information, knowledge and wisdom to One Health (Intezari *et al.*, 2016).

The inputs supporting decision making in health can be many and highly varied. In this chapter we use the **Data, Information, Knowledge** and **Wisdom** (DIKW) framework to organize and understand some of the inputs into One Health decision-making processes. The DIKW framework was selected because it has been used to understand the role of data, information, knowledge and wisdom in decision making (Intezari *et al.*, 2016), risk assessment in engineering (Aven, 2013), and in health surveillance (Berezowski *et al.*, 2020). We describe the DIKW hierarchy and the relationship between DIKW and One Health decision-making processes. Building on the description of complex health problems in Chapter 1, we begin with a refresher activity of those followed by a description of the DIKW framework. We then discuss the role of DIKW in the decision-making process by presenting three case studies as examples.

5.2 Background

5.2.1 Complexity of health problems

Health problems result from many interactions between individuals of the same and different species living within the same **complex system.** Positive and negative interactions can form feedback loops that accelerate or slow system change, making these systems difficult to predict. Complex systems have no clear boundaries, and they operate on multiple scales (see Chapters 1 and 10 for more information), resulting in health-related problems being expressed differently at different scales. Harmful health problems continue to emerge, and decision makers are required to find solutions to reduce the harm, often with insufficient understanding of the complex system they are working in. Considering this complexity, informing the decision-making process with as much useful information, knowledge and wisdom as possible can only benefit the decisions being made.

Task: This activity on **complex systems thinking** allows you to think about different connections in a system on a One Health problem, as discussed in Chapter 1. Consider a recent disease emergence such as COVID-19, Porcine Epidemic Diarrhoea, or another human, animal, plant or insect disease emergence of your choice. Can you think of some of the factors that contributed to the disease emergence and suggest how these factors could be countered to prevent or reduce the impact of the disease?

Example answer taking into consideration the re-emergence of leptospirosis in tropical countries: Leptospirosis is a disease of humans and many animal species that is caused by bacteria from the genus *Leptospira*. Infected humans and animals spread the bacteria in urine. In urban settings, rats often act as a reservoir and transmitter of the **pathogen.** The bacteria can survive for a few weeks to months in water or soil. Infection can occur by contact with urine, water, soil or food contaminated with the bacteria. It is important to consider all factors that can potentially result in increased infections and also factors that affect the vulnerability and resilience of the community to an increase in disease. We present examples as perspectives for understanding the factors that may be driving an increase in diseases.

Perspective 1 – it is a climate change issue: Re-emergence of waterborne epidemics of leptospirosis has been associated with heavy rainfall and floods. Since they are strongly driven by **climate**, leptospirosis outbreaks are predicted to increase along with climate change, especially in flood-prone areas. Many tropical countries have inadequate financial resources to mitigate flooding and standing water expected with climate change. Leptospirosis cannot be controlled until mitigation strategies and affordable infrastructure are universally available (Semenza *et al.*, 2022).

Perspective 2 – it is a disease of poverty: 'Residents of urban slums suffer from a high burden of **zoonotic diseases** due to individual, socioeconomic, and environmental factors'. There is inadequate capacity to provide basic sanitation services, as well as abundant habitat and food for rodents, which are sources of the infections. Impoverished communities often lack access to early diagnostic services, are underserviced by surveillance systems and have inadequate healthcare. Leptospirosis cannot be controlled until access to health and hygiene services is available to all, especially the most vulnerable and impoverished communities (Khalil *et al.*, 2021).

Perspective 3 – it is a biomedical issue: It remains a challenging diagnosis since it presents with marked clinical polymorphisms, clinicians must have a high degree of suspicion, and serological tests have low sensitivity. This can make early detection and containment of outbreaks a problem and can facilitate international spread of infection. A human vaccine is lacking, eliminating an option for prevention. Leptospirosis cannot be contained until better biomedical interventions are created and equitably distributed (Monteiro *et al.*, 2021).

Perspective 4 – it is a rodent control issue: Rats (*Rattus* spp.) are ubiquitous in cities globally. With increasing global urbanization, more rat–human interfaces can be expected, providing more opportunity for spillover of the pathogen into people. Rats are a key source of human infection. There is little evidence that the traditional approach of waging war on rats is working. Leptospirosis cannot be controlled until alternative management objectives that place a priority on improving the overall health of the community are adopted, instead of on eliminating rats (Lee *et al.*, 2022).

5.2.2 Benefit of One Health in health-related decision making

One Health offers a promising approach for improving our health-related decision-making processes. One Health is a transdisciplinary decision-making process that includes people from different health domains (human, animal, plant and the environment), different scientific domains, and different societal groups (Chapters 3, 4 and 10). Including such a wide range of people brings more information, knowledge and wisdom to the decision-making process than is available when single individuals or smaller groups make decisions. This can lead to a better understanding of the problem, the harm caused by the problem, and the costs, benefits and harms to all species that may result from the solutions, leading to better and more stable solutions. See Chapter 12 for more information on how to conceptualize these effects in an evaluation and Chapter 13 for guidance on economic evaluation.

Learning question: Who should be involved? Zoonotic diseases occur when a pathogen is transmitted from an animal reservoir host to a human. An example is Q fever, a disease of people and animals caused by *Coxiella burnetii*. It causes abortions in cattle, sheep and goats and can cause illness in people when they breathe in dust that has been contaminated by infected animal faeces, urine, milk and birth products. Who do you think should be involved in controlling zoonotic diseases such as Q fever?

Example answer: Below we identify some of the **actors** that we consider should be involved in Q fever control. Please note that our answer is not comprehensive. There might be other relevant stakeholders depending on the zoonotic disease under consideration, the specific aspects to be investigated, or the boundaries you set for the system.

- Farmers – farmers check their animals every day and will be the first to recognize that something is wrong with their animals. Because of their close contact with their animals, they also have a higher risk of being infected.
- Farmers' associations – farmers' associations can be relevant for the implementation of control measures. They are also important

communication channels for reaching out to farmers.

- Livestock practitioners – veterinarians are critical for the identification of disease cases. They also need to be aware of the procedure to be followed when they encounter an animal that could have the disease. Farmers trust their veterinarians, and veterinarians can play an important role in advising farmers about the correct implementation of preventive measures.
- Dairy companies – due to the risk of transmission of Q fever via unpasteurized products, the dairy industry should be aware and involved in the control of the disease.
- Veterinary and food safety authorities – these government agencies are often responsible for the design and implementation of control programmes and play a central role in maintaining animal health and food safety.
- Public health authorities – in the case of zoonotic diseases such as Q fever, public health authorities should be involved in the development of control programmes.
- Medics – it is important that medics are aware of high-risk occupations (e.g. farmers, vets), and include Q fever as a differential diagnosis (particularly given the possible severe complications).
- Wildlife associations – Q fever can be transmitted to wildlife and therefore preventive and control measures might need to be taken in order to have a holistic control programme.

Key learning points: Problems at the human, environment, animal interface can be: (i) simple, linear and have few variables to consider (e.g. a clinical decision to treat a person with a known zoonotic infection); (ii) complicated and involve several interacting variables, but in predictable ways (e.g. launching a wildlife rabies immunization programme in an area endemic for rabies); (iii) complex with multiple interacting variables that act unpredictably and cause emerging **outcomes** (e.g. forecasting geographic locations and timing of the next emerging disease). The diversity of people to involve in a One Health issue needs to be scaled to the complexity of the problem.

Often the people in place to launch actions to prevent, mitigate or control a One Health problem are found outside of the usual veterinary or medical system. The people and expertise needed to understand pathophysiology and epidemiology of diseases are not necessarily the same as the cadre of people who can create socially acceptable policies and programmes to act on the problem. For an example of a description of stakeholders to include in One Health decision making see Mazet *et al.* (2014). In Chapter 10, you can learn more about how to identify and engage different stakeholders.

Japanese Encephalitis control in Nepal: The Nepal government encouraged the development of pig farming as a means of poverty alleviation. Pigs are the intermediate host of Japanese Encephalitis, a vector-borne zoonotic infection, creating occupational health concerns for pig farmers and the risk of disease spread outside of the farming community. Nepal lacks economic resources for vaccination programmes or investment in farm biosecurity practices. Many of the pig farmers are unhoused, migrating communities with little capacity for vector control or avoidance. These communities often reside temporarily in peri-urban areas where urbanization, agriculture and forestry practices interact to inadvertently create vector habitat. This farming community has little ownership of land and limited education, requiring prevention messaging to be tailored to low levels of literacy, and accounting for gender inequities and population mobility. Treating clinical cases requires a team that can finance and deliver necessary diagnostic and therapeutic tools. Preventing clinical cases requires social marketers to reduce disinformation leading to poor human vaccine uptake. Eliminating the epidemiologic conditions that enable persistence and spread of the disease requires land-use planners, social development expertise, policy experts, entomologists, ecologists and agronomists (Dhakal *et al.*, 2012; Robertson *et al.*, 2013). See Chapter 8 for further information on the **social determinants of health.**

5.3 The Data–Information–Knowledge–Wisdom (DIKW) Framework

The DIKW framework is commonly used to understand the inputs into complex decision-making processes and how they relate to each other (for an example, see Gee and Corry, 2012). The individual components of the DIKW framework are not mutually exclusive as they overlap each other, and the framework should be considered a continuum of increasing complexity and increasing human contribution moving from the lowest level / tier (data) to the highest (wisdom) (Fig. 5.1).

Data, the foundation of the DIKW framework, are composed of symbolic representations of the real world such as numbers, letters of the alphabet, words and text. Data are created by human observation or measurement and/or recording by machines. The elements of data have little meaning, value or use on their own. They become useful only when they are processed, analysed, organized and interpreted to provide context. There are different types of data, different ways to understand data validity (Chapter 3), and there are challenges when it comes to sharing of data (Chapter 11).

Information is created when data are processed, organized, structured, analysed and interpreted. Information has meaning and value and is useful when it is created for a purpose. The purpose can often be found in the questions that the information was created to answer and, as seen in Chapter 4, will be influenced strongly by different epistemologies rooted in the traditions of a particular discipline or field. For population health management based on epidemiological principles (in both humans and animals), information most commonly answers questions relating to the current and future state of the population's health, such as what is the current amount of disease in a population, and is it changing? What are current levels of important risk factors for disease, and are they changing? Since health management is not just limited to managing disease, information may also be created to answer questions about health (see Chapter 1 for an introduction to the concepts of health and disease). For example, what are the current levels of important determinants of health, and are they changing? Has access to certain health determinants recently been limited? Additional information may be needed for One Health decision making depending on the One Health problem being addressed, the stakeholders involved, the systems and their boundaries, and the potential

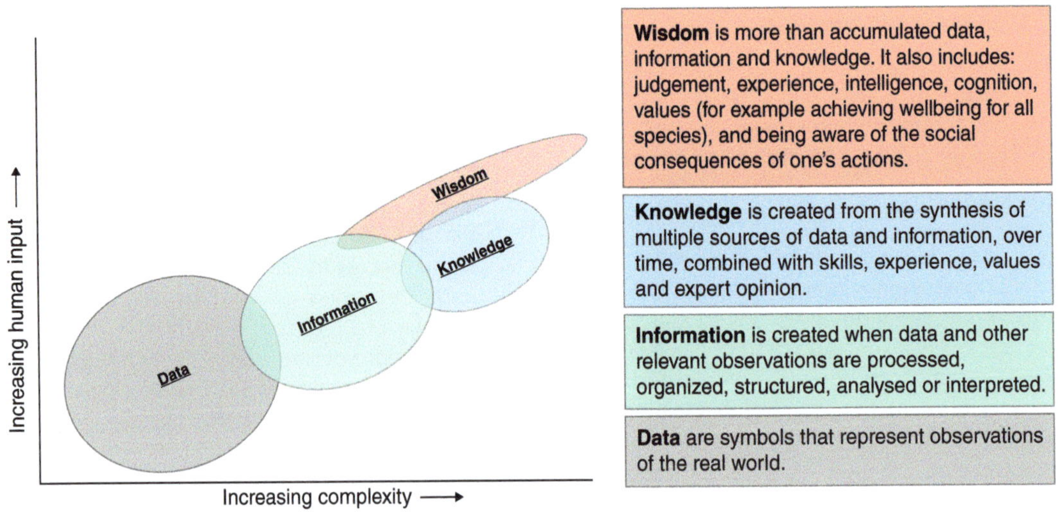

Fig. 5.1. Schematic representation of the DIKW framework, illustrating: (i) the connectedness of the DIKW components; (ii) the increasing complexity and human input moving from data to information to knowledge to wisdom; (iii) that wisdom is more than accumulated data, information and knowledge; and (iv) the decreasing quantity that is available moving from data to wisdom, as illustrated by the sizes of the ellipses. Developed by the authors.

interventions (Chapters 10 and 11). For example, we may wish to know whether there are concurrent changes in the amount of disease in multiple groups of the same or different species in the same location. We may also wish to know whether a human activity, such as a change in land use in one location, is occurring at the same time as a change in the health of local insect, plant or wildlife species. This can be important for vector-borne diseases because changes in land use can in some cases promote an increase in the population of vector species, resulting in an increase in vector-borne disease in people, terrestrial animals or birds (Lemy, 2021).

Learning question: What information is needed? Yellow Fever is a viral haemorrhagic disease that affects humans and several species of non-human primates. The disease is transmitted among populations of these species by mosquitos. Although vaccination is available, there are still periodic epidemics of Yellow Fever often within rural, forested regions in countries such as Brazil. What information would be helpful for predicting an impending epidemic of Yellow Fever in people?

Example answer: From a public health perspective, knowing the risk of human infection is essential for the timely implementation of preventive measures. Since Yellow Fever virus is transmitted by mosquitos, knowing when the virus is present in local mosquito populations is a signal that the risk of human infection has increased, and an intervention is necessary. This information can be captured in several ways. For similar diseases such as Eastern Equine Encephalitis or West Nile Virus, in countries where resources are less of a constraint on public health practice, mosquitos are often trapped in urban areas and tested for the presence of the virus. An alternative is to house chickens in cages in urban settings where they can be bitten by mosquitos and their blood tested regularly for the presence of antibodies to zoonotic pathogens. In rural Brazil, where resources are limited, these approaches may not be possible, and communities are forced to look for other signals of increased human infection risk. Since Yellow Fever also causes mortalities in non-human primates, finding dead monkeys in rural areas close to forests has been used as a signal that Yellow Fever virus may be circulating in the area. When dead monkeys are found, the local public health authorities can then either examine and test the dead monkey for evidence of Yellow Fever virus, implement vaccination programmes and/or inform communities about taking precautions to prevent mosquito bites.

Information can also be created directly by humans observing the world and mentally processing their observations, for example, processes to improve climate change preparedness (Hiwasaki *et al.*, 2014). Another example is farmers who, because they are very familiar with their animals, are often able to identify subtle disease-related changes in their animals that would not be recognized by a veterinarian. These and other non-scientifically trained people who have life experiences related to the problem at hand can be an important and often neglected source of information.

You have learned in Chapter 4 that **knowledge** is a property of people and encompasses everything a person employs to interpret and act on the world. It is created from the synthesis of multiple sources of data, observation and information over time, combined with skills, experience, emotion, values and cognitive judgement. Knowledge can be either **tacit** (contained within a person) or explicit (codified within books, web pages, newspapers, documents, etc.). A person can obtain knowledge through experience, instruction or transmission from others who have it (for example, from oral history or by reading explicit knowledge).

In Chapter 4 we saw that there is a wide variety of knowledge traditions and that there can be domineering behaviour of one over another. Appreciating and learning how to connect these different ways of generating, accepting and using knowledge is critical in One Health practice. **Indigenous Peoples**' ways of knowing (knowledge) comprises centuries of intergenerational experiences and understandings pertaining to a particular people in a particular location. The knowledge held by Indigenous Peoples is different from, but complementary to, that created through scientific research. Including Indigenous Peoples can better inform decision making.

Knowledge is critically important in decision-making processes because it provides an understanding of the importance of specific pieces of information in relation to a specific problem. With respect to disease management, knowledge is, for example, needed to make a decision about whether a surveillance signal is important or not. Knowledge is necessary to understand whether a sudden increase in the number of cases of a disease in a population is important. In disease prevention, knowledge is needed to understand whether the reduction at a population level of a factor that is associated with good health is important enough to cause a significant change in the health of a population. In both prevention and management, understanding the importance of these pieces of information is essential for deciding whether something should be done in response to the signal. The knowledge required will be case specific. It can include pathogen-specific knowledge such as whether a pathogen is likely to spread rapidly or whether it can cause significant disease. Knowledge about social and environmental circumstances will also be required, such as whether a population is likely to express behaviours in support of or against a vaccination programme, or whether a change in environmental conditions can cause an epidemic of disease in animals (Kock *et al.*, 2018). There are similar examples for non-infectious diseases. For example, knowledge about the highly addictive nature of Oxycontin (an opioid pain reliever) combined with an understanding of the social, economic and psychological factors of addiction should have been enough to predict an increase in opioid addictions and associated mortalities seen in the first wave of the opioid epidemic based on increased registrations of prescriptions for Oxycontin in the USA (Humphreys *et al.*, 2022).

Learning question: What knowledge is needed? The World Health Organization (WHO) has added 'Disease X' to its list of priority diseases (WHO, 2023). Disease X is a previously unknown disease that suddenly appears in a human population, spreads rapidly and causes significant disease and harm. When a new human disease emerges, what information **and** knowledge do you think would be helpful for deciding whether the new disease is a potential Disease X that requires a global response? Who would you involve in this decision-making process?

Example answer: There are international agreements and expectations for human, animal and plant health that unknown diseases are reported, that actions are taken on transboundary diseases, and that joint efforts should be undertaken to prevent the dissemination of pathogens. There are not, however, universally agreed thresholds for actions that can translate across species nor for non-infectious threats, such as the global spread of a new pollutant, or the spread of chronic diseases. Take, for example, climate change. It undoubtedly shares many of the characteristics of Disease X, especially when harms emerge after climate **tipping points** have been exceeded, but it has yet to provoke coordinated efforts by health agencies. The first question to consider, therefore, is which harms and to what constitute a signal for action?

To help answer this question, let us take for example the emergence of neo-tropical Cryptococcosis in British Columbia, Canada (Stephen *et al.*, 2002; Bartlett *et al.*, 2008). Unusual rates and clusters of animal cases, albeit with low case counts, were sufficient only to provoke curiosity because: (i) jurisdictional boundaries created uncertainty as to who would be responsible to investigate cases in pets or wildlife; (ii) this was not a listed disease with assigned response plans; (iii) early warning detection occurred before social or ecological harms occurred (i.e. when the only impact was individual animal deaths). Only when an animal health professional informally asked a public health colleague, connected via a professional social network, if human cases were being seen, was it recognized that this was a multi-species clustered outbreak showing a slow spatial spread. The occurrence of human cases was now the signal for an investigation; however, the small case numbers and relatively slow spread early in the disease did not inspire funders or government agencies to invest in an investigation.

Lesson 1 – In advance of Disease X occurring, there should be agreement amongst local animal and human health authorities of how disease in species for which no programme exists will be communicated, and the threshold of harm needed to warrant investigation. While a too early warning, as seen in the case of Cryptococcosis, is the best time to contain a disease, it did not cross a threshold of concern for action, allowing the pathogen to spread geographically and into another country.

Lesson 2 – Professional social networks to speed and facilitate information sharing should be established before Disease X.

As evidence mounted to pinpoint the epicentre of the disease and to demonstrate spatial expansion to new bio-geo-climatic zones and another country, it was now seen by regulatory authorities as time to act. Options for action included excluding residents and visitors from the epicentre (which was a popular local attraction), mandating disinfection of fomites seen to spread the diseases via vehicle traffic, and surveillance and disinfection of fomites before people left the epicentre. None of these actions were attractive to local government authorities or business interests. As media began to report on the disease, tourism declined and real estate sales for the area sharply dropped. This dissuaded governments in this tourism and retirement hotspot to act, allowing the disease to spread.

Lesson 3 – The capacity and willingness to act early on Disease X will require compliance of government, and at times police authorities, to bar movements or invoke other control measures. Science literacy and trust in epidemiological data may not be high in some of these groups. Leaving engagement of those empowered to enforce actions will suffer if trust and understanding must be developed in the midst of an early outbreak. Trust must be developed well before an epidemic with pandemic potential has emerged.

Lesson 4 – Media can shape public and political concern and awareness of an issue. Developing relationships with media and health communicators will be important to frame an appropriate response in the public's mind.

The knowledge integration you learned about in Chapter 4 constitutes an important foundation for achieving wisdom. **Wisdom** is more than accumulated data, information and knowledge. Wisdom also includes judgement, experience, intelligence, cognition, values and being aware of the social consequences of one's actions. Importantly, wisdom can be achieved when there is awareness that knowledge 'must be constructed via critical inquiry or through the synthesis of opposing views [...] (these constructions) are generative, offering [...] a new, more complete way to view the issue under consideration' (Awbrey and Scott, 1994). Successful knowledge integration in One Health (Chapter 4) can pave the way towards wisdom and sound decision making in the face of uncertainty. Reflexivity is an important competency to contribute towards gaining wisdom (Chapter 6). In a health context, wisdom is the ability to choose the optimum solution to a problem. An optimum solution is one that achieves the most desirable outcome(s) while minimizing unwanted and unexpected negative outcomes. Wisdom is knowing which response will be most effective and cost effective for reducing disease in the affected population while minimizing the harmful effects on other populations, species, **ecosystems** and the environment. Good decisions are just and equitable across different people, species and generations (see Chapters 10 to 13 to see how this can be operationalized in the One Health project life cycle). It is only in relatively simple situations that a single individual will have sufficient knowledge and wisdom to identify the most appropriate response. A common example is physicians and veterinarians who examine a patient (gather data) and then make a diagnosis (create information) that the person/animal being examined has a specific disease. If the physician/veterinarian has repeatedly treated similar individuals with the same condition, their training combined with wisdom gained from their experience treating the disease many times will often allow them to select an intervention that is both successful and has limited side effects. Selecting an optimal solution for more complex health problems that affect large populations, multiple species or ecosystems requires much more wisdom. It is unlikely that single individuals will have sufficient wisdom to select good solutions for these complex problems and collective wisdom achieved in a One Health community through engagement and knowledge integration may offer a better solution.

Climate change is an example of a complex global problem that is likely to affect the health of millions of people, animals, plants and ecosystems. Clear signals that global temperatures are rising have been available for many years. There is widespread recognition by the scientific community that these signals are critically important. It has taken many years, however, for some groups within human societies to begin to accept these signals as being important, and there are still sectors of society that do not recognize their importance. Deciding on what are the best solutions to slow or reverse climate change is an even greater challenge. There are some very broad strategies, such as reducing carbon emissions, that have gained widespread acceptance. But specific interventions for reducing carbon emissions vary considerably from country to country, indicating there is as yet no clear consensus about which are the best interventions. This variation suggests that the wisdom held within the decision-making groups in these countries is not yet sufficient to identify interventions that are most likely to be optimal in terms of being able to reduce carbon emissions without causing undue harm to people, animals, plants and ecosystems.

5.4 Case Studies

In the following section, we look at three case studies that show how the DIKW framework can be incorporated when taking decisions or designing interventions for complex One Health problems.

5.4.1 Case study 1 – One Health surveillance

Health surveillance is a continuous and dynamic process that generates information with the ultimate aim of helping to make decisions about health problems (El Allaki *et al.*, 2012). From the moment data are collected to the final stage of the health surveillance cycle when decisions are made, a series of steps need to be followed to ensure that actions taken are well-informed and appropriate. The DIKW framework can provide a guiding conceptual structure for health surveillance and disease-control systems. The framework can be particularly useful for those surveillance systems that aim to tackle complex health problems and that require collaboration between different domains and stakeholders.

Health surveillance has been heavily dominated by systems that focus on individual species and single diseases. Such an approach may be adequate for diseases that affect a single species, but they fail when addressing more complex health problems, such as zoonotic and emerging diseases, antimicrobial resistance, food insecurity, and impacts of climate change on the determinants of health. One of the most relevant aspects of the inability to address more complex problems is the lack of a comprehensive understanding of the system that hosts the problem, which in turn leads to unsustainable and inequitable decisions.

Surveillance monitors change and generates information useful for decision making. The time we live in is characterized by rapid change. In a constantly changing world, new information is of critical importance for adapting to changing conditions and responding with optimal actions. Managing under uncertainty and changing conditions requires new collaborations to inform decisions that are effective, and to provide a holistic view of a given problem. This will ensure that responses to health problems are not short sighted, and that they do not benefit one species to the detriment of others. Engaging the communities experiencing the problem and/or the people who need to make decisions is a useful process to understand their needs and what they value. This approach can be beneficial for the design of surveillance systems.

Learning questions: Table 5.1 presents a series of questions aimed at exploring some of the basic concepts of health surveillance. Think about the questions in the left column before looking at the example answers provided.

One Health surveillance has emerged as a method for providing some of the information needed to inform One Health approaches. One Health surveillance has been defined as 'the systematic collection, validation, analysis, interpretation of data and dissemination of information collected on humans, animals and the environment to inform decisions for more effective, evidence- and system-based health interventions' (Stärk *et al.*, 2015). For examples of One Health surveillance systems, please see Box 5.1 with a review by Bordier *et al.* (2020). With the advent of One Health surveillance, however, several challenges have arisen. For example: What is the purpose and value of the information created by combining these varied data? How do we combine the knowledge and wisdom of various stakeholders from dissimilar domains to inform the decision-making processes? How do we combine different data collected for different purposes at different frequencies and scales? How do we reconcile different thresholds for action for different segments of a One Health problem (e.g., human health vs ecosystem health)?

Table 5.1. Heath surveillance learning questions.

Learning questions	Example answers
Why are we doing surveillance?	Surveillance is purpose oriented. Its essential purpose is to create information and knowledge for health decision making that leads to action. All elements of system design and operations should be informed by its purpose and objectives. They set the scope of the system, informing issues such as who should participate, and which methods are most appropriate. However, surveillance objectives must be tempered with practical realities such as limited resources being available for surveillance of certain species, lack of value of certain species, and other pressures, such as the limited time available to operationalize surveillance in the face of an epidemic.
What issue are we going to keep under surveillance?	The issue under surveillance must be important enough to warrant management. The surveillance outputs must generate information that is desired, understandable and useful to decision makers. Are there measurable, reliable metrics that allow decision makers to estimate the size of the problem, monitor its spread, and measure the effects of an intervention?
Who / what are we going to keep under surveillance?	Careful consideration of the populations (humans, animals, vectors) to be kept under surveillance is critically important because generated results can be either a true reflection of what is happening in the population or a false reflection of what is happening resulting from a bias in the sample or attention to the wrong populations.
What are we going to look at during the surveillance activities?	Not all surveillance needs to track hazards or adverse outcomes. Social or ecological risk factors can be tracked. Even assets that keep populations well can be kept under surveillance. Different metrics will be needed to track the outcome of past situations versus prediction or prevention and preparedness planning.
Who needs to be involved?	The answer to this question is affected by two questions, 'who needs to know?' and 'how will you gather, analyse and assess your surveillance data and samples?'
How will we recognize a signal?	The goal of surveillance is to find a change. But agreement on what constitutes an actionable change can vary with the values of the involved stakeholders, confidence in established cause–effect relationships, and the implications of being wrong.
How will we know if the surveillance system is good?	Despite the growing demand for One Health surveillance there is little guidance on the necessary performance standards of One Health surveillance programmes. The dearth of performance standards and different expectations from different partners complicate attempts to show that investments and activities are meeting the expectations of public or private investors in surveillance services.

The DIKW model can provide the conceptual framework needed to help further the development and implementation of One Health surveillance systems. Surveillance systems are ongoing processes that continuously generate inputs for DIKW. Such dynamic systems are particularly useful for identifying changes in the system, such as the emergence of a new disease, and allow for decisions to be made in a constantly evolving environment.

Data collected for health surveillance systems often relate to cases of disease or exposures. The definition of a case can vary greatly, as can the methods used for identifying cases. These can range from laboratory diagnostic methods (e.g. use of a PCR test), to self-reporting of cases (e.g. report of pharmaceuticals' side effects), to prescription registries (e.g. surveillance of on-farm antimicrobial use). Case data are often accompanied by other data that provide context and help to profile cases. Examples of contextual data are date, location, age, sex, species, breed, profession, level of education, ethnic background, geographical details such as local forest cover, species diversity, and many others. In a One Health surveillance context, data will often need to be collected from several species.

Let us use the example of the One Health surveillance system implemented in Italy for West Nile Virus (WNV) and reported by Paternoster *et al.* (2017a). West Nile Virus is a mosquito-transmitted virus that affects birds, people, horses and some other mammals. Samples from avian wildlife that were found dead or shot as part of population control programmes were analysed using real-time PCR for detecting positive cases. Mosquitos that can transmit WNV were trapped during the high-risk season and screened for the virus. Suspected cases of WNV disease in horses that were reported to the veterinary authorities were tested for antibodies and the presence of the virus. Plasma, serum and cerebrospinal fluid were collected from suspected human cases and tested to determine whether they were due to WNV infections. Birds, mosquitos, horses and humans are part of the complex WNV transmission network. Because mosquitos are the main transmitters of the virus, transmission risk is seasonal, increasing in the summer during mosquito season; however, the exact date when the risk increases varies from year to year. The purpose of the surveillance system was to detect increases in the risk of WNV circulation. Collecting data from all these species was essential for detecting increasing virus transmission because all these species are interconnected within the transmission network. Sharing data across **disciplines** and **sectors** comes with various challenges. These aspects are further discussed in other chapters of this textbook.

Box 5.1. One Health surveillance systems

Bordier *et al.* (2020) conducted a systematic literature review to identify the characteristics of One Health surveillance systems, the context in which they are implemented, and the factors that might hinder or promote their creation and performance.

In their review process, 41 One Health surveillance systems were identified. The most common health hazard being surveilled was antimicrobial resistance (10/41), followed by West Nile Virus (9/41) and zoonotic diseases in general (9/41). From the 41 surveillance systems, 19 had a shared coordination between multiple institutions and 22 engaged three or more sectors in their collaboration.

The primary objectives of the One Health surveillance systems were early detection and monitoring of trends. Data sharing and analysis, collaboration for laboratory testing, and cross-sectoral notification of health events were defined as the main collaborative efforts.

As previously mentioned, data on their own have no intrinsic value. Data become **information** once they are processed and analysed. Within the context of health surveillance, case and contextual data are often combined to answer specific questions, such as: Did the number of cases increase or decrease in a given period of time? Is there a geographical clustering of cases? Are there any case characteristics that might indicate there is an increase in risk factors for the occurrence of the disease? We will use the same example as above. One of the main goals of the One Health surveillance system for WNV was the early detection of virus circulation in the environment (Paternoster *et al.*, 2017b). By analysing the data that were collected, it was possible to monitor changing risk of infection and apply adequate control measures, if necessary.

Surveillance **outputs** can be used for disease management and control. Once the surveillance system generates information, a question arises: Does an action need to be taken? This relates to **knowledge** – the capacity to understand the relevance of the information produced. Within a One Health framework, this concept is extremely relevant. Interpreting information and deciding whether an action needs to be taken requires a deep understanding of various disciplines (e.g. epidemiology, economics, human/animal/ecosystem health, etc.) and the links between the different populations (humans, animals and environment). In a One Health surveillance context, the decisions that are made should not be short-sighted but rather thought through from a systemic perspective. This may differ significantly from species-centric surveillance systems, where decision makers only need to consider one disease and the benefits and consequences for a single species. It is unlikely that a single person will have such diverse knowledge and, thus, disease control in a One Health setting requires collaboration between people with different backgrounds. Without proper knowledge, data and information generated from the surveillance system have no value for the decision-making process. Understanding the relevance of the information produced is not always straightforward, especially in a complex One Health context. Antimicrobial resistance surveillance is a good example. Trends in antimicrobial resistance in samples of indicator bacteria from livestock are monitored in many countries but understanding the significance of this information is complicated. This is particularly difficult when attempting to make inferences about the level of risk for public health from antimicrobial resistance trends seen in samples from livestock. This relates not only to the data that are collected and the information generated (e.g. which information are we trying to obtain from the data, and are the data, methods and analysis adequate for the information we want to obtain?), but also to the knowledge gaps that emerge due to the complexity of antimicrobial resistance epidemiology (e.g. what is the relevance of different sources of antimicrobial resistance for human infections?). Incorporating knowledge from various fields for decision making has several challenges, including competing priorities and different action threshold levels. Hindrances to effective collaboration are discussed in Chapters 3, 10, 11 and 16.

In the context of disease control, **wisdom** relates to the use of surveillance information, combined with knowledge from a variety of sources, to make the best possible decision. Optimal decisions should lead to solutions that yield the highest benefit to harm ratio. From a One Health perspective, maximizing benefits and reducing harm should not be limited to a single species, but rather take the whole system into consideration. The management of the COVID-19 pandemic provides an example of the role of wisdom in a health-related decision-making process. The pandemic had a broad impact on society; not only on health-related aspects, but also on the economy, the political sphere and education. It was not possible for decision makers to base their decision only on health-related information. Wisdom was required to compile the information and knowledge from various disciplines to determine which were the most appropriate measures to implement through the various stages of the pandemic. Figure 5.2 provides a schematic representation of the relationship between data, information, knowledge and wisdom in a surveillance context.

In health surveillance, data collection and analysis often take centre stage. The majority of One Health surveillance systems, however, have focused their efforts on the integration of data from various populations. While data collection and analysis have been led by analysts and epidemiologists, the role of other stakeholders in the generation of evidence should not be diminished. Data and information generated by communities, as previously described in this chapter, can have great value. For instance, observation and reporting of dead animals by hunters can be used for disease management purposes. With the emergence of the 'Internet of Things', huge amounts of data have become available, many of which are being used for secondary purposes (e.g. data about individuals' location from Google and Facebook were used to evaluate the impact of interventions and forecast disease spread during the COVID-19 pandemic; Ilin *et al.*, 2021). Data owners/collectors often have a deep understanding of the data and the information that can be generated from it. Therefore, engaging these stakeholders in the data analysis and the interpretation of information created from it can be very beneficial. Transdisciplinary methods can guide these collaborative processes, not only in the process of generating information, but also when combining knowledge and wisdom from different sectors and fields. For further information on transdisciplinarity and other collaborative approaches, see Chapter 3.

The world is interconnected and so is the health of humans, animals and the environment. In a constantly evolving world, a continuous flow of information is needed. In the context of complex health problems that link animals, humans and the environment, One

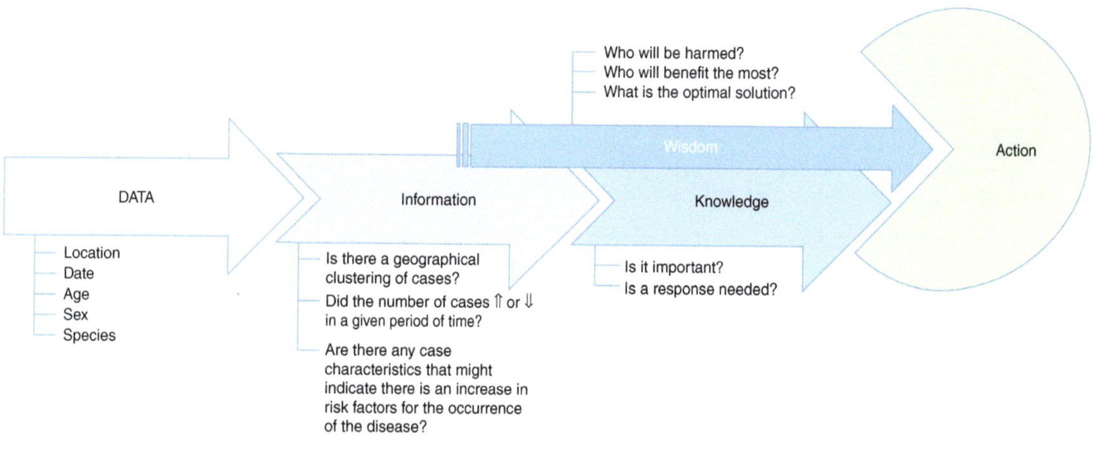

Fig. 5.2. Relationship between data, information, knowledge and wisdom in disease surveillance. Developed by the authors.

Health surveillance can collect relevant data and generate useful information. Interpreting this information to draw optimal conclusions about the importance of this information for people, animals and the environment should be done using group knowledge and wisdom from multiple stakeholders from various fields. Once a decision that an action is needed has been made, choosing the optimum action that will provide maximum benefit to the most people, animals and the environment should be done using the same group knowledge and wisdom. Figure 5.3 exemplifies, in a schematic fashion, the use of the DIKW framework for decision making in a One Health surveillance context.

The next two case studies are more descriptive, to illustrate the breadth of topics the DIKW framework can be applied to. As you read the case studies, you may consider: Which other sources of data could be tapped in to? How could the data be analysed and interpreted to generate useful information? Who may have the required knowledge and wisdom to guide the decision-making process? We have also included Fig. 5.4 (adapted from Stephen *et al.*, 2021) as a source of guiding questions for action.

5.4.2 Case study 2 – a One Health response

Climate change has become an inevitable reality. Every day we hear about erratic weather patterns, be they record-breaking heat spells, prolonged droughts or flash floods. These have an impact on all life systems within our ecosystem, and innovative One Health responses are needed to improve our resilience and allow us to adapt to climate change. Such responses can be developed within a DIKW framework, combining data and information accrued through science and technology, with traditional environmental knowledge and Indigenous wisdom. Let us look at a few examples.

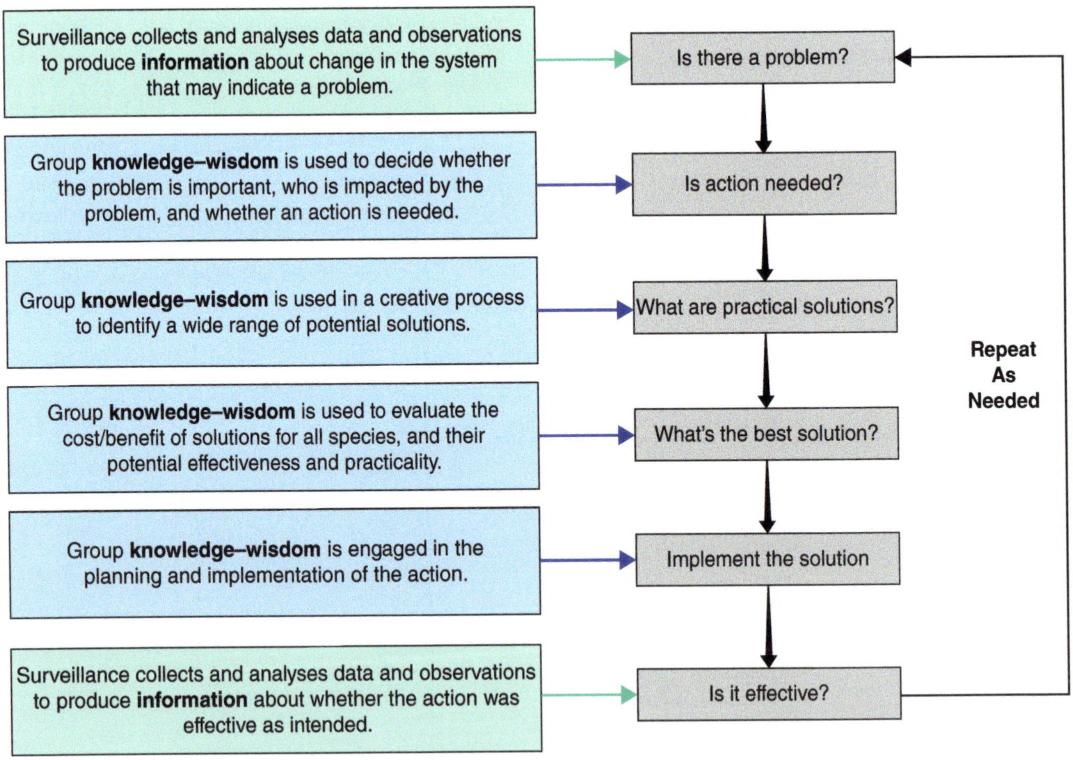

Fig. 5.3. The role of surveillance and DIKW in a One Health decision-making process. The process as presented relates to a community health problem, but it can be generalized to larger systems such as populations or ecosystems. Developed by the authors.

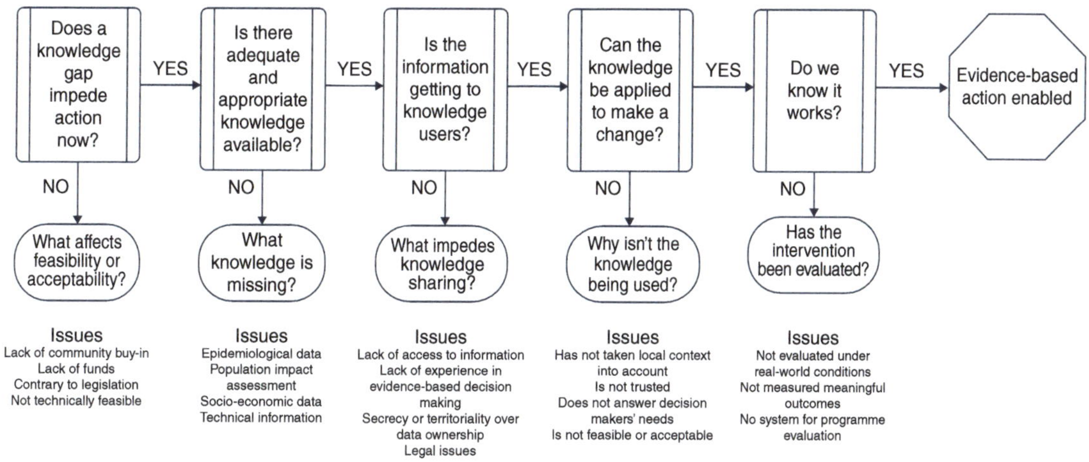

Fig. 5.4. Questions to guide a decision-making process that enables evidence-based action. Adapted from Stephen *et al.* (2021) (CC BY-SA 3.0 IGO DEED: https://creativecommons.org/licenses/by-sa/3.0/igo/).

Wildfires are becoming more frequent, and more devastating. Holistic land management is considered essential for controlling and mitigating their spread. Native American communities have traditionally employed land stewardship practices, such as wood collection and setting of intentional controlled fires, which made their landscape more resistant to uncontrolled and extreme fire events (Roos *et al.*, 2021), though this may have varied depending on the forest type. Prescribed burning and 'thinning' of the forest through selective logging was recently put into practice in the Malheur National Forest in Oregon, with a consequent decrease in the intensity and speed of wildfires (Cornwall, 2021). Another component of Indigenous land management revolved around the use of grazing ruminants to keep plant material in check, thus reducing fire fuel material. This practice, supported by research on its positive knock-on effects on biodiversity and conservation (Barry and Huntsinger, 2021), is now being reintroduced in various localities particularly prone to wildfires. This shows how current data can complement traditional knowledge to inform a One Health response that encompasses animal, human and environmental health.

Ocean Network Canada is an institution that monitors climate change and the impact it is having on the health of oceans. It employs several innovative technologies, including mobile applications, observatories and sensors, to collect real-time oceanographic data. These long-term continuous scientific data are merged with Indigenous knowledge held within coastal communities who have, for generations, depended on these same oceans for their sustenance. They have therefore learned to recognize ecological indicators of ocean health and have developed sustainable practices which respect the ocean's biodiversity (Brown, 2017). **Big data**, **information analytics**, **inter-generational knowledge** and **Indigenous wisdom** are therefore contributing to the development of ocean management practices that are evidence-based and sustainable.

Pastoralist and small-scale farming communities rely on their ecosystem for their livelihood. They have learnt to observe, and recognize, nature's patterns. They know when the weather is going to change, when it is the right time to sow seeds, or when to move their herds to the next grazing area. This knowledge has been passed on from generation to generation. It is now being harnessed through qualitative research methods, such as participatory mapping of locally relevant sites. These research methods also incorporate a gender lens, giving voice to women (Oumarou, 2019). In sub-Saharan Africa, researchers have developed systems which combine the **local technical knowledge** with **data** collected through wireless sensor networks to inform drought predictive models developed using artificial intelligence. This **information**, which is contextual and locally relevant, is relayed back to the farmers through mobile phones, allowing for a two-way communication system between local communities and scientific experts (Masinde and Bagula, 2012).

Throughout these examples we can observe a common thread. Knowledge and wisdom acquired through generations of observation of the ecosystem contribute to the interpretation and contextualization of data generated by digital technologies, which are then transformed into new information using various analytical approaches. In these examples, the past and the present come together to generate innovative solutions that can take us sustainably into the future. Can you think of other examples?

5.4.3 Case study 3 – COVID-19 and vaccine hesitancy

So far, we have seen how the different components of the DIKW framework can come together to inform and guide decisions regarding complex situations. But what happens when we have too much information? Or if some of that information is wrong? Novel and evolving situations are particularly prone to this problem. A good example is the COVID-19 pandemic and the way it was managed. Let us take a look at how the DIKW components were, and could be, incorporated within the decision-making processes.

Following the first report of COVID-19 in December 2019, **data** on the causal agent and transmission patterns were constantly generated, leading to evolving **information** on the topic. While this is to be expected given the novelty of the virus and ensuing disease, inconsistencies in the **knowledge** shared with the general public created confusion on how the disease could be transmitted and prevented (Seytre *et al.*, 2021). These inconsistencies also led to stigmatization of those people testing positive for the disease, hindering disease tracing and control practices (Chandrashekhar, 2020). There were also substantial differences in how data were collected and presented across countries, sometimes leading to a biased or under-estimation of the true disease burden (Anand *et al.*, 2021).

During the COVID-19 pandemic we also witnessed a concomitant infodemic, defined as 'too much information, including false or misleading information, in digital and physical environments during a disease outbreak' (WHO, 2021). Even when correct, an excessive amount of unfiltered information on a problem makes it hard to process and interpret. This is further complicated when that information is useless (**misinformation**) or maliciously fabricated (**disinformation**) (Zielinski, 2021). While incorrect information can be shared through multiple means, our hyper-connected environment has augmented the speed and breadth by which erroneous information can spread. Many people do not have the knowledge to evaluate correctly all the information they are exposed to, and are unable to decide which pieces of information are important to them, their families and communities. This can result in people making decisions that are not in their best interests. As an example, misinformation led to an over-reliance on antimicrobials for treatment of COVID-19, despite them not being effective against the disease (Arshad *et al.*, 2020). Misinformation also fuelled anti-vaccine sentiments (Adepoju, 2021).

Vaccine hesitancy did not start with the COVID-19 pandemic. The WHO included vaccine hesitancy as one of the top ten threats to global public health in 2019 (WHO, 2019), and vaccine refusals have been documented in different countries prior to the pandemic (Olive *et al.*, 2018; de Figueiredo *et al.*, 2020). However, the urgency to vaccinate as many people as possible to curb the spread of the coronavirus highlighted the importance of understanding underlying sources of misinformation to better manage and address them.

So how could the DIKW framework contribute to the collaborative response required to handle such a complex situation, where data are continuously being generated, our knowledge is evolving, and misinformation abounds?

While social media are often maligned as a source of misinformation, they are an important source of **crowd-generated data** that can be analysed to capture what is happening on the ground. These data can be particularly useful at the early stages of an epidemic when other data sources may not yet be available. This was evidenced by Turiel *et al.* (2021), who found that the intensity of social tweets could forecast the severity of COVID-19 and which regions would be most affected the following month. This enables better disease preparedness.

Ensuring that everyone has access to accurate and relevant **health information** can go a long way to empowering individuals to make informed health decisions (Zielinski, 2021). There are many different health information sources; some people may prefer to ask their healthcare workers (Arce *et al.*, 2021), while others may prefer to consult internet sites (Azizi *et al.*, 2017). As mentioned previously, online material may be false or unfounded, and efforts are needed to monitor more effectively what is available online by establishing safe sites for trusted information (Zielinski, 2021). Moreover, efforts are needed to improve health literacy to help people turn data into information, and information into knowledge (Naeem and Boulos, 2021).

Providing access to **knowledge** that allows people to evaluate health information is critical for enabling people to make optimal decisions that benefit themselves and their families. For example, basic knowledge on infections and their treatment can improve the general understanding and encourage adherence with preventive measures (Arshad *et al.*, 2020), while sharing knowledge of success stories of previous vaccination campaigns can help reduce vaccine hesitancy (Adepoju, 2021). Education is therefore crucial at all levels, including educating school children on basic science (Ochu *et al.*, 2021), and parents on the importance of vaccines (Albanna, 2020). All education efforts must be underpinned by effective communication strategies, with an understanding and empathy for underlying fears and beliefs (Larson, 2020).

Finally, **practical wisdom** is essential when making decisions about complex public health situations, such as the COVID-19 pandemic (Fowers *et al.*, 2021). Aristotle defined practical wisdom as 'the combination of moral will and moral skill'. It is based on experience and is an essential virtue in those problems where the context is continuously changing (Schwartz, 2009). As an example, during the early stages of the COVID-19 pandemic, when information was changing and knowledge evolved slowly, practitioners often had to rely on their practical wisdom to make decisions regarding patient treatment or triaging systems (Gill *et al.*, 2021). Trusted community members, such as village elders or church leaders, also acquire practical wisdom through their daily interactions with their community. Such practical wisdom should therefore be incorporated within any decision-making process to allow for the formulation of solutions that are culturally adapted and contextually relevant.

References

Adepoju, P. (2021) Africa is waging a war on COVID anti-vaxxers. *Nature Medicine* 27, 1122–1125. DOI: 10.1038/s41591-021-01426-2.

Albanna, A. (2020) Ideas NOT worth spreading: The psychology of vaccine hesitancy. *TED Talks*. Available at: https://www.ted.com/talks/dr_ammar_albanna_ideas_not_worth_spreading_the_psychology_of_vaccine_hesitancy (accessed 27 January 2023).

Anand, A., Sandefur, J. and Subramanian, A. (2021) Three new estimates of India's all-cause excess mortality during the COVID-19 pandemic. In: *CGD Working Paper 589*. Center for Global Development, Washington, DC, USA. Available at: https://www.cgdev.org/publication/three-new-estimates-indias-all-cause-excess-mortality-during-covid-19-pandemic (accessed 27 January 2023).

Arce, J.S.S., Warren, S.S., Meriggi, N.F., Scacco, A., McMurry, N. *et al.* (2021) COVID-19 vaccine acceptance and hesitancy in low- and middle-income countries. *Nature Medicine* 27, 1385–1394. DOI: 10.1038/s41591-021-01454-y.

Arshad, M., Mahmood, S.F., Khan, M. and Hasan, R. (2020) Covid-19, misinformation, and antimicrobial resistance. *British Medical Journal* 371, m4501. DOI: 10.1136/bmj.m4501.

Aven, T. (2013) A conceptual framework for linking risk and the elements of the Data-Information-Knowledge-Wisdom (DIKW) hierarchy. *Reliability Engineering and System Safety* 111, 30–36. DOI: 10.1016/j.ress.2012.09.014.

Awbrey, S.M. and Scott, D.K. (1994) Knowledge into wisdom: Incorporating values and beliefs to construct a wise university. *To Improve the Academy* 301. Available at: https://digitalcommons.unl.edu/podimproveacad/301 (accessed 2 September 2023).

Azizi, F.S.M., Kew, Y. and Moy, F.M. (2017) Vaccine hesitancy among parents in a multi-ethnic country, Malaysia. *Vaccine* 35, 2955–2961. DOI: 10.1016/j.vaccine.2017.04.010.

Barry, S. and Huntsinger, L. (2021) Rangeland land-sharing, livestock grazing's role in the conservation of imperiled species. *Sustainability* 13, 4466. DOI: 10.3390/su13084466.

Bartlett, K.H., Kidd, S.E. and Kronstad, J.W. (2008) The emergence of *Cryptococcus gattii* in British Columbia and the Pacific Northwest. *Current Infectious Disease Reports* 10(1), 58–65.

Berezowski, J., Carmo, L.P. and Stephen, C. (2020) Chapter 7: Building health surveillance for decision support at the animal, human, environment nexus. In: Stephen, C. (ed.) *Animals, Health and Society Health Promotion, Harm Reduction and Health Equity in a One Health World.* CRC Press, Abingdon, UK. ISBN: 9780367336226.

Bordier, M., Uea-Anuwong, T., Binot, A., Hendrikx, P. and Goutard, F.L. (2020) Characteristics of One Health surveillance systems: A systematic literature review. *Preventive Veterinary Medicine* 181, 104560. DOI: 10.1016/j.prevetmed.2018.10.005.

Brown, Q.J. (2017) The relationship between Indigenous Knowledge and Ocean Science. *TED Talks.* Available at: https://www.ted.com/talks/qatuw_as_jessica_brown_the_relationship_between_indigenous_knowledge_and_ocean_science (accessed 28 July 2021).

Chandrashekhar, V. (2020) The burden of stigma. *Science* 369, 1419–1423. DOI: 10.1126/science.abe8114.

Cornwall, W. (2021) Clearing the tinderbox. *Science* 373, 1300–1303. DOI: 10/1126/science.acx9070.

de Figueiredo, A., Simas, C., Karafillakis, E., Paterson, P. and Larson, H.J. (2020) Mapping global trends in vaccine confidence and investigating barriers to vaccine uptake: A large-scale retrospective temporal modelling study. *Lancet* 396, 898–908. DOI: 10.1016/S0140-6736(20)31558-0.

Dhakal, S., Stephen, C., Ale, A. and Joshi D.D. (2012) Knowledge and practices of pig farmers regarding Japanese encephalitis in Kathmandu, Nepal. *Zoonoses and Public Health* 59, 568–574. DOI: 10.1111/j.1863-2378.2012.01498.x.

El Allaki, F., Bigras-Poulin, M., Michel, P. and Ravel, A. (2012) A population health surveillance theory. *Epidemiology and Health* 34, e2012007. DOI: 10.4178/epih/e2012007.

Fowers, B.J., Novak, L.F., Calder, A.J. and Sommer, R.K. (2021) Courage, justice, and practical wisdom as key virtues in the era of COVID-19. *Frontiers in Psychology* 12, 647912. DOI: 10.3389/fpsyg.2021.647912.

Gee, R.E. and Corry, M.P. (2012) Patient engagement and shared decision making in maternity care. *Obstetrics & Gynecology* 120, 995–997. DOI: 10.1097/aog.0b013e31827946ac.

Gill, D., Baker, E.H. and Hitchings, A.W. (2021) We need clinical guidelines fit for a pandemic. *British Medical Journal* 373, n1093. DOI: 10.1136/bmj.n1093.

Hiwasaki, L., Luna, E., Syamsidik and Shaw, R. (2014) Process for integrating local and indigenous knowledge with science for hydro-meteorological disaster risk reduction and climate change adaptation in coastal and small island communities. *International Journal of Disaster Risk Reduction* 10, 15–27. DOI: 10/1016/j.ijdrr.2014.07.007.

Humphreys, K., Shover, C.L. *et al.* (2022) Responding to the opioid crisis in North America and beyond: Recommendations of the Stanford–Lancet Commission. *Lancet* 399, 555–604. DOI: 10.1016/S0140-6736(21)02252-2.

Ilin, C., Annan-Phan, S., Tai, X.H., Mehra, S., Hsiang, S. *et al.* (2021) Public mobility data enables COVID-19 forecasting and management at local and global scales. *Scientific Reports* 11, 13531. DOI: 10.1038/s41598-021-92892-8.

Intezari, A., Pauleen, D.J. and Taskin, N. (2016) The DIKW hierarchy and management decision-making. In: *49th Hawaii International Conference on System Sciences.* Kaloa, Hawaii, USA, pp. 4193–4201. DOI: 10.1109/HICSS.2016.520.

Khalil, H., Santana, R., de Oliveira, D., Palma, F., Lustosa, R. *et al.* (2021) Poverty, sanitation, and Leptospira transmission pathways in residents from four Brazilian slums. *PLoS Neglected Tropical Diseases* 15, e0009256. DOI: 10.1371/journal.pntd.0009256.

Kock, R.A., Orynbayev, M., Robinson, S., Zuther, S., Singh, N.J. *et al.* (2018) Saigas on the brink: Multidisciplinary analysis of the factors influencing mass mortality events. *Science Advances* 4, eaao2314. DOI: 10/1126/sciadv.aao2314.

Larson, H.J. (2020) *Stuck: How Vaccine Rumours Start – and How They Don't Go Away.* Oxford University Press, New York, NY, USA.

Lee, M.J., Byers, K.A., Stephen, C., Patrick, D.M., Corrigan, R. *et al.* (2022) Reconsidering the 'war on rats': What we know from over a century of research into municipal rat management. *Frontiers in Ecology and Evolution* 10, 813600. DOI: 10.3389/fevo.2022.813600.

Lemy, E. (2021) Deforestation and emergence of malaria: A disease of public health importance. *ACADEMIC Letters.* Available at: https://www.academia.edu/83616930/DEFORESTATION_AND_EMERGENCE_OF_MALARIA_A_DISEASE_OF_PUBLIC_HEALTH_IMPORTANCE (accessed 27 January 2023).

Masinde, E.M. and Bagula, A. (2012) ITIKI: Bridge between African indigenous knowledge and modern science of drought prediction. *Knowledge Management for Development Journal* 7, 274–290. DOI: 10.1080/19474199.2012.68344.

Mazet, J.A.K., Uhart, M.M. and Keyyu, J.D. (2014) Stakeholders in One Health. *Revue Scientifique et Technique – Office International des Épizooties* 33, 443–452. DOI: 10.20506/rst.33.2.2295.

Monteiro, M.B., de Sousa, I.E., Piteira, M., Coelho, S. and Freitas, P. (2021) Leptospirosis, a re-emerging threat. *Cureus* 13, e14295. DOI: 10.7759/cureus.14295.

Naeem, B.S. and Boulos, M.N.K. (2021) COVID-19 misinformation online and health literacy: A brief overview. *International Journal of Environmental Research and Public Health* 18, 8091. DOI: 10.3390/ijerph18158091.

Ochu, C.L., Akande, O.W., Oyebanji, O., Aderinola, O., Ogunbode, O. *et al.* (2021) 'Fighting a global war using a local strategy': Contextualism in COVID-19 response in Africa. *British Medical Journal Innovations* 7, 347–355. DOI: 10.1136/bmjinnov-2020-000637.

Olive, J.K., Hotez, P.J., Damania, A. and Nolan, M.S. (2018) The state of the antivaccine movement in the United States: A focused examination of nonmedical exemptions in states and counties. *PLoS Medicine* 15, e1002578. DOI: 10.1371/journal/pmed.1002578.

Oumarou, H. (2019) Indigenous knowledge meets science to take on climate change. *TED Talks*. Available at: https://www.ted.com/talks/hindou_oumarou_ibrahim_indigenous_knowledge_meets_science_to_take_on_climate_change?language=en (accessed 28 July 2021).

Paternoster, G., Tomassone, L., Tamba, M., Chiari, M., Lavazza, A. *et al.* (2017a) The degree of One Health implementation in the West Nile virus integrated surveillance in northern Italy, 2016. *Frontiers in Public Health* 5, 236. DOI: 10.3389/fpubh.2017.00236.

Paternoster, G., Babo Martins, S., Mattivi, A., Cagarelli, R., Angelini, P. *et al.* (2017b) Economics of One Health: Costs and benefits of integrated West Nile virus surveillance in Emilia-Romagna. *PLoS One* 12, e0188156. DOI: 10.1371/journal.pone.0188156.

Robertson, C., Pant, D.K., Joshi, D.D., Sharma, M., Dahal, M. *et al.* (2013) Comparative spatial dynamics of Japanese encephalitis and acute encephalitis syndrome in Nepal. *PLoS One* 8, e66168. DOI: 10.1371/journal.pone.0066168.

Roos, C.I., Swetnam, T.W., Ferguson, T.J., Liebmann, M.J., Loehman, R.A. *et al.* (2021) Native American fire management at an ancient wildland-urban interface in the Southwest United States. *Proceedings of the National Academy of Sciences* 118, e2018733118. DOI: 10.1073/pnas.2018733118.

Schwartz, B. (2009) Our loss of wisdom. *TED Talks*. Available at: https://www.ted.com/talks/barry_schwartz_our_loss_of_wisdom#t-48036 (accessed 27 January 2023).

Semenza, J.C., Rocklöv, J. and Ebi, K.L. (2022) Climate change and cascading risks from infectious disease. *Infectious Diseases and Therapy* 11, 1371–1390. DOI: 10.1007/s40121-022-00647-3.

Seytre, B., Barros, C., Bona, P., Fall, B., Konaté, B. *et al.* (2021) Revisiting COVID-19 communication in Western Africa: A health literacy-based approach to health communication. *American Journal of Tropical Medicine and Hygiene* 105, 708–712. DOI: 10.4269/ajtmh.21-0013.

Stärk, K.D.C., Kuribreña, M.A., Dauphin, G., Vokaty, S., Ward, M.P. *et al.* (2015) One Health surveillance – More than a buzz word? *Preventive Veterinary Medicine* 120, 124–130. DOI: 10.1016/j.prevetmed.2015.01.019.

Stephen, C., Lester, S., Black, W., Fyfe, M. and Raverty, S. (2002) Multispecies outbreak of cryptococcosis on southern Vancouver Island, British Columbia. *The Canadian Veterinary Journal = La Revue Vétérinaire Canadienne* 43(10), 792–794.

Stephen, C., Berezowski, J. *et al.* (2021) *A Rapid Review of Evidence on Managing the Risk of Disease Emergence in the Wildlife Trade*. Report Prepared for the Preparedness and Resilience Department of the World Animal Health Organization (OIE) Paris, France. Available at: https://web.oie.int/downld/WG/Wildlife/OIE_review_wildlife_trade_March2021.pdf (accessed 24 July 2024).

Turiel, J., Fernandez-Reyes, D. and Aste, T. (2021) Wisdom of crowds detects COVID-19 severity ahead of officially available data. *Scientific Reports* 11, 13678. DOI: 10.1038/s41598-021-93042-w.

WHO (2019) Ten Threats to Global Health in 2019. Available at: https://www.who.int/news-room/spotlight/ten-threats-to-global-health-in-2019 (accessed 26 July 2021).

WHO (2021) Infodemic. Available at: https://www.who.int/health-topics/infodemic#tab=tab_1 (accessed 26 July 2021).

WHO (2023) Prioritizing Diseases for Research and Development in Emergency Contexts. Available at: https://www.who.int/activities/prioritizing-diseases-for-research-and-development-in-emergency-contexts (accessed 27 January 2023).

Zielinski, C. (2021) Infodemics and infodemiology: A short history, a long future. *Revista Panamericana de Salud Pública* 45, e40. DOI: 10.26633/RPSP.2021.40.

6 In Search of Integration and Health: Reflexivity and Communities of Practice in One Health

Glen Cousquer
University of Edinburgh, Edinburgh, Scotland, UK

Contents

DOI: 10.1079/9781800623002.0007

Summary

This chapter explores the role of personal and professional reflexivity in integrative practice for One Health. In doing so, it recognizes the need to transcend Western modernist thinking in which art, ethics and science have been torn asunder. Modernist thinking is characterized by the arbitrary separation of truth, beauty and goodness and the growth of commercial and civic institutions powered by instrumental rationality, an exploitative relationship to nature and life and the accompanying bureaucracy that sustains a blind belief in progress. This chapter proposes that modernist thinking may well be the root cause of the crises we face today and argues that to address this we need a reflexive turn that recognizes how mind and body, consciousness and matter are co-dependent. This turn is needed both at the individual and collective level if we are to address the knowledge–doing gaps that characterize the global crises of our modern era. In order to fulfil the aim of nurturing an integrative approach to health, this chapter adopts an experiential approach rooted in practice. The reader is encouraged to engage in a series of reflexive intermissions and practice throughout and to reflect on these experiences. The chapter starts by emphasizing the primordial importance of attentional practice and the role of attitudes including curiosity and compassion in shaping not just our epistemologies but our ontological realities. The chapter explores how reflective practice has arisen and developed across disciplines and how it informs learning at the level of the individual, the collective (including organizations) and the wider system. Its relevance to One Health is considered before exploring a range of practices designed to nurture reflexivity, develop self-awareness, address biases and promote more equitable co-creative practice. Finally, this chapter concludes by considering the future prospects of One Health if our inter- and intra-connections, dependencies and potentialities are explored, nurtured and realized.

Attentional practice: Paying attention to tension

Please think back to the last time you were experiencing significant tension within yourself or within a team or community group. Allow that first- or third-person experience to come fully into view.

Now imagine that you were able to detach yourself, float up, see, feel and appreciate every little detail of the processes contributing to the construction of this experience.

Please pause between each short paragraph to let this reviewing exercise sink in. As you do so, please take a slow, deep, fully conscious breath to anchor yourself in the present moment. What does it feel like to breathe in deeply and oxygenate, to breathe out and let go? Please repeat this and allow yourself to feel into the flavour of this experience.

Intentionally pausing is an essential skill to nurture in becoming reflexive and integrative for it allows us to return to source and to fine tune our attentional practice: for 'We cannot know anything without attending to it, and the nature of that attention alters what we find' (McGilchrist, 2021, p. 1129). It is in pausing that we can observe how we are and how we attend and, in creating such a space, we create distance between ourselves and the tension.[1,2]

Flying over the experience, you develop a rich overview of the whole. You find yourself seeing beyond the constituent parts and see the connections between them. You can even start seeing beyond the connections and see the patterns they make.

You are able to sense where energy is flowing and is stuck. You are able to sense the emotional fabric of the situation and trace this back into the shadows each of us carry within. You are able to appreciate the depth of understanding that each participant has (or does not have) of the matter under discussion and how this inter-relates with their values, intentions, attitudes, biographies and other factors.

Floating like a weather balloon, you feel calm and collected. You bring a certain curiosity to this reflective practice, enjoying the opportunity to develop a richer, multisensory appreciation of how all these parts interrelate and make up the integrated whole.

Perhaps the experience of tension you are considering is personal to you, rooted in a personal experience. Imagine that you are able to press pause and simply feel your mind and your body interacting with the wider **environment**. Where in your body do you experience that tension? When did you first notice it? How did the tension arise and become manifest? Perhaps the experience of tension arose within you in a meeting where you struggled to contribute because of some 'sand in the system', an anxiety, a misunderstanding or some other unprocessed and unintegrated element.

Perhaps the experience of **tension** arose between others within a meeting. I, for example, am harking back to a meeting with a senior manager to express concerns about the impact of heavy workloads and lack of adequate staffing on the health and wellbeing of colleagues. I did not feel in the meeting that I was being listened to or taken seriously. The manager did not seem to have any grasp of the situation and we were clearly not familiar with each other's maps or willing to explore them. This unsettled me deeply to the point that I became reactive and any opportunity to exchange insights and compare maps was lost. I am reflecting on this now after the event and am wondering how I might have been able to network all the elements (including my inner state) better. This is **reflecting *on* practice**. Had I been able to do so in the meeting itself, rather than afterwards, I would have been **reflecting *in* practice**. The ability to pause and reflect in such ways are professional and personal competencies that we can nurture and develop throughout our careers. These competencies allow us to open to, receive and integrate feedback and evolve in response to feedback. This is true at the level of the individual; but it is also true at the level of the collective.

Have I managed to capture your curiosity, dear reader? Are you wanting to learn more about reflexivity in One Health? If so, please read on for we have only just scraped the surface.

6.1 Introduction and Aims

In the preceding section, we have encouraged you to consider how, at the level of the individual and of the collective, we can become fragmented and experience tensions as our functioning is impacted by those faulty connections and our loss of an integrated state. A synonym for **integration** is **coherence**; it is a form of oneness that has immense significance for One Health.

Coherence, whether sought at the level of the individual or group, requires the constituent parts to connect and be brought into relationship. In any system, the relational practices that constitute the whole help provide the richness of balancing feedback processes that sustain the whole. Whether the system is you or me, us or we, or the MWe proposed by interpersonal neurobiologist Dan Siegel (Siegel, 2023), attention to our relational practices is essential if we are to promote healthy functioning and integration and avoid disintegration and dysfunction. This shift in focus from objects (the parts) to relationships and processes and the way parts and wholes are co-constituted and synergize is a clear sign we are starting to think systemically.

Systems thinking requires us to shift our attention from objects to relational processes, from hierarchies to networks, from objective knowledge[3] to situational / contextual knowledge. In doing so we come to recognize that knowledge is always partial and situated and our problem statements invariably incomplete. What do you sense happening as you consider that shift in attention?[4]

What do we mean by attention? Very simply, we are able to focus our attention on internal and external aspects of our experience. **Focused attention** is one of the three pillars of mind training; the other two are **open awareness** and **kind intention** (Villamil *et al.*, 2018).

Open awareness is widely recognized within physics, neuroscience, mindfulness studies and the field of collective trauma studies as an energy state where we are connected to the field of possibility. Awareness is, however, distinct and very different from thought, which is a product of the thinking mind. The state of open awareness is rooted in the present moment (it just is) and affords us our remarkable ability to be conscious of our whole selves, our relationship with our self, our thoughts and emotions and our experiences and the relationships we co-create with others. We can draw on this awareness of our being and becoming to in-form what we do (our many practices, including our thinking practices – our doing). This ability to integrate our awareness into our healthcare practices involves us nurturing our reflexivity through the development of reflective and reflexivity practices. At this point, we hope you are feeling a little curious about how reflective and reflexivity practices may differ. **Curiosity** is a powerful ally in this work so please note down any questions that arise as you read.[5]

This chapter seeks to provide the reader with a thorough introduction to the **What?**, **Why?** and **How?** of professional reflexivity. We aim to provide an overview of the history and development of theory and practice in this area so that the reader can better appreciate **how** this field has evolved in response to practitioners' learning and development as they learn through experience to integrate the 'science' of their own inner world and the sciences of the outer world. We will then build on these antecedents to consider **why** awareness of these inter-dependencies and how to work with them is of such crucial importance in the field of One Health. This will involve exploring **why** these practices are crucially important in developing the necessary levels of individual and collective awareness and consciousness required to respond to the complex health and ecological crises humanity and the planet are confronted by in this, the middle of the first half of the 21st century. Finally, we will look at how the practitioner can develop their practices and nurture their reflexivity throughout their professional lives. This chapter therefore also aims to support intermediate and advanced practitioners in second-order reflective practice – that is to say in reflecting on their own reflective practice with a view to tending and nurturing it further.

Proficiency in reflective practice becomes something we can share with less experienced colleagues as we take on roles as mentors, coaches, tutors or facilitators. Together we can develop a richer appreciation of how reflective practice in-forms at a very fundamental level our approach to learning, to inquiry and to collaborative work. Working at this fundamental level draws on an awareness of how we direct our attention, of our attitudes in doing so, of our intentionality and core values; we thus become aware of **the source from which we operate**. The importance of values to reflective practice means that this chapter will also touch on reflexivity as an ethical practice and help the reader understand how this informs how we create and hold the space for better, more generative, conversations.

As you may already have surmised, this chapter sets out to engage the reader in an experiential manner with a view to encouraging you from the start to read in a reflexive manner. This will help you to appreciate experience as the primary way of knowing and distinguish **experiential knowing** from propositional **forms of knowing**. You will therefore encounter 'reflexive intermissions' in which you, the reader, are invited to consider and reflect on your experience; in this way, you will be invited to **reflect in practice** as you move not just through[6] but backwards and forwards in this chapter. At this point you may wish to skip ahead to Section 6.5 of this chapter, to have a look at how reflective practice can be nurtured so that you know where to go to find more support each time you take a reflexive intermission. By offering you these opportunities, we seek to engage you in a more reciprocal form of reading as you move backwards and forwards between the text and your understanding of the text and assimilate these insights and understanding into your practice. **Reciprocity** is another powerful ally in this work as it is born of openness and is key to nurturing our relational selves.

We recognize that some of the concepts and terms you are encountering in this chapter will be unfamiliar. In recognition of this, there is a definitions box (Box 6.1) for you to refer to, and terms highlighted in bold and italic are included in the glossary.

Box 6.1. Definitions

Reflexivity as attentional practice, as distinct from reflection, as expansive awareness, as a commitment to remaining flexible and open, as a commitment to becoming wise.[7]

For the purpose of this chapter, reflexivity can be defined as **an approach to living and a set of practices** that allow us to develop deeper awareness of ourselves and of our work so that this awareness informs and enhances our practice.

Reflexivity is to be distinguished from reflection. The metaphor of the reflection provided by a deep, deep pond is helpful here. The surface reflection is not the only reflection… there is always more to see and we need to pay particular attention to the invisible connections, inter-relationships and inter- and intra- dependencies that make us who we are and inform our work. When we focus on what we have learnt and our skills, we are focusing on explicit knowledge and technical proficiencies. We are not focusing on the person acquiring the knowledge and developing those skills and evolving into their highest future possibility. We can think about (reflect on) our know-what and know-how; but to know who is emerging as a person, we need to draw on awareness. This is when we become reflexive.

Reflexivity therefore requires us to engage with multiple ways of knowing (**epistemic practices**). It requires us to cultivate awareness as distinct from thought and to reconnect with the plane of possibility. We can then draw on this awareness in deciding how to act to bring about the future that is waiting to manifest itself through us.

Reflexivity is thus about becoming mindful, becoming aware, deepening our awareness of self and other and, in doing so, learning to nurture a more **expansive awareness** and an appreciation of our extended relational selves. This nurturing involves becoming mindful and heartful and, in doing so, gaining clarity about our habits of thought, our ways of acting, the boundaries and framings we adopt and the stories we tell. In Awareness-Based Systems Change work, this is described as a move from ego-system awareness (a narrow and very limited definition of the self) into eco-system awareness (a less boundaried, more generous definition of the self). As such, reflexivity can go far beyond the process of simply reflecting for it is not limited to thinking and to thought; neither is it limited to the cognitive processes that our logical / rational minds engage in.

Reflexivity is more than a skill, however; it is an extremely important practice that we should seek to develop in order to learn and grow as professionals, as individuals, community members and global citizens. In this sense it is, arguably, a way of being for it allows us to attend to and articulate our learning on a moment-by-moment-by-moment-by-moment basis. It is also a commitment to unlearning and relearning for where children learn by establishing new neural connections and therefore new neural networks, adults already have a brain full of connections. These connections can be well established and can manifest themselves as habits of thought, biases (both conscious and unconscious) and patterns of listening from habit (otherwise known as downloading). Reflexivity is thus a **commitment to remaining flexible and open**.

If reflexivity seeks to contribute to our growth and development, it is appropriate to ask what we hope to grow into. The simple answer for some may be 'wise', for the development of practical **wisdom**, or 'phronesis' allows us to be discerning and to exercise good judgement when confronted with the unique particularity and specificity of the situations we encounter. This challenges us to move beyond technical and codified responses and into a more open, virtuous engagement with the world. **Reflexivity can thus**

Continued

Box 6.1. Continued

also be defined as critical to becoming wise. For the purposes of this definition, however, we wish to emphasize that by developing the habit of reflexivity and remaining open, we are able to evolve as part of the whole. Evolving is dynamic and ongoing; it is a process. As part of this evolutionary process we can learn to process our experiences and integrate them into our being.

Integration is thus a key component of reflexivity, both in the intra-personal and inter-personal realms. Integration is an essential professional competency in One Health and can be defined as restorative health, of being whole, of being resilient, of thriving and flourishing.

Reflexive intermission: Having read the introduction and the outline of aims presented, please take a three-minute breathing space and then journal about this experience (see Practices 1 and 2 in the Practices section of this chapter).

How are you left feeling? What specific feelings are you aware of?

You might want to notice whether you are feeling engaged, energized, surprised, irritated, disengaged, confused, angry, threatened even? Please notice these feelings without judging them. If you detect any shame, please note this down too.

You might want to notice what has led you to visit the chapter. What is it you hoped to find in this chapter? Does this introduction speak to these hopes? The invitation here is to recognize the expectations you carried into the reading. Does the introduction offer other promises or opportunities and how do you feel about these?

You might also want to notice your gut reaction to self-reflection. Do you view this as introspective navel gazing, as a waste of time? Do you view it as challenging or even threatening?

Please view everything noticed as **data**. Recognize what arises. Allow it to be. Inquire into it with curiosity. Nurture the opportunity for growth it presents with compassion and kindness. To read more about the practice of RAIN, see Brach (2020).

6.2 What is Reflexivity and Reflective Practice?

In this section, we consider the history of **reflexivity** and of the development of **reflective practice** in order to propose a working definition for the purposes of this chapter, a working definition that will support the One Health professional and the wider One Health community in becoming reflexive. In doing so, we have focused on the interdisciplinary fields that have pioneered integrative approaches to working across **disciplines** and that have, in particular, integrated process philosophy, **systems thinking** and creative approaches into their praxis. The SHAPE[8] disciplines have a long history of applying process philosophy and of embracing creative and regenerative practice (Wahl, 2006, 2016). The STEM[9] disciplines and in particular the natural and medical sciences are largely unaware of the extent to which reductive thinking and analytic philosophy continues to characterize and limit their world view and therefore their contributions. If One Health is to break out of modernist thinking and move into meta-modernity, it will be challenged to learn from those fields that have been actively exploring the meta turn and regenerative **health** approaches. This historical section is therefore helpful in understanding how an interdisciplinary approach can see collaborative work arise where contributions from the arts, social sciences and humanities allow us to address the real root causes of the poly-crises we face. Such collaborative work requires us to establish new foundations and thereby become aware of how we attend, see, feel and enact our realities.

> If we wish to render transparent the true extent of the meta-crisis, to get a clear sense of how to navigate through it, then we need to thoroughly identify the foundations of the world coming undone. In order to navigate this space 'between worlds', we need a phenomenology of consciousness that can help us to trace, as it were, the underlying ontological 'structures' of the old world, the constellations of sensemaking we have relied on up until now. We should do this so that we can better recognise what the new world might be like – to re-constellate ourselves around that emergent foundation.
>
> (Jeremy Johnson quoted in Rowson, 2021, p. 31)

This section is therefore seeking to help us establish more reflexive foundations with a view to realizing the full potential of interdisciplinary collaboration. To do this we need to go back to roots.

The noun 'reflexivity' and adjective 'reflective' clearly share a common etymological root with 'reflection'. In considering what reflexivity and reflective practice might be, we offer an exploration of reflections that moves beyond the literal and very superficial definition of the word 'reflection' where light is bounced back off a surface and into 'a game of mirrors'. This game is both playful and mysterious for each mirror offers us glimpses of ourselves, our stories and who we might be, with some beams of energy bouncing off surfaces we did not even know we possessed, whilst others penetrate more deeply. We then build on this understanding to consider the history and evolving definitions of reflexivity and reflective practice in greater detail. The aim here is to understand how we can work with light and allow it to illuminate our practices and our practising.

Reflexive intermission: Are there times when you prefer metaphorical games where the purpose (the objective) remains unclear? What feelings accompany this preference?

Are you someone who finds themselves drawn to images, story, allegory and poetry as ways of conveying deeper truths? What are they able to offer us that more direct literal ways of speaking cannot offer us?

Please take this opportunity to write down your answers to these questions.

Lastly, please reflect on your relationship to certainty. How do you relate to uncertainty? What about complexity, volatility and ambiguity?

In journalling (see Practice 2, later in the chapter) about how you and uncertainty get along, you may want to consider whether this is a product of the pathological emphasis placed on nouns by the English language, compared to Indigenous languages where verbs are far more important. Verbs are fluid and dynamic, they are all about relational processes and they are better able to speak of systems, of oneness, of wholes. The hunger for certainty that characterizes Western scientific culture prefers nouns and 'facts' and this deterministic obsession with 'objectivity' and control is unhelpful when it comes to becoming reflexive and developing self-awareness.

The planetary crises we face today are characterized by VUCA (volatility, uncertainty, complexity and ambiguity) and we need to learn to relate to this. The same is true of our inner world and of the interface between our inner world and the outer world. Donna Haraway (2016) advises us that one of the most important things we must learn to do when faced with such uncertainties is to 'stay with the trouble'.

Now look back on your journalling and notice how you have articulated your account of your experience. This is an opportunity to see how you represent (i.e. re-present) your lived experience. The following notes may help you shift your perspective on your presentational practice – the ways you represent the world.

Staying with the trouble involves remaining present to the sympoietic flow of the world and its unfolding, rather than problematizing it and seeking to control it. So, if you notice yourself privileging nouns, facts and answers, focusing on quantification, on equations and on utility... this should alert us to a particular way of attending to the world and thinking. A limited and limiting way. The left hemisphere is then in the driving seat and it sees much less than the right. It is the right hemisphere that is best able to appreciate the priority of movement over the things that move, which are an abstraction from the movement. As Bergson (2007, p. 122) wrote: 'There are changes, but there are underneath the change no things which change: change has no need of support. There are movements but there is no inert or invariable object which moves: movement does not imply a mobile.' For healthcare professionals whose training arguably indoctrinates them into a way of seeing the world in order to act on it, this may be challenging to read. The abstract presentational knowing that structures these actions is adequate and sufficient within a narrow framing – that of the patient – but, sooner or later, the complexity of the system highlights the failings of such framings and how much they leave out. This is especially so when we realize how much of life has been excluded from the frame, how much of our pain at the ecocide perpetrated by the Industrial Growth System (Macy and Brown, 2014) we have shut out. Opening to our pain is required if we are to become open-systems thinkers, aligned with life and with life-sustaining systems.

Systems thinking recognizes that life is a dance, not an equation to be solved. And this is why we need metaphors and other presentational ways of knowing. Richard Boyd (1979, p. 485) pushed the use of metaphor deep into the heart of the scientific enterprise, arguing that metaphors are needed to accomplish the sorely needed task of accommodating language to the causal structure of the world. One Health will increasingly need to engage with Indigenous knowledge practices, theology and deep ecology to address the problematic **assumptions** baked into modernist thinking – in particular our assumptions about time, space and causality (Roy, 2021).

Yunkaporta (2019) proposes metaphor as bridging the gap between the abstract and the real world. Metaphor is inter-active; it is a relationship between theory and practice that we must use carefully 'because metaphors are the language of spirit and that's how we operate in our fields of existence either to increase or decrease connectedness within creation. We are the custodians who are uniquely gifted to do this work, so we need to do it consciously and with mastery, within cultural frameworks aligned with the patterns of creation' (Yunkaporta, 2019, p. 119).

The invitation here is therefore to start collecting and drawing on metaphor more in our work and especially in our shadow work. Jonathan Rowson's use of 'pickle' as a metaphor for the meta-crisis is a good place to start (Rowson, 2021). For an exploration of how metaphor can contribute to STEM subjects becoming more creative see Wonham and Wasson (2023).

The invitation is also to see light as a metaphor and to steer clear of the dazzling neon light that causes us to become frozen. The light we must carry with us into our reflective work is a kinder, flickering, gentle light. We need candlelight if we are to work in the shadows.

6.2.1 What is reflection?

Reflection can mean many things (Fig. 6.1), reflecting a multiplicity of usages, as you will discover if looking the word up in a dictionary. Reflection can be used as a noun to indicate 'that which you see' reflected back at you – the face in the mirror, the person you see. It can

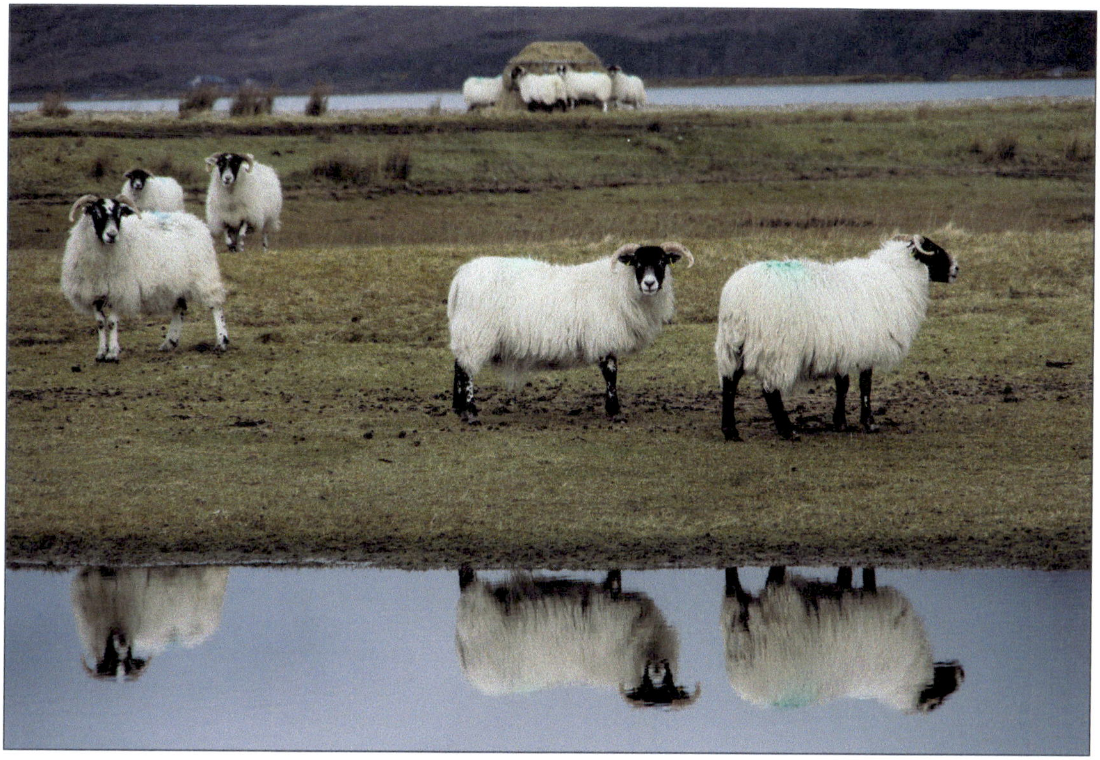

Fig. 6.1. Reflection can provide us with a mirror and new perspectives on who we are as individuals and as a flock or community of individuals. It can also help us reflect on the way(s) we move and choose to move, our behaviours, our habits and our experiences. It can also help us develop insights into the 'gaze' we bring to the world and how that informs the world we see before us. Picture credit: Glen Cousquer Photography.

also refer to the thoughts that pass through our heads: 'I reflected on my missed penalty' thus means that I thought about it and played it back in my head repeatedly. When the same experience is looped back again and again, it becomes unhealthy. Thich Nhat Hanh describes this as 'inappropriate attention' (Hanh, 2021, p. 179) because our attention is fixated on replaying what happened and our nervous system is re-traumatized every time the experience is replayed. To break free of this, we can choose to relate to our thoughts and feelings in ways that allow us to compost, metabolize and integrate the experience.

In this sense, reflections can mirror back to us our experiences so that we have an opportunity to review and make sense of what we have done – our performance. To really understand a noun, we need to take a leaf out of Indigenous languages (Goodchild, 2022) and look at the verbs and therefore stories that dynamically give rise to the noun. The invitation here is therefore to start to view the quality of reflections as a product of the penetrative, illuminating and co-creative practices that the light participates in.

Breaking through the surface reflection allows us to see and explore below the surface image and our reading of it. Jeff Brown articulates this beautifully when he writes:

> If you think your lens on reality isn't shaped by your unresolved material, you are mistaken. We will live life as projection until we live life as truth. You want to see things as they are? First you have to see yourself, as you are.
>
> (Brown, 2020, p. 39)

This is a central pillar of awareness-based systems change science and of collective trauma studies. The quantum physicist David Bohm used to say that 'thought creates the world and then says I didn't do it', which highlights our tendency to deny that the biases that lie hidden behind our actions constitute the world. Mind and matter are not separate and if we become more aware of those biases, we can quite literally co-create the world differently. As Otto Scharmer emphasizes:

> A true systems philosophy closes the feedback loop between the human being, their experience of reality, and their sense of participation in that whole cycle of awareness and enactment... The essence of systems thinking is to help people close the feedback loop between the enactment of systems on a behavioural level and its invisible source of awareness and thought.
>
> (Scharmer, 2016, p. 53)

Turning the camera back on ourselves in order to observe the source from which we operate and that in-forms our thoughts and actions allows us to appreciate the origins and histories that contribute to the image we see reflected back to us and that stabilizes it sufficiently so that it appears stable and real. A breath of wind, a diving kingfisher, a drop of rain can all break the pattern of thought and allow new patterns and networks to form.[10] Understood in this way, we are reminded that we are not our thoughts and are not who we see in the mirror. There is not just one reading; indeed, there is so much more that could be explored when considering who we are, our work and the experiences we have. We can think of this in terms of the depth of reflection and therefore of awareness we can access.

Accessing these depths requires us to cross certain thresholds and access deeper social fields of awareness; to do so, however, requires us to approach this work with curiosity and compassion.

Reflexive intermission: When introducing yourself, how do you usually do so? Please write out a typical line of introduction. Now read that line back to yourself and ask yourself how you feel about the way it sums you up.

How much of the 'you' that you know is missing? What have you excluded? How might the way you present yourself change according to who you are presenting yourself to? How does how you present yourself affect how you meet[11] with others?

You may want to consider how your parents introduce you. Are there differences in how your mother and/or father introduce you? How would you prefer them to introduce you?

What insights are you gaining about the descriptors that we carry that can come to define and even limit us and behind which we may hide?[12]

What insights are you gaining about who you are and how you are (how you show up)?

This short section has explored understandings of reflection and proposes that there are both physical and mental practices that give rise to our reflection and that they inform each other for the reflection interacts dynamically with the ways it is perceived. In the same way that the weather can ruffle a reflection, our own inner weather system interacts with the reflection. This realization highlights the importance of **right attitude** in learning to become reflexive.

6.2.2 Reflecting with curiosity and compassion

It is quite possible, and indeed likely, that some readers may be left feeling decidedly uncomfortable at the suggestion that they may not know themselves as well as they think. You may also be left feeling threatened and defensive. This section therefore explores why we need to cultivate compassion and curiosity when developing reflexivity. This is the kind attitude that complements curious inquiry, referred to earlier.

The ego is very good at defending itself and it is quite natural for a strong fight–flight–freeze reaction to be elicited when 'we' feel threatened in this way. The collective second person (we) is used here to emphasize that this is a universal reaction that we all share and can get curious about together. The word ego is often defined as the 'I' that is capable of referencing the self and making decisions. It is the part of each of us that is engaged in self-justification. This is a defensive behaviour that we can notice and observe. In doing so we start to notice other parts of ourselves…

Having recognized this common defensive (i.e. fear-based) reaction, it makes sense to acknowledge early in this chapter that this reaction is a product of our individual and collective nervous systems seeking to protect us. In reacting to rather than reflecting on the fear, our systems shut down essential feedback loops and this leads us to cut ourselves off from feedback. This represents a shift into closed systems thinking and leads people to seek to control and exert 'power over' a system, which further blocks feedback (Macy and Brown, 2014, pp. 56–61).

Why does this happen? The simple answer is because we are afraid. Our fear feeds a cycle of absencing[13] and this denial can get in the way of reflective work, both at the level of the individual and in group work. So what can we do about this? There are two attitudes or virtues (you may want to think of these as habits[14]) that can help here. The first is curiosity, the second compassion. Each habit serves as a way for us to navigate a common block to our learning and growth. Habit forming involves habit breaking though, and it is useful to recognize that in shifting our attention from answers to questions we have to suspend judgement; we have to engage a non-judgemental attitude. This suspension of the judging dualistic mind (Scharmer, 2016, pp. 125–138) allows us to engage with curiosity and to see beyond our habits of thought. Learning to engage with curiosity allows us to move across the threshold into a social field where we are engaging in inquiry; we are literally living life as inquiry and are open to being surprised. The threshold we must cross in order to reflect with compassion requires us to suspend cynicism – the habitual view that feelings should be suppressed and denied. This will feel counterintuitive to many healthcare professionals colonized and indoctrinated by a culture of dispassionate rational thinking.

We have suggested that reflective work involves 'looking at ourselves'. This can be understood as a U-turn, a subtle shift of our awareness from our thoughts to our senses. In refocusing on sensory moment-by-moment experience we are able to suspend the mind and connect with consciousness. This stillness allows us to observe the habits of thought of our minds and recognize that we are not our thoughts.

For many of us who have not developed a practice of cultivating conscious awareness, this distinction between thought and awareness may be unfamiliar, mystical even.

Reflexive intermission:

The last[15] word you read was 'mystical'…

Please use this prompt to record your gut reaction to that word.

What did your judging mind say in reaction to that term?

Are you able to suspend judgement and engage with curiosity?

What role is there for the mystical and for non-dualistic thinking in reflective practice and indeed in One Health?

Many of us default to judging ourselves: to weighing our strengths and our weaknesses, to asking ourselves what we could do better, how to improve and progress. That is the judging mind at work. Developing our reflexivity requires us to notice the mind's chatter and, in listening to ourselves with curiosity and compassion, we can restore our peace and freshness. This allows our two intelligences to support each other. Many of us may not be familiar with this crucial distinction that allows us to move from reflective thinking into reflexivity but it is a distinction that lies at the heart of all the world's wisdom traditions. As the Sufi poet Rumi points out, there are two kinds of intelligences:[16]

One acquired,
as a child in school memorises facts and concepts
from books and from what the teacher says,
collecting information from the traditional sciences
as well as from the new sciences.

With such intelligence you rise in the world.
You get ranked ahead or behind others
in regard to your competence in retaining
information. You stroll with this intelligence
in and out of fields of knowledge, getting always more
marks on your preserving tablets.

There is another kind of tablet, one
already completed and preserved inside you.
A spring overflowing its springbox. A freshness
in the centre of the chest. This other intelligence
does not turn yellow or stagnate. It's fluid,
and it doesn't move from outside to inside
through conduits of plumbing-learning.

This second knowing is a fountainhead
from within you, moving out.

Engaging with wonder and curiosity allows us to tap into this second form of knowing. When we allow ourselves to be surprised by who we are, we give in to wonder, recognizing that we cannot see the whole. There is always an element of mystery but to reflect in this way, we have to suspend judgement and embrace ourselves with kindness and compassion.

Reflexive intermission: Are you inclined to follow this invitation or is some disinclination making itself felt? Are you rebelling against it, rejecting it? Notice in this moment what this invitation prompts in you.

This may present us with an opportunity to appreciate whether we are approaching the questions offered in the Reflexive Intermissions with curiosity and a willingness to be surprised.

You may notice a need for unambiguous answers, a tendency to seek certainty, clear categories and finalities. Often this is underlain by a judgement about how things ought to be that encroaches on our freedom to evolve freely.

Our reflections can thus provide us with opportunities to see more of the whole, more of who we are and might be and to integrate these insights compassionately into our ongoing development. This is an act of nurturing for it seeks to nurture growth rather than to stunt it; something we are keen to emphasize here before we go on to present an overview of the history and development of reflective practice.

6.2.3 A brief historical overview of reflective practice

The development of reflective learning and reflective practice that has accompanied different practitioners' explorations of how people learn and hone their craft means there is now a vast body of literature, spanning a wide range of disciplines and professions. These range from the people professions such as social work, counselling, teaching and ministry (Gibbs, 1988; Bondi, *et al.*, 2011; Dana, 2020) as well as from:

- high performance sports (Thelwell and Dicks, 2019);
- organizational learning (Argyris and Schön, 1974, 1978, 1996; Senge, 2006; Cunliffe, 2009; Scharmer, 2016; Cunliffe and Easterby-Smith, 2017);
- outdoor education (Higgins and Nicol, 2002; Greenaway *et al.*, 2015; Parry and Allison, 2021);
- ecotourism (Christie and Mason, 2003);
- music (Zander and Zander, 2000);
- architecture (Schön, 1983, 1987);
- nursing and health / social care (Esterhuizen and Howatson-Jones, 2019);
- awareness-based Action Research (Scharmer, 2016, 2018b); and
- conflict resolution work and collective trauma studies (Hübl, 2020).

We wish to acknowledge that much if not all of this work draws heavily on centuries old wisdom traditions from across the world. In this short section, we provide a brief overview of some of the key work that has informed the recent development of this field. This is offered very much as background for readers to follow up on, if interested, for we recognize that it is not possible or appropriate here to provide either a definitive or comprehensive account of reflective practice.

Donald Schön (1930–1997) is widely recognized, together with Chris Argyris, as one of the pioneers of reflective practice in the 21st century. It is highly likely that Schön's training in different disciplines, including both philosophy and music, made of him an early trans-disciplinarian. Given that One Health seeks to nurture transdisciplinarity, it is worth saying a little more about the various influences and ideas that came together in Schön's work and helped to establish reflective practice as a key characteristic of professionalism. We will then build on this understanding of foundational influences and ideas to draw the reader's attention to a critically important distinction that emerged from this work and has come to characterize advanced reflective practice – that of 'single loop' and 'double loop' learning. This distinction will then be carried through into the next section of this chapter where we encourage One Health professionals to reflect not just on their experiences but on the system, paradigm or silo that they may be caught up in and need to transcend in order to access a social field ripe with co-creative potential.

Schön's PhD work focused on the pragmatic philosophy of John Dewey who is widely viewed as the father of experiential education (Dewey, 1933). Dewey's work is central to outdoor adventure education where learners of all ages are taken out of their familiar environments for what can be profoundly transformative experiences. The lessons learnt from these experiences are typically surfaced through reviewing processes (Greenaway *et al.*, 2015) such that they can be integrated back into everyday life. There is significant overlap between outdoor education and other forms of transformative learning, whether aimed at organizations and how they foster learning communities or the rehabilitation of persons suffering with addiction or who have offended.

Donald Schön's first book was called *Displacement of Concepts* (1963). It was concerned with how categories are deployed to examine things without subjecting the categories and the practices of attributing categories to scrutiny. In 1970, he was invited to deliver the Reith Lectures in London. He chose to focus on 'change and industrial society' and this subsequently became the central focus of his 1971 classic text *Beyond the Stable State* in which he argues that change is a fundamental feature of modern life and that we therefore need to develop social systems that can learn and adapt to such changes.

He argued that stable states do not endure, and that society and all of its institutions are in **continuous** processes of transformation. This alerts us to the effort we invest in establishing and maintaining such states and our expectations that new stable states will endure for our own lifetimes. Faced with this inevitability we are challenged to respond to change by seeking to guide (or accompany), influence and perhaps even manage these transformations and to invest in developing our capacity to do so, both at the level of the individual and in our institutions. We are thus challenged to become more nimble and adept at learning. This does not limit itself to transforming institutions, in response to changing needs and situations; there is a need to go further and create and develop institutions which are 'learning systems', capable of facilitating their own continuing transformation. The relevance of this work to lifelong learning at the first-person (individual), second-person (other individuals) and third-person (the group, collective or organization) level and to addressing the global challenges that humanity is gradually becoming aware of, is hopefully becoming clearer.

Two important contributions to reflective learning theory and practice arose in the two decades that followed. In 1975, Kolb and Fry published their experiential learning cycle (Fig. 6.2). In 1988, the American psychologist and sociologist Graham Gibbs published his classic work *Learning by Doing*, in which he introduces a reflective cycle (Fig. 6.3) that encourages people to think more systematically about their experiences, whether during a specific activity, event or other situation. These two cycles are really good practices for the reader to try out if they are new to reflective work. A particularly valuable activity I use when teaching reflective work is to apply this cycle to a specific piece of feedback they have received. Try it now if you like.

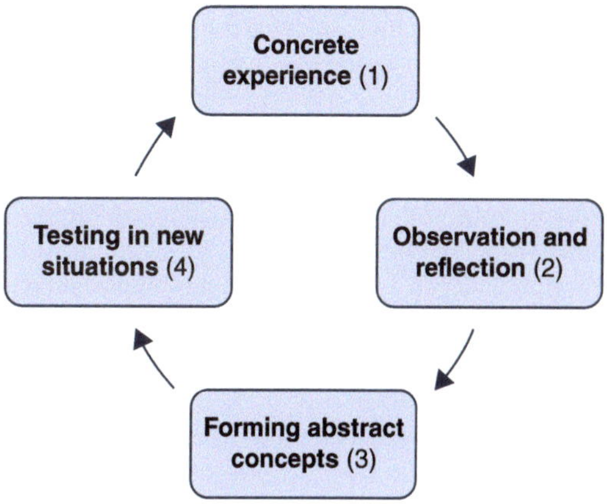

Fig. 6.2. The Experiential Learning Cycle (developed by author based on Kolb and Fry, 1975).

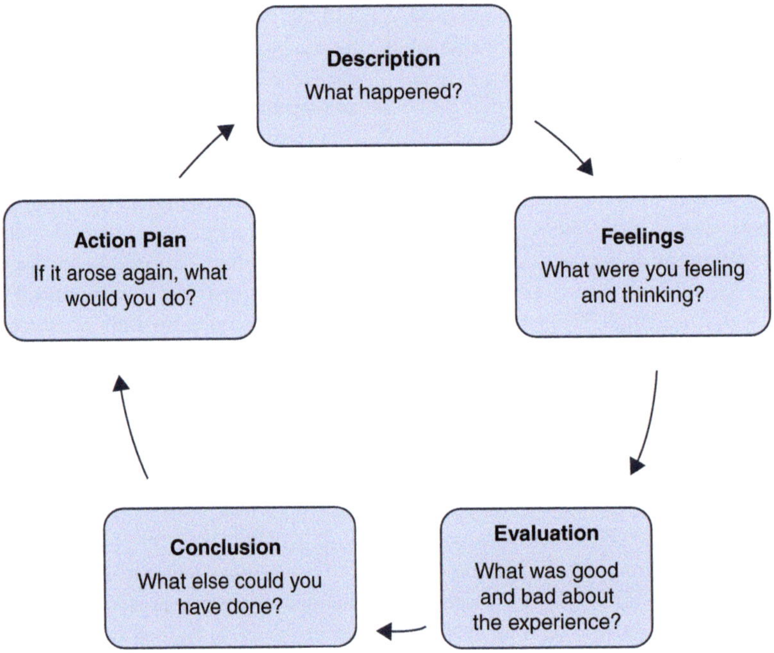

Fig. 6.3. Gibbs' (1988) reflective model (developed by author based on Gibbs, 1988).

Reflective intermission:

What piece of feedback have you chosen to reflect on?

Have you captured the key factual details associated with this situated experience? These might include where you were when receiving the feedback, who delivered it, how it was delivered.

Have you captured in detail the feelings that accompanied this experience? Are you struggling to find the words to describe the emotional landscape that the facts are set in? Where do you feel that you are blocked or getting stuck? Would it help to traffic light the feedback, drawing on green/amber/red to characterize how challenging the feedback was? Is this a familiar experience? Has it occurred before?

What would you like to inquire into? Can you articulate a series of questions that help you to feel into the experience and see it less literally and more holistically?

What would you like to playfully explore next? Maybe there are some assumptions that you want to test? Maybe you want to inquire into where a reaction originated from? Maybe you weren't listening to your own needs, including your energy levels and what drains them... Maybe the feedback leaves your sense of worthiness diminished. If this is the case, there are practices[17] that you might explore to address the trance of unworthiness we can all fall victim to.

A crucially important development is the recognition of the importance of feelings and emotion as part of who we are and what we do. The omission of the affective (felt) dimension of experience is, arguably, a legacy of the objectivist methodologies that the positivist sciences have promulgated. In promoting a dispassionate, supposedly neutral and objective science, positivism has led to a disconnect between mind and body that is now recognized as a crisis or pandemic of disconnection and one of the driving factors behind the mental health pandemic we are living through (Hübl, 2020). This is also, according to many thinkers, one of the most significant root causes of the anthropogenic crises we see today and is reflected in the oft-used saying 'In order to heal, we need to feel'.

A particularly valuable development of this kind of reflective cycle has emerged from Roger Greenaway's lifelong commitment to developing the art and practice of reviewing (Greenaway *et al.*, 2015). As part of his work, he developed the Four Es or Four Fs model – see Practice 3 in the section on practices.

This section on the history of the development of reflective practice, whilst brief, cannot be completed without mentioning the epistemic practices emphasized as learning **outcomes** in the UNESCO Learning for Sustainability agenda and in Theory U. In 1996, a UNESCO commission under the leadership of Jacques Delors proposed four pillars that education should rest on (Sobe, 2021). The commission recognized the need to 'simultaneously provide maps of a world in constant turmoil and a compass that will enable people to find their way in it' and proposed **learning to know, learning to do, learning to be** and **learning to live together** as four fundamental factors that, together, could guide education across the human lifespan. The shift in focus from reflection to reflexivity, both at the level of the individual and the collective, is evident here. Learning to be is a form of first-person reflexivity and informs third-person reflexivity when groups, teams, communities and collectives start developing their own collective intelligence.

With the development of **Theory U** by Otto Scharmer, an approach to the development of individual and organizational reflexivity emerged that emphasized self-reflexivity and self-transcendence as epistemic practices that we can access through the development of deep listening. This is, arguably, one of the most advanced practices available to reflective practitioners and leaders today. It builds on the work of Martin Buber, Johan Galtung and others (Scharmer, 2016, 2018a, b) to develop an approach based on deep listening practices that confront us with our blind spot – knowledge of the source from which action originates, whether at the level of self or the level of community, organizations or other collective groups. In particular, it develops our awareness of the origins of structural and attentional violence and how they give rise to trauma in the system.

Theory U is fast becoming a research approach and practice for delivering transformational change and has been taken up globally, including by the UN, as a way to equip people with the competencies needed to deliver systems change. It thus provides an incredibly powerful example of how trauma-sensitive reflective practices can be used in research to deliver transformative change. Such research is often termed awareness-based Action Research or awareness-based systems change. These advanced reflexive approaches are essential if we are to find a third way past the two predominant strategies that have historically characterized the unfolding environmental and social breakdowns evident in the climate and biodiversity crises, political paralysis and corruption, spreading poverty and the failures of mainstream educational, healthcare, business and government institutions. These strategies are muddling through and fighting back. Muddling through is the strategy that seeks technical fixes to problems that have barely been understood at a systemic level; muddling through therefore preserves the status quo because it does not address root causes. Fighting back seeks to take us back to an earlier social and moral order. Theory U offers a radically different approach that taps into our collective intelligence and capacity to create the world anew. As such, it is profoundly innovative and is suited to the collaborative approach One Health can develop when working collaboratively and synergistically across the arts, humanities and sciences to deliver the emergent future.

Key to this advanced reflective approach is the growing awareness that the shift into deeper levels of listening allows us to access social fields where there is greater scope for change and for emergent futures to be nurtured. Much of the conversation that characterizes science is locked into what Scharmer describes as Level 1 listening (downloading) and Level 2 listening, also known as debate or **technical dialogue**. At Level 1 listening, we listen for what we want to hear and are not open to disconfirming information. A shift into Level 2 listening requires us to suspend our habits of judgement and be open to curiosity. The promise offered by learning to practise **genuine dialogue** (Level 3 listening) is that we become more adept at crossing a threshold into a social field where we engage empathically and can attune to others. This allows us to avoid **mismeetings**, which commonly arise when we are not communicating openly and fully. In mismeetings, energy and information do not flow freely across boundaries. When listening at Level 3, we are fully integrated at an interpersonal level, and this provides us with richer data and a deeper awareness of the system we are confronted with. This means that we are working with a richer, more complete understanding of the problem statement and of the possibilities available to us. A further deepening is possible when we connect to the present moment (the **I-Now**) and become aware of the future that is calling to us because it wants to emerge through us. This shift takes us into Level 4 listening (**generative dialogue**) and can perhaps best be experienced when we are resting in a fully integrated stillness and are thereby connecting with the field of possibility and engaging with emergent complexity. An example of applying Theory U in practice will be presented later in this chapter.

Reflective intermission:

In your experience, what are the consequences of making decisions without empathy?

1. Write a short descriptive account of what happened.
2. Describe how empathy was excluded.
3. How did you feel about this?
4. What were the consequences?
5. How might you have included empathy and what might have arisen as a result?
6. What is the difference between empathy and compassion and why is compassion science so important if we are to address the planetary challenges we face?

Reflective intermission:

How do you create time and space for contemplation in your life?

1. When are you most calm and collected?
2. What practices do you consciously draw on to gather your awareness and become fully present to what is?
3. What attitudes do you bring to these moments of being with what is?
4. What drags you away from the moment?

Noticing and journalling about specific experiences of being dragged away from the moment can help us to observe them and reflexively evolve our relationship with the habits of thought that hijack us. It becomes possible to watch the inner weather system within as thoughts and feelings arise in the mind and move through, much as clouds (the outer weather system) move across the sky.

6.2.4 Single and double loop learning and reflection

We would like to close this section by pointing out that it is possible to step out of the system and develop a perspective on how we are conceptualizing and engaging with the system. In the case of reflexivity, it is possible to step back and reflect on our reflective practice. This creates a second loop of learning that can inform the development of our reflective practice.

The rest of this chapter will explore the why and the how of reflective practice and the reader will develop a sense that there are many reasons why reflexivity is a crucially important competency for the One Health professional to nurture and that there is no one truth or one way of being reflexive.

6.3 Why is Reflexivity Important in General?

There are so many possible ways of presenting the importance and value of reflexivity and there is no comprehensive answer here. We have chosen to emphasize a number of key elements, including:

1. Individual learning and the integration of our inner and outer worlds.
2. Collective or organizational learning and the establishment of resonance across nervous systems and the importance of developing collective awareness in group work.
3. The development of systems thinking / approaches to complex challenges.

6.3.1 Individual learning

According to Thomas Hübl (2020, 2023), one of the challenges of our time is to facilitate the conversation between inner and outer science. This can be perhaps best appreciated by seeing how these two sciences inform and in-form each other. By developing our ability to direct our attention inwards to take stock of how our inner state informs how we are and how this, in turn, informs our ways of seeing and contributing, we can establish greater resonance with ourselves and bring this into our relational practices as relational beings.

Reflective intermission:

Inner and outer attention: When confronting an external challenge, what internal challenges arise for you? How are they related and how do you choose to work with them?

When working collaboratively, do you create time and safe spaces to explore these inner challenges? Do these spaces feel genuinely safe?

According to Dr Christina Bethell, professor at the Johns Hopkins University School of Public Health, we can think of inner science as an ability to enter into relational experience with awareness. She refers to this as 'mentalization' and describes mentalization as:

> the ability to feel yourself and know you're feeling yourself on purpose and the ability to sense another person on purpose, and sense whether that other person senses that you're sensing them – or to sense whether that person is able to sense that you're sensing them.
>
> (Hübl, 2020, p. 23)

This definition emphasizes the reciprocal nature of deep listening when genuine meeting has been achieved. Such listening arises from receptivity and does not therefore require language because genuine dialogue is possible across cultures and indeed species (Cousquer, 2023). In seeking to understand this, it is helpful to go back to current understanding in physics of the nature of reality and the fact that reality arises from energy flow. It is only the receiver of the energy who translates that energy into information (Siegel, 2023). When we are open to listen fully to propositional ideas, to feeling and to the present moment and can do so collectively, the potential for learning is immense. This, however, has to be experienced for we can only know about such creativity through opening to the future that seeks to become manifest through us and that will author us. In the next section, we say a little bit about how mentalization can inform collective, community and organizational learning.

6.3.2 Collective learning

Building on our growing proficiency in 'learning to be', we can expand this from the first-person work into the second- and third-person realms by learning to be, live and work together. Developments in collective learning have arisen both in the fields of community building and organizational learning.

One of the foremost authorities on community building is Dr Scott Peck, who identified four clear stages to successful building of genuine community, or 'One Community' (Peck, 2015). These stages are pseudocommunity, chaos, emptiness and true community and are outlined further below:

- **Pseudocommunity:** This is the stage where people pretend to have a balanced and open friendship with one another, and cover up their differences by acting as if the differences do not exist. Pretending differences do not exist can never directly lead to True Community. For those working to facilitate collective learning, the goal is to maintain open communication and a commitment to celebrating diversity. This will help members of the collective minimize the time spent in this pretend state and stage of community.
- **Chaos:** When pseudocommunity fails to work, the members start falling upon each other, giving vent to their mutual disagreements and differences. This is a period of chaos and gives rise to the realization that differences cannot simply be ignored. Chaos may appear counterproductive, but it is the first genuine step towards community building.
- **Emptiness:** After chaos comes emptiness. At this stage, the people learn to empty themselves of those ego-related factors that are preventing their entry into Community. Emptiness is a challenging process to undergo because it involves the death of a part of the individual (ego). It is essential, however, to the emergence of a more relational way of being and to Community.
- **True Community:** Having worked through emptiness, members of the Community are in complete empathy with each other: there is a greater degree of tacit understanding, acceptance and forgiveness. Underlying intentions are clear, and the level of mutual respect and self-compassion is such that disagreements are never shaming or taken personally.

Otto Scharmer has outlined a similar four-stage process in organizational learning as the shift from ego to eco is nurtured through the development of deep listening skills. This shift enables and involves a shift in energy and information flow and therefore of structure as organizations evolve from hierarchies to networks (Scharmer and Yukelson, 2015). This social technology has been applied within healthcare reform (Scharmer, 2016) and a wide range of other **sectors**, including education (Souza and Muniandy, 2014; Smith *et al.*, 2020). The parallels between Peck's four steps of community building and the evolution from organization 1.0 to organization 4.0 are very striking. This, however, is unsurprising because these shifts are rooted in vertical literacy both at the level of the individual and the collective.

6.3.3 Systems thinking

The singular importance of systems thinking has become apparent as we have come to recognize the damage caused by reductive ways of thinking and acting in the world. Stephen Harding (2006, p. 38) captures the need to find consilience between a reductive approach and a systems approach:

> Reductionism works very well if we want to design things like cars and computers, but its success is more limited in areas such as biology, ecology or in the realm of human social life, where complex non-linear interactions are the norm. In these areas we need to apply a different style of thinking which builds on and incorporates reductionism whilst moving beyond it. Physicist Fritjof Capra points out that this new approach, which he calls 'systems thinking', involves shifting our focus from objects to processes and relationships, from hierarchies to networks and from objective knowledge to contextual knowledge.
>
> What does this mean? A key insight in systems thinking is that we can understand a great deal more about a system if we focus on the patterns of relationships between the parts rather than on the parts themselves as isolated entities. We come to realize that the properties of the parts depend upon how they relate to each other and to the larger whole they help to constitute.

Since then, systems thinking has emerged as a key element within a growing number of areas of study including farming and agriculture (Bawden, 1991), animal **welfare** (Cousquer and Haounati, 2022; Luke *et al.*, 2023; Cousquer, 2020, 2023) and deep ecology, with their emphasis on relational thinking and power literacy. Joanna Macy is particularly articulate in this area, emphasizing the crucial importance of appreciating the difference between power-over and power-with as part of the development of such literacy (Macy and Brown, 2014, pp. 137–159). Power over blocks feedback and leads to the deadening of hearts and minds. Developing our power literacy is therefore one of the most crucially important things we can do in nurturing our humanity and promoting flourishing. Power and vertical literacy thus lie at the heart of reflexivity and awareness-based systems change (Cousquer, 2023; Cousquer *et al.*, 2024).

6.4 Why is Reflexivity Important in One Health?

In this section we would like to explore and consider why both the capacity to reflect and reflexivity are crucial for One Health approaches. To situate and contextualize this discussion, it is helpful to remind the reader of the family of approaches that possess this One Health character. We then build on this to consider educational approaches and ethics in and for One Health. This allows us to articulate some meaningful reasons for proposing that reflexivity is an essential One Health competency.

6.4.1 One Health approaches

There are many One Health approaches, but the most commonly referred to are One Health, **EcoHealth**, **Planetary Health**, **Conservation Medicine** and **One Welfare**. These fields claim that their main emphasis is on **inter-** or **transdisciplinarity** both in research projects and in implementations in society.[18] Interdisciplinary and transdisciplinary approaches to global challenges are seen across a range of areas of study and are, arguably, more holistic and integrated in those areas with a long history of integrating different ways of knowing into their approaches. Such areas include Human Geography, Regenerative Design (Wahl, 2016) and Education and Sustainability Studies. The latter has contributed particularly to the development of the field of inter- and transdisciplinary research (Toomey *et al.*, 2015; Vienni-Baptista *et al.*, 2023). Learning for sustainability has benefited in particular from the integration of deep ecology approaches and systems thinking (Macy and Brown, 2014), which explicitly seek to deliver systems change and have therefore deliberately and comprehensively integrated reflexivity as a fundamental skill required to work in this area.

Another central emphasis in One Health approaches is the interconnectedness between humans, other-than-human animals, plants and **ecosystems** (Degeling *et al.*, 2019; Lerner and Zinsstag, 2021). As One Health evolves and becomes more transdisciplinary through its engagement with fields that have been developing their own approaches to integration and the challenges of living together, most notably perhaps, peace studies, interpersonal neurobiology, eco-feminism and eco-theology, the very notion of interconnectedness will evolve. This is perhaps best captured by the work of Thich Nhat Hanh (2017, p. 45) who proposes that:

> … not only the human body, but all phenomena are empty of a permanent, separate self … The insight of interbeing is that nothing can exist by itself alone, that each thing exists only in relation to everything else.

> The insight of impermanence is that nothing is static, nothing stays the same. Interbeing means emptiness of a separate self, however, impermanence also means emptiness of a separate self. Looking from the perspective of space we call emptiness 'interbeing'; looking from the perspective of time, we call it impermanence.

Awareness of who we are in relation to everything, what Canguilhelm (2012, p. 17) refers to as our social, psychological and biological frameworks, or *milieu*, is a lifelong question for us all to live into and explore. As we do so, we may come to realize that we are not just interconnected but intraconnected (Siegel, 2023). This exploration is very much part of the reflexive journey we are on and allows us to make sense of our relationships to ourselves and others, whether of our own species or other species (Cousquer, 2023).

There are understandably many differences between the different approaches in terms of their **ontologies**, their values, scope and aspirations (see Lerner and Berg, 2015 for some of these approaches), but they are all concerned with exploring health, healing and integration in its various forms. The key underlying principles of One Health, according to the OHHLEP, endorse the importance of reflexivity to put One Health into practice (Adisasmito *et al.*, 2022):

1. Recognizing the stewardship and responsibility of humans to change behaviours to adopt sustainable solutions clearly is a mandate to reflect and learn.
2. The claim for **equity** between sectors and disciplines requires for all to reflect on relationships and boundaries existing in our societies.
3. Acknowledging the intrinsic value of all living things raises a high benchmark for ethical behaviour and imposes that we assess our habits in relation to this principle.
4. Integrating traditional[17] forms of knowledge and a broad representative array of perspectives requires that we overcome prejudices and expand our awareness.

Having considered the evolving form of One Health and its aspiration to integrate responsibility, equity, respect and openness into a more holistic approach to the health challenges we face, we consider how we can educate for these and recognize the need to decolonize society, science and education if we are to deliver the emergent future that will move us beyond reproducing the old and muddling through. As Scharmer points out, the next frontier of science is bias, which is why reflexivity is so vital if we are to embrace the great turning that will move us from the industrial-growth society to a life-sustaining society (Macy and Brown, 2014).

6.4.2 Education

In tertiary education critical thinking is recognized as a skill to master and a vital part of the framework for curricula in the health sciences (Bozorgmehr *et al.*, 2011). The emphasis within undergraduate teaching is on explicit knowledge and on acquisition of that knowledge and the necessary technical skills to work in the profession. This is perhaps a product of the overloaded curricula and the emphasis on testing knowledge retention and students' ability to work with that knowledge. It is when working with knowledge and applying it in specific situations that critical thinking skills are developed. This is the reflection that students will be most familiar with.

Reflection is thus part of critical thinking and becomes especially important when drawn on as part of a One Health approach where many collaborators have different disciplinary and educational backgrounds. Parkes *et al.* (2012) state that education is a crucial component in building the field of Ecohealth. One of the outcomes of their analysis describes one aspect of reflexivity, the ability to be challenged in views and values and learning for oneself from other perspectives:

> Learning beyond individuals or isolated projects – new levels of impact become possible when collective experiences create opportunities for learning and exchange that would not otherwise have been possible, while leaving individuals feeling challenged, valued, enabled, motivated, and better equipped to engage with new types of challenges.
>
> (Parkes *et al.*, 2012, p. 249)

In seeking to work across disciplines, One Health has had to consider to what extent there is added value in collaborating in inter- or transdisciplinary ways and in bringing in new, often disruptive perspectives (Lerner and Berg, 2015; Lerner and Zinsstag, 2021). There are claims that One Health approaches need that added value, otherwise its claims to work across disciplines are weak (Rüegg *et al.*, 2018; Lerner and Zinsstag, 2021). The extent to which this inter- or transdisciplinarity is evidenced in work that claims to be One Health varies, reflecting the challenges that professionals experience in breaking out of their silos and working across disciplines. To help with this, Lerner and Berg (2015) proposed an interdisciplinary matrix for reflection on these matters, which could be helpful in the operationalization of One Health (Fig. 6.4).

This example illustrates the dominance in One Health of human and veterinary medicine. One Health is not limited to these fields, however, and there is

One Health aspect	Interdisciplinary	Veterinary medicine	Human medicine	Biology	...
Theory					
Concepts					
Methods					
Instruments					
Data					
...					

Fig. 6.4. The interdisciplinary matrix adapted from Lerner and Berg (2015) proposes a framework for evaluating different aspects of One Health (e.g. reading scientific papers or policy documents as well as planning research projects or implementations to achieve health) according to whether the aspect is interdisciplinary or belongs to a specific discipline. Depending on subject, further aspects or disciplines could be added or omitted.

growing recognition of the need for a dialogue between the various sciences and other academic disciplines, including the arts and humanities. This, however, requires that dialogical proficiency be developed. As previously emphasized, there is a widespread tendency within many fields to see debate (Level 2 listening) as synonymous with dialogue (Level 3 listening). As Martin Buber's life work has demonstrated, the shift into genuine meeting and dialogue involves an opening of the heart in addition to an opening of the head (Scharmer, 2016; Cousquer, 2023). This is therefore something to be emphasized in educational training for One Health.

Such training initiatives will need to recognize that, in order to work across disciplines and contribute to any inter- or transdisciplinary research project, it is essential to have a detailed awareness of the ontological and epistemological practices that have informed our training and our partial views of the world. There is therefore an urgent need for the biases in One Health arising from the dominance of a group of traditional (medical) disciplines to be recognized. These disciplines are rooted in an objectivist methodological paradigm, which means that they are at odds with disciplines that have integrated interpretivist and creative, constructivist and enacted methodologies (Hinchliffe, 2008). Training in methodological approaches (as distinct from methods) is therefore essential if the health of systems is to be informed by a comprehensive understanding of systems thinking and complexity theory. Such training will allow collaborators to appreciate the relative merits of different ontological and epistemological starting points.

As part of educational curricula development within One Health, there will therefore be a need to recognize how much professionals may need to unlearn. A school of unlearning as well as a school of learning may thus be needed. This is where an emphasis on reflexivity and on the development of vertical literacy and higher-level proficiencies may pay dividends. Otto Scharmer's work has repeatedly revisited the need for our pedagogical practice to deliver the intellectual, emotional and spiritual intelligences (Scharmer, 2009, pp. 447–449) required for us to bridge the ecological, social and spiritual divides we face in today's world (Scharmer, 2016). He has argued that, where the scholastic university was characterized by its teaching (its transmission of knowledge) and the classical concept of the university by the unity of teaching and research (knowledge acquisition and knowledge production), there is a need for us to reinvent our educational institutions around the interplay of a more comprehensive ecology of knowledge that leads to civilizational renewal (Scharmer, 1995, 2009, 2018a, b; Scharmer and Kaufer, 2000, 2013). This third way recognizes the importance of self-reflective and self-transcending **epistemologies** and the need for universities to integrate not just research and teaching but also transformative change into their teaching so that we no longer reproduce the 'same old same old' but can intuit and deliver healthier emergent futures (Peschl and Fundneider, 2014). This is about recognizing the need for a paradigmatic shift from autopoietic (self-reproducing) to sympoietic (co-evolving with) approaches. Donna Haraway (2016, p. 33) has alerted us to the fact that many systems are mistaken for autopoietic when they are really sympoietic and that:

> ... this point is important for thinking about rehabilitation (making livable again) and sustainability amid the porous tissues and open edges of damaged but still ongoing living worlds, like planet earth and its denizens in current times being called the Anthropocene.
>
> (Haraway, 2016, p. 33)

Universities as organizations therefore need to fundamentally revisit their understanding of social responsibility in terms of our practices of connecting and the connections we make, make possible, nurture and deny. Interconnections are everywhere and yet the human exceptionalism and boundaried individualism that have come to characterize the culture that emerged from the imperializing 18th century largely blind us to our interconnections and interdependencies with natural systems and the ecosystem services they provide. Haraway challenges us to ask ourselves:

> What happens when the best biologies of the 21st century cannot do the job with bounded individuals plus contexts, when organisms plus environments, or genes plus whatever they need, no longer sustain the overflowing richness of biological knowledges, if ever they did?
>
> (Haraway, 2016, p. 30)

Universities are challenged to update their own understanding of who we are as a community of inter-related co-evolving beings and recognize that we are a part of nature rather than apart from nature, that our own **wellbeing** is deeply entangled with the wellbeing of our ecosystem. This involves recognizing that we inter-are with nature (Hanh, 2021), that we are intra-connected (Siegel, 2023) and that we need to be afforded opportunities to encounter nature and fall in love with it again, thereby rediscovering biophilia (Cousquer, 2022; 2024). Any move towards interbeing and intraconnection involves the nurturing of and teaching for vertical literacy, but for rekindling of the flame of learning, universities themselves need to take responsibility for reimagining themselves and develop their own vertical literacy (Scharmer, 2018a, b):

> The lack of vertical literacy is the main problem in our universities and schools today. Talk to experienced CEOs and CPOs (chief people officers) of major companies and ask them what they need. They commonly say: people, teams, and leaders that can make our organization thrive in a world of VUCA (volatility, uncertainty, complexity, ambiguity). By that, I believe they mean people and capacities that can take their organization into the 4.0 world in which they respond to disruption by co-sensing and co-shaping the future. Then go to universities and talk to faculty and deans of management and engineering schools. Many, maybe most, are rather illiterate when it comes to vertical development. They think mostly in terms of horizontal development – for example, about adding another skill here or another app or course there. They do not think in terms of upgrading the entire educational OS – of our students, our learners, and our societal systems.
>
> (Scharmer, 2018a, b)

What might this operating software upgrade for greater vertical literacy consist of? There are no ready-made answers to this for universities need to explore how teaching and research can partner with and be informed by the life-sustaining future we need. Currently, we are teaching for a society that has become increasingly **anthropocentric** and egocentric, that is to say disconnected from the living and therefore the real world. We are learning about the world out there rather than learning how to co-sense and co-create a new world through our own self-, collective and organizational transformation. Much of this is due to the failure of universities (with a few notable exceptions) to embrace the inner and outer dimensions of learning through reflexivity, Action Research and awareness-based systems change (Arnold and Schön, 2021). This involves embodied practice and the concomitant development of somatic awareness and emotional literacy. It is this emotional literacy that equips us to develop both self-reflexive and self-transforming knowledge. Universities could facilitate this learning at the first-person (individual) and second-person (group) level; they could also open to and engage with this themselves, to a much greater degree, ultimately allowing students to study how they themselves can change the institution and the society they are part of. Awareness of this shift in pedagogy is reflected in the Learning for Sustainability guidance produced by the Quality Assurance Agency for Higher Education and Advance HE. This recognizes that, in addition to supporting students and staff to develop the knowledge, competencies and ability to pursue sustainable visions of the future, we also need to develop their appreciation of 'the complexity of our world, the "wicked problems" that continuously emerge, and how they can personally and professionally contribute to positive change' and need to challenge, support and enable students to 'co-design solutions and drive change for sustainability' (QAA and Advance HE, 2021, p. 9).

The guidance goes on to explain how universities must engage with the sustainability challenges in a comprehensive way, involving students, staff (including non-academic members of staff from the professional services team) and the wider community. This can lead to all parties:

> … questioning their own and societies' ways of thinking, ways of practicing and ways of being, which is central to a transformational learning experience. This can be unsettling at first, but is the start of a transformative journey that can lead to a more sustainable future.
>
> (QAA and Advance HE, 2021, p. 20)

We close this section with a short foray into the relationship between ethics and reflexivity.

6.4.3 The integration of ethics into One Health

Reflexivity is also crucial in ethics. This is a common strand in most ethical theories that one needs to reflect on one's own opinion in ethical matters, other conflicting opinions and try to overcome obstacles that arise. Also, ethics is more or less always collective, considering interrelations in groups of humans, with animals or nature. Ethics related to One Health issues is a fairly new field and has not yet been formalized as central to One Health approaches, although it should in the future (Degeling *et al.*, 2019). In a pluralistic ethical world where one has to consider ethics in individuals, populations and ecosystems as well as among different species, ethical reflexivity is still something to develop in the context of One Health approaches.

One example when reflexivity is implemented in ethical guiding documents is the Code of Ethics developed by the International Society of Ethnobiology (ISE). Ethnobiologists gather traditional and Indigenous knowledge about biodiversity that could help save species and ecosystems. In these efforts the Code of Ethics deals with how to interact with local and Indigenous communities. One central aspect in the code is mindfulness, which is defined as a kind of reflexivity as 'a continual willingness to evaluate one's own understandings, actions, and responsibilities to others' (Tunón *et al.*, 2016).

6.5 Nurturing and Developing Your Reflective Practice

This section of the chapter provides you with a selection of practices and exercises that can contribute to and help you develop your reflective practice. They each contribute in different ways and I have tried to provide insights into the value of these contributions whilst recognizing that reflective work is deeply personal and unique to the individual.

Whilst many of the practices offered below are suitable for reflective practitioners of all levels, we recognize that it is important to signpost those that can serve as 'entry points' for professionals with minimal or limited experience. I further recognize that becoming reflexive is accompanied inevitably by some discomfort if only because we are opening ourselves up to feedback, to learning and to transformation. This can feel threatening and we need to be compassionate towards ourselves and our fellow practitioners in order to identify appropriate levels of challenge. A key question for us then to consider is the nature of an 'appropriate challenge' (Fig. 6.5) and the attitude we adopt in exploring our stretch zone such that you become comfortable entering that zone, whilst also remaining alert to when you stray too close to the panic zone.

Reflective intermission:

Nurturing is about tending and befriending. How good a friend are you to yourself? Please use this prompt to write down a few lines about how you look out for yourself and nourish your whole self (body, mind and soul).

- Are there any essential needs that you have fallen into the habit of neglecting?
- What nourishes your body, mind and soul and how do you supply this 'compost'?
- When do you allow yourself to slow down and to shift from doing into being?
- What practices anchor you and allow you to feel grounded and experience equanimity?

Figure 6.6 offers some gentle suggestions to help the reader develop their reflective practice with an emphasis on journalling as a way of engaging with reflexivity. We then offer you a series of practices and exercises that you can explore and familiarize yourself with. Practices 1–3 are entry-level practices. Practice 1, for example, supports some of the prompts presented in the first

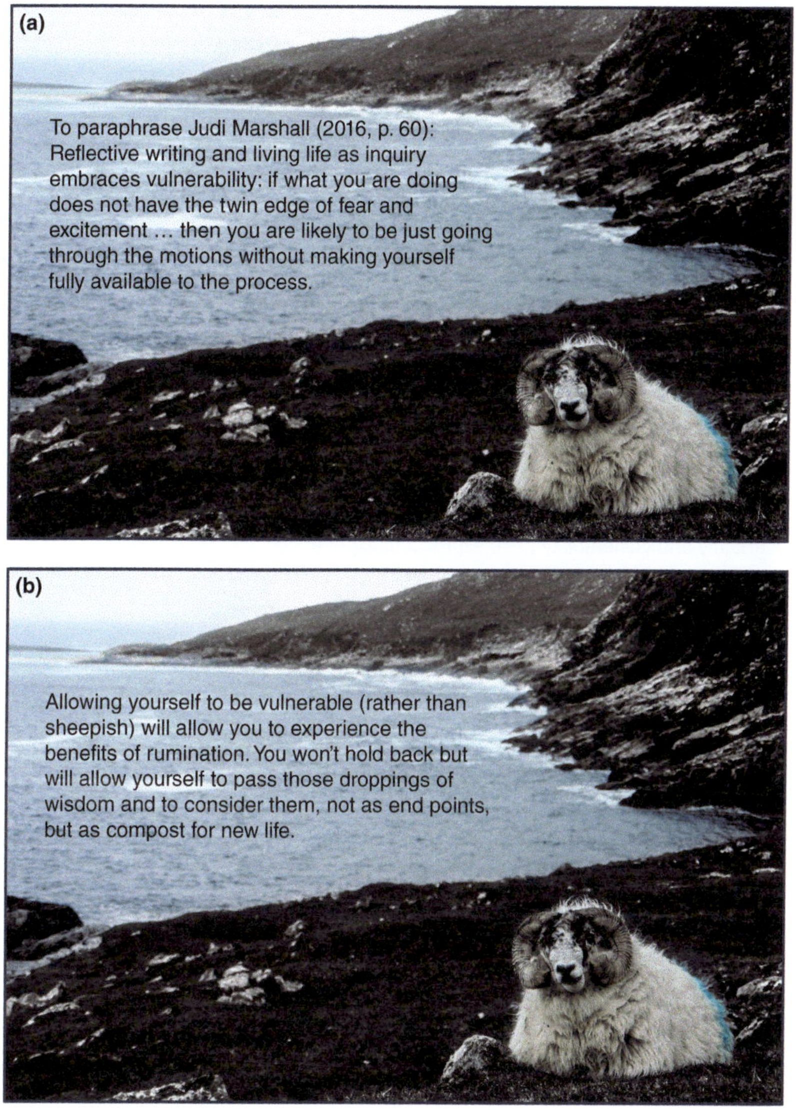
(a)
To paraphrase Judi Marshall (2016, p. 60): Reflective writing and living life as inquiry embraces vulnerability: if what you are doing does not have the twin edge of fear and excitement ... then you are likely to be just going through the motions without making yourself fully available to the process.
(b)
Allowing yourself to be vulnerable (rather than sheepish) will allow you to experience the benefits of rumination. You won't hold back but will allow yourself to pass those droppings of wisdom and to consider them, not as end points, but as compost for new life.

Fig. 6.5. **(a)** The armour we all carry both weighs us down and makes it difficult to listen to feedback. If we shut ourselves off from this feedback, we deny ourselves the possibility of learning, growth and flourishing. Picture credit: Glen Cousquer Photography. **(b)** To ruminate engages the whole body system in a digestive practice that allows us to digest not just food but other forms of nourishment. We can digest our experiences and the thoughts and emotions that accompany those experiences. This allows the lessons of these experiences (whether formative or traumatic) to be integrated into the whole. Picture credit: Glen Cousquer Photography.

panel of Figure 6.6 and will help you to develop your awareness of the value of having access to contemplative time / space and how to create this.

Practices 4–7 are more advanced. Once familiar with the insights a practice can bring and how to integrate these insights into your life and work, you can start exploring other practices. In time, you will have amassed a toolbox of different practices (tools) and a rich awareness of their value when faced with different situations.

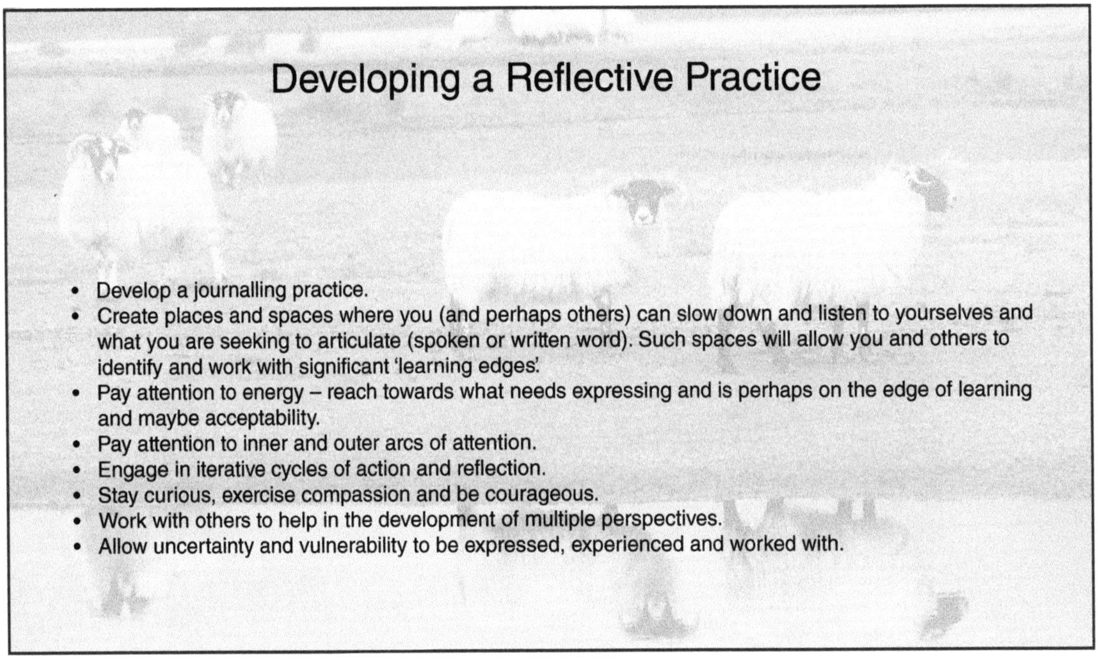

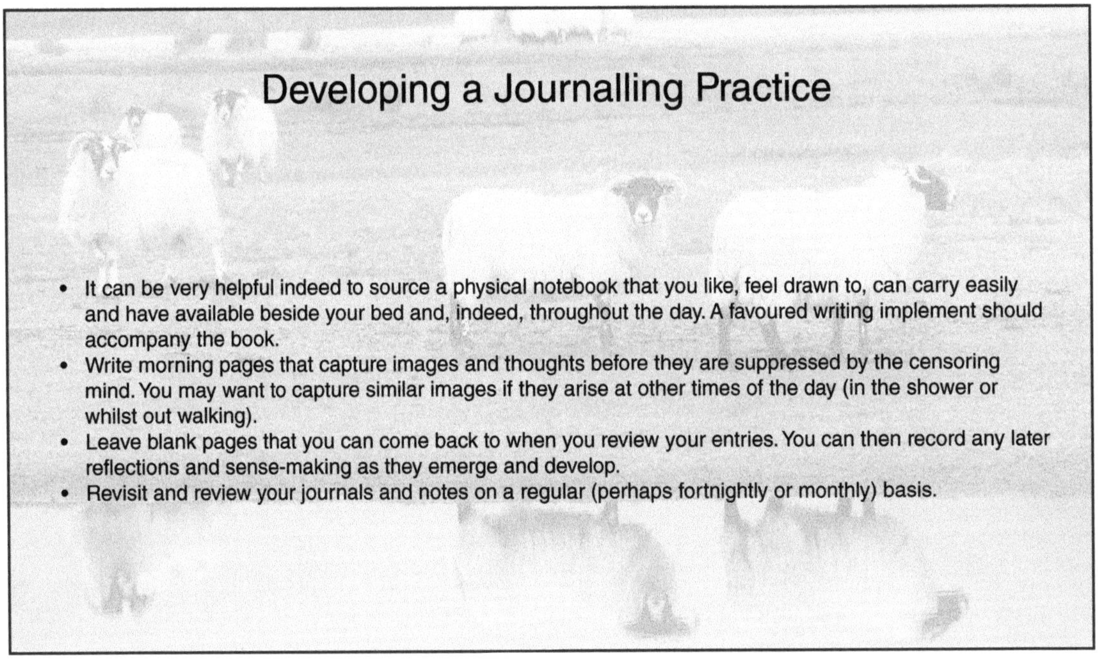

Fig. 6.6. Developing a reflective practice can start with journalling. Here some prompts are offered to get you started. Journalling can be a powerful tool to adopt during a project as it will provide you with a regular opportunity to reflect and to capture those reflections. These entries in a journal can then be reviewed at the end of the project and written up into a reflective report. Picture credit: Glen Cousquer Photography.

Practice 1: Working with your nervous system to prepare the ground for reflexivity

One of the most important things to seek and nurture in reflexive work is a sense of internal spaciousness. This kind of space allows us to witness our relational processes, including our thinking and our feeling, to be conscious in the moment. This is very different from the tight claustrophobic spaces that we experience when our sympathetic nervous system is triggered and our body is flooded by the fight–flight emotions.

Space is, as they say, 'the last frontier', a frontier or threshold that affords us so much possibility because it allows us to slow down, to suspend, to relax and to become more present. So often, we are absent and our absencing means that our availability is diminished. It might be that a situation has triggered us and caused our thinking to spin off into worrying about the past, planning or problem solving. This is the doing mode and is very distinct from the being mode. Being mode allows us to be present with what is and to be so with kindness and compassion. This 'presencing' allows us to reconnect to our breath, to our bodies, to the moment and to the now and to the infinite possibilities that present themselves in the now.

Accessing this sense of spaciousness is something we can learn to cultivate and that can provide us with more information about the situation (understood in the fullest sense, with both internal and external components) we are confronted with whilst also providing us with an opportunity to suspend interfering information. Interfering information here is information that arises when a fight–flight response is triggered and we are left feeling frustrated, angry or fearful.

We all know that this sympathetic response does not prime us for social engagement. Instead, it primes us for fight or flight depending on whether anger or fear get the upper hand. How then do we work with our nervous systems to prime ourselves for reflexivity both at the individual level and at the group level? This is where polyvagal theory comes in and can help us reflexively appreciate how to connect with our own selves and to tune into our nervous system and stabilize it. This can be understood as finding resonance or falling into our own rhythm. Proficiency in this practice then opens up the possibility of stabilizing and attuning collective consciousness so that group resonance becomes possible.

For the purposes of this chapter, we just want to focus on those practices that allow us to reconnect with ourselves. A number of anchors are classically used to establish this kind of awareness and inner calmness. These include the breath and the body, as well as sound.

The invitation here is therefore for you to cultivate one or more practices that allow you to return to the breath, the body, to nature or to some other present-moment anchor. What is your go-to and how do you create time and space for this in your life on a daily basis?

One option mentioned early in this chapter was the three-minute breathing space (see Reflexive intermission, p. 117). Here is a short three-step practice you can slot into key moments of your daily routine. It is a perfect introductory practice suitable for beginners as well as being something we can all draw on. It is designed to allow us to step out of autopilot and to reconnect with the present moment.

Step 1 – Become Aware

Deliberately adopt an erect and dignified posture and ask yourself what body sensations are here. What moods and feelings are here? What thoughts are going through my mind?

Step 2 – Gathering

Redirect your attention to focus on the sensations of breathing. In doing so allow the mind to settle on the breath wherever you are feeling it most vividly. Allow yourself to tune into the full experience as the inbreath gives way to the outbreath, following them for their full duration.

Step 3 – Expanding

Having gathered your attention to the breath, allow it to expand outwards, allowing it to take in the sensations in the body as a whole, your posture, energy field, facial expressions and anything else that presents itself in the present moment.

Practice 2: Journalling

Journalling can allow us to tap into our unfiltered stream of consciousness and to allow it to flow. This can be aided by writing with our non-dominant hand sometimes.

Allow yourself to write, to doodle, to draw connections and to observe the flow of expression and inquiry as it appears on the page.

Don't overthink … don't think … just write…

It can help to carry a notebook on a walk and to capture ideas as they arise direct from the experience of being in nature (Fig. 6.7).

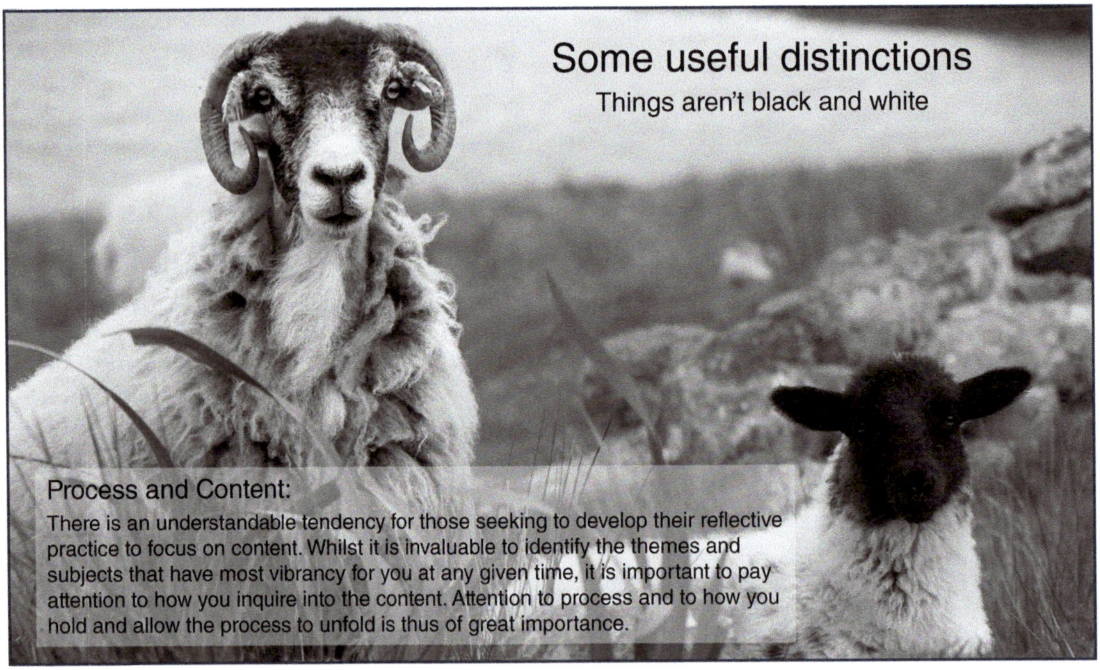
Some useful distinctions
Things aren't black and white
Process and Content:
There is an understandable tendency for those seeking to develop their reflective practice to focus on content. Whilst it is invaluable to identify the themes and subjects that have most vibrancy for you at any given time, it is important to pay attention to how you inquire into the content. Attention to process and to how you hold and allow the process to unfold is thus of great importance.

Fig. 6.7. The process and practices of journalling are more important than the content. This is about choosing a focus and trusting the process. Insights then emerge. Picture credit: Glen Cousquer Photography.

Practice 3: Reviewing an experience

The invitation here is to develop a habit of reviewing an experience in order to make sense of it. Reviewing can be undertaken during or after an experience and can be undertaken in both structured and unstructured ways. The following is a recommended structured practice for reviewing called the 4Fs or 4Es. The 4Es or 4Fs model is a beautifully simple and easy to implement practical tool / approach that was developed by Roger Greenaway and is supported by a range of materials that he has developed over the course of a long career in reviewing and facilitation. Please visit his website to access these resources.

- **Step 1: Facts / Experience** – describe what happened as factually as you can.
- **Step 2: Feelings / Emotions** – articulate / express how you felt about the experience.
- **Step 3: Findings / Examine** – inquire into and explore the whole experience.
- **Step 4: Futures / Explore** – consider how you might act on these findings in the future.

Practice 4: Reviewing feedback

For those readers undertaking further study and receiving formal feedback on formative and summative assessments, it can be really helpful to review that feedback. The following practice is offered as a way of evolving your relationship to feedback.

1. Set your attitude: bring kindness and compassion to the process.
2. Set your intention clearly.
3. Nurture positive psychology by focusing on the positives and capturing what you are grateful for and why.
4. Reframe any negative feedback as a learning opportunity and remind yourself that the cracks are where the light comes in.
5. Produce a summary table of the most significant feedback from an assignment, course or programme of study.
6. Apply a 4Fs review process to each of these bits of feedback.
7. Identify one particularly significant bit of feedback to explore in greater depth. Follow your curiosity here.
8. Revisit your intention.

You are likely to find that as you learn to practise vulnerability, you develop what Brené Brown describes as a 'strong back soft belly' (Brown, 2017, pp. 153–154). You are likely to become aware of where and when you armour up and the extent to which that armour weighs you down. You are more likely to find yourself exploring the puppy move where you roll over onto your back and expose your belly, not as a submissive move but as a reciprocal opening to playful mutuality – to the exchange of feedback.

When you give feedback, it is worth assuming the process is two-way rather than one-way and to follow the same eight-step process above so that it is intentionally informed and is more likely to be well received. A helpful question here is to ask ourselves whether we are encouraging curiosity and compassion.

Practice 5: Reflective essay writing

A good way of writing reflections is to choose one or a number of 'critical' event(s) – this does not necessarily mean something that has gone wrong, but something that you are curious about, is significant for you, has had an effect on you at the time and subsequent to the event. It is useful to include the context of the event, timing and who was involved, then you can clarify the incident for discussion. This clarification should not exclude the affective dimensions of the experience, which is why a 4Fs model is so helpful as it includes this as an explicit aspect of the experience. In moving into inquiry, you may find it helpful to develop a thematic analysis. Potentially useful categories include: concerns; thoughts; feelings; accomplishments; difficulties; satisfying and disturbing aspects; importance. Pay attention for threshold concepts, moments or insights that transform your framing of the experience and that are relevant to learning and changes to future practice.

- Choose a critical experience, episode or focus. This would be something that stands out for you, e.g. a successful or unsuccessful learning incident, a problem presented to you, which may have made an emotional **impact**.

1 Describe the incident to include:
- When and where it happened.
- What actually happened (who said or did what)?
- What you were thinking and feeling at the time and just after the incident?
- What were the significant factors?

2 Interrogate your description to include:
- Why did this incident stand out?
- What was going on?
- Did you bring personal bias or a particular mindset to the event?
- Could you have interpreted this event differently from another point of view?
- What alternative framings change the narrative arc in a helpful way?
- What can you learn from the episode about the context, your colleagues and yourself?
- Is there any useful theory you can apply to this incident?

3 Ongoing Critical Incident Analysis
- Find a friend or colleague to:
    - Share your account of the episode
    - Discuss your interpretation
- Modify your analysis, where necessary, in the light of peer suggestion, advice and perspective.
- This can be done as part of a coaching circle in which deep listening is practised.

Practice 6: Critical thinking and the production of SMART targets

This practice is included for those who like to have a focus on outcomes. When you reflect on something, you turn thoughts over in your mind and will reach certain conclusions or form further questions. The following series of questions help structure a reflective process that can allow you to think critically about your experience with a view to forming future SMART targets. In doing so, you should include your own and other people's feelings and consider 'negative' as well as 'positive' experiences.

1. What happened? Give detail of the action or event.
2. How did I feel? How did other people feel? How did people respond?
3. What is/are my objective view(s) about what happened and the 'causes'?
4. What can I learn from this?
5. What improvements can I make for my own learning?

6. What do I need to do to achieve these improvements?
7. What are my SMART (Specific, Measurable, Achievable, Relevant and Time-bound) targets?
8. How does this relate to the wider context of my work?

This series of questions can be a good starting place for people who think logically and systematically about the task or challenge in front of them. It is worth noting, however, that this is a starting point rather than an end-point and a practice that focuses very much on holding means up to scrutiny rather than considering more deeply the ends we seek.

It is also worth noting that SMART objectives have been questioned. The original acronyms are provided below together with Rubin's (2002) account of how they have slipped and can mean many things to many people. These additional definitions are offered to help you reflect on how the original SMART acronym has been and can be interpreted.

- **S**pecific (simple, sensible, significant).
- **M**easurable (meaningful, motivating).
- **A**chievable (action-oriented, accountable, as-if-now, agreed, agreed-upon, actionable, assignable agreed, attainable).
- **R**elevant (reasonable, realistic and resourced, results-based, reviewable, relative, rewarding, reasonable, results-oriented, relevant to a mission).
- **T**ime bound (time based, time limited, time/cost limited, timely, time sensitive, toward what you want, truthful).

Practice 7: Metaphor, poetry and other forms of presentational knowing

The more we know the less we see. Our education systems take the beginner's mind with its ability to connect with the field of possibility and superimpose a conceptual way of knowing the world that biases and limits our ability to see fully. This is why decolonizing One Health is so important if we are to break free from silo thinking rather than evolve into slightly bigger silos, the silo thinking of which then becomes our new ideology. As Scharmer (2009) so clearly emphasizes, bias is the next frontier of science and it is a reflexive frontier. Dan Siegel (2023, pp. 54–55) alerts us to the 'ways we've learned to perceive reality, including how to construct a solo self' and how they 'filter what we sense into what we perceive in a top-down construction of the world'. He goes on to emphasize that it is because of this that we are 'humbled and inspired to do the hard work of being open to learning from different ways of seeing, different ways of knowing, than what we were originally taught'.

We need to learn to let go of conceptual knowledge and to become aware of how conceptual knowledge can filter our sensations into limited perceptions. Humility is key here, which is perhaps why Ed Schein became so interested in humble inquiry (Schein, 2013) and why Action Research emphasizes how humility can help to address epistemic justice issues and encourage us to delay the shift into abstract conceptual knowledge. The four ways of knowing developed by Heron and Reason (1997) propose that we engage more with experiential and presentational knowing as a way of better engaging with propositional and practical knowing. Propositional knowing is here understood to encompass abstract, conceptual and theoretical epistemologies (knowledge practices).

Metaphor and poetry are two forms of presentational knowing that do not seek to pin down concepts in a definitive framework. As such they remain truer to the experience and to the wide range of potential interpretations available to us. Drawing on metaphor and poetry and integrating it into our work can allow us to see beyond the academy and beyond our own training in science and medicine.

The invitation here is therefore to bring metaphor and poetry into your writing, drawing either on the work of others or writing our own poetry. This allows us to see things afresh for, as Pakman (2000, p. 3) reminds us when writing about Donald Schön's own interest in metaphor, it came to 'grow years later toward his elaborations on "generative metaphor," and its role in allowing us to see things anew'.

Soil and soul are metaphorically aligned, for example, and remind us of the common route of humus and human. Donna Haraway thus reminds us that post-humanist work is about composting:

> Human as humusities has potential if we could chop and shred human as Homo, the detumescing project of a self-making and planet-destroying CEO. Imagine a conference not on the Future of the Humanities in the Capitalist Restructuring University, but instead on the Power of the Humusities for a Habitable Multispecies Muddle. (Haraway, 2016, p. 32)

Where poetry is concerned, you may wish to integrate readings into workshops and into your journalling and writing. Here is an example of a poem I draw on frequently. It is called 'The Pedagogy of Conflict' by Pádraig Ó Tuama:[20]

When I was a child,
I learned to count to five
one, two, three, four, five.
but these days, I've been counting lives, so I count

one life
one life
one life
one life
one life

because each time
is the first time
that that life
has been taken.

Legitimate Target
has sixteen letters
and one
long
abominable
space
between
two
dehumanising
words.

The work undertaken by presentational knowledge forms happens in the shadows; it is largely invisible to us but by bringing our attention to bear on it, we can draw on it and invite it to in-form who we are becoming. This is why I bring it into workshops and encourage poems and songs that speak to a complex issue we are unable to fully comprehend to be shared. Try it and see where it leads you.

Practice 8: Ego to Eco

As you explore your relational self and move from being highly defended and heavily armoured towards a more open receptive being, you will have opportunities to reflect on the emergence of an ecological self. This is a lifelong journey of awakening that involves the unfolding of the deeper structures of the human psyche through individuation, identification and initiation. It can be thought of in many different ways, but it is perhaps best summarized as the second half of life in which we come to recognize that we are inextricably connected to and interdependent with something much larger than ourselves. Thich Nhat Hanh's practice of interbeing (Hanh, 2021) and Dan Siegel's wheel of awareness and notion of intraconnection (Siegel, 2023) are particularly relevant to any exploration of the shift from ego to eco (Cousquer, 2022).

The invitation here is therefore to explore Level 3 and Level 4 listening through a range of sensing and presencing practices and to reflect on how you evolve as you explore these aspects of an extended self. Two suggested activities here are empathy walks[21] and wheel of awareness meditation.[22]

In research this is a key part of our methodological approach for we can choose to deny any relationship with the objects of our research or to actually become with them and evolve into higher possibilities (Fig. 6.8). See Cousquer (2023) for further discussion.

The invitation here is therefore to consider and journal about who you are becoming in any given situation. You can consider this exercise in the first or third person. This represents an opportunity to engage with the epistemic practices of learning to be and learning to be together that are at the heart of learning for sustainability (QAA and Advance HE, 2021).

Practice 9: Reflexivity in Research

As discussed in the previous practice, reflexivity is essential to good research because it recognizes the situated nature of all knowledge. As the philosopher and historian of science and medicine Georges Canguilhelm reminds us: 'scientific notions and practices are constructed thanks to an empirical and conceptual back and forth, but coalesce around theoretical systems that tend to become reductive and rigid' (Canguilhelm, 2012, p. 6). He goes on to argue that positivist stances are ideological systems that 'tend to be self-enclosed and tend to produce norms of their own in order to formulate, validate and defend what they perceive as their own truths'.

Given that One Health seeks to be transdisciplinary and open to many ways of knowing, it is essential that all One Health research be reflexive. This starts with routinely recognizing one's positionality and continues by integrating a reflexive practice into our research approaches.

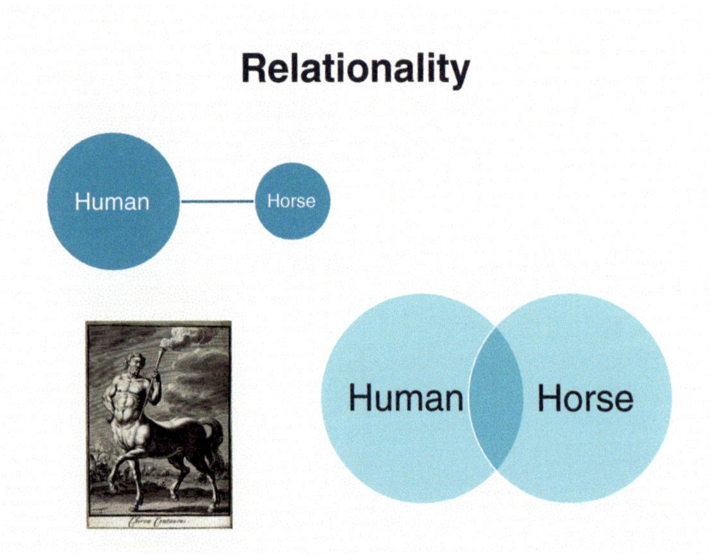

Fig. 6.8. It is very easy for researchers to view the object of research as independent of them. In objectifying the object of research, it becomes impossible to meet genuinely with the other. Othering arises through this distancing and this is a form of colonial domination. It is violence, a form of terrorism that we are only just waking up to. Genuine partnering requires a turning to the *I-Thou* such that both researcher and the object of research can be transformed by the encounter and grow transcendentally into a higher potential. In the example illustrated here, horse and human develop their potential to become with. The centaur thus emerges metaphorically and literally. Developed by author. Picture source: Chiron. Etching. Wellcome Collection. Public Domain Mark. (https://wellcomecollection.org/works/dfpaywet Creative Commons Attribution 4.0 International license).

The invitation here is to write a positionality statement that captures the many elements that in-form your contributions to One Health. This includes your sociocultural background, ethnicity, **gender**, preferred pronouns, neurodiversity, educational background, professional background and theoretical beliefs, and anything else that gives rise to your world view.

Here are a few considerations to include in your positionality and reflexivity sections:

- Identify your positionality at the planning stage, before starting the research, and revisit it regularly throughout the research process (Holmes, 2020).
- Be aware that your positionality may change during your project and is not static. Reflecting on your relationship to your research question, the context within which your research is situated and the people you engage with will help you become aware of how this can evolve.
- Make use of your fieldwork journal to consider your reflexivity journal. This will support you in capturing and reflecting on what arises while collecting and interpreting / analysing data (Braun and Clarke, 2013).

Writing a positionality statement benefits from setting aside the time to consider, craft, edit and revise your statement (Holmes, 2020). It is also worth noting that Braun and Clarke (2013) encourage researchers to revisit their statement by weaving their positionality and reflexivity throughout their thesis chapters, rather than having one positionality statement at the beginning. This allows you to write your reflexivity into your work.

6.6 Conclusion and Future Perspectives

This chapter has considered the nature of reflective practice and distinguished it from reflexivity, which draws on awareness-based practice to develop meta-cognition. It has emphasized why we need to create safe spaces for ourselves and others when engaging in this vulnerable work, which can threaten the ego and be resisted. Kindness and compassion are essential attitudes to reflexive work, as is power literacy. Attention to the unfolding of the maturing individual and collections of individuals can thus be nurtured.

It is important to realize that this unfolding is an alchemical process that cannot be forced, for the butterfly cannot be freed from the chrysalis but emerges as a result of process. This is why there is a need to develop and trust a range of practices that can in-form our growth, development and flourishing.

Reflexivity is essential if we are to develop communities of practice, learning, inquiry and co-creation that can sustain One Health and sustainability. A range of practices have been proposed that will support this development and further reading is available via the reference list, weblinks and endnotes.

We trust you can find inspiration for your ongoing growth and reflexive development in this account of reflexivity, which has emphasized the need for experiential knowing and learning over conceptual knowing because concepts block our ability to transcend ourselves and seek more sustainable and healthier ways of being and being with. Sustainability is synonymous with integrating whatever food we are offered (whether this be food we eat, feedback we are offered, experiences and traumas we have to process). Learning for sustainability and integration has thus been emphasized throughout this chapter, and this has been informed by a trauma-sensitive approach that is recognized as essential to the healing of individual, generational and collective trauma. This integrative practice therefore is another aspect of One Health that readers are encouraged to engage with and assimilate into their personal and professional practice.

Acknowledgements

As the author of this chapter, I would like to thank Barbara Häsler, Simon Ruegg, Henrik Lerner, Ann Sterckz and Hans Keune for their feedback on an early draft. This input was invaluable in shaping its development and evolution. I also owe an immense debt of gratitude to a number of people who have nurtured my own development as a reflective practitioner, most notably Pete Allison, Roger Greenaway, David Carr and Eva Pomeroy. Lastly, I wish to thank Geoffrey Baines for introducing me to Theory U and for nurturing my development as an awareness-based change maker and to Avinash Bansode who has overseen my training as a mindfulness teacher.

Notes

[1] Please refer to the three-minute breathing space in the Reflexive intermission on p. 117 for suggestions on how to develop this practice further.

[2] As Viktor Frankl (1946) reminds us, 'between the stimulus and response, there is a space. And in that space lies our freedom and power to choose our responses. In our response lies our growth and our freedom.'

[3] Please refer to Chapters 4 and 5 where knowledge practices are explored in different ways.

[4] You may also want to notice if there is some resistance or perhaps a sense of surprise or even relief. Notice whatever comes up, note it down so that you can revisit it and perhaps journal on this.

[5] Please refer to Journalling in the Practices section of this chapter (Practice 2) for suggestions on how to take note and explore further.

[6] For many of us there may be an assumption that we read from left to right and start to finish. Where does this originate from? Have you ever stopped to consider how linear our practices are and explored what might be involved in breaking free of left-hemisphere thinking and in embracing the spiralling flow of life?

[7] Krista Tippett's exploration of wisdom through the On Being project has brought together a collection of interviews and insights from across global society into what it means to be human, how we want to live and who we will be together (Tippett, 2016).

[8] Social Science, Humanities and Arts for People and the Economy. See the British Academy for more: https://www.thebritishacademy.ac.uk/this-is-shape/.

[9] Science, technology, engineering, and mathematics (STEM) is an umbrella term used to group together the distinct but related technical disciplines of science, technology, engineering, and mathematics.

[10] For those wanting to read more about our ways of seeing and how to take appearance(s) more seriously, please read Bortoft (1996, 2012).

[11] We will be discussing the difference between mismeeting and genuine meeting later in the chapter.

[12] According to Brené Brown (2012): 'Vulnerability is not weakness, and the uncertainty, risk, and emotional exposure we face every day are not optional. Our only choice is a question of engagement. Our willingness to own and engage with our vulnerability determines the depth of our courage and the clarity of our purpose; the level to which we protect ourselves from being vulnerable is a measure of our fear and disconnection.'

[13] Absencing also arises through other emotional responses including judgement. Recognizing that we are judging and therefore dividing that which is whole is a key skill the One Health professional must develop.

[14] A habit arises from how we direct our attention and how this focus informs our mind's thinking practices and therefore our habits of thought.

[15] It is anticipated that the word 'even' did not register in the same way as the word 'mystical' and that you may not have noticed that the last word was actually 'even'.

[16] Translation by Coleman Barks, from *The Essential Rumi* (1995, p. 175).

[17] Please see: https://www.tarabrach.com/reflection-recognizing-trance/ https://www.tarabrach.com/awakening-from-the-trance/

[18] See Chapter 3 on interdisciplinarity and transdisciplinarity for a more in-depth exploration.

[19] The term traditional can imply 'conservative' and as such it may be important to distinguish Indigenous knowledge from traditional knowledge. First Nations or Indigenous knowledge is rooted in a very different ontology and cosmology from Western cultures. They recognize the value of other ways of knowing and are typically animistic and emphasize interconnection to a significant degree. In the West, the emphasis on rationality and the rejection of spirituality and mysticism have tended to limit our world view.

[20] Pádraig Ó Tuama, Part III of 'The Pedagogy of Conflict' from *Sorry for Your Troubles* (Canterbury Press, 2013) used with permission of the poet and the publisher.

[21] https://www.u-school.org/empathy-walk

[22] https://drdansiegel.com/wheel-of-awareness/

References and Further Reading

Adisasmito, W.B., Almuhairi, S., Behravesh, C.B., Bilivogui, P., Bukachi, S. A. *et al.* (2022) One Health: A new definition for a sustainable and healthy future. *PLOS Pathogens*, 18(6), e1010537. DOI: 10.1371/journal.ppat.1010537.

Argyris, C. and Schön, D. (1974) *Theory in Practice: Increasing Professional Effectiveness.* Jossey-Bass, San Francisco, California.

Argyris, C. and Schön, D. (1978) *Organizational Learning: A Theory of Action Perspective.* Addison Wesley, Reading, Massachusetts.

Argyris, C. and Schön, D. (1996) *Organizational Learning II: Theory, Method and Practice.* Addison Wesley, Reading, Massachusetts.

Arnold, R. and Schön, M. (2021) The reflexible person. *Journal of Awareness-Based Systems Change* 1(2), 51–71. DOI: 10.47061/jabsc.v1i2.971.

Bawden, R. J. (1991) Systems thinking and practice in agriculture. *Journal of Dairy Science* 74(7), 2362–2373. DOI: 10.3168/jds.s0022-0302(91)78410-5.

Bergson, H. (2007) [1911] *The Creative Mind.* Dover, New York.

Bondi, L., Carr, D., Clark, C. and Clegg, C. (2011) *Towards Professional Wisdom: Practical Deliberation in the People Professions.* Ashgate Publishing, Farnham, UK.

Bortoft, H. (1996) *The Wholeness of Nature.* Lindisfarne Books, USA.

Bortoft, H. (2012) *Taking Appearance Seriously.* Floris Books, Edinburgh, UK.

Boyd, R. (1979) Metaphor and theory change: What is a 'metaphor' a metaphor for? In: Ortony, A. (ed.) *Metaphor and Thought.* Cambridge University Press, Cambridge, UK.

Bozorgmehr, K., Saint, V.A. and Tinnemann, P. (2011) The 'global health' education framework: A conceptual guide for monitoring, evaluation and practice. *Globalization and Health* 7(1), 8. DOI: 10.1186/1744-8603-7-8.

Brach, T. (2020) *Radical Compassion: Learning to Love Yourself and Your World with the Practice of RAIN.* Penguin Random House, London.

Braun, V. and Clarke, V. (2013) *Successful Qualitative Research: A Practical Guide for Beginners.* Sage, London.

Brown, B. (2012) *Daring Greatly: How the Courage to be Vulnerable Transforms the Way We Live, Love, Parent, and Lead.* Penguin Random House Audio Publishing Group, New York.

Brown, B. (2017) *Braving the Wilderness: The Quest for True Belonging and the Courage to Stand Alone.* Penguin Random House, New York.

Brown, J. (2020) *Hearticulations: On Love, Friendship and Healing.* Enrealment Press, Ontario, Canada.

Canguilhelm, G. (2012) *Writings on Medicine.* Fordham University Press, New York.

Christie, M.F. and Mason, P.A. (2003) Transformative tour guiding: Training tour guides to be critically reflective practitioners. *Journal of Ecotourism* 2(1), 1–16, DOI: 10.1080/14724040308668130.

Cousquer, G. (2020) One Health, systems thinking, actor-network theory and the delivery of emergent futures for working equine welfare. *Veterinary Practice Today.* Available at: https://www.research.ed.ac.uk/en/publications/one-health-systems-thinking-actor-network-theory-and-the-delivery (accessed 25 July 2024).

Cousquer, G.O. (2022) *Becoming Unfrozen: Seeing, Sensing, and Presencing to Better Face and Respond to Ecological Crises.* The University of Edinburgh: Teaching Matters. Available at: https://www.teaching-matters-blog.ed.ac.uk/becoming-unfrozen-seeing-sensing-and-presencing-to-better-face-and-respond-to-ecological-crises/ (accessed 25 July 2024).

Cousquer, G. (2023) From domination to dialogue and the ethics of the between: Transforming human-working equine relationships in mountain tourism. *Austral Journal of Veterinary Sciences* 55(1), 35–60. DOI: 10.4067/S0719-81322023000100035.

Cousquer, G. (2024) *Wild Places, Wild Encounters: Exploring Edinburgh's Living Landscape.* Whittles Publishing.

Cousquer, G. and Haounati, A. (2022) Action Research with and for pack mules. *Journal of Awareness-Based Systems Change* 2(2), 109–139. DOI: 10.47061/jasc.v2i2.4621.

Cousquer, G., Norris, E., Lurz, P., Vander Meer, E., and Gurnell, J. (2024) Hedgerows for hedgehogs and campus biodiversity. *Journal of Awareness-Based Systems Change* 4(1), 101–126. https://doi.org/10.47061/jasc.v4i1.7544.

Cunliffe, A.L. (2009) Reflexivity, learning and reflexive practice. In: Armstrong, S.J. and Fukami, C.V. (eds) *The SAGE Handbook of Management Learning, Education and Development*. Sage Publications, London, pp. 405–418. DOI: 10.4135/9780857021038.n21.

Cunliffe, A.L. and Easterby-Smith, M. (2017) From reflection to practical reflexivity: Experiential learning as lived experience. In: Reynolds, M. and Russ, V. (eds) *Organizing Reflection*. Routledge, London, pp. 44–60.

Dana, D. (2020) *Polyvagal Exercises for Safety and Connection*. Norton and Company, New York.

Degeling, C., Dawson, A. and Gilbert, G.L. (2019) The ethics of One Health. In: Walton, M. (ed.) *One Planet, One Health*. Sydney University Press, Australia, pp. 65–84.

Dewey, J. (1933) *How We Think*. D.C. Heath, New York.

Esterhuizen, P. and Howatson-Jones, L. (2019) *Reflective Practice in Nursing*. Sage Publications, London.

Frankl, V.E. (1946) *Man's Search for Meaning*. Beacon Press, Boston, Massachusetts.

Gibbs, G. (1988) *Learning by Doing: A Guide to Teaching and Learning*. FEU, London.

Goodchild, M. (2022) Relational systems thinking: The Dibaajimowin (story) of re-theorizing 'systems thinking' and 'complexity science'. *Journal of Awareness-Based Systems Change* 2(1), 53–76. DOI: 10.47061/jabsc.v2i1.2027.

Greenaway, R., Vaida, B. and Lepure, C. (2015) *Active Reviewing: A Guide for Facilitators and Teachers*. CreateSpace Independent Publishing Platform.

Hanh, T.N. (2017) *The Other Shore*. Parallax Press, San Francisco, California.

Hanh, T.N. (2021) *Zen and the Art of Saving the Planet*. Penguin Books, London.

Haraway, H. (2016) *Staying with the Trouble: Making kin in the Chthulucene*. Duke University Press, Durham, North Carolina.

Harding, S. (2006) *Animate Earth*. Chelsea Green Publishing, New York.

Heron, J. and Reason, P. (1997) A participative enquiry paradigm. *Qualitative Inquiry* 3(3), 274–294.

Higgins, P. and Nicol, R. (2002) *Outdoor Education: Authentic Learning in the Context of Landscapes*. Kinda Education, Kisa, Sweden.

Hinchliffe, S. (2008) *Geographies of Nature: Societies, Environments, Ecologies*. Sage Publications, London.

Holmes, A.G.D. (2020) Researcher positionality – A consideration of its influence and place in qualitative research – A new researcher guide. *Shanlax International Journal of Education* 8(4), 1–10.

Hübl, T. (2020) *Healing Collective Trauma: A Process for Integrating our Intergenerational and Collective Wounds*. Sounds True, Boulder, Colorado.

Hübl, T. (2023). *Attuned*. Sounds True, Boulder, Colorado.

Kolb, D.A. and Fry, R.E. (1975) Toward an applied theory of experiential learning. In: Cooper, C. (ed.) *Theories of Group Processes*. John Wiley & Sons, New York.

Lerner, H. and Berg, C. (2015) The concept of health in One Health and some practical implications for research and education: What is One Health? *Infection Ecology & Epidemiology* 5(1), 25300. DOI: 10.3402/iee.v5.25300.

Lerner, H. and Zinsstag, J. (2021) Towards a healthy concept of health. In: Zinsstag, J. *et al.* (eds) *One Health: The Theory and Practice of Integrated Health Approaches* (2nd edn). CABI, Wallingford, UK, pp. 52–56.

Luke, K.L., McAdie, T., Warren-Smith, A.K., Rawluk, A. and Smith, B.P. (2023) Does a working knowledge of learning theory relate to improved horse welfare and rider safety? *Anthrozoös* 36, 703–719. DOI: 10.1080/08927936.2023.2166713.

Macy, J. and Brown, M. (2014) *Coming Back to Life: The Updated Guide to the Work That Reconnects*. New Society Publishing, Gabriola Island, B.C., Canada.

Marshall, J. (2016) *First Person Action Research Living Life as Inquiry*. Sage Publications Ltd. https://uk.sagepub.com/en-gb/eur/first-person-action-research/book228121

McGilchrist, I. (2021) *The Matter with Things: Our Brains, our Delusions, and the Unmaking of the World*. Perspectiva Press, London.

Pakman, M. (2000) Thematic foreword: Reflective practices: The legacy of Donald Schön. *Cybernetics & Human Knowing* 7(2–3), 5–8.

Parker, P. (2020) *The Art of Gathering: How We Meet and Why It Matters*. Penguin Books, London.

Parkes, M.W., Charron, D.F. and Sánchez, A. (2012) Better together: Field-building networks at the frontiers of ecohealth research. In: Charron, D.F. (ed.) *Ecohealth Research in Practice: Innovative Applications of an Ecosystem Approach to Health*. Springer, pp. 231–253.

Parry, J. and Allison, P. (2021) *Experiential Learning and Outdoor Education: Traditions of Practice and Philosophical Perspectives*. Routledge, London.

Peck, M.S. (2015) *The Different Drum*. Random House, London.

Perry, S.A.B. (2021) Participatory feeling: Re-visioning transformative learning theory through Heron's whole person perspective. *Adult Education Quarterly* 71(4), 074171362110167. DOI: 10.1177/07417136211016779.

Peschl, M. F. and Fundneider, T. (2014) Evolving the future by learning from the future (as it emerges)? Toward an epistemology of change. *Behavioral and Brain Sciences* 37(4), 433–434. DOI: 10.1017/s0140525x13003245.

Pomeroy, E. and Oliver, K. (2018) Pushing the boundaries of self-directed learning: Research findings from a study of u.lab participants in Scotland. *International Journal of Lifelong Education* 37(6), 719–733. DOI: 10.1080/02601370.2018.1550447.

QAA and Advance HE (2021) *Education for Sustainable Development Guidance | Advance HE*. Available at: https://www.advance-he.ac.uk/knowledge-hub/education-sustainable-development-guidance (accessed 26 August 2024).

Rowson, J. (2021) Tasting the pickle: Ten flavours of meta-crisis and the appetite for a new civilisation. In: Rowson, J. and Pascal, L. (eds) *Dispatches from a Time Between Worlds: Crisis and Emergence in Metamodernity*. Perspectiva Press, London, pp. 15–51.

Roy, B. (2021) Time, change and causality: Notes towards a metamorphosis of mind. In: Rowson, J. and Pascal, L. (eds) *Despatches from a Time Between Worlds: Crisis and Emergence in Metamodernity*. Perspectiva Press, London, pp. 53–70.

Rubin, R. (2002) Will the real SMART goals please stand up. *The Industrial-Organizational Psychologist* 39(4), 26–27.

Rüegg, S.R., Nielsen, L.R., Buttigieg, S.C., Santa, M., Aragrande, M. *et al.* (2018) A systems approach to evaluate One Health initiatives. *Frontiers in Veterinary Science* 5. DOI: 10.3389/fvets.2018.00023.

Rūmī, J.a.-D.M. (1995) *The Essential Rumi* (C. Barks, Trans.). Harper, San Francisco.

Scharmer, C.O. (1995) *Reflexive Modernisierung des Kapitalismus als Revolution von innen*. Pöeschel, Stuttgart, Germany.

Scharmer, C.O. (2009) *Theory U: Leading from the Future as It Emerges* (1st edn). Berrett-Koehler, San Francisco, California.

Scharmer, C.O. (2016) *Theory U: Leading from the Future as It Emerges* (2nd edn). Berrett-Koehler, San Francisco, California.

Scharmer, C.O. (2018a) *Education is the Kindling of a Flame: How to Reinvent the 21st-Century University*. Available at: https://www.huffpost.com/entry/education-is-the-kindling-of-a-flame-how-to-reinvent_b_5a4ffec5e4b0ee59d41c0a9f (accessed 31 March 2023).

Scharmer, O. (2018b) *The Essentials of Theory U: Core Principles and Applications*. Berret-Koehler, Oakland, California.

Scharmer, C.O. and Kaufer, K. (2000) Universities as the birthplace for the entrepreneuring human being. *Reflections: The SOL Journal on Knowledge, Learning, and Change*, MIT Press, Massachusetts.

Scharmer, C.O. and Kaufer, K. (2013) *Leading from the Emerging Future: From Ego-System to Eco-System Economies* (1st edn). Berrett-Koehler, San Francisco, California.

Scharmer, O. and Yukelson, A. (2015) Theory U: From ego-system to eco-system economies. *The Journal of Corporate Citizenship* 58, 35–39. DOI: 10.9774/GLEAF.4700.2015.ju.00005.

Schein, E. (2013) *Humble Inquiry: The Gentle Art of Asking Instead of Telling*. Berrett-Koehler, San Francisco, California.

Schön, D. (1971) *Beyond the Stable State*. Random House, New York.

Schön, D. (1983) *The Reflective Practitioner: How Professionals Think in Action*. Temple Smith, London.

Schön, D. (1987) *Educating the Reflective Practitioner: Toward a New Design in Teaching and Learning in the Professions*. Jossey Bass, San Francisco.

Senge, P. (2006) *The Fifth Discipline: The Art and Practice of the Learning Organisation*. Random House, London.

Siegel, D. (2023) *Intraconnected: Mwe (Me + We) as the Integration of Self, Identity and Belonging*. W.B. Norton, New York.

Smith, S., Mason, J. and Bowden, M. (2020) Local wisdom in regenerative teacher practices. *Australian Journal of Teacher Education* 45(9), 92–104. DOI: 10.14221/ajte.2020v45n9.6.

Sobe, N.W. (2021) Reworking four pillars of education to sustain the commons. *UNESCO Futures of Education Ideas LAB*. Available at: https://en.unesco.org/futuresofeducation/ideas-lab/sobe-reworking-four-pillars-education-sustain-commons.

Souza, P.D. and Muniandy, B. (2014) The heart of education is the education of the heart. In: *The Heart of Education: Learning to Live Together; Selected Papers Presented at the 16th UNESCO-APEID International Conference*. UNESCO, Paris.

Thelwell, R. and Dicks, M. (2019) *Professional Advances in Sports Coaching: Research and Practice*. Routledge, Abingdon, Oxon.

Tippett, K. (2016) *Becoming Wise: An Inquiry into the Mystery and Art of Living*. Corsair, London.

Toomey, A., Markusson, N., Adams, E. and Brockett, B. (2015) GSDR 2015 Brief Inter-and Trans-disciplinary Research: A Critical Perspective. Available at: https://sdgs.un.org/sites/default/files/documents/612558-Inter-%2520and%2520Trans-disciplinary%2520Research%2520-%2520A%2520Critical%2520Perspective.pdf (accessed 26 August 2024).

Tuama, P.Ó. (2013) *Sorry for Your Troubles*. Canterbury Press, London.

Tunón, H., Kvarnstrom, M. and Lerner, H. (2016) Ethical codes of conduct for research related to Indigenous Peoples and local communities – Core principles, challenges and opportunities. In: Drugge, A.-L. (ed.) *Ethics in Indigenous Research: Past Experiences, Future Challenges*. Umeå University, Sweden, pp. 57–80.

UNESCO (2017) *Education for Sustainable Development Goals: Learning Objectives*. Available at: https://unesdoc.unesco.org/ark:/48223/pf0000247444.

Vienni-Baptista, B., Fletcher, I. and Lyall, C. (2023) *Foundations of Interdisciplinary and Transdisciplinary Research*. Bristol University Press, Bristol, UK.

Villamil, A., Vogel, T., Weisbaum, E. and Siegel, J.D. (2018) Cultivating well-being through the three pillars of mind training: Understanding how training the mind improves physiological and psychological well-being. *OBM Integrative and Complementary Medicine* 4(1), 1–16. DOI: 10.21926/obm.icm.1901003.

Wahl, D.C. (2006) Design for human and planetary health: A transdisciplinary approach to sustainability. In: *Management of Natural Resources, Sustainable Development and Ecological Hazards*, Vol. 99. DOI: 10.2495/rav060281.

Wahl, D.C. (2016) *Designing Regenerative Cultures.* Triarchy Press, Charmouth, UK.

Wonham, M. and Wasson, C. (2023) Molluscs, morphology, and metaphor in Pablo Neruda's STEAMiest poem. *Invertebrate Biology* 142(1). DOI: 10.1111/ivb.12393.

Yunkaporta, T. (2019) *Sand Talk: How Indigenous Thinking can Save the World.* HarperCollins Publishers, New York.

Zander, B. and Zander, R. (2000) *The Art of Possibility: Transforming Personal and Professional Life.* Harvard Business School Press, Cambridge, Massachusetts.

Suggested Web Resources

The General Medical Council (GMC) The reflective practitioner: guidance for doctors and medical students is available at: https://www.gmc-uk.org/education/standards-guidance-and-curricula/guidance/reflective-practice/the-reflective-practitioner---guidance-for-doctors-and-medical-students.

Roger Greenaway's website devoted to reviewing practices is available at: https://reviewing.co.uk/_site.htm.

To listen to Pádraig Ó Tuama in conversation with Krista Tippett and his recital of his poem 'A Pedagogy of Conflict' please visit: https://onbeing.org/programs/padraig-o-tuama-this-fantastic-argument-of-being-alive/.

7 Biodiversity Conservation, Ecosystem Services and One Health

Barry J. McMahon[1,6], Cyril Caminade[2], Daniele de Meneghi[3,6], Caoimhe Doyle[1], Julie Garnier[4,6], Martin Hitziger[5,6], Hans Keune[6,7], Richard Kock[6,8], Claire Martin[1], Grace Patterson[9] and K. Marie McIntyre[6,10]

[1]UCD School of Agriculture & Food Science, University College Dublin, Dublin, Ireland; [2]Earth System Physics Department, The Abdus Salam International Centre for Theoretical Physics, Trieste, Italy and Institute of Infection, Veterinary and Ecological Sciences, University of Liverpool, Liverpool, UK; [3]Department of Veterinary Sciences, University of Turin, Turin, Italy; [4]Odyssey Conservation Trust, Bakewell, UK; [5]Section of Epidemiology, Vetsuisse Faculty, University of Zurich, Switzerland; [6]Network for Ecohealth and One Health (NEOH); [7]Faculty of Medicine and Health Sciences, Department of Family Medicine and Population Health, Chair Care and the Natural Environment, University of Antwerp, Antwerp, Belgium; [8](in retirement) Independent Scholar, Kent, UK and Chief Editor on Research Directions One Health; [9]Department of Population Medicine, Ontario Veterinary College, University of Guelph, Guelph, Canada; [10]Modelling, Evidence and Policy Group, School of Natural and Environmental Sciences, Newcastle University, Newcastle, UK

Contents

DOI: 10.1079/9781800623002.0008

Chapter Overview

Elevator pitch

The understanding and the management of biodiversity is key to the management of our ecosystems. This understanding can enable us to better manage food production, water regulation, climate change and the spillover of infectious disease and zoonoses. One Health and Ecohealth approaches can facilitate an improved appreciation of how connected these challenges are, therefore enabling us to manage them.

Book objectives the chapter relates to

☑ 1. Understand what One Health and Ecohealth mean
☑ 2. Think in a One Health and Ecohealth way
☑ 3. Apply One Health and Ecohealth in their professional and personal life
☑ 4. Know how to share One Health and Ecohealth knowledge
☑ 5. Integrate One Health and Ecohealth knowledge actively
☑ 6. Acquire or enhance core One Health competencies

One Health competencies covered

☑ 1. Effective communication
☑ 2. Collaborative and resilient working
☑ 3. Systems understanding
☑ 4. Transdisciplinarity
☑ 5. Social, cultural and gender equity and inclusiveness
☑ 6. Collective learning and reflective practice
☑ 7. One Health concepts
☐ 8. Theoretical and methodological pluralism
☑ 9. Harnessing uncertainty, paradox and limited knowledge

Learning outcomes

1. Understand the concept of biodiversity conservation and ecosystem services.
2. Obtain an appreciation of the importance of biodiversity and its connectedness to global environmental challenges such as food security, water regulation, climate change and emergence of infectious diseases.
3. Value biodiversity conservation as a mechanism to acquire One Health competencies.
4. Explain how biodiversity can impact disease emergence in what is referred to as the dilution effect or the amplification effect.

Summary

In this chapter, you will first learn what the term 'biodiversity' means, and why the food system is reliant on the resources it provides. Second, you will gain an understanding of our ability to produce food under a variety of different circumstances, using a set of biotic and abiotic resources directly and indirectly related to animal, human, plant and ecosystem health; this creates resilience in our food system. Third, you will be trained in the definition of ecosystem services, and the link between biodiversity and ecosystem services in tackling global environmental challenges such as food security, water regulation, climate change and emergence of infectious diseases. Using examples, throughout the chapter, you will learn about potential actions and solutions using One Health approaches that will help to maintain good biodiversity and ecosystem services, whilst sustaining resilient food systems and tackling other global environmental challenges.

7.1 Introduction

The concept of **ecosystem services** has significant history, starting with the work of, for example, Costanza *et al.* (1997), and has developed over time. In the European Union (EU), the concept of **nature-based solutions** was coined in 2015 (European Commission, 2015). Within the Intergovernmental Science-Policy Platform on Biodiversity and Ecosystem Services (IPBES), a similar concept was developed years later: nature contributions to people (Diaz *et al.*, 2018). It recognizes the interdependence of **climate**, **ecosystems** and **biodiversity**, and human societies; the value of diverse forms of **knowledge**; and the close linkages between climate change adaptation, mitigation, ecosystem health, human **wellbeing** and sustainable development (IPCC, 2023). These concepts share a common foundation: they recognize the value of nature for human wellbeing, but they have distinct focuses and scopes. Ecosystem services emphasize the specific benefits that ecosystems provide to humans, nature-based solutions centre on utilizing nature to address societal challenges, and **nature contributions to people** encompass the multifaceted ways in which nature enriches human lives beyond material benefits. These concepts are explained in more detail later in the chapter.

So, how about **health** within these concepts? Health was taken into account quite prominently in 2005 in the Millennium Ecosystem Assessment (MEA). In ecosystem services and similar concepts, consideration of health took longer, and, until recently, much of the emphasis has been on physical human health, where there are many ways in which nature and biodiversity, i.e. the variety of all living things, can contribute to human wellbeing. Until recently, 'ecology' in the health sector often had limited reference to nature, but instead referred to the social or societal **environment** of a patient (White and Walker, 1997; Hoffmann *et al.*, 2019). Nature was only to a limited extent considered in health, e.g. primary healthcare (Lauwers *et al.*, 2020), and even the concept of 'green prescription' (i.e. refers to a prescription of 'nature-based activities' that a medical professional can give to a patient) initially had few links with nature, but mainly referred to environmental pollution and climate change challenges, lifestyle and non-medicinal prescriptions (Swinburn *et al.*, 1997; Patel *et al.*, 2011; Anderson *et al.*, 2015). A prominent exception is the WHO Ottawa Charter on Health Promotion (WHO, 1986), which highlights the importance of a balanced ecosystem: 'The fundamental conditions and resources for health are peace, shelter, education, food, income, a stable ecosystem, sustainable resources, social justice and equity. Improvement in health requires a secure foundation in these basic prerequisites.'

There is no equivalent charter explicitly for animals as comprehensive as the Ottawa Charter for Health Promotion. Other frameworks exist for animal **welfare** and wellbeing (e.g. the Five Freedoms, the five domains) and serve as important guiding principles to ensure that animals are treated ethically and provided with living conditions necessary to sustain their wellbeing (Webster, 2001). Animals are not commonly discussed in nature-based concepts and are not a key target in nature contributions to people. There is, however, recognition of the importance of healthy ecosystems in supporting and contributing to the wellbeing of animal populations, whether wild or domesticated species. Protecting and enhancing animal health contributing to maintain the overall health and functionality of ecosystems and the services they provide to humans and the environment, and this is not a new concept (Evan and Leighton, 2014).

Apart from this example, the (more tangible) negative drivers relating to environment like pollution have dominated the human health narrative. In One Health, until recently, there has been relatively little integrated discussion on the positive and negative relationship between ecosystems and biodiversity. In fact, until recently, animal health, human health and ecosystem health interests have been largely working in distinct silos (McIntyre *et al.*, 2018; Keune *et al.*, 2017, 2022), even though conceptual convergence of **Ecohealth**, **One Health** and **Planetary Health** occurred in the research community. Chapter 2 provides an overview of the meaning of these different integrated health approaches spanning the health of people, animals and ecosystems, how they have evolved, and what the integration points and differences are.

7.2 Conceptualizing the Links Between Human Health and the Environment

It is important to recognize that human, animal and ecosystem health are interconnected, and that the degradation of ecosystems has significant negative impacts on human and animal health. Protecting and restoring ecosystems is vital to safeguard human health and promote sustainable development.

Ecosystems provide essential water and foods contributing to life. Additionally, they provide services by acting as natural purifiers, filtering the air and water, regulating infectious disease and, in general, providing a clean and safe environment. Moreover, forests regulate the climate by sequestering carbon dioxide and mitigating climate change effects (Foley *et al.*, 2005; McIntyre *et al.*, 2018). Biodiversity within ecosystems helps with pollination, pest and disease control, soil fertility and nutrient cycling, and climate regulation (Keith *et al.*, 2016). Ecosystems offer livelihood opportunities, such as gathering, hunting, fishing and farming, and material for making tools and building shelter for humans and livestock; they thus contribute to economic prosperity (Romanelli *et al.*, 2015). Access to natural environments positively impacts mental wellbeing, reducing stress and anxiety. Ecosystems also hold cultural and spiritual significance, fostering a sense of belonging. They provide natural resources and medicinal plants, supporting traditional and modern medicine.

While many of the points above also apply to animals (e.g. feed, shelter, clean air and water, climate regulation, reduction of stress), there are few conceptualizations and studies of these linkages for animal health in the way that they have been done for humans. Indeed, animals are also seen as providers of these services to humans. This is complicated by the fact that 'animals' is an all-encompassing term that includes the animal kingdom, which is incredibly diverse, including humans, ranging from tiny microscopic organisms like plankton to the largest creatures on Earth, such as whales and elephants. It includes a wide array of species of various shapes, sizes, behaviours and ecological roles, inhabiting diverse environments across the globe, from terrestrial ecosystems to oceans, freshwater bodies and the air. Thus, when talking about the links between animals and ecosystems, it may make sense to specify which animals' taxa are referred to.

The multiple linkages between ecosystem services and health can be conceptualized in different ways. For example, the concept of ecosystem services highlights the ways in which ecosystems support human needs, preferences and economic activities; the value and importance of these services are primarily assessed from a human-centric perspective (McIntyre *et al.*, 2018). While this approach has been instrumental in making the link between nature and human wellbeing more tangible and relevant to decision makers and the general public, critics of the **anthropocentric** view argue that it overlooks and undervalues the intrinsic value of nature and the rights of non-human species. The impact of the **Anthropocene** on biodiversity and ecosystem services can be seen through the loss of 69% in wild vertebrates' biomass since 1970 (Westveer *et al.*, 2022) and the global loss of ecosystem services from 1997 to 2011 due to land-use change were estimated at US$4.3–20.2 trillion per year (Costanza *et al.*, 2014). Ecosystems have value and importance beyond their **utility** to humans, and their protection is essential to maintain the planet's biodiversity and ecological integrity independently of humans and animals (Jackson *et al.*, 2013a).

As the understanding of the value of nature evolves, efforts are being made to incorporate non-anthropocentric perspectives, such as **BIOCENTRISM** and **ECOCENTRISM**, into discussions on ecosystem services. These perspectives acknowledge the intrinsic value of nature and the interconnectedness of all living beings, recognizing that the wellbeing of ecosystems is essential for the wellbeing of all species.

Task: Compare Fig. 7.1 and Fig. 7.2. Figure 7.1 was developed before the start of the COVID-19 pandemic (Hartig *et al.*, 2014), and Fig. 7.2 afterwards (Marselle *et al.*, 2021). Have a look at the different linkages of biodiversity and nature and health. What are the similarities? What are the differences? What does COVID-19 have to do with these differences? What are the implications of these differences?

Example answer: The similarities include that both figures have almost the same structures and conceptual configuration, and numerous authors are common to both. The differences are that Fig. 7.1 focuses on nature-related health benefits, whereas Fig. 7.2 also includes health benefits and related health risks.

Perhaps the COVID-19 pandemic has heightened awareness of zoonoses and nature's threats to human health.

The implications are that figures demonstrate the change in the concept through time (from 2014 to 2021) with respect to how humans view nature and health. More importantly, the figures show how conservationists will need to communicate how zoonoses are part of wild systems and humans need to accept this as a biological reality.

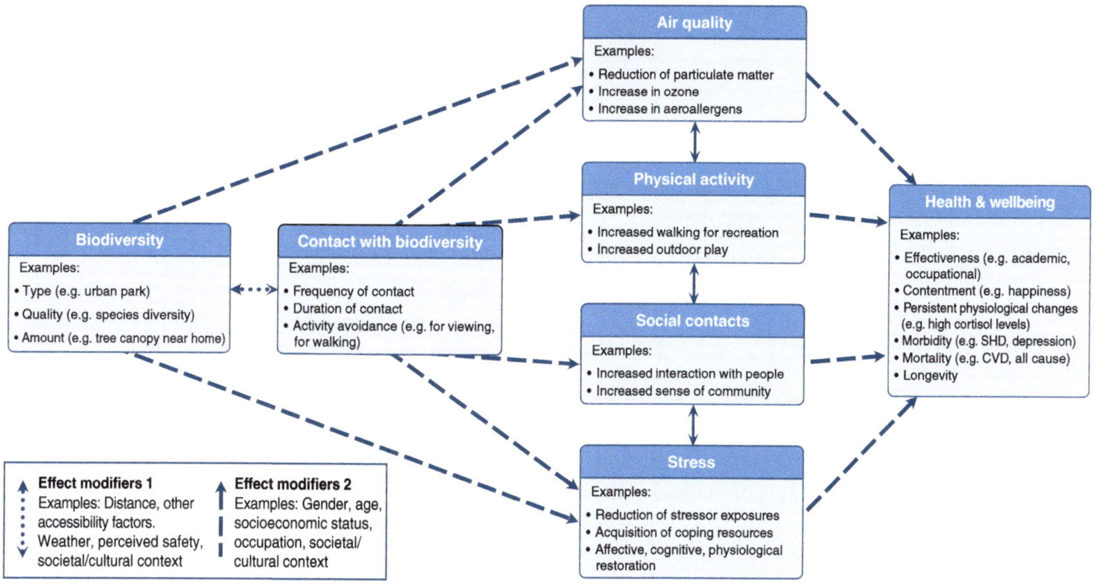

Fig. 7.1. Four pathways that the natural environment can influence the health of the wider human population. Adapted from Hartig *et al.* (2014).

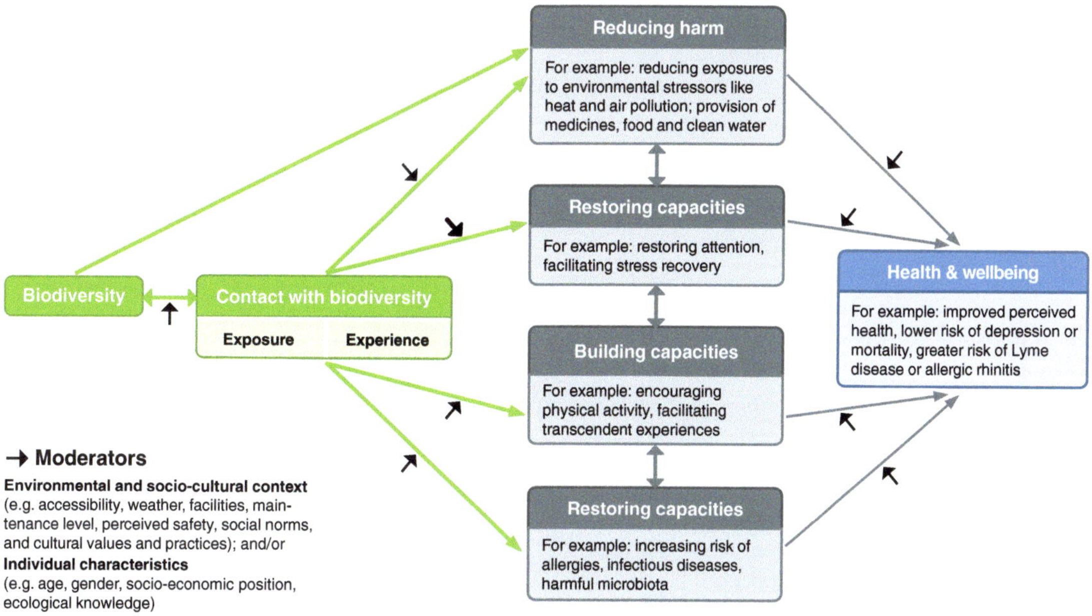

Fig. 7.2. The pathways linking biodiversity to human health and wellbeing. Four domains of pathways linking biodiversity and health involve contact with biodiversity. Adapted from Marselle *et al.* (2021) (CC BY 4.0 DEED: https://creativecommons.org/licenses/by/4.0/).

As illustrated in Chapter 15, the **Sustainable Development Goals** (SDGs) promote sustainable practices, conservation efforts and ecosystem-based approaches and aim to safeguard and enhance ecosystem services, thereby advancing sustainable development on a global scale. However, there are important trade-offs between those and other goals that for example aim to enhance production and enhance growth.

Learning question: Many people argue that nature and biodiversity should have priority over everything else given that it supports life for everything and everyone on the planet. What is your view on this and why?

Example answer: One perspective is that we should protect biodiversity as a priority since all living forms of life depend on resilient ecosystems.

The other approach is that we should prioritize human health because humans have the consciousness to manage biodiversity resources for many species on the planet.

Applications of One Health or Ecohealth, in this respect, would be that human, animal, plant and ecosystem health are interconnected and, therefore, the health of each is directly or indirectly related to one another, suggesting that there is equal importance given to biodiversity, human health and domestic animal health.

A side note to this discussion is that humans are part of biodiversity because we are a species that is part of the ecological community on the planet. The recent ecological evidence would indicate that we are the most influential species.

Extinction occurs when species disappear entirely from the Earth, and it is currently happening at an unprecedented rate, often referred to as the '**sixth mass extinction**' or 'biodiversity crisis'. Human activities, such as deforestation, habitat destruction, overexploitation of natural resources, pollution, climate change and introduction of invasive species, have significantly accelerated the rate of extinction. As a result, countless plant and animal species are disappearing, leading to the loss of vital ecological functions, genetic diversity and potential resources for human use. The ramifications of extinction are profound and far-reaching, disrupting ecosystems, jeopardizing food and water security, and affecting human livelihoods and health. Additionally, the disappearance of species can lead to the loss of potential sources for scientific discoveries and future adaptations to environmental challenges (Wilson, 1992).

Another major concern is pollution. It refers to the release of harmful substances or contaminants into the environment, causing adverse effects to many living organisms, ecosystems and human health. These substances are, usually but not always, sourced from human activities. Pollution comes in various forms: air pollution, which involves harmful gases and particles emitted from vehicles, industries and fossil fuel combustion; water pollution, which contaminates water bodies with chemicals, sewage and industrial waste; and soil pollution, which degrades soil quality through the accumulation of harmful substances like pesticides and heavy metals. Other types include noise pollution, light pollution and thermal pollution. Pollution has severe consequences, such as ecosystem degradation, biodiversity loss, air pollution-related respiratory problems, contaminated water supplies, **soil degradation**, habitat destruction and animal health issues such as disruption of endocrine functions. Addressing pollution is crucial for safeguarding the environment (Manisalidis *et al.*, 2020).

Climate change refers to the long-term alteration of Earth's climate patterns due to human activities, primarily the excessive emission of greenhouse gases. The risks associated with climate change are numerous and diverse. Rising temperatures lead to heatwaves, wildfires and sea-level rise, threatening coastal communities and ecosystems. Extreme weather events like hurricanes, heavy rainfall and droughts are becoming more frequent and severe. Ecosystems and biodiversity are disrupted, affecting species distribution and migration. Food and water security are at risk due to changes in agricultural productivity and water availability. Health issues, economic losses and social disruptions also result from climate change. Addressing these risks requires global cooperation, mitigation efforts to reduce emissions, and adaptation measures to build resilience to climate impacts. Urgent action is essential to secure a sustainable future for humanity and the planet (Box 7.1).

In the next sections, these important topics are dealt with one by one. For each, the value and importance of the ecosystem services are described, followed by the problem description, drivers of the problem, as well as ongoing and potential actions and solutions.

Box 7.1. Triple Planetary Crisis

Triple Planetary Crisis is what the UN refer to as the three main interlinked issues that humanity faces, namely biodiversity loss, pollution and climate change. In addition, humans are the main drivers of these issues.

The UN has organized programmes, conventions and frameworks to manage the triple planetary crisis as the implications of these issues are pressing for the planet and humanity. More information is available on the UN website (https://unfccc.int/blog/what-is-the-triple-planetary-crisis).

7.3 Breakdown of the Main Problems the Earth is Facing

7.3.1 Biodiversity loss and one of its key drivers: food production

7.3.1.1 The cultural value of ecosystem services of biodiversity

In terms of direct impacts on human health, biodiversity in green spaces has a significant effect on human mental health and wellbeing, both directly and indirectly (Carrus *et al.*, 2015). Positive links with biodiversity are most evident when assessing species richness and mental wellbeing relationships (Marselle *et al.*, 2019). Local studies have associated plant and bird abundance with positive influences on reflection, mental health and mental wellbeing (Dallimer *et al.*, 2012; Fuller *et al.*, 2007; Cox *et al.*, 2017). The abundance of a taxonomic group may be more noticeable by people than the number of species, given that most people cannot distinguish between species (Dallimer *et al.*, 2012). There are several theoretical frameworks linking the influence of nature and biodiversity to our wellbeing. Attention-restoration theory proposes that natural settings are mentally restorative, offering opportunities for reflection and recovery from mental fatigue due to focused attention on cognitive tasks (Kaplan and Kaplan, 1989). Stress-reduction theory suggests that encounters with natural environments will have a stress-reducing or restorative influence (Ulrich *et al.*, 1991). The sense of place framework suggests that the positive relationship between people and greenspaces is an emotional bond associated with specific locations (Altman and Low, 1992), or a sense of identity through association with a place (Proshansky *et al.*, 1983).

Human cultures have co-evolved with the environment. Cultural landscapes are the result of enduring and intricate human–nature interactions (Tieskens *et al.*, 2017; Assandri *et al.*, 2018). Cultural landscapes promote provision of cultural ecosystem services as set out in the Millennium Ecosystem Assessment (2005) (Tengberg *et al.*, 2012), i.e. the 'non-material benefits people gain from ecosystems, such as spiritual, religious, aesthetic and cultural values (Millennium Ecosystem Assessment, 2005).

Biodiversity conservation also contributes to the preservation of spiritual identity. An example of this can be seen in the spiritual and religious significance of vultures in Parsi communities in India. The ancient Parsi religion holds earth, fire and water sacred and, to avoid contaminating them, Parsis dispose of their dead by placing them in 'Towers of Silence', where the corpses are left exposed in the open for vultures to rapidly strip the bones of flesh (Markandya *et al.*, 2008). The decline in vulture populations means that human corpses are no longer being adequately disposed of using this method, impacting the spiritual service provided at the Towers of Silence (Prakash *et al.*, 2003).

The importance of the cultural, spiritual and religious values that are tied to biodiversity cannot be overstated. Owing to their intangible nature, however, they are often difficult to quantify and to integrate into economic evaluations (Plieninger *et al.*, 2015). These services are essential for human quality of life and must be conserved to protect the cultural identity of past, present and future generations.

Task: Think about where and how you grew up and where and how you live now. Was / is there a natural environment with abundant biodiversity that allows you to explore forests, underwater worlds and observe wildlife? Is nature talked about in your community or integrated into daily life or even worshipped or referred to in religion? Have you had formal or informal education that has covered biodiversity? How did all these things shape your knowledge and awareness of biodiversity? Has it changed over time and how? Were there any critical moments that influenced this change?

Example answer: Below is an account from a woman in Australia who is 27 years of age. Your story may look very different, and this is absolutely fine because this is about exploring your relationships to biodiversity, where every person's story is different. The example below shows resilience, awareness of transdisciplinary approaches and reflexivity.

From a young age, my life was intricately tied to the ocean. Living in a coastal village, my parents were skilled divers who relied on the sea for their livelihood as diving instructors. As soon as I could swim, I wanted to accompany my parents on their underwater journeys. I marvelled at the beautiful creatures living underwater and while enjoying the multiple different fish, corals, and turtles, I never thought much about biodiversity and it was not something talked about at school either. For years, I used diving as a recreational activity while getting trained and working in it. One summer when visiting my parents, I decided to swim out to one of my favourite coral reefs from my childhood. The once impressive coral reefs bore scars of coral bleaching, with patches of pale and lifeless structures. Plastic debris and discarded fishing tackle marred the otherwise pristine seafloor. My heart sank, as I realized that human actions were taking such a visible toll on the very biodiversity that fascinated me. Not immediately, but during the weeks that followed, something inside me started to shift. At first, I didn't know what it was that bothered me - the destruction of beauty? Not having a place my children could explore in the same way? My own thoughtless behaviour? As the week passed by, I started to feel that I was angry - with myself - for taking things for granted and not educating myself properly. I started to feel a strong sense of responsibility and it was at that point that I decided to approach local politicians in an attempt to communicate the importance of the coral, not only as a natural resource, but also its value as a cultural, societal resource as well as its natural beauty. All the time I was reading and beginning to understand how sensitive coral is and how it needs to be managed for sustainable use. After verbal and written communication with various politicians and local stakeholders (including those who rely on tourism activities and diving centres, like my parents), I realized that this was a value conflict where various stakeholders have different views on how resources should be managed. The disagreement was between those who wish to protect the biodiversity in the seas and those who wish to exploit resources for excessive economic gain. While I could never understand those who wish to exploit a beautiful resource, like coral, for economic gain, I have learned to sit on a local working group with a range of stakeholders in order to find resolutions to our differences with the aim of integrating our views and working together towards a shared solution towards using and pursuing the coral at the same time. This process has enabled me to accept and work with a range of different views, which are unlike mine, on this issue (reflexivity). My working group and I have also come to accept that we can influence activities at a local scale but other factors, such as increasing ocean temperatures, are beyond our influence, although they have impact on the health of the coral.

7.3.1.2 The problem: mass extinction

The Earth is currently undergoing a rapid, massive loss of biodiversity, heralding the sixth mass extinction event in the planet's history. During the past century, there has been a loss of vertebrate species at a rate 100 times higher than natural background extinction rates (Ceballos *et al.*, 2015), and rates of extinction and reduction of species abundance among invertebrates are at least as severe as among vertebrates (Dirzo *et al.*, 2014). Ongoing biodiversity loss is driven largely by human activity (Ceballos *et al.*, 2015) and will result in ecological changes that will limit future ecosystem resource availability. Current estimates indicate that human impact on the environment and biodiversity is demonstrated by the loss of 69% of the world's vertebrate biomass since 1970 (Westveer *et al.*, 2022), and more than a million plant and animal species are threatened with extinction (Díaz *et al.*, 2019). Although some of the functional implications for biodiversity loss are obvious, e.g. ecosystem services, Box 7.2 describes some less obvious associations between overall biodiversity and humans. Again, it should be noted that there are region variations where the USA and Europe have disproportionally liability for biodiversity loss and climate change.

7.3.1.3 The drivers: anthropocentric and Capitalocene role in biodiversity loss, food production and global land-use changes

Human activity drives ecological loss and accelerated extinction via overexploitation of ecosystem resources, habitat destruction, introduction of invasive species and climate change (Dirzo *et al.*, 2014). Although we cannot compare or equate the responsibility of a rural subsistence female farmer in Mozambique with a giant producer of food from Brazil, we should be aware of the **CAPITALOCENE**, which is a system that not only accumulates capital, but drives extinction; see Moore (2017) for more details. We will discuss this in broader terms.

Box 7.2. Biodiversity (old friends) hypothesis

According to the biodiversity hypothesis (Hanski *et al.*, 2012), contact between people and microbial biodiversity is important for human health, especially in childhood. Chronic human health conditions associated with urban lifestyles are on the rise (Dye, 2008). One of the main challenges in this field of research is unravelling the importance of the specific quality of exposure to nature elements (Frumkin *et al.*, 2017) and biodiversity (Aerts *et al.*, 2018). Enhanced immune functioning emerges as one promising candidate of a central pathway between nature and human health (Kuo, 2015). Plants, animals and humans are colonized by microorganisms (microbiota) and exposed to countless others (Flandroy *et al.*, 2018). The microbiota affect the development and function of essentially all organic systems from organ to ecosystem, protecting against pathogenic microorganisms and toxins. Genetics and lifestyle factors, including contact with the natural environment, affect the composition of the microbiota, influencing all host health. Humans, animals and plants share similar relationships with microbes. For example, research demonstrates the influence of environmental microbial ecosystems on the microbiota and human health of organisms and indicates links between environmental and internal microbial diversity and good human health, and this is the case with other species. Recently, results suggested a link is emerging between environmental microbial biodiversity, the microbiome and positive effects on immunological and other health outcomes in the children (Roslund *et al.*, 2021; Gisler *et al.*, 2021). Especially during childhood, exposure to specific microorganisms and/or a diverse environmental microbiome has been associated with a lower risk of developing inflammatory conditions, such as allergies, asthma and rheumatoid arthritis (Ege *et al.*, 2011; Fyhrquist *et al.*, 2014; Sandhya *et al.*, 2016; Kirjavainen *et al.*, 2019), although the exact relationship is yet to be elucidated.

Many of these drivers are directly or indirectly related to food production. Biodiversity forms the basis of the ecosystem services which are essential to sustain agriculture and human wellbeing (Convention on Biological Diversity, 2008), and biodiversity and agriculture are strongly intertwined.

In recent decades, global biodiversity has been degraded at an unprecedented rate (Ceballos *et al.*, 2015) because of worldwide population growth and the increased consumption of natural resources (Jackson *et al.*, 2007). The homogenization of agricultural production systems, chiefly due to intensification of practices, is one of the greatest causes of agrobiodiversity loss, predominantly through genetic erosion and increasing levels of genetic vulnerability for specialized livestock and crops (Convention on Biological Diversity, 2008). This has impacted the production of food, fuel and raw materials, alongside the provision of ecosystem services.

In the past 60 years, 32% of the global land area has been impacted by land-use change (for example, from forest to cropland), with most of that change due to agricultural intensification (Winkler *et al.*, 2021). Today, agriculture uses 50% of habitable land, with 77% of agricultural land devoted to livestock grazing or animal feed production, and 23% used by all other crops (Ritchie and Roser, 2013). Management and financial decisions for much of the land used for agriculture are focused on their globalized ownership, reflecting little sensitivity to biodiversity or the viability of local communities.

Land-use change is directly linked to losses in biodiversity (Newbold *et al.*, 2015), which occur through a variety of mechanisms including habitat loss and **habitat fragmentation**. Tropical deforestation in Brazil for beef and soy production (Dirzo *et al.*, 2014) has famously led to habitat loss. Fragments of remaining tropical rainforest are broken up by tracts of land for cattle grazing areas and crop production, disrupting natural wildlife movement patterns. Similar processes of land-use change, through linear infrastructure (roads and railway) development within the savannah and steppe landscapes of Central Asia, have impacted on biodiversity, e.g. the population of saiga antelopes, *Saiga tatarica*, has crashed dramatically in recent years for many reasons, including habitat fragmentation and isolation (UNEP, 2017; Wetzel, 2022).

Modern agricultural production systems can be highly intensive and extractive, managing the ecosystems of agricultural land to produce maximum yields of a single commodity (DeFries and Nagendra, 2017) while devaluing existing biodiversity and ecosystem services (defined gains acquired by humankind from surroundings ecosystems) that the land previously provided, such as flood alleviation. Overgrazing, deforestation, insufficient crop rotation and conventional tilling methods can all contribute to soil degradation and soil loss, which reduce the capacity of the land to support plant life (Jie *et al.*, 2002). Excess application of fertilizers, pesticides and antimicrobials can also upset terrestrial and aquatic ecosystems and have contributed to substantial decreases in pollinator species in recent years (Potts *et al.*, 2010). Loss of pollinator insects, needed for 75% of the world's human food crops, will reduce future crop yields and exacerbate the need for more intensive practices to grow the same amount of food (Dirzo *et al.*, 2014). Indeed, the management of the domestic honeybee, *Apis mellifera*, appears to have direct and indirect negative impacts on wild bee pollinators (Elbgami *et al.*, 2014; Pirk *et al.*, 2017).

Increases in agricultural land use occurred in response to the need to feed the rapidly expanding global population. This reached 1 billion in 1803, and then 2 billion 124 years later (Roser *et al.*, 2013). The population has since increased by 1 billion approximately every 16 years, up to the current 8.1 billion. Rising concerns around how to feed this population have led to estimates that the total global food demand may increase by 35–56% from 2010 to 2050 (van Dijk *et al.*, 2021). The worldwide burden of obesity coupled with undernutrition in the global south indicates that the challenge is not only to produce sufficient calories, but to distribute them equitably to meet diverse nutritional needs (Swinburn *et al.*, 2019). Opinions vary, however, on the best way to meet these needs while preserving biodiversity.

7.3.1.4 Current and potential actions and solutions to reduce biodiversity loss from food production

Sustainable intensification and changing dietary patterns

Some analysts suggest that ecosystem-conscious '**sustainable intensification**' will allow us to produce more food while protecting biodiversity (Holt *et al.*, 2016). Such approaches are increasingly discussed across government, industry and non-governmental organization sectors. These approaches would require multifunctional land use, integrated pest management to reduce pesticide use, and development of high-yield, environmentally resilient strains of crops, among other approaches (Holt *et al.*, 2016; Crist *et al.*, 2017). However, it is unclear as to what extent and how quickly agricultural land use can realistically be optimized in this way. This approach will also increase the upfront cost of food production, so food producers will require economic or regulatory incentives to enact these changes.

Other analyses suggest that shifting global dietary patterns and minimizing food waste will allow us to feed a growing population without further intensification of food production. These approaches again rely on incentivizing relatively small but influential societal groups to make fundamental changes to global food systems (Crist *et al.*, 2017). The growing global middle class is increasing demand for meat and processed foods, two classes of foods that draw heavily on commodity crops such as soy, sugar and corn and, in the case of processed foods, are of poor nutritional value. Overconsumption of both meat and processed foods must be reduced in favour of diverse, plant-based diets to have a chance at feeding the future global population at current food production levels, as has the use of alternative and surface efficient protein sources, e.g. chicken (Eshel *et al.*, 2014). Gender also has to be taken into consideration when addressing this challenge because gender differences exist in meat consumption (Ritzel and Mann, 2021).

Reframing biodiversity protection in economic terms

Underpinning these approaches (and others not discussed here) to feed the world is a need to reframe biodiversity protection in economic terms. Powerful transnational food corporations hold major influence with governance groups and are allowed to pass the societal and environmental costs of food production on to the public at large to maximize their own profit (Swinburn *et al.*, 2019). Consumers often live far from the ecosystems being directly impacted, and this decoupling reduces the likelihood that consumers will place economic or political pressure on responsible parties (DeFries and Nagendra, 2017). Economic **valuation** of **ecosystem services** (Chapter 13) can raise public awareness of the value of different ecosystems and provide the information needed to hold transnational food corporations to account for their practices and potentially facilitate consumer behavioural change towards more environmentally sustainable production systems. Ecosystem services valuation may also be used to create regulations that shift market dynamics and convince food producers that it is in their own economic interest to pursue ecosystem-sensitive practices. One estimate suggests that, per hectare per year, the value of terrestrial ecosystem services ranges from US$149 for cropland, to $376 for grassland, $3251 for tropical forest and $23,952 for wetland (Li *et al.*, 2019). Such valuations make it clear that the price of sacrificing diverse ecosystems for the diminishing returns of modern food production systems is too high to bear.

Empowering communities and using community-based/traditional knowledge

Considering the interlinked environmental, health and climate crises, which indicates the great acceleration of human actions and impacts into the Anthropocene, conservation and restoration of biodiversity have become the top priorities in delivering UN Sustainable Development Goals. In addition, the specific component of the Anthropocene needs to be acknowledged and addressed, i.e. Capitalocene, which is a system that not only accumulates capital, but drives extinction (Moore *et al.*, 2017).

Protected areas represent the most widely used tool for safeguarding biodiversity and there is no doubt that granting legal protection to areas of high conservation and biodiversity value is essential to defend vital natural resources (Watson *et al.*, 2014). However, the physical separation of people and nature upon which the original concept of national parks was created in the USA, and later exported to other continents, has contributed to a belief system that views humans and nature as separate entities. Communities have different conceptions and relations to nature according to class, gender, education level, origin, country of birth and residence, culture, religion, amongst others, and farmers, fishermen and fisherwomen, hunters and gatherers do not have the same relation to nature and biodiversity as urban communities since their interactions are different. Siloed perspectives that separate humans from nature and biodiversity are partly responsible for the ill-health of the planet and of people, and the call for a holistic One Health perspective for health and the environment. In addition, this view ignores geographic factors. For example, there are different compositions and configurations of land uses in various parts of the world where, for example, in North and South America there is greater separation between agricultural and biodiversity in national parks, often referred to as land-sparing, and alternative situations such as in Europe, where the integration of production agriculture and biodiversity is more prevalent (Fischer *et al.*, 2014; Kremen, 2015), referred to as land-sharing. This debate has been divisive and often seems to ignore the fact that, in the Anthropocene, the planet is composed of a set of cultural landscapes rather than pristine natural landscapes. In relation to the land-sparing and the land-sharing debate, there are a range of factors like geography and socio-economic factors that influence decision making around food security, biodiversity and land scarcity.

As there is now a move towards the protection of 30% of the planet Earth (both terrestrial and marine), much more consideration needs to be given to Indigenous Peoples and Local Communities (IPLCs) living in biodiverse areas and ecologically intact landscapes (Dinerstein *et al.*, 2020). There are at least 370 million people who define themselves as Indigenous; descendants of people who inhabited countries before the time of conquest or colonization. It is estimated that Indigenous Peoples manage or have tenure rights over a quarter of the world's terrestrial surface, intersecting with about 40% of all terrestrial protected areas or ecologically intact landscapes; their involvement in meeting local and global conservation goals is essential (Garnett *et al.*, 2018). There are, however, serious concerns about the rights of IPLCs, as many communities surrounding protected areas have been unable to access their ancestral lands or utilize the natural resources they contain, which impacts their subsistence, traditions and culture. Spatial and social marginalization of IPLCs from their land creates a sense of bio-cultural dislocation, contributing to poorer health and social outcomes for Indigenous versus non-Indigenous populations (Anderson *et al.*, 2016; Garnier *et al.*, 2020).

Biodiversity conservation and restoration efforts need to recognize and support community stewardship and rights-based approaches, promoting the unique environmental knowledge and management practices of IPLC groups (Garnier *et al.*, 2020). Biodiversity loss is most critical in economically poor, but biodiversity-rich countries of the global south, where a whole range of ecosystems are being (have been) destroyed or irretrievably altered, as it is in the case of Africa. The experiences (successes and failures) gained by local institutions and individuals involved in biodiversity conservation in Africa have been reviewed by Bennun *et al.* (1995). By acknowledging that their health and wellbeing, way of life, values and belief systems are entirely dependent on their holistic relationship with nature, IPLCs have developed locally adapted management systems which can deliver remarkable conservation outcomes, often better than protected areas without Indigenous Peoples (Schuster *et al.*, 2019). Conservation actions need to be co-designed with all **stakeholders** and to combine enhanced understanding from One Health approaches with traditional environmental knowledge to ensure **sustainability**. For example, Indigenous Peoples' food systems are often extremely diverse, representing vital knowledge repositories on what a healthy and resilient diet with minimal environmental impacts might look like.

Around 80% of the world's population is estimated to use traditional medicine (Ekor, 2014), both through cultural preference and because of lack of access to Western healthcare. In addition, within the veterinary field, traditional medicine (ethnoveterinary) practices are well known, especially in the global south (McGaw and Abdalla, 2020). Traditional medicines derived from plants and animals are drawn from biodiverse environments by IPLCs but are often under threat from broader environmental destruction or increasing demand. The efficacy of these medicines and the pressure placed on these plants and animals may be at odds. The WHO has created a Global Centre for Traditional Medicine to develop a body of reliable evidence and data on traditional medicine practices and products. Many of these medicinal products are also of interest for pharmaceutical research (WHO, 2019a). Importantly, Tu Youyou was awarded the prestigious Nobel Prize in Physiology or Medicine in 2015 for her discovery of artemisinin from the leaves of *Artemisia annua*. This plant-based drug has significantly reduced the mortality rates for patients affected by malaria and has been a significant breakthrough in Tropical Medicine. This type of medical practice and knowledge can be closer to caring for nature and biodiversity conservation targets (Kassam *et al.*, 2010; Unnikrishnan and Suneetha, 2012; Barata *et al.*, 2016), but may also result in unsustainable use (IPBES, 2022).

Using an interdisciplinary approach for agrobiodiversity

Biodiversity is the foundation of agriculture, and greater biodiversity in complex landscapes potentially enhances agricultural production by providing **ecosystem resilience**, which enhances human wellbeing (Estrada-Carmona *et al.*, 2022). While biodiversity is crucial for agricultural production and food security, traditional agricultural practices encourage biodiversity, whereas modern practices do not facilitate species richness or diversity to the same extent, meaning that additional resources are needed to encourage biodiversity. Traditional farming methods have a reliance on manual labour with older techniques used to grow crops and livestock husbandry, with fertility often provided by manures. There is a closer link to the seasonal climate as production is closely linked to natural resources and temperatures. Traditional farming emphasizes the importance of crop diversity, rotation and intercropping to maintain soil fertility and pest control naturally, with a strong connection often developed between the land and communities (Pretty *et al.*, 2005).

Regenerative agriculture is a holistic approach to farming that aims to restore and enhance the health of agroecosystems by improving soil health and fostering sustainable agricultural practices. This includes activities such as holistic grazing, cover cropping, crop rotation, minimal soil disturbance and integrated pest management. Regenerative agriculture aims to improve soil structure, increase water retention and promote biodiversity (O'Donoghue *et al.*, 2022).

Agrobiodiversity encompasses the genetic, species and ecosystem diversity of mammals, plants and microorganisms, and is the result of the interactions between these and management practices developed over millennia by farmers to cultivate crops and rear animals (Jackson *et al.*, 2013a, b; Convention on Biological Diversity, 2008). Furthermore, agrobiodiversity can provide plausible solutions to challenges posed by climate change, pests and diseases by offering genetic resources for crop improvement and innovation. Box 7.3 summarizes key aspects of agrobiodiversity.

Agrobiodiversity incorporates socio-cultural, economic and environmental elements, and is sustained in a mutually beneficial feedback loop (Fig. 7.3). It is essential for the provision of food and raw materials and performs the ecosystem services necessary to sustain human life. Moreover, the genetic diversity of agrobiodiversity enables species to adapt to environmental shifts, allowing for their evolution in response to, for instance, drought or frost, alongside disease, pests and parasites. This is imperative in the face of ever-looming climate change. The evolution of biodiversity, and hence our survival, hinges on this genetic diversity.

Agriculture faces two main challenges regarding biodiversity:

- Sustaining food production, agrobiodiversity and ecosystem services; and
- Mitigating the negative effects of agricultural management practices on biodiversity.

Box 7.3. Aspects of agrobiodiversity (based on Convention on Biological Diversity, 2008)

1. Genetic variation:
Genetic variation is the foundation of global food production (Soumya *et al.*, 2021). Globally, genetic diversity in livestock is steadily decreasing due to selective plant and animal breeding and the harmonizing effects of globalization (Soumya *et al.*, 2021). Species selection leads to an increased abundance of a limited number of wild terrestrial species, with domesticated (food-producing) species creating a major shift in vertebrate biomass composition since the beginning of the Agricultural Revolution (Smil, 2003). Resilience to, for example, pandemics is created through biodiversity and critical decision makers in the public and private sectors, at local and global level, sticking to the idea that a major increase in biodiversity can be enabled by reacting to acute crises instead of developing systems resilience (Lomborg, 2001).
2. Ecosystem services and the organisms that support them (Foley *et al.*, 2011; McIntyre *et al.*, 2018). These services include:
   - Food production
   - Forest production
   - Nutrient cycling
   - Pest and disease regulation
   - Pollination, pollution and sediment regulation
   - Maintenance of the hydrological cycle, erosion control
   - Climate regulation and carbon sequestration
   - Infectious disease mediation
3. Abiotic factors
   - Local climatic and chemical factors
   - The physical structure and functioning of ecosystems
4. Socio-economic and cultural dimensions: Agrobiodiversity is moulded by human activities and management practices. These dimensions include:
   - Traditional and local knowledge of agrobiodiversity
   - Cultural factors and participatory processes
   - Gender equity
   - Agricultural landscape-related tourism

To address these challenges, agriculture must consider different drivers of change and how they are contributing to the balance of sustainable food production and agrobiodiversity loss (Fig. 7.4).

It is vitally important that interdisciplinary and transdisciplinary approaches are used to protect our agrobiodiversity and safeguard food security. The economic, socio-economic and cultural value of biodiversity must be considered when developing and modernizing agricultural practices (Jackson *et al.*, 2007). Agrobiodiversity has been shaped by generations of farmers, and local and traditional knowledge and culture passed down in farming communities is central to the protection and management of agrobiodiversity (Convention on Biological Diversity, 2008). Moreover, the gender dimension of agrobiodiversity needs to be integrated since very often women have broad ethnobotanical knowledge that they use for harvesting, growing and conserving wild plants, which will help to improve resilience in difficult times (Garnier *et al.*, 2020).

Creating biodiverse environments to promote mental health and wellbeing

Policy makers and landscape planners should consider supporting biodiverse environments to promote mental health and wellbeing in the community (Methorst *et al.*, 2021). Protection of habitats to promote high species richness will not only help conservation goals, but it will additionally improve human health and wellbeing (Cook *et al.*, 2019).

The EKLIPSE project systematically reviewed the effects of specific types and characteristics of urban and

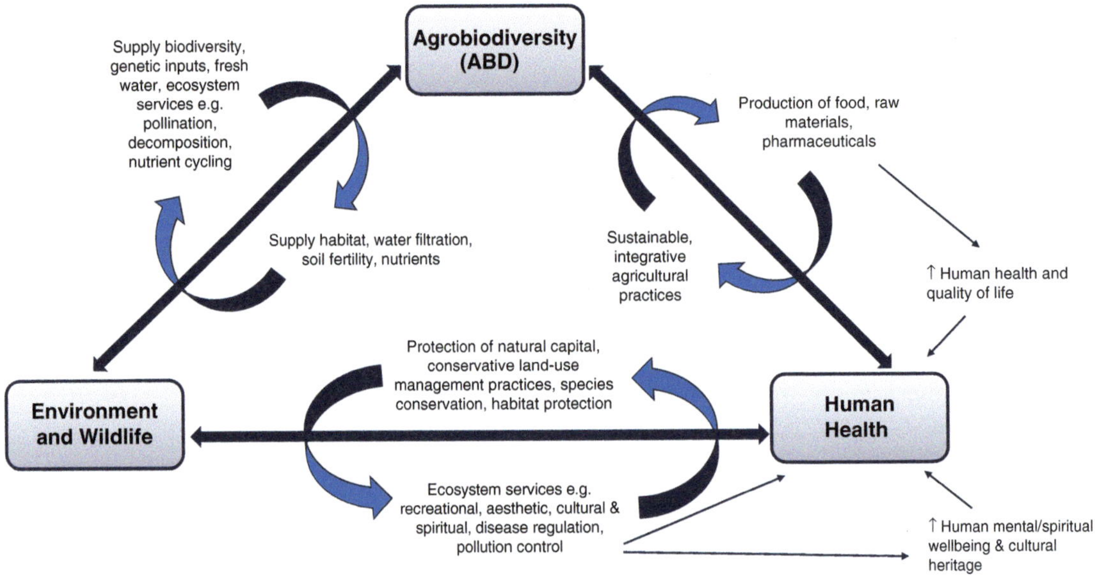

Fig. 7.3. The mutually beneficial relationships that exist between agrobiodiversity, the environment and wildlife, and human health, and the positive feedback loops that are created when the ecosystem services supported by these relationships are conserved. Developed by authors based on Scherr and McNeely (2007), Clark *et al.* (2014), Couvillion (2017) and Thatcher and Milner (2014).

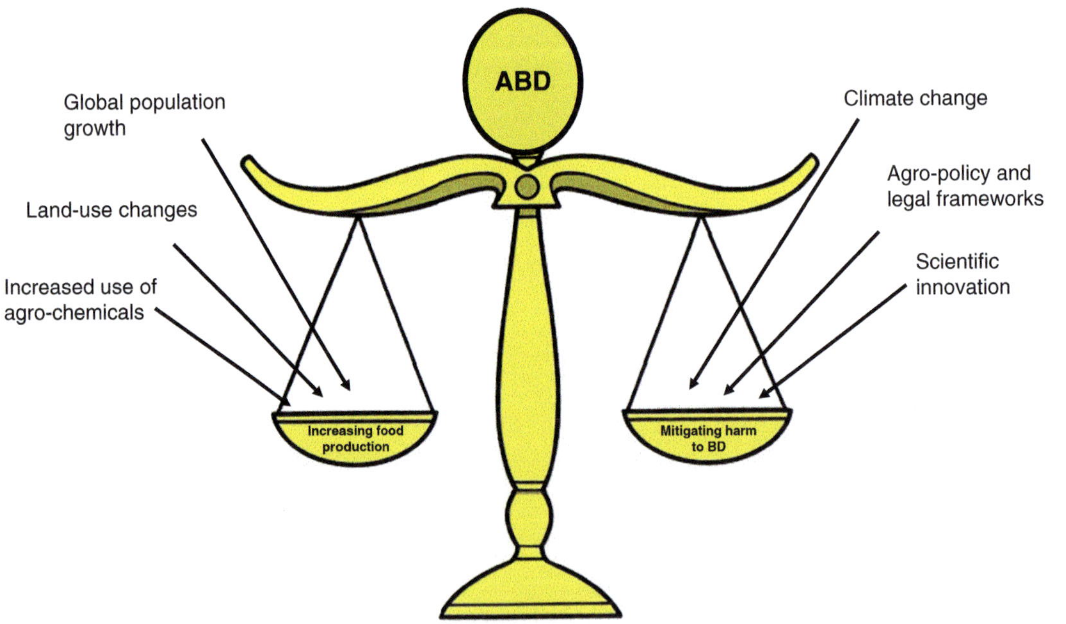

Fig. 7.4. The balance to be struck between sustainable increased food production and the mitigation of harm to biodiversity as a whole. ABD, agrobiodiversity. Developed by the author (Caoimhe Doyle).

peri-urban blue spaces on mental health and wellbeing (Beute, 2020). No firm conclusions regarding mental health and wellbeing effects on specific types and characteristics of urban and peri-urban blue spaces could be drawn. The EKLIPSE systematic review on those associations (Beute, 2020) did identify enough scientific studies to confirm findings on the mental health benefits of green spaces, for all types of green space considered in the literature. Yet, the review could not identify clear-cut, generalizable findings regarding specific types and characteristics of urban and peri-urban green space. The extensive review could not find a gold standard for a particular green space type or characteristic which works best for everyone, everywhere, and at every time. This heterogeneity may result from differences in exposure duration, in experiences (see also Bratman *et al.*, 2019), and among target groups. This leads to a recommendation of a variety of green space types to capture all potential users, needs and activities with a gender perspective since women and men present different sensitivities and expectations related to urban green spaces. Beute *et al.* (2020) stress the need to look at the effects of experienced, or perceived, biodiversity compared to objectively measured biodiversity; not all insects or plants may be perceived by green space visitors. Different studies show different outcomes, indicating that objective biodiversity levels may have more pronounced effects than how the green space visitors perceive biodiversity.

Task: In this section, you have learned about the value of biodiversity, the problem and drivers of biodiversity loss, and several actions that could help to reduce the problem including sustainable intensification, changing dietary patterns, empowering Indigenous Peoples' practices and knowledge, using interdisciplinary approaches for agrobiodiversity and creating green spaces. Thinking about a wider system, consider how these different actions and solutions interact, where they could be mutually beneficial and where there may be challenges.

Example answer: In a progressive agricultural initiative, a community in Costa Rica successfully achieved sustainable intensification by adopting interdisciplinary approaches for agrobiodiversity. By using ecological knowledge with modern farming techniques, they not only increased crop yields but also preserved the region's rich biodiversity. This transformation enabled them to shift their dietary patterns towards a healthier and more sustainable plant-based diet, reducing their reliance on livestock farming. Furthermore, they empowered Indigenous Peoples' practices and knowledge, integrating their traditional farming methods with modern agricultural innovations. As a result, the community not only thrived economically but also preserved their cultural heritage and integrity while creating lush green spaces that served as vibrant areas for biodiversity conservation, education and recreation. This approach serves as a model for sustainable agriculture and community development (Shaver *et al.*, 2015).

7.3.2 Disruptions to water, soil and air

7.3.2.1 Ecosystem services of freshwater, soil and air

Soil, water and air are intricately linked components of the Earth's environment, forming essential cycles that sustain life and maintain the health of ecosystems. The water cycle connects these three elements, as rainwater and surface water interact with the soil, infiltrating it to recharge groundwater and nourish plants. Through transpiration, plants release water vapour into the atmosphere, contributing to cloud formation and precipitation, continuing the cycle.

Freshwater systems play a fundamental role in the global water cycle – regulating and maintaining ecosystem services to supply, purify and protect freshwater resources (United Nations, 2021).

These services include:

- Water purification by trapping, processing and transforming pollutants, toxins and heavy metals present in water, thereby maintaining water quality for drinking and domestic use.
- Decomposition and cycling of nutrients, e.g. nitrogen and phosphorus through freshwater and terrestrial systems by aquatic plants and algae.
- Flood control by regulating the frequency and magnitude of runoff and flooding through water interception and storage.

- Erosion prevention, e.g. soil retention by using bankside vegetation, reed beds, riparian zones and wetlands.
- Carbon sequestration within living plant tissue and decomposed vegetation in waterlogged systems, helping to regulate carbon dioxide levels in the atmosphere.
- Regulation of local climate via evaporation over freshwaters and wetlands.
- Acting as fire breaks to regulate wildfire spread (MEA, 2005).

Soil serves as a crucial reservoir for water, retaining moisture in its pore spaces, influencing plant growth, microbial activity and nutrient availability. The nutrient cycling that occurs in the soil impacts plant health and productivity, affecting air quality through processes like photosynthesis and respiration. Soil acts as a reservoir for nutrients, and various microorganisms help to break down organic matter and release essential nutrients like nitrogen, phosphorus and potassium. This nutrient cycling supports plant growth and provides the foundation for healthy and productive ecosystems. Soil is the primary medium for growing crops and supporting both plant and animal agriculture, thereby sustaining human societies. Soil acts as a natural filter, removing impurities and contaminants from water as it percolates through the soil layers (McBratney *et al.*, 2014). This filtration process helps to improve water quality and ensure the availability of clean water for ecosystems and human use. Additionally, soil's ability to store and release water helps regulate water flow, reducing the risk of floods and droughts. Soil also plays a significant role in the exchange of greenhouse gases with the atmosphere, as certain microbes produce and consume gases like carbon dioxide, methane and nitrous oxide. Soil erosion can lead to sedimentation in water bodies, affecting water quality and aquatic ecosystems. Additionally, soil acts as a sink for certain air pollutants, filtering and trapping them before they reach the atmosphere.

The atmosphere is critical for the air we breathe. Plants, algae and some bacteria convert carbon dioxide into oxygen during photosynthesis, providing the primary source of breathable oxygen for all aerobic organisms, including humans and animals. The atmosphere absorbs and regulates the levels of carbon dioxide in the atmosphere. It helps to disperse pollutants and contaminants released into the air by human activities and natural processes, thereby reducing the immediate impact of pollutants on local ecosystems and populations. Finally, it plays a significant role in regulating the Earth's climate (McBratney *et al.*, 2014).

7.3.2.2 The problems: loss of soil, water and air quality

The decline in soil biodiversity, including beneficial microorganisms and soil-dwelling organisms, impacts soil health and nutrient cycling, affecting plant growth and ecosystem functioning. With a disruption of the intricate web of interactions that support soil fertility, there are problems of reduced agricultural productivity, degraded natural habitats and increased vulnerability to environmental stressors. Erosion leads to loss of fertile topsoil and sedimentation in water bodies. Desertification worsens environmental and food security challenges. Soil pollution poses risks to ecosystems, human health and food safety. Biodiversity loss disrupts the intricate web of interactions that support soil fertility, leading to reduced agricultural productivity, degraded natural habitats and increased vulnerability to environmental stressors. Conserving and restoring biodiversity is essential for maintaining healthy and fertile soils.

Biodiversity in freshwater ecosystems is in danger. Freshwater vertebrate species have declined more than twice as steeply as terrestrial or marine populations (WWF, 2018; Tickner *et al.*, 2020). Rivers, lakes and inland wetlands cover less than 1% of Earth's surface, and yet house approximately one-third of vertebrate species and 10% of all species (Strayer and Dudgeon, 2010). Climate change has impacted sensitive mountain ecosystems and associated biodiversity (Schmeller *et al.*, 2022), and ongoing modifications to high-mountain freshwater ecosystems may also have significant impacts on human wellbeing and livelihoods (Schmeller *et al.*, 2018). The biodiversity threat to these systems is clear with 29,500 freshwater-dependent species so far assessed for the IUCN Red List, and 27% of these threatened with extinction (IUCN, 2019).

Access to clean water is a necessity for human health (WHO, 2019b). Biodiversity of an ecosystem is fundamental in cleaning and purifying water that contributes to ecosystem health. It does so by supporting the provisioning and regulatory ecosystem services that maintain water quality (Marselle *et al.*, 2021; MEA, 2005). Contaminated water and poor sanitation are linked to transmission of diseases such as cholera, hepatitis A, typhoid and polio (WHO, 2019b). Symptoms such as diarrhoea are potentially indicative of a range of potential waterborne **pathogens**, including zoonoses like cryptosporidium, leptospirosis, vibriosis and amoebae. According to the Millennium Ecosystem Assessment, although ecosystems can be a source of impurities in freshwater, they also filter and decompose organic wastes introduced into waters (MEA, 2005).

Biodiversity loss and degradation of ecosystems, however, undermine the provisioning and regulatory services that ecosystems carry out to maintain access to safe, fresh water; this increases the transmission of infectious diseases (Everard *et al.*, 2020) and affects men and women differently as well since women and girls, for example, are responsible for fetching water in seven out of ten households without supplies on the premises, according to WHO. For instance, frequent handwashing has been identified as a key action required to slow the spread of COVID-19 (UNICEF, 2020). This suggests that undermining an ecosystem's ability to provide fresh water plays a significant role in the potential spread of infectious diseases (Everard *et al.*, 2020).

Air pollution arises from the release of harmful substances into the atmosphere, leading to adverse effects on health and the environment. It poses severe health risks, particularly in urban areas where concentrations of pollutants are higher. Short-term exposure to pollutants can lead to respiratory and cardiovascular issues, exacerbate asthma, and cause acute respiratory infections. Long-term exposure has been linked to chronic respiratory diseases, heart disease, lung cancer and even adverse effects on brain health. Acid rain, smog and ground-level ozone harm ecosystems, soils and the built environment. Another significant concern is air pollution's contribution to climate change (see the next section).

7.3.2.3 The drivers: human activity and food production

Human activity impacts water quantity and quality. Natural landscapes being lost to urbanization, industry and agriculture, mismanagement of our resources, combined with climate change, is devastating our global ecosystems, undermining their ability to provide essential freshwater services. This, in turn, threatens our health and the health of our natural environments (United Nations, 2021).

Unsustainable agricultural practices, such as excessive use of chemical fertilizers and pesticides, monoculture farming and intensive tillage, lead to soil degradation and nutrient depletion. Deforestation and land conversion for urbanization and industrial purposes disrupt natural ecosystems, reducing the protective cover of vegetation and exposing soil to erosion. Overgrazing by livestock in fragile ecosystems can lead to soil compaction and loss of vegetative cover. Additionally, pollution from industrial activities, improper waste disposal and mining operations can contaminate soils with heavy metals and harmful chemicals, rendering them unsuitable for agricultural use. The spread of toxins in soils, related to the dioxin accident in Seveso, Milan in 1979, was aggravated by heavy rainfall conditions during the autumn of 1976 (Cerlesi *et al.*, 1989). Land use and fertilizer applications have a significant impact on earthworms, which are pivotal for soil health (Singh *et al.*, 2019). The physical and chemical properties of soil can impact human health. For example, climate change has led to changes in soil microbial community composition, impacting soil functionality (Singh *et al.*, 2019; Cavicchioli *et al.*, 2019). This results in reduced capacity to produce food, directly impacting humankind, but also indirectly influencing higher trophic life-forms via changes to microorganism populations.

The primary sources of air pollution include industrial emissions, vehicular exhaust, burning of fossil fuels, agricultural activities, and natural phenomena like wildfires and volcanic eruptions. These activities release pollutants such as particulate matter (PM), nitrogen oxides (NOx), sulfur dioxide (SO_2), volatile organic compounds (VOCs), ozone (O_3) and carbon monoxide (CO) into the air. But almost all of the global population – 99% – breathe in polluted air according to WHO; a growing body of evidence suggests women are among the worst affected and breathing in pollutants is linked to, among other impacts, worsening maternal health outcomes (Mitku *et al.*, 2023).

Task: The drivers are manifold and interconnected and can be difficult to explain. To practise your One Health communication skills, summarize these drivers and their interconnectivity for the soil, air and water problems in a way suitable for a five-year-old child.

Example answer: Hey there, little buddy! Let me explain some things in a fun way! You know how we need water to drink and for plants and animals to live? Well, sometimes, what we do can make it hard for the Earth to have enough clean water. When people build big cities, factories and farms, it can change the land and water. And because of things like climate change, some places may not get enough rain, which makes it even harder for the Earth to have good water for us and all the animals. Soil is like the Earth's special blanket for plants to grow. But sometimes, when people do not take care of the land, the soil gets hurt. Using too many chemicals on farms and cutting down too many trees can make the soil not feel good. Even animals like earthworms that help the soil can get sad. We need to look after the Earth and make sure the soil stays healthy so we can grow yummy food and help all the little creatures. The air we breathe is so important! But sometimes, things we do like using too many cars or factories can make the air not very clean. This is called air pollution. It is like having too much dust in the air, and it can make people and animals feel sick. We need to be kind to the Earth and find ways to keep the air clean, so everyone can be happy and healthy.

Remember, we can be superheroes for the Earth by being careful with water, soil and air. Let's protect our home and all the animals and plants that live here!

7.3.2.4 Current and potential actions and solutions to reduce disruptions to water, soil and air

Water purification and waste treatment

Improve water quality to sustain aquatic life: The EU Urban Waste Water Treatment Directive (https://environment.ec.europa.eu/topics/water/urban-wastewater_en) is credited with the reduction of sewage production and demonstrates how legislation and policy can facilitate behavioural change. In Singapore, the regulation of polluting industries resulted in the relocation of pollution from pig and duck farms while encouraging business and development along the waterfront. Another example is in Lake Taupo, New Zealand, where catchment scale nitrogen caps, farmer permits and the establishment of a trust fund to help farmers reduce nitrogen have resulted in diffuse pollution from grassland agriculture. Other methods for freshwater improvement include the use of market-based incentives to reduce pesticides and fertilizer use, exemplified by cotton and sugarcane farming in India and Pakistan. While in China, floodplains have been restored along the Yangtze River that have improved water quality for fisheries and biodiversity in the form of a nature-based solution (Tickner *et al.*, 2020).

Protect and restore critical habitats: An example of the successful designation and management of a protected area is the 825,000 ha Bita River Basin in Colombia, which is designated as a Ramsar site. Another example of land-use planning for ecosystem services is the New York City Watershed Agreement, which resulted in improved land-use planning to protect and restore ecosystem services and planning in the Catskills–Delaware watersheds. Finally, habitat restoration of floodplain wetlands has been restored along the lower Danube River because of an international agreement between Bulgaria, Romania, Moldova and Ukraine (Tickner *et al.*, 2020).

Prevent and control non-native species invasions into waterways: The identification and control of introduction pathways for non-native carp species into the Great Lakes of North America has been a combination of risk assessment, prohibition of live fish transport and electrical barriers. Control and eradication of established invasive non-native species has been effective in Australia with weed species, e.g. *Mimosa pigra*, where managed areas limited the spread compared to unmanaged areas (Tickner *et al.*, 2020).

Soil security

Soil security is motivated by sustainable use of soil resources and focuses on the maintenance and improvement of global soil resources to produce food (McBratney *et al.*, 2014). Soil stewardship can act as the nexus for the integration of ecosystem services, One Health and good soil stewardship, improving the delivery of a range of ecosystem services including resilience in food production and disease mediation (Foley *et al.*, 2005; Keith *et al.*, 2016). For example, van Elsas *et al.* (2012) have demonstrated that increased diversity of the soil microbial community has controlled invasion by an *Escherichia coli* strain, indicating a relationship between soil stewardship, biodiversity and potential disease regulation. Another example highlights how improving soil structure and physical resilience could mediate disease (and possibly improve fertility) where leptospirosis outbreaks are linked to flooding. Poor soil hydrology and erosion mobilize bacteria into waterways (Raghavan *et al.*, 2012), while flood mitigation is a regulating ecosystem service (McBratney *et al.*, 2014) provided by well-structured soils. Therefore, soil management, as part of sustainable agricultural practices and elsewhere, will protect soil functioning, benefiting the delivery of ecosystem services as well as human, animal and ecosystem health (Purvis *et al.*, 2012).

Learning question: Can you think of actions and solutions that would help to improve soil, water and air quality simultaneously?

Example answer: Improving soil, water and air quality simultaneously requires an integrated approach that considers the interconnectedness of these elements. Implementing agroecological practices, like crop rotation, cover cropping and minimum tillage, can enhance soil health by increasing organic matter, reducing erosion, and minimizing the need for chemical fertilizers and pesticides. This boosts crop productivity but can also prevent soil runoff. Water quality in nearby rivers and streams can be improved. Planting trees and maintaining vegetative buffer strips can additionally help filter pollutants from runoff, further enhancing water quality. Further, adopting clean energy sources and reducing industrial emissions can reduce air pollution, benefiting human health, animal health and the environment. Integrated approaches like these address our challenges around soil, water and air quality, and promote a harmonious and sustainable coexistence among these critical components of our ecosystem.

7.3.3 Climate change

7.3.3.1 The function of climate

Climate refers to the long-term average of weather conditions in a particular region over an extended period, typically ranging from decades to centuries. It encompasses various elements of the atmosphere, such as temperature, precipitation, humidity, wind patterns and atmospheric pressure, which collectively define the climate of a specific area.

Climate plays a fundamental role in shaping the environment and influencing various natural processes, ecosystems and human activities.

7.3.3.2 The problem: future climate according to the IPCC

The International Panel on Climate Change (IPCC) reports that climate models indicate an increase in global mean surface air temperature relative to 1990 of about 3°C, with a likely range of 2.5°C to 4°C, by 2100 (IPCC, 2021a). Average global temperature has already increased by 1.09°C (0.95 to 1.20°C) from 1850–1900 to 2011–2020. Larger increases have been observed over land – 1.59°C (1.34 to 1.83) – than over the ocean – 0.88°C (0.68 to 1.01). Global mean sea level has increased by 0.20 m (0.15–0.25) between 1901 and 2018, and average sea level is expected to rise by 0.28–0.55 m by 2100 under the very low greenhouse gas (GHG) scenario and 0.63–1.01 m under the most extreme scenario (IPCC, 2021a). However, sea-ice melting is a nonlinear process; a complete melting of Greenland could add a further 7 m to sea-level rises. Some models suggest that the Greenland ice sheet could collapse with a further +1.5°C of warming, and this could happen as soon as 2030 (Lenton *et al.*, 2019; Ripple *et al.*, 2022). Other important **tipping points** include potential dieback of the Amazon rainforest, modification of the North Atlantic oceanic circulation, melting of the Antarctic ice sheet, coral reef die-off, changes in boreal forests and permafrost thawing (Lenton *et al.*, 2019). Global warming will lead to an increase in the occurrence of extremely hot days and a decrease in the occurrence of extremely cold days (IPCC, 2021a). The IPCC estimates that every additional 0.5°C of global warming causes clearly discernible increases in the intensity and frequency of extremes, including heatwaves and heavy precipitation, as well as agricultural and ecological droughts in some regions. Warmer temperatures will lead to a more vigorous hydrological cycle, causing more severe droughts and flooding (IPCC, 2021b). Sustained rapid climate change could shift the competitive balance of species, leading to the upsetting of ecosystem balances, and forest diebacks, as well as alteration in the terrestrial uptake and release of carbon, exacerbating further changes in climate (IPCC, 2021a).

Changes in climate can cause direct and indirect mediated impacts on ecosystem, human, animal (both domestic and wild) and plant health (Pecl *et al.*, 2017).

Changes in temperature including heat and cold waves have direct impacts upon organisms (Glaser *et al.*, 2016), and climate change can alter the distribution of species (Harley 2011; Dyderski *et al.*, 2017), and the resilience of community infrastructures, with knock-on effects on food security, disease transmission and carbon sequestration (Pecl *et al.*, 2017; see Box 7.4 for an example). Sea-level rise, drought and flooding can also influence the health of ecosystems and organisms, through direct as well as disease-related impacts, such as from vector-borne (McIntyre *et al.*, 2017; Caminade *et al.*, 2018), waterborne (McIntyre *et al.*, 2017; Levy *et al.*, 2018), soilborne (McIntyre *et al.*, 2017; Delgado-Baquerizo *et al.*, 2020), and foodborne transmission routes (McIntyre *et al.*, 2017) or from water-quality changes linked to **land-use change** and pollutants (Dunn *et al.*, 2015). Reduced rainfall and increased temperatures can lead to drought, causing forest fires and other air quality issues (Fiore *et al.*, 2012), leading to respiratory disease. Men and women are also impacted differently by climate change whether through a more difficult access to resources they are responsible for, such as water, or during extreme weather events when women can be considerably more impacted than men (Bagnol *et al.*, 2015; Garnier *et al.*, 2020). The threshold for vulnerability within populations may change depending upon their age, demographic and socio-economic structure; communities are not equally affected in terms of access to healthcare including vaccinations and other preventive measures against disease (dos Santos *et al.*, 2019), but also including mental health issues associated with climate change (Cianconi *et al.*, 2020). Poorer populations are more likely to become climate refugees and to need to migrate but may be less able to cope with such changes (Schmidt, 2015).

Changes in climate can have direct impacts upon the health of humans, animals and the environment. Climate change can also have indirect effects upon organisms, increasing stresses upon populations, but also upon natural and anthropogenic infrastructures including ecosystems and public health facilities, e.g. medical clinics (Boyce *et al.*, 2016). For humans, climate change can impact wellbeing but also livelihoods, probably reducing individuals' socio-economic status by changing their likelihood of being impacted by disease. For animals, drought will lead to a reduction in biodiversity and therefore availability of food sources, reducing the health status of wildlife populations, encouraging chronic non-infectious disease impacts and propagating infectious disease transmission (Morand and Lajaunie, 2021). Droughts can also influence the proximity of various animals (wild and domestic) to scarce water

Box 7.4. Climate change and pathogen emergence

Climate change does not happen in isolation; however, it is one of many factors that influence (as well as being influenced by) the health of our environment, through ecosystem services. This was illustrated perfectly in research that examined the factors affecting the emergence and re-emergence of human pathogens (Woolhouse and Gowtage-Sequeria, 2005); emergence is driven by many different parameters, so it is vital that One Health approaches are used to aid control. There are a number of factors causing pathogen emergence and re-emergence including land use, agricultural intensification, socio-economic factors, human demographics, human behaviour, ecological factors, poor human health, hospitals and medical procedures, pathogen evolution (e.g. development of antimicrobial drug resistance and increased virulence of pathogens), contamination of food sources or water supplies, international travel, failure of public health programmes and international trade (Jones *et al.*, 2008; Jones *et al.*, 2013; Olson *et al.*, 2015). Climate change was ranked the tenth most important factor influencing the development of vector-borne disease (Woolhouse and Gowtage-Sequeria, 2005). Multifaceted solutions to climate change require internationally established understanding; for example, the Shared Socio-economic Pathways (SSPs) are part of a scenario framework established by the climate change research community to help integrate analyses of future climate impacts, vulnerabilities, adaptation and mitigation (Riahi *et al.*, 2017). The SSP is a framework to describe an alternative trend in the evolution of society and ecosystems over a century timescale, in the absence of climate change or climate policies. The current Representative Concentration Pathway (RCP) is a set of four pathways of land use and emissions of air pollutants and greenhouse gases that span a wide range of future outcomes through 2100 (van Vuuren *et al.*, 2014). Emission scenarios are now coupled with SSPs within the RCP-SSP framework (O'Neill *et al.*, 2016, 2020).

points, further increasing the risk of disease transmission, including zoonoses. A prime example is the enhanced transmission of West Nile virus in California during drought periods (Paull *et al.*, 2017).

7.3.3.3 The drivers of climate change

Climate change is primarily driven by human activities (i.e. anthropogenically driven), with the main drivers being greenhouse gas emissions from burning fossil fuels for energy, industrial processes and deforestation. The burning of coal, oil and natural gas releases significant amounts of carbon dioxide (CO_2) into the atmosphere, while other activities like agriculture and livestock farming produce methane (CH_4) and nitrous oxide (N_2O) emissions. Deforestation and land-use changes release stored carbon into the atmosphere, reducing the capacity of trees to act as carbon sinks. Industrial activities and waste management also contribute to greenhouse gas emissions, as well as the release of aerosols that can have cooling and warming effects on the climate. Additionally, land degradation can release carbon stored in the soil into the atmosphere. These human-induced activities disrupt the Earth's climate system, leading to many of the problems described above. Calculate your own environmental footprint at https://footprint.wwf.org.uk. Note there are tips on how to reduce your footprint on the site.

7.3.3.4 Current and potential actions and solutions to prepare for and mitigate climate change

Efforts to mitigate climate change involve reducing greenhouse gas emissions, transitioning to renewable energy sources, promoting sustainable land-use practices, transforming food production, and adopting circular economy principles to address the drivers of climate change and build a more sustainable future for the planet. As mentioned in previous sections, it should be acknowledged that there are region variations where the USA and Europe have disproportionally liability for climate change.

Learning question: To mitigate the effects of the climate crisis, many actions are necessary and they are urgently needed now to protect future generations and allow them to have decent living conditions. However, the size of the task and the large uncertainty around what exactly will happen can lead to active dissociation and inaction.

Active dissociation from climate change refers to a conscious or intentional avoidance of engaging with or acknowledging the reality of climate change and its impacts. It involves distancing oneself mentally or emotionally from the issue, often as a coping mechanism to reduce feelings of anxiety, guilt or helplessness associated with the overwhelming nature of the problem.

Have you encountered the problem or seen it in others? How did that feel or how did you perceive it in others? What steps can you take to avoid feeling overwhelmed and paralysed into a state of inaction?

Example answer: While active dissociation may provide temporary relief from climate change-related anxiety, it can hinder collective efforts to address the problem effectively. Acknowledging and confronting the reality of climate change is essential for promoting awareness, fostering collective action, and finding sustainable solutions to mitigate its impacts. Active dissociation in high-profile individuals, such as politicians, can be extremely disheartening as it is clear that all countries and all levels of society need to take ownership of the problem in order to bring about meaningful solutions.

Encouraging open dialogue, providing accessible information, and fostering a sense of community and shared responsibility can help you and others to move from a state of dissociation to active engagement and positive action on climate change. A transdisciplinary and multidisciplinary approach could enable improved communication and knowledge exchange. Certainly, harnessing the expertise of sociologists and psychologists in conjunction with climate scientists and modellers could be an effective method to encourage individuals to deal with the scale of the challenge as well as provide advice on how we can make a behavioural change as individuals, e.g. eat less red meat, use public transport. This could help remove the sense of individual powerlessness and encourage positive action.

Preparing for climate change

We can best prepare for climate impacts by using research tools that incorporate life-cycle analysis with a gender perspective to understand the impact of changes in climate, including the following:

- Resultant physiological responses of organisms.
- Changes to chronic non-infectious and infectious diseases in terms of morbidity, mortality and the wellbeing of populations.
- Impacts on organism community infrastructures.
- Determinants which will influence future weather patterns including extreme weather events.

Simple, affordable planning responses are aided if we can most effectively identify strategies to improve community resilience; environmental hazards, including exposure to pollutants; and mechanisms of surveillance and preparedness for disease including preventive measures. To achieve this, a One Health approach is required to:

1. Precisely define the problems associated with climate change, creating large-scale horizon scanning mechanisms to help identify emerging trends, new developments and gaps in our current knowledge and understanding (e.g. Woolhouse and Gowtage-Sequeria, 2005; Jones *et al.*, 2008; Mawdsley *et al.*, 2009; Fiore *et al.*, 2012; Dunn *et al.*, 2015; McIntyre *et al.*, 2017).
2. Characterize variables involved in creating climate impacts (e.g. CEOS, 2011).
3. Conduct a gender analysis (Bagnol *et al.*, 2015; Garnier *et al.*, 2020).
4. Forecast future effects of climate on health and associated uncertainties (e.g. Caminade *et al.*, 2012; Liu-Helmersson *et al.*, 2014; Caminade *et al.*, 2014; Tjaden *et al.*, 2021; Guis *et al.*, 2011; Colón-González *et al.*, 2021; Romanello *et al.*, 2022).
5. Develop preventive and preparedness understanding and measures against these effects (e.g., Suk *et al.*, 2014; Riahi *et al.*, 2017).
6. Provide a system-wide transformation of all systems, including food systems, to avoid climate disaster (Rushton *et al.*, 2021; UNEP, 2022).

So, what is horizon scanning and how can you use it? **HORIZON SCANNING** is the systematic examination of information sources to detect early signs of important developments (Hines *et al.*, 2019). It is used to identify, assess and prioritize trends (or innovations) in a timely manner so that decision makers such as policy makers are best informed on emerging or re-emerging issues. Horizon scanning projects often use qualitative or semi-quantitative framework methods, utilizing the opinions of experts to provide evidence for policy makers to help decide where to focus resources or further information gathering. Such mechanisms can work well; however, limited resources mean that only a small number of trends (or innovations) can be prioritized for further work.

If we examine the efforts to transform the food system to prepare for future climate change scenarios, we can look at UN Food System Summits; the latest was in July 2023. Some current and future solutions include selection of climate smart varieties of crops, reducing food waste and food loss, promoting plant-based diets and aiming to achieve this by appropriate policies and regulations. One Health is likely to facilitate an improved impact when implementing these changes to the food system.

Learning questions: The impacts of changes in climate have become more obvious in your country, with the emergence and re-emergence of Chikungunya, Zika, West Nile, Yellow Fever and Visceral Leishmaniasis, which are caused by vector-borne pathogens. Modelling exercises are often used to identify what is going to happen to a certain pathogen causing disease now and in the future; these exercises are complex and expensive to develop.

Your government is worried about the diseases that are emerging, and what to do about them. They want to understand which diseases (caused by which pathogens) might be a problem, to know when to spend available financial resources on surveillance for the diseases, healthcare for when they happen, preventive measures such as bed nets, interventions such as vaccination, and control of aspects of the environment to reduce disease spread (e.g. making sure there is no standing water near people's houses). Your government appoints you as an expert in horizon scanning. They task you with developing a plan to identify which diseases should be looked at in more detail, before making further decisions.

Develop a plan for what your horizon scanning process will do, and how you will undertake the project. What evidence will you look at? Who will you involve in the process (if anyone else)? What **discipline**(s) will the other people you involve have experience of? At what point(s) during the life cycle of the pathogens will you examine evidence for? How will you assess differences in the evidence? In your plan, think about using a systems understanding, transdisciplinary approaches, and how you will harness uncertainty, paradox and limited knowledge.

Example answer: The ENHANCE project was developed to identify which infectious diseases and pathogens that cause impacts were most important in Europe when thinking about climate change (McIntyre *et al.*, 2010). It examined how realistic the threat to human and animal health from climate change actually was (McIntyre *et al.*, 2010), using objective, repeatable evidence-based methods. Of all infectious diseases, it prioritized those with the greatest potential impact using a proxy. Studying these in greater detail, it identified those which are sensitive to climate drivers, e.g. changes in temperature or rainfall, and identified their characteristics: were certain groups of pathogens most likely to be climate sensitive, and were they transmitted in specific ways (McIntyre *et al.*, 2017)? This involved developing a big data resource describing infectious pathogens, their hosts, vectors, and where they occur, by mining information from published sources (McIntyre *et al.*, 2014a; Wardeh *et al.*, 2015). A proxy for the impact of pathogens or diseases in humans or domestic animals (McIntyre *et al.*, 2014b) was based upon the Hirsch index (or H-index), which describes for a group of keywords or phrases the number of published papers and number of times these are cited; where the two are equal, this indicates the technical productivity and apparent scientific impact of the pathogen. The H-index score for diseases correlates well with metrics of disease impact such as disability-adjusted life-year (DALY) estimates (McIntyre *et al.*, 2011), health-adjusted life-years (Cox *et al.*, 2014), years-of-life-lost (Cox *et al.*, 2014), year-equivalents-of-reduced-function (Cox *et al.*, 2014), but also for Atlantic salmon (*Salmo salar*), changes in diseases in salmon stocks and national country-level concerns on infections (Murray *et al.*, 2016). For the pathogens with the greatest apparent impact, the research literature was systematically reviewed and scored for evidence linking pathogens to climate drivers. Final scores including the data distribution around these scores were calculated. The results suggest that zoonotic pathogens (transmitted between humans and animals) are much more likely to have at least one climate driver (e.g. be sensitive to changes in rainfall) than either human-only or animal-only pathogens. Certain pathogens are also associated with certain transmission routes, for example foodborne and waterborne pathogens are more likely to be zoonotic than non-zoonotic and directly transmitted pathogens are much less likely to be non-zoonotic than zoonotic. Some pathogens have much greater numbers of climate drivers, e.g. the helminth *Fasciola hepatica*, which causes liver fluke and is a concern in livestock, the zoonotic bacteria *Bacillus anthracis*, which causes anthrax, and zoonotic *Borrelia burgdorferi*, which causes emerging tick-borne Lyme disease. The study concluded that a large proportion of infectious pathogens are sensitive to climate drivers and therefore likely to be impacted by climate change. The best estimates of the impact of disease come from the global burden of disease (GBD) study, which includes quantification of deaths, long-term illness and disability caused by disease (GBD, 2019). For pathogens studied in both the GBD and ENHANCE, 37% of disability-adjusted-life-years were likely to change with changes in climate, e.g. diarrhoeal disease caused by foodborne and waterborne transmission is one of the highest causes of early death and disability in humans, particularly in poorer populations; many diarrhoeal pathogens are highly sensitive to climate change (McIntyre *et al.*, 2017). Once published, the results of the study were used by government and international agencies to prioritize which diseases to look at in more detail; they also appeared in policy documents published by the Food and Agriculture Organization of the United Nations, and were also reported by news outlets, to highlight the most important emerging diseases.

North and south dialogue and identification of pathways/climate justice

Low- and middle-income individuals and communities, which have contributed least to climate change, are the most affected by the consequential natural catastrophes. Developing countries have said that Western countries, which industrialized much earlier, are responsible for the bulk of the environmental damage, GHG emissions and therefore for global warming. This process has often been at the expense of the global south. Countries from the south have been demanding climate compensation from richer countries. Those who have generally contributed less to climate change are the most vulnerable. Regional contributions to global human-caused GHG emissions continue to differ widely with Northern America bearing the greatest liability per capita and Southern Asia bearing the lowest per capita. In addition, there are sectoral variations with respect to contributions with approximately 34% of net global GHG emissions coming from the energy **sector**, 24% from industry, 22% from transport and 6% from buildings (https://report.ipcc.ch/ar6syr/pdf/IPCC_AR6_SYR_LongerReport.pdf).

Gender issues and inclusiveness

Climate change has the greatest impact on sections of the population, in all countries, that are most reliant on natural resources for their livelihoods and/or who have the least capacity to respond to natural hazards (e.g. droughts, landslides, floods and hurricanes). Women commonly face higher risks and greater burdens from the impacts of climate change in situations of poverty, and the majority of the world's poor are women. Women's unequal participation in decision-making processes and labour markets compounds inequalities and often prevents women from fully contributing to climate-related planning, policy making and implementation (https://unfccc.int/gender). Some examples are listed:

1. Social, economic, legal, cultural and political factors influence how men and women impact the environment.
2. Men and women experience different health risks which are interconnected with gender inequality.
3. Human, animal and plant diseases impact men and women differently.
4. Biological differences between men and women influence differences in exposure, infection rates and mortality rates of men and women during their life cycle (Bagnol *et al.*, 2015).

The participation of men and women in decision making at the international level is unequal, with women representing only one third of the leaders sitting at the Bureau of the COP28 (https://unfccc.int/documents/636729).

Data show that women tend to be under-represented in decision-making bodies at all levels (international, national and local). As well as not taking part in political decisions affecting the planet, the nation or their community, women are often unable to make decisions relating to their own health. The under-representation of women at decision-making level means that their views, needs and knowledge are not taken into account. Under the right conditions, more women in decision-making positions will ensure better governance for all. Conversely, the lack of women in decision-making positions reflects a failure to recognize the diverse needs of citizens in public policy.

Most interventions are designed without the participation or even consultation of women:

- Women's knowledge and problems are not taken into consideration.
- Interventions impact nature in ways that women are not always conscious of and that do not provide solutions to women's constraints and needs.
- Interventions are thus more likely to employ men, give them more access to resources, power and knowledge, and reinforce power inequities.

The effects of climate change are not the same for men and women because of their different access to resources such as education, information, capital, access to land, wood and income. Women generally have less access to resources than men, which makes them more vulnerable to climate change (https://www.uil.unesco.org/en/lifelong-learning/gender-equality).

Men and women are affected differently by poverty and food security, two aspects linked to climate change. While young men tend, in some regions, to be attracted by the rural migration, women tend to stay.

As the main users of natural resources, women have an in-depth understanding of their environment, and their knowledge of biodiversity can be extensive. It is mainly women who manage plant biodiversity, at the interface between wild and cultivated species. Women gather and manage wild plants and gardens. They are herbalists and healers; they are the guardians of the entire seed cycle, from selection, cleaning and storage to identifying the seeds to be planted each season. In this way, they make the link with human nutrition and health (Howard, 2003).

The increase in the world's population and associated activities (e.g. increased deforestation, intensive food production, resource extraction and global travel) and the resulting state of the planet (e.g. global warming, loss of biodiversity) will lead to the emergence of new infectious diseases, probably zoonoses, with a pandemic risk if governments, health authorities and citizens do not act on these phenomena in a more systemic manner. The role of women in this debate is essential.

7.3.4 Biodiversity and infectious disease

7.3.4.1 The problem: infectious disease emergence and biodiversity

When we look at the ratio of relative biomasses of humans, domestic mammals and wild mammals there has been a dramatic change in the last 50–70 years. There used to be greater balance between the three but now the planet is utterly dominated by domestic mammals and humans (Smil, 2011) and we have noted a 69% decline in wild vertebrates since 1970 (Westveer *et al.*, 2022), which compounds the evidence regarding the decline in mammals. This reduced biodiversity index has also been linked with increased zoonotic spillover because there are more humans potentially in contact with wild areas, increasing the human–wildlife interface.

Infectious disease involves the interactions between species, including the hosts, pathogens, vectors and organisms with which these species interact (Keesing *et al.*, 2010). Shifts in biodiversity may potentially impact both the emergence and transmission of infectious diseases (Keesing *et al.*, 2010). While small alterations to biodiversity in an ecosystem with a high level of functional redundancy may lead to only small changes in ecosystem function (Jones *et al.*, 1994; Power *et al.*, 1996), the possibility of significant losses of function increases with increasing species loss and a reduction in redundancy (Naeem *et al.*, 1994). It is predicted that species will aggregate in new combinations at high elevations, in biodiversity hotspots, and in areas of high human population density in Asia and Africa, causing cross-species transmission of viruses an estimated 4000 times. Owing to their unique dispersal ability, bats account for most of the novel virus sharing (Luis *et al.*, 2013) and are likely to share viruses along evolutionary pathways that will facilitate future emergence in humans. Notably, this ecological transition may already be underway, and holding warming under 2°C within the 21st century will not reduce future virus sharing. There is an urgent need to pair viral surveillance and discovery efforts with biodiversity surveys tracking the range shifts of species, especially in tropical regions that contain the most zoonoses and are experiencing rapid warming (Carlson *et al.*, 2022).

Men and women impact their environment differently and are also impacted differently by it. **Sex** and **gender** are interacting variables[1] and may be involved in the transmission and acquisition of diseases and in the success or failure of treatments or interventions. Hence the importance of taking them into account in research, with the aim of reducing sex- and gender-related inequalities in the management of health problems and improving the wellbeing of people, regardless of their sex and gender. Sex and gender have an impact on exposure to environmental, infectious or other types of risks, and therefore on susceptibility or resistance to infectious diseases, and on the type and effectiveness of responses, particularly in health interventions.

The incidence, duration and severity of disease are influenced by both sex and gender in two different ways. On the one hand, sex and gender directly influence vulnerability, exposure to pathogens and response to disease, three key elements of the transmission model. These in turn help determine incidence, duration and severity of disease. On the other hand, sex and gender indirectly influence incidence, duration and severity through interactions with health interventions that affect vulnerability, exposure and response to disease.

Due to the differences between men and women in many aspects of life in all societies, it is important to understand how men and women face disease at all stages (prevention, diagnosis, treatment and recovery). Exposure to environmental, infectious or other types of risks are gender-related, because men and women use the environment in different ways.[2] They have different access to resources (e.g. natural resources, financial resources, agricultural inputs and education). They do not have the same kind of control over resources (e.g. not the same property rights, not the same decision-making power). Moreover, they do not derive the same benefits from the resources. In addition, men and women are affected differently by the environment and diseases (plant, animal and human). Gender norms increase inequalities in access to health. Because they do not always have access to the same information, financial resources or autonomy to decide whether to go to the hospital or to a traditional doctor, for example, men and women behave differently when they are ill.

Sex and gender intersect with other forms of discrimination that impact on health. Different groups of women and men, in particular the most excluded such as those who are victims of racism, those living in poverty, the homeless, displaced persons, refugees, migrants, people with disabilities, Indigenous Peoples, lesbian, gay, bisexual, transgender, queer or questioning people, and intersex people, as well as all those facing discrimination, are at greater risk of being left behind in accessing the response to the disease, including testing, treatment, social protection and care.[3]

7.3.4.2 The drivers of infectious disease emergence related to biodiversity loss

The link between infectious disease and levels of biodiversity has been investigated (e.g. Ostfeld, 2009; Roberts and Heesterbeek, 2018; Vadell *et al.*, 2019). Evidence exists for both the dilution effect, which states that in an ecosystem with a diverse host community, a pathogen would have a lower probability of finding a highly competent host, and, for a vector-borne disease, be transmitted to a suitable vector, i.e. increased biodiversity is associated with a reduction in the risk of infectious disease (Ostfeld and Keesing, 2000; Schmidt and Ostfeld, 2001; Keesing *et al.*, 2010; Civitello *et al.*, 2015; Halliday and Rohr, 2019); and the amplification effect, which predicts biodiversity to be positively correlated with disease risk, as it results in an increased abundance of pathogen sources for a competent host (Pagán *et al.*, 2012; Salkeld *et al.*, 2013; Luis *et al.*, 2018; Rohr *et al.*, 2020).

Until recently, ecosystems supporting naturally biodiverse habitats were considered to provide a larger pool of novel, potentially infectious pathogens (Jones *et al.*, 2008; Wood *et al.*, 2017; Keesing and Ostfeld, 2021). This creates the assumption that species-richness in an ecosystem lends itself to a diversity of pathogens, which in turn must be a risk factor for infectious disease emergence (Ostfeld and Keesing, 2017). However, it has also been shown that, under some conditions, high biodiversity in an ecosystem can both decrease the transmission of newly emerging diseases and decrease the transmission of already established diseases (Keesing *et al.*, 2010; Civitello *et al.*, 2015).

Biodiversity loss can influence infectious diseases transmission by altering:

1. The abundance of the host or vector.
Example: West Nile virus is a mosquito-transmitted virus for which several species of bird, including passerines species, function as hosts. In the USA, research identified strong correlations between increased human risk or incidence of West Nile encephalitis and low avian diversity (Ezenwa *et al.*, 2006; Allan *et al.*, 2008; Swaddle and Calos, 2008). Communities with low avian diversity tend to be dominated by species that amplify the virus, which causes high infection frequency in mosquitoes and people, while communities with higher avian diversity contain more species that are less competent as hosts (Keesing *et al.*, 2010).

2. The behaviour of the host, vector, or parasite.
Example: Schistosomiasis is an infection caused by a parasitic worm that inhabits freshwater ecosystems in subtropical and tropical regions. Within a biodiverse community, one of these parasitic worms is more likely to enter an unsuitable intermediate host, which reduces the probability of a subsequent human infection by 25–99% (Laracuente *et al.*, 1979).

3. The condition of the host or vector.
Example: In experimental rice fields in China, rice plants in genetically diverse mixtures had drier leaves because the mixture changed microclimatic conditions. Consequently, researchers saw a decreased prevalence in rice blast fungus infection in these diverse fields (Zhu *et al.*, 2005).

Although the networks linking biodiversity, disease and the functioning of ecosystems are complex and may be context dependent (Marselle *et al.*, 2021), anthropogenic activities are clear drivers of infectious disease emergence and transmission, altering the force of infection (FOI) for diseases (Foley *et al.*, 2005; Keesing *et al.*, 2010; McMahon *et al.*, 2018; Everard *et al.*, 2020; Marselle *et al.*, 2021). FOI is defined as the rate at which susceptible individuals become infected per unit time and is used to compare different diseases or transmission in different risk groups (McMahon *et al.*, 2018). Established pathways for disease transmission have been described for the Anthropocene (Crutzen and Stoermer, 2000), and human activities have degraded ecosystem services, including disease regulation and suppression, by removing the natural barriers to transmission. They have also impacted the provision of fresh water, which is essential for hygiene to prevent human-to-human disease transmission (Everard *et al.*, 2020). Some commentators, e.g. Rob Wallace, believe that human behaviour in the form of big farms, free-trade agreements, global capital circuits and deforestation cause these epidemics. Perhaps these activities are at the core of the problem and the biodiversity elements are symptoms.

7.3.4.3 Current and potential actions and solutions to avoid infectious disease emergence related to biodiversity loss

The Millennium Ecosystem Assessment (2005) classification of ecosystem services recognizes Human Disease Regulation as being central to the regulation of health and human wellbeing (MEA, 2005). Moreover, it also acknowledges that there is evidence that altering ecosystems can have 'important consequences for human well-being' including facilitating disease emergence and directly changing the abundance of human pathogens (MEA, 2005; Everard *et al.*, 2020). Additionally, in 2020, the United Nations Environment Programme (UNEP) determined that greater biodiversity hinders rapid pathogen spread, while anthropogenic habitat modification or alteration of ecosystem biodiversity produces conditions that facilitate disease emergence and spread (UNEP, 2020).

Infectious diseases such as COVID-19 and Ebola, alongside vector-borne diseases such as malaria, dengue fever, Zika, schistosomiasis, visceral leishmaniasis and tick-borne encephalitis, all have wildlife origins (Müller *et al.*, 2019; Ahmad *et al.*, 2020; Marselle *et al.*, 2021). Infectious disease epidemics involve interactions between organisms, and they are facilitated by the disturbance or degradation of an ecosystem, including unsustainable and exploitative habitat modification, urban expansion and agricultural intensification (Barouki *et al.*, 2021).

Land use and agricultural change are major drivers of zoonotic disease (Jones *et al.*, 2013). However, the context of disease emergence appears all important (McMahon *et al.*, 2018), and there is considerable divergence of opinion around the subject (Kock and Caceres-Escobar, 2022). By altering the structure of ecosystem components, humans may be changing vector or host populations, shifting population dynamics and composition, and altering the services provided by the regulatory functions of ecosystems (Lugassy *et al.*, 2019).

Points to consider with zoonoses emergence:

- Numerous diseases in humans originated in vertebrate mammals and this is likely to continue in the future.
- Ecological, evolutionary perspectives can provide valuable insights into zoonotic disease-control programmes.
- Transdisciplinary collaboration, including but not limited to clinicians, public health scientists, ecologists and disease ecologists, veterinarians, and economists, is necessary for effective management of emergence and spread of zoonoses.
- As land-use change is such a critical driver of zoonoses emergence, perhaps we have now reached a point where an ecological impact assessment, like an environmental impact assessment, should be required to limit diseases emergence (McMahon *et al.*, 2018).
- It also appears that, in conjunction with other ecosystem services, the disease regulatory service of biodiversity demonstrates why biodiversity should be conserved for prevention of **zoonotic disease** in many circumstances.

Learning questions: What is your opinion of the biodiversity dilution and amplification hypotheses? How should this information inform local, national and global biodiversity conservation? How would you develop research activity that reflects a more balanced approach to the components of One Health?

Example answer: The biodiversity dilution and amplification hypotheses are context dependent and influenced by numerous factors such as pathogen type, reservoir host and geography. One example of this variability is Lyme disease where in the USA it appears that the dilution hypothesis holds true, whereas in Europe the amplification hypothesis is more plausible (McMahon *et al.*, 2018). The differences are due to details in disease ecology factors and this understanding coupled with communication between clinicians, public health scientists, ecologists and disease ecologists could result in more informed public health measures being in place.

With respect to biodiversity conservation, the role that biodiversity plays in disease emergence should not be taken in isolation; this is particularly the case with a One Health approach. If there is a dilution effect, we should still value other ecosystem services like the provision of food or regulation of climate. This holistic and One Health approach is even more important where there may be an amplification effect; perceived negative attributes of biodiversity should not take away from the potential overall positive services provided by well-functioning ecosystems (see Box 7.3, part 2, for a range of potential ecosystem services).

Global health would benefit from the inclusion of the appropriate discipline (e.g. human medicine, veterinary medicine, disease ecology) at the conception stage or at the beginning of One Health projects, with continued consultations in the process, through to conclusion. With respect to biodiversity and One Health, an understanding and management of specific ecosystem services in relation to the priorities (e.g. food production within agricultural ecosystems) is required. The vision of a balanced One Health project studying an agricultural ecosystem would involve balance between ecosystem services related to food production, forest production, biodiversity, climate regulation, water regulation and infectious disease mitigation (see Foley *et al.*, 2005; McIntyre *et al.*, 2018; Rushton *et al.*, 2021).

7.4 Conclusions

- There is a clear connection between biodiversity conservation, ecosystem services and One Health.
- Biodiversity is core to the management of global environmental challenges such as food security,

water regulation, climate change and emergence of infectious diseases.

- In order to implement a One Health approach comprehensively, biodiversity management needs to be understood and valued with a gender perspective.
- With respect to infectious diseases, a problem to which the One Health approach was initially applied, biodiversity can impact on disease emergence by what is referred to as the dilution or amplification effects.

Notes

[1] See: https://www.inserm.fr/information-en-sante/dossiers-information/genre-et-sante

[2] See: https://www.unep.org/topics/gender

[3] See: https://www.unfpa.org/sites/default/files/resource-pdf/COVID-19_Preparedness_and_Response_-_UNFPA_Interim_Technical_Briefs_Gender_Equality_and_GBV_23_March_2020_.pdf

References

Aerts, R., Honnay, O. and Van Nieuwenhuyse, A. (2018) Biodiversity and human health: Mechanisms and evidence of the positive health effects of diversity in nature and green spaces. *British Medical Bulletin* 127, 5–22. DOI: 10.1093/bmb/ldy021.

Ahmad, T., Khan, M., Haroon, Musa, T., Nasir, S. *et al.* (2020) COVID-19: Zoonotic aspects. *Travel Medicine and Infectious Disease* 36, 101607. DOI: 10.1016/j.tmaid.2020.101607.

Allan, B., Langerhans, R., Ryberg, W., Landesman, W., Griffin, N. *et al.* (2008) Ecological correlates of risk and incidence of West Nile virus in the United States. *Oecologia* 158, 699–708. DOI: 10.1007/s00442-008-1169-9.

Altman, I. and Low, S.M. (1992) *Place Attachment: Human Behavior and Environment.* Plenum Press, New York.

Anderson, I., Robson, B., Connolly, M., Al-Yaman, F., Bjertness, E. *et al.* (2016) Indigenous and tribal peoples' health (The Lancet–Lowitja Institute Global Collaboration): A population study. *The Lancet* 388, 131–157. DOI: 10.1016/s0140-6736(16)00345-7.

Anderson, Y., Taylor, G., Grant, C. *et al.* (2015) The green prescription active families programme in Taranaki, New Zealand 2007–2009: Did it reach children in need? *Journal of Primary Health Care* 7, 192. DOI: 10.1071/hc15192.

Assandri, G., Bogliani, G., Pedrini, P. and Brambilla, M. (2018) Beautiful agricultural landscapes promote cultural ecosystem services and biodiversity conservation. *Agriculture, Ecosystems and Environment* 256, 200–210. DOI: 10.1016/j.agee.2018.01.012.

Bagnol, B., Alders, R. and McConchie, R. (2015) Gender issues in human, animal and plant health using an ecohealth perspective. *Environment and Natural Resources Research* 5, 62–76.

Barata, A.M., Rocha, F., Lopes, V. and Carvalho, A.M. (2016) Conservation and sustainable uses of medicinal and aromatic plants genetic resources on the worldwide for human welfare. *Industrial Crops and Products* 88, 8–11. DOI: 10.1016/j.indcrop.2016.02.035.

Barouki, R., Kogevinas, M., Audouze, K., Belesova, K., Bergman, A. *et al.* (2021) The COVID-19 pandemic and global environmental change: Emerging research needs. *Environment International* 146, 106272. DOI: 10.1016/j.envint.2020.106272.

Bennun, L.A., Aman, R.A. and Crafter, S.A. (eds) (1995) Conservation of biodiversity in Africa: Local initiatives and institutional roles. *Proceedings of a conference held at the National Museums of Kenya, 30 August - 3 September 1992.* National Museums of Kenya, Nairobi, Kenya.

Beute, F., Davies, Z., de Vries, S., Glanville, J., Keune, H. *et al.* (2020) Types and characteristics of urban and peri-urban blue spaces having an impact on human mental health and wellbeing: Systematic review: An EKLIPSE Expert Working Group report. EKLIPSE, EU.

Boyce, R., Reyes, R., Matte, M. *et al.* (2016) Severe flooding and malaria transmission in the Western Ugandan highlands: Implications for disease control in an era of global climate change. *Journal of Infectious Diseases* 214, 1403–1410. DOI: 10.1093/infdis/jiw363.

Bratman, G.N., Anderson, C.B., Berman, M.G., Cochran, B., de Vries, S. *et al.* (2019) Nature and mental health: An ecosystem service perspective. *Science Advances* 5, eaax0903. DOI: 10.1126/sciadv.aax0903.

Caminade, C., Kovats, S., Rocklov, J., Tompkins, A., Morse, A. *et al.* (2014) Impact of climate change on global malaria distribution. *Proceedings of the National Academy of Sciences* 111, 3286–3291. DOI: 10.1073/pnas.1302089111.

Caminade, C., McIntyre, K. and Jones, A. (2018) Impact of recent and future climate change on vector-borne diseases. *Annals of the New York Academy of Sciences* 1436, 157–173. DOI: 10.1111/nyas.13950.

Caminade, C., Medlock, J., Ducheyne, E., McIntyre, K., Leach, S. *et al.* (2012) Suitability of European climate for the Asian tiger mosquito *Aedes albopictus*: Recent trends and future scenarios. *Journal of the Royal Society Interface* 9, 2708–2717. DOI: 10.1098/rsif.2012.0138.

Carlson, C.J., Albery, G.F., Merow, C., Trisos, C.H., Zipfel, C.M. *et al.* (2022) Climate change increases cross-species viral transmission risk. *Nature* 607, 555–562. DOI: 10.1038/s41586-022-04788-w.

Carrus, G., Scopelliti, M., Lafortezza, R., Colangelo, G., Ferrini, F. *et al.* (2015) Go greener, feel better? The positive effects of biodiversity on the well-being of individuals visiting urban and peri-urban green areas. *Landscape and Urban Planning* 134, 221–228.

Cavicchioli, R., Ripple, W.J., Timmis, K.N., Azam, F., Bakken, L.R. *et al.* (2019) Scientists' warning to humanity: Microorganisms and climate change. *Nature Reviews Microbiology* 17, 569–586. DOI: 10.1038/s41579-019-0222-5.

Ceballos, G., Ehrlich, P.R., Barnosky, A.D., García, A., Pringle, R.M. and Palmer, T.M. (2015) Accelerated modern human–induced species losses: Entering the sixth mass extinction. *Science Advances* 1(5), e1400253. DOI: 10.1126/SCIADV.1400253.

Cerlesi, S., Di Domenico, A. and Ratti, S. (1989) 2,3,7,8-tetrachlorodibenzo-p-dioxin (TCDD) persistence in the Seveso (Milan, Italy) soil. *Ecotoxicology and Environmental Safety* 18(2), 149–64. DOI: 10.1016/0147-6513(89)90076-6.

CEOS C. (2011) CEOS Earth Observation Handbook. In: Eohandbook.com. Available at: http://www.eohandbook.com/eohb2011/climate_variables.html (accessed 17 April 2022).

Cianconi, P., Betrò, S. and Janiri, L. (2020) The impact of climate change on mental health: A systematic descriptive review. *Frontiers in Psychiatry* 11, 74. DOI: 10.3389/fpsyt.2020.00074.

Civitello, D., Cohen, J., Fatima, H., Halstead, N., Liriano, J. *et al.* (2015) Biodiversity inhibits parasites: Broad evidence for the dilution effect. *Proceedings of the National Academy of Sciences* 112, 8667–8671. DOI: 10.1073/pnas.1506279112.

Clark, N.E., Lovell, R., Wheeler, B.W., Higgins, S.L., Depledge, M.H. and Norris, K. (2014) Biodiversity, cultural pathways, and human health: A Framework. *Trends in Ecology and Evolution* 29, 198–204. DOI: 10.1016/j.tree.2014.01.009.

Colón-González, F.J., Sewe, M.O., Tompkins, A.M., Sjödin, H., Casallas, A. *et al.* (2021) Projecting the risk of mosquito-borne diseases in a warmer and more populated world: A multi-model, multi-scenario intercomparison modelling study. *The Lancet Planetary Health*. DOI: 10.1016/s2542-5196(21)00132-7.

Convention on Biological Diversity (2008) What is agricultural biodiversity? In: *Convention on Biological Diversity*. Available at: https://www.cbd.int/agro/whatis.shtml (accessed 5 March 2022).

Cook, P.A., Howarth, M. and Wheater, C.P. (2019) Biodiversity and health in the face of climate change: Implications for public health. In: Marselle, M.R., Stadler, J., Korn, H., Irvine, K.N. and Bonn, A. (eds) *Biodiversity and Health in the Face of Climate Change*. Springer International Publishing, Cham, pp. 251–281. DOI: 10.1007/978-3-030-02318-8_11.

Costanza, R., d-Arge, R., de Groot, R., Farber, S., Grasso, M. *et al.* (1997) The value of the world's ecosystem services and natural capital. *Nature* 387(6630), 253–260. DOI: 10.1038/387253a0.

Costanza, R., de Groot, R., Sutton, P., van der Pleog, S., Anderson, S.J. *et al.* (2014) Changes in the global value of ecosystem services. *Global Environmental Change* 26, 152–158.

Couvillion, L. (2017) Habitat loss, agrobiodiversity, and incidental wildlife loss. In: Steier, G. and Patel, K. (eds) *International Farm Animal, Wildlife and Food Safety Law*. Springer, Cham. DOI: 10.1007/978-3-319-18002-1_24.

Cox, R., McIntyre, K., Sanchez, J., Setzkorn, C., Baylis, M. and Revie, C. (2014) Comparison of the index scores among pathogens identified as emerging hazards in North America. *Transboundary and Emerging Diseases* 63, 79–91. DOI: 10.1111/tbed.12221.

Cox, D., Shanahan, D., Hudson, H., Plummer, K., Siriwardena, G. *et al.* (2017) Doses of neighborhood nature: The benefits for mental health of living with nature. *BioScience* 67(2), p.biw173.

Crist, E., Mora, C. and Engelman, R. (2017) The interaction of human population, food production, and biodiversity protection. *Science* 356(6335), 260–264. DOI: 10.1126/SCIENCE.AAL2011.

Crutzen, P. and Stoermer, E. (2000) The 'Anthropocene'. *The Future of Nature* 479–490. DOI: 10.12987/9780300188479-041.

Dallimer, M., Irvine, K., Skinner, A., Davies, Z., Rouquette, J. *et al.* (2012) Biodiversity and the feel-good factor: Understanding associations between self-reported human well-being and species richness. *BioScience* 62(1), 47–55.

DeFries, R. and Nagendra, H. (2017) Ecosystem management as a wicked problem. *Science* 356(6335), 265–270. DOI: 10.1126/SCIENCE.AAL1950.

Delgado-Baquerizo, M., Guerra, C., Cano-Díaz, C., Egidi, E., Wang, J. *et al.* (2020) The proportion of soil-borne pathogens increases with warming at the global scale. *Nature Climate Change* 10, 550–554. DOI: 10.1038/s41558-020-0759-3.

Díaz, S., Settele, J., Brondízio, E.S., Ngo, H.T., Agard, J. *et al.* (2019) Pervasive human-driven decline of life on Earth points to the need for transformative change. *Science* 366(6471). DOI: 10.1126/science.aax3100.

Díaz, S., Pascual, U., Stenseke, M. *et al.* (2018) Assessing nature's contributions to people. *Science* 359, 270–272. DOI: 10.1126/science.aap8826.

Dinerstein, E., Joshi, A.R., Vynne, C., Lee, A.T.L., Pharand-Deschênes, F., Franca, M. *et al.* (2020) A 'global safety net' to reverse biodiversity loss and stabilize Earth's climate. *Science Advances*. DOI: 10.1126/sciadv.abb2824.

Dirzo, R., Young, H.S., Galetti, M., Ceballos, G., Isaac, N.J.B. and Collen, B. (2014) Defaunation in the Anthropocene. *Science* 345(6195), 401–406. DOI: 10.1126/SCIENCE.1251817.

dos Santos, M., Howard, D., Kruger, P., Banos, A. and Kornik, S. (2019) Climate Change and Healthcare Sustainability in the Agincourt Sub-District, Kruger to Canyons Biosphere Region, South Africa. *Sustainability* 11, 496. DOI: 10.3390/su11020496.

Dunn, S., Towers, W., Dawson, J., Sample, J. and McDonald, J. (2015) A pragmatic methodology for horizon scanning of water quality linked to future climate and land use scenarios. *Land Use Policy* 44, 131–144. DOI: 10.1016/j.landusepol.2014.12.007.

Dyderski, M., Paź, S., Frelich, L. and Jagodziński, A. (2017) How much does climate change threaten European forest tree species distributions? *Global Change Biology* 24, 1150–1163. DOI: 10.1111/gcb.13925.

Dye, C. (2008). Health and urban living. *Science* 319, 766–769. DOI: 10.1126/science.115019.

Ege, M.J., Mayer, M., Normand, A.-C., Genuneit, J., Cookson, W.O. *et al.* (2011) Exposure to environmental micro-organisms and childhood asthma. *New England Journal of Medicine* 364, 701–709. DOI: 10.1056/nejmoa 1007302.

Ekor, M. (2014) The growing use of herbal medicines: Issues relating to adverse reactions and challenges in monitoring safety. *Frontiers in Pharmacology* 4, 177. DOI: 10.3389/fphar.2013.00177.

Elbgami, T., Kunin, W.E., Hughes, W.O. and Biesmeijer, J.C. (2014) The effect of proximity to a honeybee apiary on bumblebee colony fitness, development, and performance. *Apidologie* 45, 504–513. DOI: 10.1007/s13592-013-0265-y.

Eshel, G., Shepon, A., Makov, T. and Milo, R. (2014) Land, irrigation water, greenhouse gas, and reactive nitrogen burdens of meat, eggs, and dairy production in the United States. *Proceedings of the National Academy of Sciences* 111, 11996–12001. DOI: 10.1073/pnas.1402183111.

Estrada-Carmona, N., Sánchez, A.C., Remans, R. and Jones, S.K. (2022) Complex agricultural landscapes host more biodiversity than simple ones: A global meta-analysis. *Proceedings of the National Academy of Sciences* 119, e2203385119. DOI: 10.1073/pnas.2203385119.

European Commission, Directorate-General for Research and Innovation (2015) Towards an EU research and innovation policy agenda for nature-based solutions and re-naturing cities: Final report of the Horizon 2020 expert group on 'Nature-based solutions and re-naturing cities' (full version), Publications Office. Available at: https://data.europa.eu/doi/10.2777/479582 (accessed 19 December 2022).

Evan, B.R. and Leighton, F.A. (2014) A history of One Health. *Revue Scientifique et Technique* 33, 413–420.

Everard, M., Johnston, P., Santillo, D. and Staddon, C. (2020) The role of ecosystems in mitigation and management of Covid-19 and other zoonoses. *Environmental Science and Policy* 111, 7–17. DOI: 10.1016/j.envsci.2020.05.017.

Ezenwa, V., Godsey, M., King, R. and Guptill, S. (2006) Avian diversity and West Nile virus: Testing associations between biodiversity and infectious disease risk. *Proceedings of the Royal Society B: Biological Sciences* 273, 109–117. DOI: 10.1098/rspb.2005.3284.

Fiore, A., Naik, V., Spracklen, D., Steiner, A., Unger, N. *et al.* (2012) Global air quality and climate. *Chemical Society Reviews* 41, 6663. DOI: 10.1039/c2cs35095e.

Fischer, J., Abson, D.J., Butsic, V., Chappell, M.J., Ekroos, J. *et al.* (2014) Land sparing versus land sharing: Moving forward. *Conservation Letters* 7, 149–157. DOI: 10.1111/conl.12084.

Flandroy, L., Poutahidis, T., Berg, G. *et al.* (2018) The impact of human activities and lifestyles on the interlinked microbiota and health of humans and of ecosystems. *Science of the Total Environment* 627, 1018–1038. DOI: 10.1016/j.scitotenv.2018.01.288.

Foley, J.A., Ramankutty, N., Brauman, K.A. *et al.* (2011) Solutions for a cultivated planet. *Nature* 478, 337–342. DOI: 10.1038/nature10452.

Foley, J., DeFries, R., Asner, G., Barford, C., Bonan, G. *et al.* (2005) Global Consequences of Land Use. *Science* 309, 570–574. DOI: 10.1126/science.1111772.

Frumkin, H., Bratman, G.N., Breslow, S.J., Cochran, B., Kahn Jr, P.H. *et al.* (2017) Nature contact and human health: A research agenda. *Environmental Health Perspectives* 125(7), 075001. DOI: org/10.1289/EHP1663.

Fuller, R.A., Irvine, K.N., Devine-Wright, P., Warren, P.H. and Gaston, K.J. (2007) Psychological benefits of green space increase with biodiversity. *Biology Letters* 3, 390–394.

Fyhrquist, N., Ruokolainen, L., Suomalainen, A., Lehtimäki, S., Veckman, V. *et al.* (2014) Acinetobacter species in the skin microbiota protect against allergic sensitization and inflammation. *Journal of Allergy and Clinical Immunology* 134, 1301–1309.e11. DOI: 10.1016/j.jaci.2014.07.059.

Garnett, S., Burgess, N., Fa, J., Fernández-Llamazares, Á., Molnár, Z. *et al.* (2018) A spatial overview of the global importance of Indigenous lands for conservation. *Nature Sustainability* 1, 369–374. DOI: 10.1038/s41893-018-0100-6.

Garnier, J., Savić, S., Boriani, E., Bagnol, B., Häsler, B. and Kock, R. (2020) Helping to heal nature and ourselves through human-rights-based and gender-responsive One Health. *One Health Outlook* 2, 22. DOI: 10.1186/s42522-020-00029-0.

GBD 2019 Diseases and Injuries Collaborators (2019) Global burden of 369 diseases and injuries in 204 countries and territories, 1990–2019: A systematic analysis for the global burden of disease study 2019. *The Lancet* 396, 1204–1222. DOI: 10.1016/s0140-6736(20)30925-9.

Gisler, A., Korten, I., de Hoogh, K. *et al.* (2021) Associations of air pollution and greenness with the nasal microbiota of healthy infants: A longitudinal study. *Environmental Research* 202, 111633. DOI: 10.1016/j.envres.2021.111633.

Glaser, J., Lemery, J., Rajagopalan, B., Diaz, H., García-Trabanino, R. *et al.* (2016) Climate change and the emergent epidemic of CKD from heat stress in rural communities: The case for heat stress nephropathy. *Clinical Journal of the American Society of Nephrology* 11, 1472–1483. DOI: 10.2215/cjn.13841215.

Guis, H., Caminade, C., Calvete, C., Morse, A., Tran, A. and Baylis, M. (2011) Modelling the effects of past and future climate on the risk of bluetongue emergence in Europe. *Journal of the Royal Society Interface* 9, 339–350. DOI: 10.1098/rsif.2011.0255.

Halliday, F. and Rohr, J. (2019) Measuring the shape of the biodiversity-disease relationship across systems reveals new findings and key gaps. *Nature Communications*. DOI: 10.1038/s41467-019-13049-w.

Hanski, I., von Hertzen, L., Fyhrquist, N., Koskinen, K., Torppa, K. *et al.* (2012) Environmental biodiversity, human microbiota, and allergy are interrelated. *Proceedings of the National Academy of Sciences* 109, 8334–8339. DOI: 10.1073/pnas.1205624109.

Harley, C. (2011) Climate change, keystone predation, and biodiversity loss. *Science* 334, 1124–1127. DOI: 10.1126/science.1210199.

Hartig, T., Mitchell, R., de Vries, S. and Frumkin, H. (2014) Nature and health. *Annual Review of Public Health* 35, 207–228. DOI: 10.1146/annurev-publhealth-032013-182443.

Hines, P., Hiu Yu, L., Guy, R.H. *et al.* (2019) Scanning the horizon: A systematic literature review of methodologies. *BMJ Open* 9, e026764. DOI: 10.1136/bmjopen-2018-02676.

Hoffmann, K., Ristl, R., George, A., Maier, M. and Pichlhöfer, O. (2019) The ecology of medical care: Access points to the health care system in Austria and other developed countries. *Scandinavian Journal of Primary Health Care* 37, 409–417. DOI: 10.1080/02813432.2019.1663593.

Holt, A. R., Alix, A., Thompson, A. and Maltby, L. (2016) Food production, ecosystem services and biodiversity: We can't have it all everywhere. *Science of the Total Environment* 573:1422–1429. DOI:10.1016/J.SCITOTENV.2016.07.139.

Howard, P. (2003) *Women and Plants: Gender Relations in Biodiversity Management and Conservation*. Zed Books, London.

IPBES (2022) Intergovernmental Science-Policy Platform on Biodiversity and Ecosystem Services (IPBES) Summary for Policymakers of The IPBES Thematic Assessment Report On The Sustainable Use Of Wild Species (2022), Intergovernmental Science-Policy Platform on Biodiversity and Ecosystem Services (IPBES).

IPCC (2021a) Climate change 2021: The physical science basis. In: Masson-Delmotte, V., Zhai, A., Pirani, P., Connors, S.L. and Péan, C. (eds) *Contribution of Working Group I to the Sixth Assessment Report of the Intergovernmental Panel on Climate Change*. Cambridge University Press, Cambridge, UK.

IPCC (2021b) Summary for policymakers. In: Masson-Delmotte, V., Zhai, P., Pirani, A., Connors, S.L., Péan, C. *et al.* (eds) *Climate Change 2021: The Physical Science Basis. Contribution of Working Group I to the Sixth Assessment Report of the Intergovernmental Panel on Climate Change*. Cambridge University Press, Cambridge, UK.

IPCC (2023) Sections. In: Core Writing Team, Lee, H. and Romero, J. (eds) *Climate Change 2023: Synthesis Report. Contribution of Working Groups I, II and III to the Sixth Assessment Report of the Intergovernmental Panel on Climate Change*. IPCC, Geneva, Switzerland, pp. 35–115, DOI: 10.59327/IPCC/AR6-9789291691647.

IUCN (2019) The IUCN Red List of Threatened Species. Available at: https://www.iucnredlist.org/ (accessed 22 October 2022).

Jackson, L., Pascual, U. and Hodgkin, T. (2007) Utilizing and conserving agrobiodiversity in agricultural landscapes. *Agriculture, Ecosystems and Environment* 121, 196–210. DOI: 10.1016/j.agee.2006.12.017.

Jackson, L.E., Daniel, J., McCorkle, B., Sears, A. and Bush, K.F. (2013a) Linking ecosystem services and human health: The Eco-Health Relationship Browser. *International Journal of Public Health* 58, 747–755.

Jackson, L., Brussaard, L., de Ruiter, P., Pascual, U., Perrings, C. and Bawa, K. (2013b) Agrobiodiversity. *Encyclopedia of Biodiversity* 126–135. DOI: 10.1016/b978-0-12-384719-5.00233-1.

Jie, C., Chen, J.-Z., Tan, M.-Z. and Gong, Z.-T. (2002) Soil degradation: A global problem endangering sustainable development. *Journal of Geographical Sciences* 12(2), 243–252.

Jones, B.A., Grace, D., Kock, R., Alonso, S., Rushton, J. *et al.* (2013) Zoonosis emergence linked to agricultural intensification and environmental change. *Proceedings of the National Academy of Sciences* 110, 8399–8404. DOI: 10.1073/pnas.1208059110.

Jones, C., Lawton, J. and Shachak, M. (1994) Organisms as ecosystem engineers. *Oikos* 69, 373. DOI: 10.2307/3545850.

Jones, K., Patel, N., Levy, M., Storeygard, A., Balk, D. *et al.* (2008) Global trends in emerging infectious diseases. *Nature* 451, 990–993. DOI: 10.1038/nature06536.

Kaplan, R. and Kaplan, S. (1989) *The Experience of Nature: A Psychological Perspective*. Cambridge University Press, Cambridge, UK.

Kassam, K.-A., Karamkhudoeva, M., Ruelle, M. and Baumflek, M. (2010) Medicinal plant use and health sovereignty: Findings from the Tajik and Afghan Pamirs. *Human Ecology* 38(6), 817–829. DOI: 10.1007/s10745-010-9356-9.

Keesing, F. and Ostfeld, R. (2021) Impacts of biodiversity and biodiversity loss on zoonotic diseases. *Proceedings of the National Academy of Sciences* 118, e2023540118. DOI: 10.1073/pnas.2023540118.

Keesing, F., Belden, L., Daszak, P., Dobson, A., Harvell, C. *et al.* (2010) Impacts of biodiversity on the emergence and transmission of infectious diseases. *Nature* 468, 647–652. DOI: 10.1038/nature09575.

Keith, A.M., Schmidt, O. and McMahon, B.J. (2016) Soil Stewardship as a nexus between ecosystem services and One Health. *Ecosystem Services* 17, 40–42. DOI: 10.1016/j.ecoser.2015.11.008.

Keune, H., Flandroy, L., Thys, S., De Regge, N., Mori, M. *et al.* (2017) The need for European OneHealth/EcoHealth networks. *Archives of Public Health* 75, 64. DOI: 10.1186/s13690-017-0232-6.

Keune, H., Payyappallimana, U., Morand, S. and Rüegg, S.R. (2022) One Health and biodiversity. *Transforming Biodiversity Governance* 93–114. DOI: 10.1017/9781108856348.006.

Kirjavainen, P.V., Karvonen, A.M., Adams, R.I., Taubel, M., Roponen, M. *et al.* (2019) Farm-like indoor microbiota in non-farm homes protects children from asthma development. *Nature Medicine* 25, 1089–1095. DOI: 10.1038/s41591-019-0469-4.

Kock, R. and Caceres-Escobar, H. (2022) *Situation Analysis on the Roles and Risks of Wildlife in the Emergence of Human Infectious Diseases*. Gland, Switzerland. DOI: 10.2305/iucn.ch.2022.01.en.

Kremen, C. (2015) Reframing the land-sparing/land-sharing debate for biodiversity conservation. *Annals of the New York Academy of Sciences* 1355, 52–76. DOI: 10.1111/nyas.12845.

Kuo, M. (2015) How might contact with nature promote human health? Promising mechanisms and a possible central pathway. *Frontiers in Psychology* 6. DOI: 10.3389/fpsyg.2015.01093.

Laracuente, A., Brown, R. and Jobin, W. (1979) Comparison of four species of snails as potential decoys to intercept schistosome miracidia. *The American Journal of Tropical Medicine and Hygiene* 28, 99–105. DOI: 10.4269/ajtmh.1979.28.99.

Lauwers, L., Bastiaens, H., Remmen, R. and Keune, H. (2020) Nature's contributions to human health: A missing link to primary health care? A scoping review of international overview reports and scientific evidence. *Frontiers in Public Health* 8, 52. DOI: 10.3389/fpubh.2020.00052.

Lenton, T.M., Rockström, J., Gaffney, O., Rahmstorf, S., Richardson, K. *et al.* (2019) Climate tipping points – too risky to bet against. *Nature* 575, 592–595. DOI: 10.1038/d41586-019-03595-0.

Levy, K., Smith, S.M. and Carlton, E.J. (2018) Climate change impacts on waterborne diseases: Moving toward designing interventions. *Current Environmental Health Reports* 5, 272–282. DOI: 10.1007/s40572-018-0199-7.

Li, Y., Tan, M. and Hao, H. (2019) The impact of global cropland changes on terrestrial ecosystem services value, 1992–2015. *Journal of Geographical Sciences* 29(3), 323–333. DOI: 10.1007/S11442-019-1600-7.

Liu-Helmersson, J., Stenlund, H., Wilder-Smith, A. and Rocklöv, J. (2014) Vectorial capacity of Aedes aegypti: Effects of temperature and implications for Global Dengue Epidemic potential. *PLoS ONE*. DOI: 10.1371/journal.pone.0089783.

Lomborg, B. (2001) *The Sceptical Environmentalist: Measuring the Real State of the World*. Cambridge University Press, Cambridge, UK.

Lugassy, L., Amdouni-Boursier, L., Alout, H., Berrebi, R., Boëte, C. *et al.* (2019) What is the evidence that ecosystem components or functions have an impact on infectious diseases? A systematic review protocol. *Environmental Evidence* 8, 4. DOI: 10.1186/s13750-019-0147-5.

Luis, A.D., Hayman, D.T., O'Shea, T.J., Cryan, P.M., Gilbert, A.T. *et al.* (2013) A comparison of bats and rodents as reservoirs of zoonotic viruses: Are bats special? *Proceedings of the Royal Society B: Biological Sciences* 280, 20122753. DOI: 10.1098/rspb.2012.2753.

Luis, A.D., Kuenzi, A.J. and Mills, J.N. (2018) Species diversity concurrently dilutes and amplifies transmission in a zoonotic host–pathogen system through competing mechanisms. *Proceedings of the National Academy of Sciences* 115, 7979–7984. DOI: 10.1073/pnas.1807106115.

Manisalidis, I., Stavropoulou, E., Stavropoulos, A. and Bezirtzoglou, E. (2020) Environmental and health impacts of air pollution: A review. *Frontiers in Public Health* 8, 14. DOI: 10.3389/fpubh.2020.00014.

Markandya, A., Taylor, T., Longo, A., Murty, M., Murty, S. and Dhavala, K. (2008) Counting the cost of vulture decline – An appraisal of the human health and other benefits of vultures in India. *Ecological Economics* 67, 194–204. DOI: 10.1016/j.ecolecon.2008.04.020.

Marselle, M.R., Martens, D., Dallimer, M. and Irvine, K.N. (2019) Review of the mental health and well-being benefits of biodiversity. In: Marselle, M., Stadler, J., Korn, H., Irvine, K. and Bonn, A. (eds) *Biodiversity and Health in the Face of Climate Change*. Springer, Cham. DOI: 10.1007/978-3-030-02318-89.

Marselle, M., Hartig, T., Cox, D., de Bell, S., Knapp, S. *et al.* (2021) Pathways linking biodiversity to human health: A conceptual framework. *Environment International* 150, 106420. DOI: 10.1016/j.envint.2021.106420.

Mawdsley, J.R., O'Malley, R. and Ojima, D.S. (2009) A review of climate-change adaptation strategies for wildlife management and biodiversity conservation. *Conservation Biology* 23, 1080–1089. DOI: 10.1111/j.1523-1739.2009.01264.x.

McBratney, A., Field, D.J. and Koch, A. (2014) The dimensions of soil security. *Geoderma* 213, 203–213. DOI: 10.1016/j.geoderma.2013.08.013.

McGaw, L.J. and Abdalla, M.A. (2020) Ethnoveterinary medicine. In: McGaw, L.J. and Abdalla, M.A. (eds) *Ethnoveterinary Medicine: Present and Future Concepts*. Springer, Cham, Switzerland, p. 435. DOI: 10.1007/978-3-030-32270-0.

McIntyre, K., Setzkorn, C., Baylis, M., Waret-Szkuta, A., Caminade, C., Morse, A. *et al.* (2010) Impact of climate change on human and animal health. *Veterinary Record* 167, 586–586. DOI: 10.1136/vr.c5523.

McIntyre, K., Hawkes, I., Waret-Szkuta, A., Morand, S. and Baylis, M. (2011) The H-index as a quantitative indicator of the relative impact of human diseases. *PLoS ONE* 6, e19558. DOI: 10.1371/journal.pone.0019558.

McIntyre, A.K., Setzkorn, C., Wardeh, M., Hepworth, P., Radford, A. and Baylis, M. (2014a) Using open-access taxonomic and spatial information to create a comprehensive database for the study of mammalian and avian livestock and pet infections. *Preventive Veterinary Medicine* 116, 325–335. DOI: 10.1016/j.prevetmed.2013.07.002.

McIntyre, B.K., Setzkorn, C., Hepworth, P., Morand, S., Morse, A. and Baylis, M. (2014b) A quantitative prioritisation of human and domestic animal pathogens in Europe. *PLoS ONE* 9, e103529. DOI: 10.1371/journal.pone.0103529.

McIntyre, K., Setzkorn, C., Hepworth, P., Morand, S., Morse, A. and Baylis, M. (2017) Systematic assessment of the climate sensitivity of important human and domestic animals pathogens in Europe. *Scientific Reports* 7, 7134. DOI: 10.1038/s41598-017-06948-9.

McIntyre, K.M., Volger, B., Chantziaras, I., Coelho, A.C., Díez, J.G. *et al.* (2018) Assessing the ecological dimensions of One Health. In: Rüegg, S.R., Häsler, B. and Zinsstag, J. (eds) *Integrated Approaches to Health: A Handbook for the Evaluation of One Health*. Wageningen Academic Publishers, The Netherlands, pp. 126–169. DOI: 10.3920/978-90-8686-875-9.

McMahon, B.J., Morand, S. and Gray, J.S. (2018) Ecosystem change and zoonoses in the anthropocene. *Zoonoses and Public Health* 65, 755–765. DOI: 10.1111/zph.12489.

Methorst, J., Bonn, A., Marselle, M., Böhning-Gaese, K. and Rehdanz, K. (2021) Species richness is positively related to mental health – A study for Germany. *Landscape and Urban Planning* 211, 104084.

Millennium Ecosystem Assessment (MEA) (2005) Ecosystems and human well-being: Biodiversity synthesis. World Resources Institute, Island Press, Washington, DC. Available at: https://www.millenniumassessment.org/en/index.html (accessed 6 March 2022).

Mitku, A.A., Zewotir, T., North, D., Jeena, P., Asharam, K. *et al.* (2023) Impact of ambient air pollution exposure during pregnancy on adverse birth outcomes: Generalized structural equation modeling approach. *BMC Public Health* 23, 45. DOI: 10.1186/s12889-022-14971-3.

Moore, J.W. (2017) The capitalocene – Part I: On the nature and origins of our ecological crisis. *The Journal of Peasant Studies* 44, 594–630.

Morand, S. and Lajaunie, C. (2021) Outbreaks of vector-borne and zoonotic diseases are associated with changes in forest cover and oil palm expansion at global scale. *Frontiers in Veterinary Science* 8, 661038. DOI: 10.3389/fvets.2021.661063.

Müller, R., Reuss, F., Kendrovski, V. and Montag, D. (2019) Vector-Borne Diseases. *Biodiversity and Health in the Face of Climate Change* 67–90. DOI: 10.1007/978-3-030-02318-8_4.

Murray, A., Wardeh, M. and McIntyre, K. (2016) Using the H-index to assess disease priorities for salmon aquaculture. *Preventive Veterinary Medicine* 126, 199–207. DOI: 10.1016/j.prevetmed.2016.02.007.

Naeem, S., Thompson, L., Lawler, S., Lawton, J. and Woodfin, R. (1994) Declining biodiversity can alter the performance of ecosystems. *Nature* 368, 734–737. DOI: 10.1038/368734a0.

Newbold, T., Hudson, L.N., Hill, S.L., Contu, S., Lysenko, I. *et al.* (2015) Global effects of land use on local terrestrial biodiversity. *Nature* 520(7545), 45–50. DOI: 10.1038/nature14324.

O'Donoghue, T., Minasny, B. and McBratney, A. (2022) Regenerative agriculture and its potential to improve farmscape function. *Sustainability* 14(10), 5815. DOI: 10.3390/su14105815.

O'Neill, B.C., Tebaldi, C., van Vuuren, D.P., Ering, V., Friedlingstein, P. *et al.* (2016) The Scenario Model Intercomparison Project (ScenarioMIP) for CMIP6. *Geoscientific Model Development* 9, 3461–3482. DOI: 10.5194/gmd-9-3461-2016.

O'Neill, B.C., Carter, T.R., Ebi, K., Harrison, P.A., Kemp-Benedict, E. *et al.* (2020) Achievements and needs for the Climate Change Scenario Framework. *Nature Climate Change* 10, 1074–1084. DOI: 10.1038/s41558-020-00952-0.

Olson, S.H., Benedum, C.M., Mekaru, S.R., Preston, N.D., Mazet, J.A.K. *et al.* (2015) Drivers of emerging infectious disease events as a framework for digital detection. *Emerging Infectious Diseases* 21, 1285–1292. DOI: 10.3201/eid2108.141156.

Ostfeld, R. (2009) Biodiversity loss and the rise of zoonotic pathogens. *Clinical Microbiology and Infection* 15, 40–43. DOI: 10.1111/j.1469-0691.2008.02691.x.

Ostfeld, R. and Keesing, F. (2000) Biodiversity series: The function of biodiversity in the ecology of vector-borne zoonotic diseases. *Canadian Journal of Zoology* 78, 2061–2078. DOI: 10.1139/z00-172.

Ostfeld, R. and Keesing, F. (2017) Is biodiversity bad for your health? *Ecosphere*. DOI: 10.1002/ecs2.1676.

Pagán, I., González-Jara, P., Moreno-Letelier, A., Rodelo-Urrego, M., Fraile, A. *et al.* (2012) Effect of biodiversity changes in disease risk: Exploring disease emergence in a plant-virus system. *PLoS Pathogens* 8, e1002796. DOI: 10.1371/journal.ppat.1002796.

Patel, A., Schofield, G.M., Kolt, G.S. and Keogh, J.W.L. (2011) General practitioners' views and experiences of counselling for physical activity through the New Zealand green prescription program. *BMC Family Practice* 12, 119. DOI: 10.1186/1471-2296-12-119.

Paull, S.H., Horton, D.E., Ashfaq, M. *et al.* (2017) Drought and immunity determine the intensity of West Nile virus epidemics and climate change impacts. *Proceedings of the Royal Society B: Biological Sciences* 284, 20162078. DOI: 10.1098/rspb.2016.2078.

Pecl, G., Araújo, M., Bell, J., Blanchard, J., Bonebrake, T. *et al.* (2017) Biodiversity redistribution under climate change: Impacts on ecosystems and human well-being. *Science* 355, eaai9214. DOI: 10.1126/science.aai9214.

Pirk, C.W., Crewe, R.M. and Moritz, R.F. (2017) Risks and benefits of the biological interface between managed and wild bee pollinators. *Functional Ecology* 31, 47–55. DOI: 10.1111/1365-2435.12768.

Plieninger, T., Hartel, T., Martín-López, B., Beaufoy, G., Bergmeier, E. *et al.* (2015). Wood-pastures of Europe: Geographic coverage, social–ecological values, conservation management, and policy implications. *Biological Conservation* 190, 70–79. DOI: 10.1016/j.biocon.2015.05.014.

Potts, S.G., Biesmeijer, J.C., Kremen, C., Neumann, P., Schweiger, O. and Kunin, W.E. (2010) Global pollinator declines: Trends, impacts and drivers. *Trends in Ecology and Evolution* 25(6), 345–353. DOI: 10.1016/J.TREE.2010.01.007.

Power, M., Tilman, D., Estes, J., Menge, B., Bond, W. *et al.* (1996) Challenges in the Quest for Keystones. *BioScience* 46, 609–620. DOI: 10.2307/1312990.

Prakash, V., Pain, D., Cunningham, A., Donald, P., Prakash, N. *et al.* (2003) Catastrophic collapse of Indian white-backed *Gyps bengalensis* and long-billed *Gyps indicus* vulture populations. *Biological Conservation* 109, 381–390. DOI: 10.1016/s0006-3207(02)00164-7.

Pretty, J., Toulmin, C. and Williams, S. (2005) Sustainable intensification in African agriculture. *International Journal of Agricultural Sustainability* 3(1), 1–23. DOI: 10.3763/ijas.2010.0583.

Proshansky, H.M., Fabian, A.F. and Kaminoff, R. (1983) Place-identity: Physical world socialization of the self. *Journal of Environmental Psychology* 3, 57–83.

Purvis, G., Downey, L., Beever, D., Doherty, M.L., Monahan, F.J., Sheridan, H. and McMahon, B.J. (2012) Development of a sustainably-competitive agriculture. In: Lichtfouse, E. (ed.) *Agroecology and strategies for climate change: Sustainable agriculture reviews.* Springer, Berlin, p. 35–65. DOI: 10.1007/978-94-007-1905-7_3.

Raghavan, R.K., Brenner, K.M., Higgins, J.J., Hutchinson, J.M.S. and Harkin, K.R. (2012) Evaluations of hydrologic risk factors for canine leptospirosis: 94 cases (2002–2009). *Preventive Veterinary Medicine* 107, 105–109. DOI: 10.1016/j.prevetmed.2012.05.004.

Riahi, K., van Vuuren, D., Kriegler, E., Edmonds, J., O'Neill, B. *et al.* (2017) The shared socioeconomic pathways and their energy, land use, and greenhouse gas emissions implications: An overview. *Global Environmental Change* 42, 153–168. DOI: 10.1016/j.gloenvcha.2016.05.009.

Ripple, W.J., Wolf, C., Gregg, J.W., Levin, K., Rockström, J. *et al.* (2022) World scientists' warning of a climate emergency. *BioScience* 72, 1149–1155. DOI: 10.1093/biosci/biac083.

Ritchie, H. and Roser, M. (2013) Land Use. Our World in Data. Available at: https://ourworldindata.org/land-use (accessed 29 July 2024).

Ritzel, C. and Mann, S. (2021) The old man and the meat: On gender differences in meat consumption across stages of human life. *Foods* 10(11), 2809. DOI: 10.3390/foods10112809.

Roberts, M. and Heesterbeek, J. (2018) Quantifying the dilution effect for models in ecological epidemiology. *Journal of the Royal Society Interface* 15, 20170791. DOI: 10.1098/rsif.2017.0791.

Rohr, J.R., Civitello, D.J., Halliday, F.W., Hudson, P.J., Lafferty, K.D. *et al.* (2020) Towards common ground in the biodiversity–disease debate. *Nature Ecology and Evolution* 4, 24–33. DOI: 10.1038/s41559-019-1060-6.

Romanelli, C., Cooper, D., Campbell-Lendrum, D., Maiero, M., Karesh, W.B. *et al.* (2015) *Connecting Global Priorities: Biodiversity and Human Health: A State of Knowledge Review.* WHO/CBD, p. 344.

Romanello, M., Di Napoli, C., Drummond, P., Green, C., Kennard, H. *et al.* (2022) The 2022 report of the Lancet countdown on health and climate change: Health at the mercy of fossil fuels. *The Lancet* 400, 1619–1654. DOI: 10.1016/s0140-6736(22)01540-9.

Roser, M., Ritchie, H. and Ortiz-Ospina, E. (2013) World Population Growth – Our World in Data. Available at: https://ourworldindata.org/world-population-growth (accessed 29 July 2024).

Roslund, M.I., Puhakka, R., Nurminen, N., Oikarinen, S., Siter, N. *et al.* (2021) Long-term biodiversity intervention shapes health-associated commensal microbiota among urban day-care children. *Environment International* 157, 106811. DOI: 10.1016/j.envint.2021.106811.

Rushton, J., McMahon, B.J., Wilson, M.E., Mazet, J.A.K. and Shankar, B. (2021) A food system paradigm shift: From cheap food at any cost to food within a One Health framework. *NAM Perspectives.* Commentary, National Academy of Medicine, Washington, DC. DOI: 10.31478/202111b.

Salkeld, D.J., Padgett, K.A. and Jones, J.H. (2013) A meta-analysis suggesting that the relationship between biodiversity and risk of zoonotic pathogen transmission is idiosyncratic. *Ecology Letters* 16, 679–686. DOI: 10.1111/ele.12101.

Sandhya, P., Danda, D., Sharma, D. and Scaria, V. (2016) Does the buck stop with the bugs? An overview of microbial dysbiosis in rheumatoid arthritis. *International Journal of Rheumatic Diseases* 19(1), 8–20. DOI: 10.1111/1756-185X.12728.

Scherr, S.J. and McNeely, J.A. (2007) Biodiversity conservation and agricultural sustainability: Towards a new paradigm of 'ecoagriculture' landscapes. *Philosophical Transactions of the Royal Society B: Biological Sciences* 363, 477–494. DOI: 10.1098/rstb.2007.2165.

Schmeller, D.S., Loyau, A., Bao, K., Brack, W., Chatzinotas, A. *et al.* (2018) People, pollution and pathogens – global change impacts in mountain freshwater ecosystems. *Science of the Total Environment* 622–623, 756–763. DOI: 10.1016/j.scitotenv.2017.12.006.

Schmeller, D.S., Urbach, D., Bates, K., Catalan, J., Cogălniceanu, D. *et al.* (2022) Scientists' warning of threats to mountains. *Science of the Total Environment* 853, 158611. DOI: 10.1016/j.scitotenv.2022.158611.

Schmidt, K. (2015) Social inequality and international migration related to climate stressors: The case of Mexico. *Advances in Global Change Research* 117–128. DOI: 10.1007/978-3-319-25796-9_8.

Schmidt, K. and Ostfeld, R. (2001) Biodiversity and the dilution effect in disease ecology. *Ecology* 82, 609–619. DOI: 10.1890/0012-9658(2001)082[0609:batdei]2.0.co;2.

Schuster, R., Germain, R., Bennett, J., Reo, N. and Arcese, P. (2019) Vertebrate biodiversity on indigenous-managed lands in Australia, Brazil, and Canada equals that in protected areas. *Environmental Science and Policy* 101, 1–6. DOI: 10.1016/j.envsci.2019.07.002.

Shaver, I., Chain-Guadarrama, A., Cleary, K.A., Sanfiorenzo, A., Santiago-García, R.J. *et al.* (2015) Coupled social and ecological outcomes of agricultural intensification in Costa Rica and the future of biodiversity conservation in tropical agricultural regions. *Global Environmental Change* 32, 74–86. DOI: 10.1016/j.gloenvcha.2015.02.006.

Singh, J., Schädler, M., Demetrio, W., Brown, G.G. and Eisenhauer, N. (2019) Climate change effects on earthworms – a review. *Soil Organism* 91(3), 114–138. DOI: 10.25674/so91iss3pp114.

Smil, V. (2003) *The Earth's Biosphere: Evolution, Dynamics, and Change*. MIT Press, Cambridge, Massachusetts.

Smil, V. (2011) Harvesting the biosphere: The human impact. *Population and Development Review* 37(4), 613–636. DOI: 10.1111/j.1728-4457.2011.00450.x.

Soumya, N., Mondal, S. and Lakhan Singh, R. (2021) *Emerging Issues in Climate Smart Livestock Production*. Elsevier, The Netherlands. DOI: 10.1016/c2019-0-04196-9.

Strayer, D.L. and Dudgeon, D. (2010) Freshwater biodiversity conservation: Recent progress and future challenges. *Journal of the North American Benthological Society* 29, 344–358. DOI: 10.1899/08-171.1.

Suk, J., Ebi, K., Vose, D., Wint, W., Alexander, N. *et al.* (2014) Indicators for tracking European vulnerabilities to the risks of infectious disease transmission due to climate change. *International Journal of Environmental Research and Public Health* 11, 2218–2235. DOI: 10.3390/ijerph110202218.

Swaddle, J. and Calos, S. (2008) Increased avian diversity is associated with lower incidence of human West Nile infection: Observation of the dilution effect. *PLoS ONE* 3, e2488. DOI: 10.1371/journal.pone.0002488.

Swinburn, B.A., Kraak, V.I., Allender, S., Atkins, V.J., Baker, P.I. *et al.* (2019) The global syndemic of obesity, undernutrition, and climate change: The Lancet commission report. *The Lancet* 393(10173), 791–846. DOI: 10.1016/S0140-6736(18)32822-8.

Swinburn, B.A., Walter, L.G., Arroll, B., Tilyard, M.W. and Russell, D.G. (1997) Green prescriptions: Attitudes and perceptions of general practitioners towards prescribing exercise. *British Journal of General Practice* 47, 567–569.

Tengberg, A., Fredholm, S., Eliasson, I., Knez, I., Saltzman, K. and Wetterberg, O. (2012) Cultural ecosystem services provided by landscapes: Assessment of heritage values and identity. *Ecosystem Services* 2, 14–26. DOI: 10.1016/j.ecoser.2012.07.006.

Thatcher, A. and Milner, K. (2014) Green ergonomics and green buildings. *Ergonomics in Design: The Quarterly of Human Factors Applications* 22, 5–12. DOI: 10.1177/1064804613516760.

Tickner, D., Opperman, J.J., Abell, R., Acreman, M., Arthington, A.H. *et al.* (2020) Bending the curve of global freshwater biodiversity loss: An emergency recovery plan. *BioScience* 70, 330–342. DOI: 10.1093/biosci/biaa002.

Tieskens, K., Schulp, C., Levers, C., Lieskovský, J., Kuemmerle, T. *et al.* (2017) Characterizing European cultural landscapes: Accounting for structure, management intensity and value of agricultural and forest landscapes. *Land Use Policy* 62, 29–39. DOI: 10.1016/j.landusepol.2016.12.001.

Tjaden, N., Cheng, Y., Beierkuhnlein, C. and Thomas, S. (2021) Chikungunya beyond the tropics: Where and when do we expect disease transmission in Europe? *Viruses* 13, 1024. DOI: 10.3390/v13061024.

Ulrich, R., Simons, R., Losito, B., Fiorito, E., Miles, M. and Zelson, M. (1991) Stress recovery during exposure to natural and urban environments. *Journal of Environmental Psychology* 11, 201–230. DOI: 10.1016/s0272-4944(05)80184-7.

UNEP (2017) Saiga antelopes on the brink of extinction. Available at: https://www.unep.org/news-and-stories/story/saiga-antelopes-brink-extinction (accessed 19 December 2022).

UNEP (2020) Coronaviruses: Are they here to stay? UN Environment Programme (UNEP). Available at: https://www.unep.org/news-and-stories/story/coronaviruses-are-they-here-stay (accessed 29 July 2024).

UNEP (2022) Emissions gap report 2022: The closing window – Climate crisis calls for rapid transformation of societies. Available at: https://www.unep.org/emissions-gap-report-2022 (accessed 17 November 2022).

UNICEF (2020) Everything You Need to Know About Washing Your Hands to Protect Against Coronavirus (COVID-19). Available at: https://www.unicef.org/thailand/coronavirus/everything-you-need-know-about-washing-your-hands-protect-against-coronavirus-covid-19 (accessed 2 July 2021).

United Nations (2021) Water and ecosystems: UN-Water. Available at: https://www.unwater.org/water-facts/water-and-ecosystems (accessed 22 October 2022).

United Nations (2023) COP28: UN Climate Change Conference – United Arab Emirates 2023. Available at: https://unfccc.int/cop28 (accessed 7 August 2024).

Unnikrishnan, P.M. and Suneetha, M.S. (2012) Biodiversity, traditional knowledge and community health strengthening linkages. UNU-IAS, Yokohama, Japan.

Vadell, M., Gómez Villafañe, I. and Carbajo, A. (2019) Hantavirus infection and biodiversity in the Americas. *Oecologia* 192, 169–177. DOI: 10.1007/s00442-019-04564-0.

van Dijk, M., Morley, T., Rau, M.L. and Saghai, Y. (2021) A meta-analysis of projected global food demand and population at risk of hunger for the period 2010–2050. *Nature Food* 2, 494–501. DOI: 10.1038/s43016-021-00322-9.

van Elsas, J.D., Chiurazzi, M., Mallon, C.A., Elhottova, D., Krištufek, V. and Salles, J.F. (2012) Microbial diversity determines the invasion of soil by a bacterial pathogen. *PNAS* 109, 1159–1164. DOI: 10.1073/pnas.1109326109.

van Vuuren, D.P., Kriegler, E., O'Neill, B.C., Ebi, K.L., Riahi, K. *et al.* (2014) A new scenario framework for climate change research: Scenario matrix architecture. *Climatic Change* 122, 373–86.

Wardeh, M., Risley, C., McIntyre, M., Setzkorn, C. and Baylis, M. (2015) Database of host-pathogen and related species interactions, and their global distribution. *Scientific Data* 2, 150049. DOI: 10.1038/sdata.2015.49.

Watson, J.E., Dudley, N., Segan, D.B. and Hockings, M. (2014) The performance and potential of protected areas. *Nature* 515, 67–73. DOI: 10.1038/nature13947.

Webster, A.J. (2001) Farm animal welfare: The five freedoms and the free market. *The Veterinary Journal* 161, 229–237. DOI: 10.1053/tvjl.2000.0563.

Westveer, J., Freeman, R., McRae, L., Marconi, V., Almond, R.E.A., and Grooten, M. (2022) *A Deep Dive into the Living Planet Index: A Technical Report*. WWF, Gland, Switzerland.

Wetzel, C. (2022) Saiga antelopes have increased 10-fold after mass die-off in 2015. *New Scientist*. Available at: https://www.newscientist.com/article/2333567-saiga-antelopes-have-increased-10-fold-after-mass-die-off-in-2015/ (accessed 19 December 2022).

White, P.S. and Walker, J.L. (1997) Approximating nature's variation: Selecting and using reference information in restoration ecology. *Restoration Ecology* 5, 338–349. DOI: 10.1046/j.1526-100x.1997.00547.x.

WHO (1986) Ottawa Charter for Health Promotion. Available at: https://www.who.int/teams/health-promotion/enhanced-wellbeing/first-global-conference (accessed 29 July 2024).

WHO (2019a) *WHO Global Report on Traditional and Complementary Medicine 2019*. Available at: https://apps.who.int/iris/handle/10665/312342 (accessed 19 December 2022).

WHO (2019b) *Drinking-Water*. Available at: https://www.who.int/news-room/fact-sheets/detail/drinking-water (accessed 29 June 2021).

Wilson, E.O. (1992) *The Diversity of Life*. W.W. Norton and Company, New York and London.

Winkler, K., Fuchs, R., Rounsevell, M. and Herold, M. (2021) Global land use changes are four times greater than previously estimated. *Nature Communications* 12(1), 1–10. DOI: 10.1038/s41467-021-22702-2.

Wood, C., McInturff, A., Young, H., Kim, D. and Lafferty, K. (2017) Human infectious disease burdens decrease with urbanization but not with biodiversity. *Philosophical Transactions of the Royal Society B: Biological Sciences* 372, 20160122. DOI: 10.1098/rstb.2016.0122.

Woolhouse, M. and Gowtage-Sequeria, S. (2005) Host range and emerging and reemerging pathogens. *Emerging Infectious Diseases* 11, 1842–1847. DOI: 10.3201/eid1112.050997.

WWF (2018) *Living Planet Report – 2018: Aiming Higher*. Grooten, M. and Almond, R.E.A. (eds) WWF, Gland, Switzerland.

Zhu, Y., Fang, H., Wang, Y., Fan, J., Yang, S., Mew, T. and Mundt, C. (2005) Panicle blast and canopy moisture in rice cultivar mixtures. *Phytopathology* 95, 433–438. DOI: 10.1094/phyto-95-0433.

8 Social Determinants of Health at the Human–Animal–Ecosystem Interface

Natalia Cediel Becerra[1,2], María Guerra-Zúñiga[3], Ana Maria Castro[1], Alexander Navas Panadero[1], Nathaly Jimenez[4] and Roseanna Collins[5]

[1]*Faculty of Agricultural Sciences, Universidad de La Salle, Bogotá, Colombia;* [2]*Network for Ecohealth and One Health (NEOH);* [3]*Department of Public Health, School of Medicine, Universidad de Valparaíso, Valparaiso, Chile;* [4]*Association, Amazona, Putumayo, Colombia;* [5]*UK Health Security Agency, London, UK*

Contents

 Principles of One Health for a better planet (eds B. Häsler, A. Tvarijonaviciute and S. Savić)
DOI: 10.1079/9781800623002.0009

Chapter Overview

Elevator pitch

The Social Determinants of Health (SDH) concept is used to examine the linkages between human health outcomes and the socio-economic conditions in which people are born, grow, work, live and age. The SDH are directly linked to health inequities (unfair and avoidable differences in health status) seen within and between countries. We suggest that including One Health and Ecohealth principles in the study of SDH can improve the awareness that health disparities are present along the whole human–animal–environmental (HAE) interface, affecting all three components and highlighting their interdependence. We explain how the One Health agenda can be an equity agenda and highlight the synergy between One Health and Agroecology.

Book objectives the chapter relates to

☐ 1. Understand what One Health and Ecohealth mean
☑ 2. Think in a One Health and Ecohealth way
☐ 3. Apply One Health and Ecohealth in their professional and personal life
☐ 4. Know how to share One Health and Ecohealth knowledge
☑ 5. Integrate One Health and Ecohealth knowledge actively
☑ 6. Acquire or enhance core One Health competencies

One Health competencies covered

☐ 1. Effective communication
☐ 2. Collaborative and resilient working
☑ 3. Systems understanding
☑ 4. Transdisciplinarity
☑ 5. Social, cultural and gender equity and inclusiveness
☐ 6. Collective learning and reflective practice
☐ 7. One Health concepts
☐ 8. Theoretical and methodological pluralism
☐ 9. Harnessing uncertainty, paradox and limited knowledge

After having worked through this chapter, you will be familiar with the SDH, the concept of equity and how equity can be promoted through an SDH lens. Additionally, you will be able to apply systems understanding to identify relevant One Health elements and their relationships, interactions and patterns, which lead to health disparities and inequities worldwide. Ultimately, this chapter aims to instill an appreciation of approaches used to understand socio-ecological systems.

Learning outcomes

1. Understand the Social Determinants of Health concepts and their importance under a One Health approach.
2. Discern how the Social Determinants of Health influence One Health implementation at national and local level.
3. Identify the role of socio-economic status in determining health outcomes at the human–animal–ecosystem interface.
4. Recognize the impact of health inequity at the human–animal–ecosystem interface.
5. Give examples of challenges and successes addressing the socio-economic aspects of health at the human–animal–ecosystem interface.

Summary

This chapter illustrates the concept of Social Determinants of Health (SDH) as the drivers of health inequities experienced by certain population groups owing to socio-economic factors. In the first part, you will find a description of three existing models highlighting their limits around the human–animal–ecosystem (HAE) interface and their importance when analysing the implementation of One Health in several countries. You will get to know the paradoxical reality of Indigenous Peoples who have a belief system rooted in a closer connection to animals and nature and their intrinsic respect of relationships with all forms of life creating a better ground for wellbeing and holistic health, but who also face structural inequalities that prevent them from enjoying basic human rights such as health access, education, clean water and peaceful surroundings. Next, you will engage with a reflection about SDH using a One Health/Ecohealth lens to highlight the advantages of systems science to better explain reality and be aware of the avoidable barriers for social groups when formulating, implementing, monitoring or evaluating health projects. You get to know some principles that can be used when planning inclusive stakeholder engagement to achieve equity, inclusiveness and diversity and get an opportunity to apply the theory in practical exercises.

8.1 Social Determinants of Health

8.1.1 Introduction to the concept Social Determinants of Health (SDH)

Health follows a social gradient, meaning the higher the social position, the better the health. The social gradient in health is not confined to those in poverty; it is a continuum that extends across all levels of the social hierarchy. This means that as one moves down the social ladder or experiences lower levels of socio-economic advantage, health tends to worsen at each step. Several authors in literature report that individuals with higher social status or higher socio-economic positions tend to have better health **outcomes** compared to those with lower social status or lower socio-economic positions. These findings include not only physical health but also mental health across all age ranges (García *et al.*, 2018; Williams *et al.*, 2018; Green *et al.*, 2021; Barnett *et al.*, 2023).

To understand the causes of this gradient, a conceptual, multilevel model called **Social Determinants of Health** (SDH) was created to examine the linkages between human health outcomes and the socio-economic conditions in which people are born, grow, work, live and age, and the wider set of forces and **systems** shaping the conditions of daily life (Marmot and Wilkinson, 2006; Marmot, 2011). SDH – including **gender**, poverty, unequal access to healthcare, lack of education, stigma and racism – are underlying, contributing factors of health inequities (the unfair and avoidable differences in health status) seen within and between countries (Williams and Cooper, 2019; Balaj *et al.*, 2021). These factors disproportionately burden low- and middle-income countries (LMICs), as well as marginalized populations around the world: women, rural, mobile and livestock-dependent communities, **Indigenous Peoples**, Afro-descendants, etc. Tackling these socio-economic inequalities in health requires an understanding of how an individual's social position influences disease risk; thus, the effect of social position can be mediated by causes that are unevenly distributed across social groups and/or interact with social position (Diderichsen *et al.*, 2019).

8.1.2 Health equity

Talking about differences in health is not the same as talking about health inequities. When it is stated that there are differences in health among human beings, this refers to any variation in qualities or attributes between people or population groups (e.g. the body mass index of an individual or the prevalence of a certain disease in a country). When the word inequity or disparity in health is used, however, what is referred to is an unfair difference (Arcaya *et al.*, 2015). The SDH are the major drivers of health inequities – to expand on the earlier definition, these can be described as the unfair, avoidable and remediable differences systematically experienced by certain population groups due to socio-economic factors. These differences in health are the result of decision-making processes, **policies**, **social norms** and structures that build systematic, preventable and unnecessary injustices into all levels of society – therefore strategies must be proposed to reverse them (WHO *et al.*, 2006).

HEALTH EQUITY is 'when everyone has the opportunity to attain their full health potential' and no one is 'disadvantaged from achieving this potential because of their social position or other socially determined circumstance' (Braveman and Gruskin, 2003). This includes ensuring equity for every child from the start of their life, encompassing healthier **environments**, adequate nutrition and education, fair employment and decent working conditions, social protection across the life course and universal healthcare. Where people live and work, their race, ethnicity and gender can impact their mental and physical health; health in turn is affected by factors such as affordable, adequate housing and employment – these are the upstream causes of health. To make such progress, decided actions must be taken to address global inequities in the distribution of power, money and resources: 'the social injustice that is killing on a grand scale' (Marmot, 2011); to make such progress, decided actions must be taken to address global inequities in the SDH.

Health equity primarily focuses on addressing disparities and promoting fairness in health outcomes among human populations. It is a concept rooted in social justice and human rights, aiming to ensure that all individuals have equal opportunities to achieve good health and **wellbeing**, regardless of their social, economic or cultural backgrounds.

8.1.3 One Health

Although a human-centred concept at its core, the principles of health equity – fairness, justice, respect and compassionate care – extend to the treatment of animals. Referred to as 'animal **welfare**', this concept seeks to ensure the wellbeing of animals through prevention of unnecessary suffering, and the promotion of health and a good quality of life, both under human care and in their natural environments. By adopting a One Health approach and considering the wellbeing of both humans and animals, societies can strive for a more holistic and ethical approach to health and welfare, recognizing the interconnectedness of all living beings and their shared environments. This concept is explored in more detail below.

8.1.4 Influential models of the Social Determinants of Health

In 1991, Dahlgren and Whitehead were commissioned to prepare a policy-friendly report on policies and strategies to promote equity in health for the World Health Organization Regional Office for Europe. They formulated a rainbow-like model that conceptualizes the main determinants of health for the whole population and brought attention to the interconnection between health with environmental, cultural and socio-economic conditions. Its holistic view combined with its relative simplicity made it accessible and understandable. Furthermore, the authors highlighted that the determinants of health in the rainbow can be health promoting (salutogenic), protective (e.g. a vaccine) or health-damaging (Dahlgren and Whitehead, 2021).

This model broadened horizons and encouraged people to think beyond health services and the health **sector** in local environments and society as a whole. It has proved to be particularly helpful conceptually for professionals and policy makers operating in diverse sectors outside the health sector (Dahlgren and Whitehead, 2021). It allocates ownership and responsibility to each sector to develop and implement its own strategies for promoting health and reducing inequalities based on the reality in that sector. This model allowed many professionals to look at inequitable health outcomes from a multidimensional perspective, i.e. the product of a set of factors that go beyond human biology.

In the past five decades, there have been several visual models to represent the social determinants of health in different countries. In fact, the concept of health determinants began to appear in the public debate after the findings of the Lalonde report in Canada in 1974, who, as Minister of Health at the time, surprised the Canadian state by stating that the great burden of disease and death in that country was due to four determinants: human biological, lifestyle, environmental and healthcare systems factors (Villar, 2011). Of these four factors, lifestyle and environmental factors were the most important in determining the mortality at that time, providing a milestone for the health promotion movement, which became a pivotal principle of current public health globally (Tulchinsky and Lalonde, 2018). He wrote the New Perspective on the Health of Canadians, a document widely regarded as a groundbreaking document recognizing that other strategies beyond biomedical methods and health insurance for medical and hospital care are needed to improve the health of a population. Health promotion became the only feasible public health activity when the HIV/AIDS epidemic storm arrived in the 1980s when there were no effective biomedical measures available. Health promotion provided some useful measures such as education, and condom and syringe distribution in high-risk groups to reduce the spread of the disease, until effective antiretroviral drugs became available in the late 1990s (Tulchinsky and Lalonde, 2018).

Another important milestone in the SDH path was the contributions of Wilkinson and Marmot, who provided solid evidence regarding the influence of social determinants on human health. A person in a better social, economic and cultural position is in an advantageous situation with respect to another person who is less favoured in these aspects, thus producing a gradient in health indicators. Sir Michael Marmot, Research Professor of Epidemiology and Public Health, University College, London, led a famous research group on health inequalities for some 30 years. His work highlighted the importance of improving people's living conditions, hygiene and diet as highly beneficial to their general health and wellbeing. Due to his leadership, he was the Chair of the Commission on Social Determinants of Health set up by the World Health Organization in 2005 (Tulchinsky and Lalonde, 2018).

A new model was formulated by the Commission on Social Determinants of Health (Solar and Irwin, 2010). This model was composed of structural, intermediate and proximal determinants. They considered health as a universal human aspiration and a basic human need. Their work focused on the fundamental structures of social hierarchy and the socially determined conditions these create in which people grow, live, work and age (Marmot and Wilkinson, 2006). This was called the 'causes of the causes' of health inequality. These issues together influenced the international consensus on the Millennium Development Goals and the **Sustainable Development Goals** (Marmot and Wilkinson, 2006; Tulchinsky and Lalonde, 2018). The Commission on Social Determinants of Health placed urgent action to ensure fair health at the heart of the public health movement at the beginning of the century (Solar and Irwin, 2010).

Another model called the socio-ecological framework was first suggested by Broffenbrenner in the 1970s as an ecological systems theory and was later redefined by McLeroy and colleagues as a framework to promote health-related behavioural change (McLeroy *et al.*, 1988). This is a model for health promotion that focuses attention on both individual and social environmental factors as targets for health promotion interventions. It addresses the importance of interventions directed at changing interpersonal, organizational, community and public policy, factors that support and maintain unhealthy behaviours. The model assumes that appropriate changes in the social environment will produce changes in individuals, and that the support of individuals in the population is essential for implementing environmental changes (McLeroy *et al.*, 1988). The Social-Ecological Model (SEM) is a valuable tool for understanding and addressing complex issues related to disease prevention. The SEM is a theoretical framework that examines human behaviour by considering the hierarchical interactions of biological systems. It conceptualizes these interactions as a multi-level hierarchy centred around the individual. The SEM has proven effective in developing and enhancing disease prevention programmes, providing insights into the various factors that influence prevention efforts (Palomares Velosa *et al.*, 2022).

In Fig. 8.1, a modified figure of the social determinants of health is presented.

Human and canine rabies in Latin America: Let us have a look at an example focused on **zoonotic diseases**, which are caused by harmful germs like viruses, bacteria, parasites and fungi. These germs can be transmitted between people and animals and can cause illness from mild to serious and even death (Centers for Disease Control and Prevention, 2021). The World Health Organization has described about 200 known zoonoses (World Health Organization, 2020). One of the most important zoonoses in Latin America is the rabies virus. This disease is still circulating in dogs in Bolivia, Guatemala, Haiti and the Dominican Republic, and this cycle accounts for 100% of human lethal rabies cases (Pan American Health Organization, 2018). With respect to individual and lifestyle factors, which are placed at the centre of the model, young age is an attribute that plays against the risk of contracting the disease. Between 60% and 70% of rabies cases occur between the ages of 5 and 15 years. This background is not the only one that influences the occurrence of human rabies, as the model indicates. In less economically developed countries, such as the Southern Cone countries, there are vast rural regions far away from healthcare centres (territorial factor), rabies vaccination programmes face greater difficulties in achieving optimal coverage of this pathology (public policy) and veterinary care of pets is poor (cultural and economic aspect) (Arechiga *et al.*, 2014). Thus, according to the Swedish model, an 8-year-old boy or girl living in the most remote Andean regions of his or her province in Bolivia, born into an impoverished family and having a pet dog, has a higher risk of contracting rabies than the same 8-year-old child living in the capital of his or her country (La Paz), with an urban health centre near his or her home, vaccinated against the disease, born into a family with greater economic resources and who, if he or she has a pet, is more likely to have the necessary veterinary care. Neither human health nor animal health is assured in scenarios of lower economic resources.

The effects of COVID-19 on different social groups: Let us look at the COVID-19 infection, hospitalization and mortality impact worldwide. The World Health Organization published a report in 2021 with evidence showing that people with better living and working conditions, better education, more social capital and better access to health services have been better able to implement containment measures (World Health Organization, 2021).

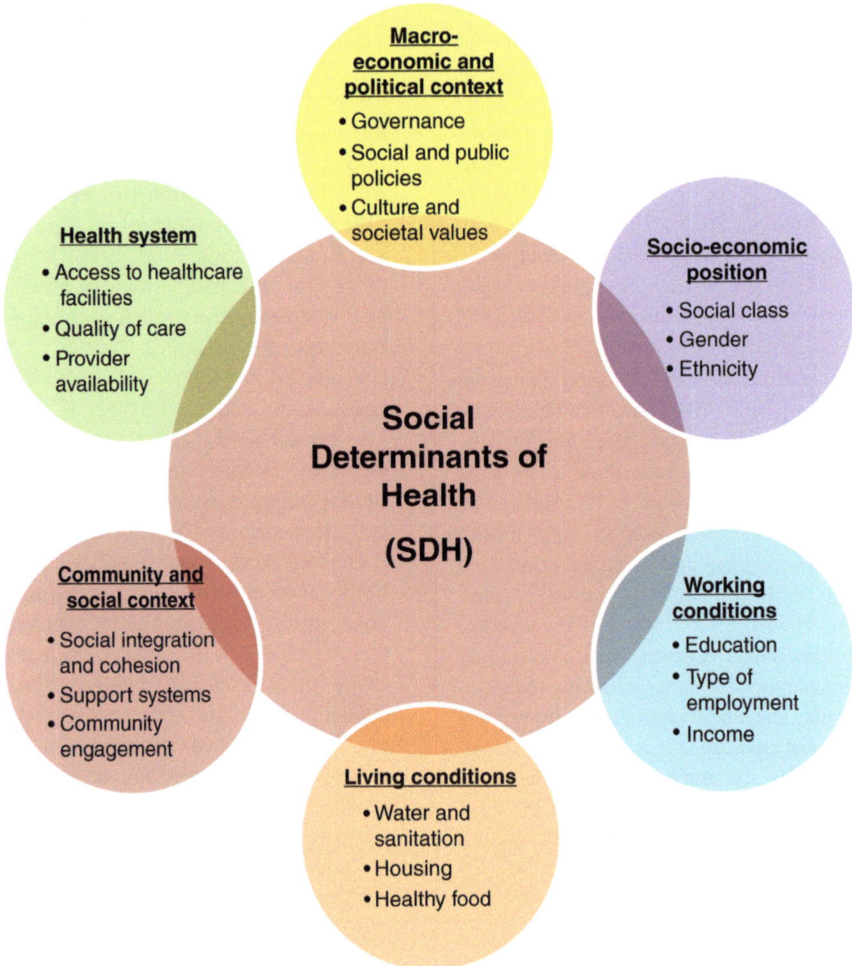

Fig. 8.1. Overview of Social Determinants of Health. Developed by the authors based on information from Dahlgren and Whitehead (2021) and Solar and Irwin (2010).

Which groups were more affected during the COVID-19 pandemic?
Groups that have experienced increased rates of COVID-19 morbidity and mortality include: (i) poorer people; (ii) marginalized ethnic minorities, including Indigenous Peoples; (iii) low-paid essential workers; (iv) migrants; (v) populations affected by emergencies, including conflicts; (vi) incarcerated populations; and (vii) homeless people. These results can be explained by unfavourable social determinants of health for these social groups as they have higher rates of chronic disease that increase their risk of poor outcomes from COVID-19, greater exposure to the COVID-19 virus, lesser capacity to adhere to public health and social measures, and poorer access to health services for treatment and vaccination (World Health Organization, 2021).

Disadvantaged populations face daily living and working conditions that result in heightened susceptibility and exposure to SARS-CoV-2, as well as obstacles to the implementation of public health and social measures. The specific social determinants that have driven these inequities include: (i) poverty and deprivation; (ii) imposed mobility of low-paid workers in precarious employment; (iii) lack of social protection; (iv) crowded housing; (v) poor protection at work and low occupational health standards; (vi) unequal legal or residential status; (vii) stigmatization (migrants); (viii) unequal access to acceptable public health information; and (ix) inequitable access to affordable treatment, prevention and vaccination (World Health Organization, 2021).

What were the additional health impacts due to overstretched health services, service disruptions and isolation?

- Decreased use of health services because of fear of infection and service disruptions particularly affected disadvantaged communities. Disruptions of services increased inequity in care for both non-communicable and communicable diseases and also for populations living with HIV/AIDS.
- Isolation worsens mental health and deteriorates health behaviours of disadvantaged groups. Stress, boredom or isolation resulting from social distancing and closures increased drug taking. Studies of mental health during COVID-19 in a large, nationally representative, cross-sectional survey in the UK found that women and young people had higher risks of general psychiatric disorders and loneliness. A longitudinal study confirmed both these findings and also found a greater impact in minority ethnic groups (World Health Organization, 2021).
- Mental health and wellbeing of lower-educated, female front-line workers was particularly impacted. There is evidence that nursing and support staff, frequently women with fewer years of education, had a higher incidence of associated health problems than medical staff. Other studies showed that female front-line healthcare workers and nurses had higher rates of depression and insomnia than male medical staff (e.g. in China and Spain) (World Health Organization, 2021).

8.1.5 Social Determinants of Health in Indigenous groups

There is a body of scientific evidence that shows health disparities are greater among racial and ethnic social groups (Devakumar *et al.*, 2022). It is crucial for the purpose of this chapter to recognize that historic systems and structures of power and oppression together with discrimination have shaped health policy and practice and are the root causes of health inequities in many countries and between countries (Devakumar *et al.*, 2022). Denying this would mean denying history. In this next section, we will transcend and make deeper, wider and more integrative reflections on how to address the social determinants of health in Indigenous communities with a focus on Latin America.

Most Latin American and Caribbean Indigenous populations – more than 800 Indigenous Peoples with a population of around 58 million people representing 10% of the total population – are imposed with habitat degradation, resource over-exploitation and forest fragmentation as their natural environment has been altered through the introduction of non-native species of animals and plants and through human interventions and changes that have coincided with the political and cultural changes that accompanied colonization of the North and South American continent, first by Europeans and later by American settlers (Cruz, 2018). The definitions of health of Indigenous Peoples include the environment as a central aspect (earth, water, volcanoes, rivers, sun, moon). For example, in the worldview of the Mapuche people (one of the ten ethnic groups originating in Chile) the concept of health is linked closely to the environment. The Mapuche are affected by everything that happens in nature; when the balance is somehow broken, the relationships between beings are affected. If someone breaks the balance by violating the laws of nature, they suffer the consequences of the imbalance they have caused in the form of both physical and spiritual illness. The rupture of harmony in the network of relationships occurs in various situations, for example, when the environment within the family is one of discord, there are fights between neighbours, there is no food for animals, sacred places and the beings that inhabit them are not respected, nature is consciously damaged. When this happens, the disorders and imbalances created by the individual have consequences on health (Marileo, 2002, cited in Díaz *et al.*, 2004).

When considering the determinants of health in the frameworks above, environment is a determinant of health. Having unhealthy environments will produce risk of illness. Many societies consider the linkages between physical, mental and spiritual health. However, what seems to be fundamentally different in Indigenous Peoples is the concept of harmony and balance with the direct consequences of one's actions, of disturbing the balance.

Focusing on another Latin American example on gender (for an explanation on gender, see Chapter 9), another social determinant of health, we can describe how Indigenous women's worldviews, perspectives and wisdom, and their concept of health and survival, constitute a collective and individual inter-generational continuum encompassing a holistic perspective, which incorporates four dimensions of life: spiritual, intellectual, physical and emotional. For them, health is viewed as the harmonious coexistence of human beings with nature, with themselves, and with others in pursuit of wellbeing (Del Popolo *et al.*, 2014). Unfortunately, structural gender inequities like poorer access to land, agricultural inputs, credit, education, extension and other services compared to men, as well as gender-determined roles and responsibilities in collecting water, firewood and other cooking fuels, and unpaid care roles reinforce gender inequities and create worse health indicators and outcomes not only for their families and communities, but also for their animals. For example, women in Indigenous Peoples and rural communities in Colombia have higher maternal morbidity and mortality rates, unwanted pregnancy, sexual abuse derived from structural violence and lack of access to culturally sensitive health services (Polanco *et al.*, 2021; Aviles, 2018, cited in Cediel *et al.*, 2022).

Many Indigenous women argue that land grabbing, deforestation, extraction and privatization of natural resources have worsened their position in recent decades, indicating that the lack of **gender equity** in society mirrors the lack of **biodiversity** conservation and natural resource protection. Despite Indigenous women's unique contribution to maintaining safe environments, achieving food security and enhancing the spiritual wellbeing of society, their impact has been overshadowed by structural and historical social determinants, such as lower access to and control of land compared to men, limited education opportunities blocking them from finding better jobs, lack of access to financial aid and poorer access to healthcare services creating higher rates of mortality due to preventable conditions during pregnancy (Cediel *et al.*, 2022). The arrival of COVID-19 in most Latin American countries exacerbated existing problems of hunger, poverty, gender gaps and health inequities.

Thus, Indigenous Peoples with their quest for harmony have what it takes to inhabit and respectfully care for nature and contribute to a better life where they are and with whom they are. They are role models for a coherent human project capable of responding to the needs of survival respecting life in all its forms through the five specific vows that the African peasant, philosopher and agroecologist Pierre Rabhi proposes to us (Rabhi, 2013):

1. Recreate human and ecological structures.
2. Reconsider the organization of the territory.
3. Revalue the microeconomy and the artisan.
4. Educate children with values of cooperation and complementarity.
5. Awaken sensitivity to beauty and respect for life.

We can learn from Indigenous Peoples to listen and to understand nature's intrinsic wisdom and order, to respect all forms of life connecting our own nature to the global fabric and to behave in a more sustainable way, allowing the next seven generations to experience the beauty, richness and health that are brought by biodiversity and protected natural resources.

Task: The examples above show the idea of harmony and balance and how all health is connected. Think about how these Indigenous Peoples' worldviews have the potential to inform the One Health principle of balance in **socio-ecological systems** and summarize your key points.

Example answer: Please note that the example answer given below is not exhaustive and that you will probably have come up with additional points that are equally valid.

- Indigenous Peoples' worldviews that emphasize the importance of balance and interconnectedness in health can significantly inform and enrich the One Health principle of balance in socio-ecological systems in modern societies. By integrating these perspectives, modern societies can adopt a more holistic and inclusive approach to health that considers not only the physical and social components but also the mental, environmental, vegetal and animal aspects of wellbeing. All life is interconnected and so is our health.
- Holistic approach: Indigenous worldviews consider health as a multifaceted concept that involves the harmony of various interconnected elements. This holistic perspective aligns with the One Health principle, which recognizes the interdependence of human, animal and environmental health. By embracing this holistic approach, modern societies can integrate **knowledge** from diverse **disciplines** to address health challenges comprehensively and sustainably.

- Connection to nature: Indigenous Peoples' worldviews acknowledge the profound connection between human health and the natural world. They recognize the importance of respecting and living in harmony with the environment, vegetal and animal realms. Incorporating this perspective into the One Health approach reinforces the significance of safeguarding **ecosystems** and biodiversity to promote human and animal wellbeing.
- Cultural respect and diversity: Indigenous worldviews value cultural diversity and the unique perspectives each community brings to health and wellbeing. Embracing cultural respect and understanding can enhance the One Health principle's effectiveness, as it encourages collaboration and co-creation of solutions that are contextually relevant and inclusive.
- Long-term **sustainability**: Indigenous Peoples' worldviews often prioritize the sustainability of resources and practices. Integrating this perspective into the One Health principle encourages a focus on long-term ecological balance and resilient socio-ecological systems that support the health of current and future generations.
- Indigenous knowledge systems: Indigenous Peoples have accumulated centuries of traditional knowledge about ecosystems, medicinal plants and animal behaviour. Recognizing and valuing these knowledge systems can enrich the evidence base for One Health initiatives, leading to more effective and culturally appropriate interventions.
- Community-centred approaches: Indigenous worldviews emphasize the importance of community involvement in decision-making processes. Applying community-centred approaches in One Health initiatives ensures that local voices and perspectives are taken into account, leading to better-designed interventions and improved health outcomes.

By embracing Indigenous Peoples' worldviews, the One Health principle can evolve into a more inclusive, culturally sensitive and sustainable approach to addressing health challenges in modern societies. It encourages a deeper appreciation for the interconnectedness of all living beings and the environment, and reinforces the importance of maintaining harmony and balance in socio-ecological systems for the wellbeing of all.

Indigenous populations can lend inspiration to policy through their traditional ecological knowledge, community-based governance and sustainable practices. Learning from their insights can lead to more inclusive and contextually relevant policies that promote harmony, balance, participation and intergenerational equity in socio-ecological systems.

8.1.6 Conceptualizing Social Determinants of Health using a One Health/Ecohealth lens

A first criticism of the Dahlgren and Whitehead SDH model (presented more than 30 years ago) is its **anthropocentric** perspective, i.e. a worldview that places human beings at the centre of consideration or gives them primary importance in relation to other living beings and the environment. In other words, human needs come first at the expense of a balanced coexistence between human beings with multiple animal and plant species on Earth – all in intimate relationships and interdependence. A second criticism is the unidirectionality from the upper layers to the centre of the model, denying or conceptually making invisible the effects of human action on the higher levels of the model (Fig. 8.1). Socio-economic, cultural, environmental systems and human lifestyles change and influence structures in a dialogic relationship and vice versa. They are not unidirectional, much less static. Faced with this, it is worth asking if there is a better model that fits these complexities in a new order of ideas. The original Dahlgren and Whitehead SDH model does not address environmental drivers of inequity of poor health and does not consider the interconnectedness among the health conditions of humans with other living beings such as animals (domestic and wildlife), plants and ecosystems (Rabhi, 2013). One Health and Ecohealth approaches provide the necessary elements for an updated framework.

During the past three decades, a growing scientific movement has emerged to promote and advocate for One Health and Ecohealth approaches to health. An ecosystem approach recognizes that health and wellbeing are the result of complex and dynamic interactions between determinants, and between people, social and economic conditions, and ecosystems. The conditions of ecosystems are also affected by a dynamic process of interactions, often determined by the social and economic activities of people (Charron, 2012), as described in Chapter 7 on biodiversity. The development of ecosystem approaches to health has been influenced by several other movements and ideas over the last 40 years, including the ecosystem approach developed by the International Joint Commission for transboundary water management in Canada, sustainable development, health promotion, ecosystem health, eco-epidemiology, Latin American social medicine, and the wider public health movement in Europe. Social, cultural and economic activities of people – from local household decisions to national policies and international treaties and systems – are occurring within ecosystems while determining human health and shaping the relationships people have with ecosystems (Charron, 2012).

This thinking is well captured in the conceptual framework of socio-ecological systems that integrates social and ecological components into a unified system to understand the interactions and interdependencies between human societies and their surrounding environment. It emphasizes the dynamic and complex relationships between people, communities, ecosystems and the natural world. In a socio-ecological system, the social component refers to human communities, cultures, economies, institutions and behaviours, while the ecological component includes the natural environment, ecosystems, biodiversity and natural processes. Key characteristics include interconnectedness, feedback loops, resilience and adaptation. In brief, social determinants are not enough to understand and acknowledge the complexity of health within populations in an interconnected world; we need to extend to also cover environment, politics, economics and behavioural determinants.

8.2 The Equity Agenda in One Health

Many international agencies are battling with the task of trading off and balancing multiple outcomes, such as community nutrition, health, livestock production and environmental protection (see also Chapter 15 on Sustainable Development Goals). One of the key principles of One Health is equity among different populations or, in other words, a One Health agenda can be considered an equity agenda.

Equity between the health of animals, people and the environment refers to the fair and just distribution of resources, opportunities and wellbeing among these interconnected components of the ecosystem. It recognizes that the health and wellbeing of animals, humans and the environment are deeply intertwined and that the health of one can impact the health of the others (One Health High-Level Expert Panel: OHHLEP *et al.*, 2022). Better livestock health will only lead to better health for animals and humans if health equity is also promoted and the interdependence of human, livestock and ecosystem health is recognized. Unconnected and 'one sectoral' approaches to managing the health of people, livestock and environments are failing to meet today's complex health challenges and are proving to be unsustainable. Thus, One Health is a pathway to synergistically addressing health and sustainability (Kock *et al.*, 2018; Garnier *et al.*, 2020).

Livestock health cannot be promoted or sustained without equal attention being paid to the health of local communities, broader society and ecosystems. We already know that persistent inequities cause some people to be systematically disadvantaged in their capacity to improve the health of their animals and themselves. Low- and middle-income countries (LMICs) are threatened by deteriorated animal health which impacts human health. According to Stephen and Parmley (2022):

> To tackle inequity, we must understand and address how health issues – livestock as well as human – variously affect different population groups. Ensuring people today and tomorrow have fair opportunities to access the health benefits from livestock requires purposely engaging with and supporting sectors of society that are systematically disadvantaged, including women, rural communities and poor people.

But how can we achieve equity in One Health projects, programmes and policies? It is crucial to first understand which **stakeholders** – people, groups or communities – are at risk of being excluded, and what are the specific opportunities and barriers to their inclusion. To ensure a project, programme or policy has equity, inclusive stakeholder engagement to achieve social and gender is recommended using the following principles (Global Infrastructure Hub, 2023):

- Identify and engage with all relevant stakeholders, including those who may be traditionally marginalized or underrepresented.
- Provide opportunities for stakeholders to provide feedback and share their perspectives.
- Ensure communication is clear and accessible to all stakeholders, regardless of language and ability.
- Use a variety of engagement methods to ensure that all stakeholders have an opportunity to participate.
- Consider the potential impacts of decisions on all stakeholders and take steps to mitigate any negative impact.

In Chapter 10 on the project life cycle, you can learn more about the process of inclusive stakeholder engagement.

8.3 Applying the Theoretical Knowledge

8.3.1 Activity neighbourhood and social dynamics

Task: Take a picture from your neighbourhood that captures the interlink(s) between inequity and health at the human–animal–ecosystem interface. Describe the social dynamics at play.

Example answer 1: Please note that the example answer may be completely different from what you have chosen and that is fine, because each context is different.

High-rise buildings that are architectural marvels have replaced nature. However, access to green space is a need that is currently treated like a privilege. Thus, an indoor garden on top of one of the high-rise buildings was created to give people a place to relax and recharge surrounded by the calming and restorative effects of plants (Fig. 8.2). Exposure to greenery is a valuable resource to people – even if it is indoors with no useful effects for the biodiversity / nature in the area. Critics of the place argue that it reinforces inequalities, as access is controlled and restricted, rollerblades, bikes, scooters and skateboards are banned, and 'proper' conduct is expected from visitors. Thus, it limits the opportunity of having a space where people from all social groups can be and meet – this example seems to be a place where only certain groups are allowed, thereby contributing to marginalization.

Example answer 2: The picture shows the living conditions where people can be bitten by bats owing to the type of housing (Fig. 8.3). There are several reports describing the common factors in most human rabies outbreaks in the Amazon Region of Brazil and Perú. Some contributory factors include: occur in small population groups, generally in remote rural areas; outbreak localities (when information is available) had experienced a change in the type of human productive process taking place there, such as a gold rush, deforestation or withdrawal of domestic animals; all the communities had poor living conditions, including precarious housing; none of the communities had access to health services offering rabies prophylactic treatment; nor did the inhabitants know how rabies is transmitted (Schneider *et al.*, 2009). The Indigenous populations are at greater risk of acquiring the disease and also of dying from it because of the lack of good healthcare access to receive the treatment. Social determinants of health in these cases create higher mortality rates in vulnerable Indigenous groups that could be preventable.

8.3.2 Applied example: agroecology and activity

In Box 8.1 a synthesis of agroecology is presented. **Agroecology** is an example of an expanded and holistic framework unifying environmental and social determinants. Please read it and then engage with the task after the box.

Task: Read the example below on an agroecological transition and list the social and environmental determinants of health and their interconnections. If you like graphical visualizations, you may want to produce an overview diagram.

Food production in the context of climate change: a view from a transition towards agroecology in Northern Colombia: The new **climate** scenarios

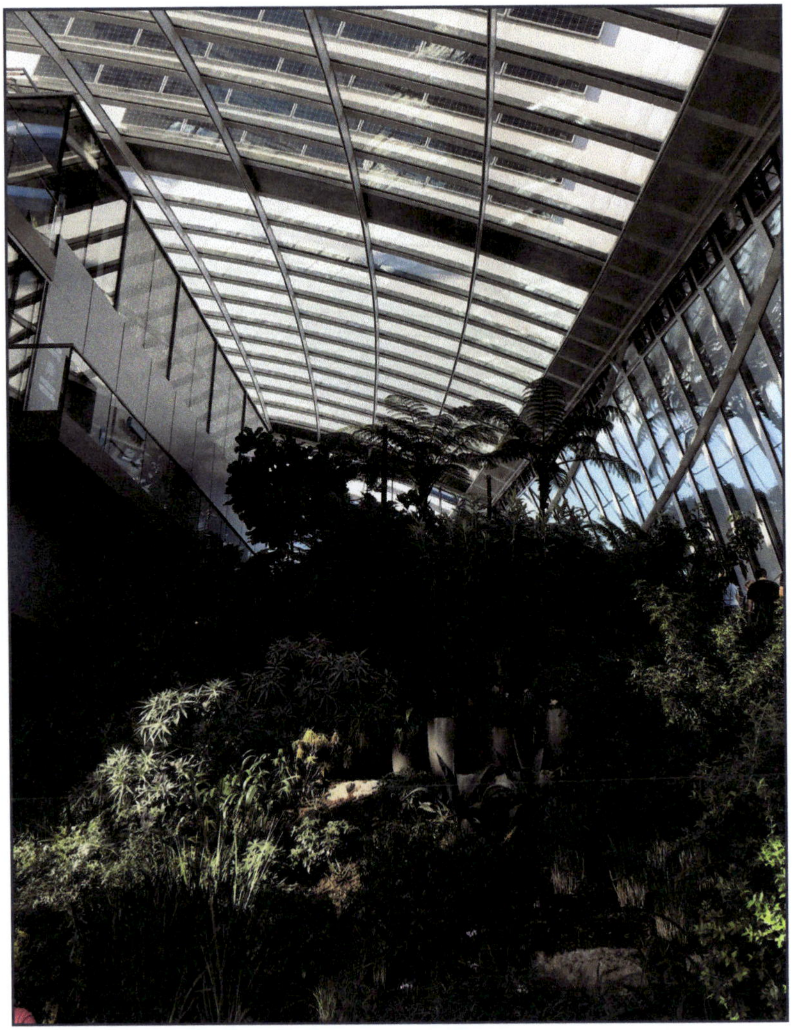

Fig. 8.2. The Sky Garden in London, UK. Source/ picture credit: Barbara Häsler.

will cause a strong reduction in food production, especially in dry areas, affecting small producers to a greater extent (Altieri and Nicholls, 2008), increasing hunger and creating food insecurity (Field *et al.*, 2014). Animal production systems will be affected by reducing the productive and reproductive efficiency of animals (González and Wing Ching, 2018) and increasing the risk for the presentation of other diseases or intoxications.

Sustainable production systems that mitigate climate change and foster resilience must be developed (Caron *et al.*, 2018), which should be driven by policies that favour knowledge and capacities in social infrastructure to change production models (Abayineh and Belay, 2017). The importance of food systems for sustainable development lies in the nexus between food security, nutrition and human health, ecosystem viability, climate change and social justice (Caron *et al.*, 2018).

The northern zone of Colombia has dry to very dry tropical forest ecosystems. In these ecosystems, rainfall is low and concentrated in some months, while in others the drought is prolonged, affecting food production for animals and people; this problem is becoming more acute under the new scenarios of climate variability and change (Fig. 8.4).

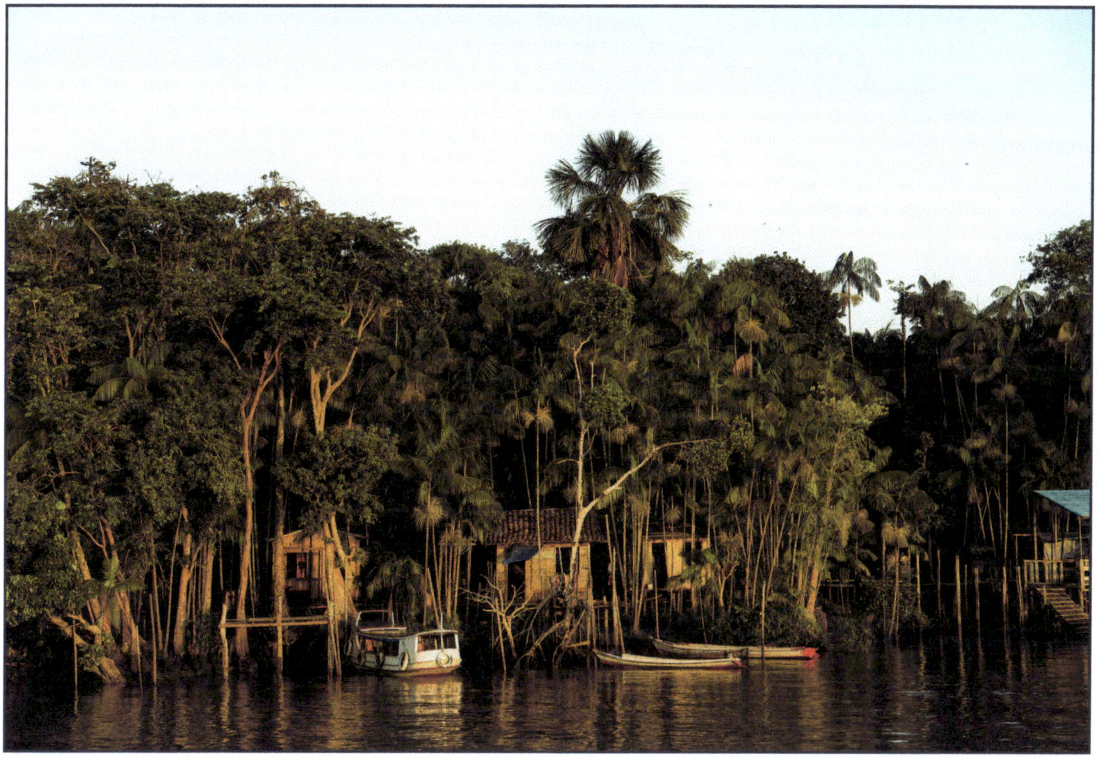

Fig. 8.3. Traditional Amazonian dwelling. Picture credit: Francisco Chaves, Wikimedia, unmodified (CC BY 2.0 DEED, https://creativecommons.org/licenses/by/2.0).

Box 8.1. Agroecology unites ecosystem health, social determinants, and socio-ecological systems

Agroecology can be understood as a scientific discipline, a set of agricultural practices and a social movement (Wezel *et al.*, 2020). As a science, agroecology studies processes and cause–effect relationships on agricultural land, and uses ecological concepts and principles for the design and management of sustainable agroecosystems, in which external inputs are replaced by natural processes (Gliessman, 2016). The object of research is the functionality of the entire agroecosystem with its multiple interconnections. As a practice, agroecology is a set of specific local and cultural methods that utilize, preserve and enhance biological and ecological processes in agricultural production. At their core is the promotion of positive interactions and synergies between plants, animals, soil, water and the agri-food system. Agroecological farming systems place a strong focus on diversification, e.g. through practices such as mixed cropping and intercropping, agroforestry, silvopasture, use of the locally adapted seeds and animal breeds, biological pest control and management, green manure, among others. As a social movement, agroecology provides the foundation for a way for people to know and control their development processes, and therefore their health and welfare, and can be a farmers' group working for food security, sovereignty and autonomy. Alternatively, it can be a more political movement of the local population for rural development. Or it can be a farmers' group movement for extending alternative agriculture through social partnerships to better respond to ecological and environmental challenges within relatively specialized agricultural production systems (Wezel *et al.*, 2020).

Continued

Box 8.1. Continued.

It incorporates 13 principles (Wezel *et al.*, 2020) aimed at promoting sustainable agriculture and enhancing functional biodiversity in agroecosystems. These principles include recycling resources, reducing input reliance, improving soil and animal health, maintaining diversity, fostering ecological synergy, economic diversification, co-creation of knowledge, promoting social values and diets, ensuring fairness, enhancing connectivity between producers and consumers, supporting land and resource governance, and encouraging participation in decision making.

The goal of agroecology is to prevent problems rather than simply curing them, similar to the approach in human health. By applying these principles, agroecosystems can function in harmony, leading to the overall wellbeing and proper functioning of the ecosystem.

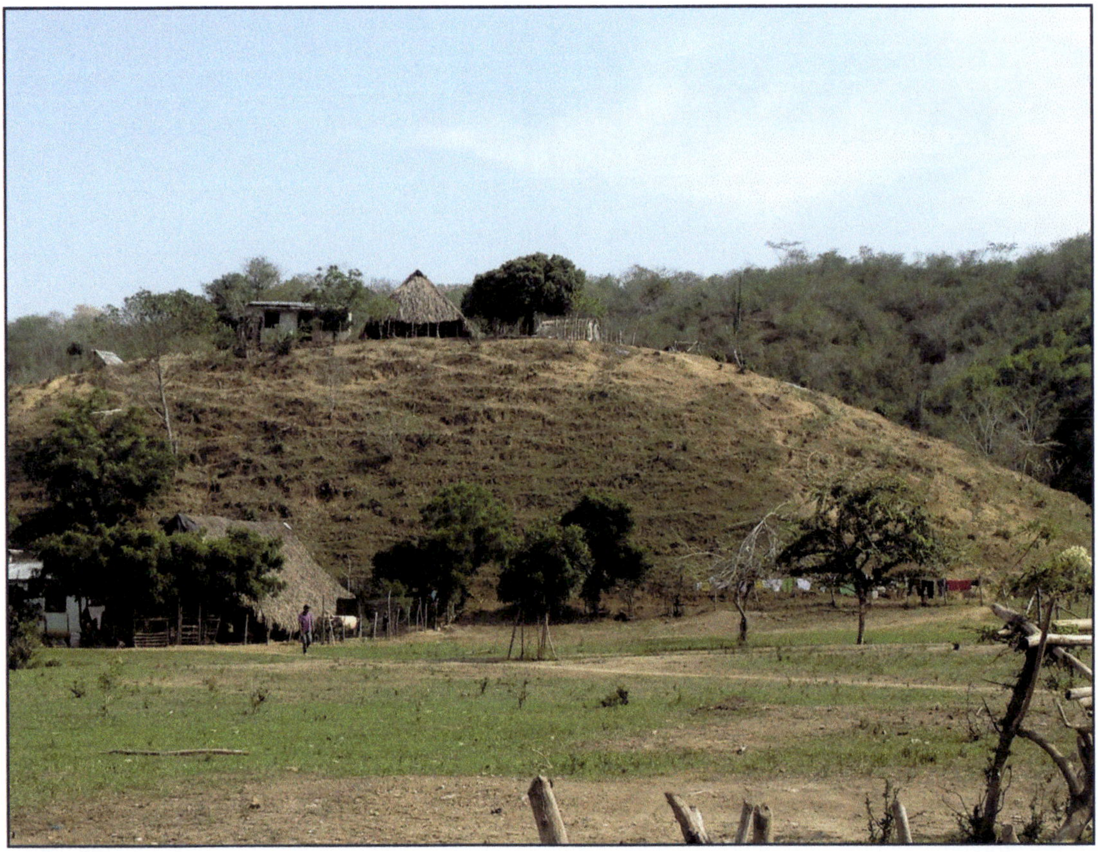

Fig. 8.4. Widespread soil loss in tropical dry forest ecosystems in northern Colombia. Picture credit: Authors' own collection (Alexander Navas).

The loss of tree cover due to deforestation has generated strong soil erosion processes that affect soil productivity. In addition, the reduction in the water catchment capacity of the ecosystems and people's activities has generated low water availability and quality, which affects the living conditions of animals and people, increasing the risk factors for malnutrition and disease. There are different social triggers that have generated changes in community relations in the region; for example, there are women who are in charge of all the productive tasks because the men migrate in search of work to obtain economic resources for the

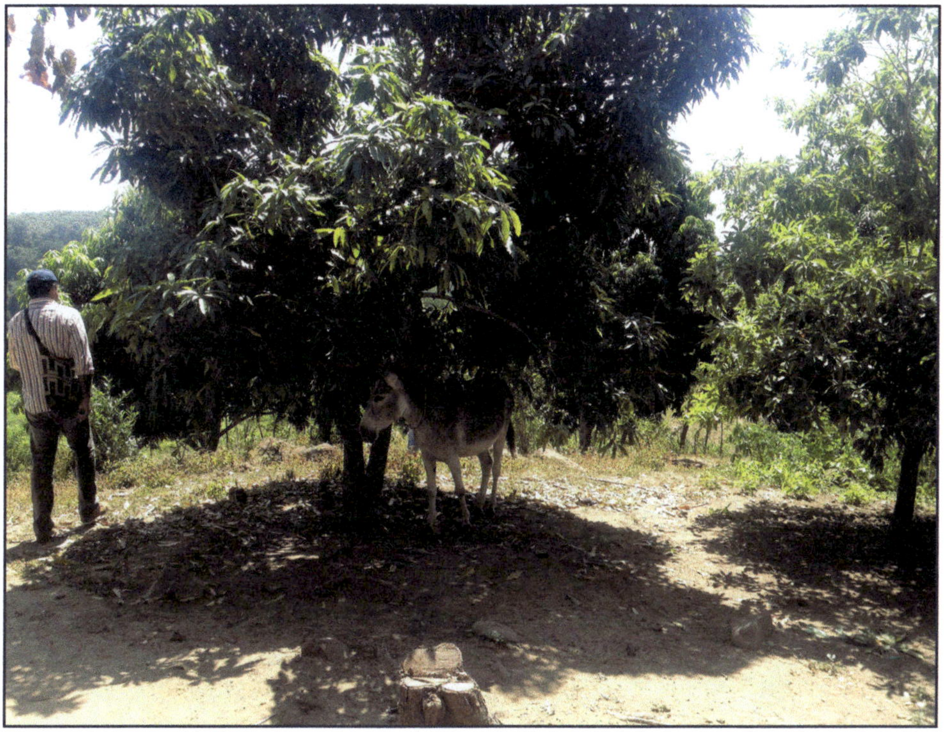

Fig. 8.5. Family gathering of food and water for animals and people in tropical dry forest ecosystems in northern Colombia. Picture credit: Authors' own collection (Alexander Navas).

family; in other cases there are elderly men on the properties because the living conditions have generated the migration of women and children to urban centres. It is also common to observe children or families that move several kilometres a day in search of water and food for the animals and people (Fig. 8.5).

Agroecology allows the development of agriculture in harmony with the environment, favouring the relations and development of the communities in the territory (Hecht, 1999); it also seeks to provide solutions to local problems from the union between local ancestral and scientific knowledge. For example, some producers know well the behaviour of the climate, the changes that have occurred in recent years and their effect on agricultural or daily work in the territory, and they also know which agroecological practices allow them to adapt to these climatic conditions (Navas, 2022), as well as the natural resources and biodiversity present in the ecosystems.

Some producers in the northern part of Colombia initiated an agroecological reconversion process in which local knowledge was gathered from community workshops and the exchange of knowledge of agroecological practices was facilitated. This allowed changes to be made in the farms over time, based on soil improvement, capture, retention and storage of rainwater, diversification of food production for animals and people, and conservation of food for critical times (Figs 8.5 and 8.6). In addition, new family and community dynamics were generated in the territory, because the reconverted farms became agroecological beacons where producers in the area can demonstrate that by using local resources, and with organizational processes, each member can contribute to improving the family's living conditions. These changes made it possible to improve food sovereignty and security, reduce risk factors for malnutrition and disease, generate economic resources and recover the health of the ecosystem. Another benefit of this agroecological transition is that neither women

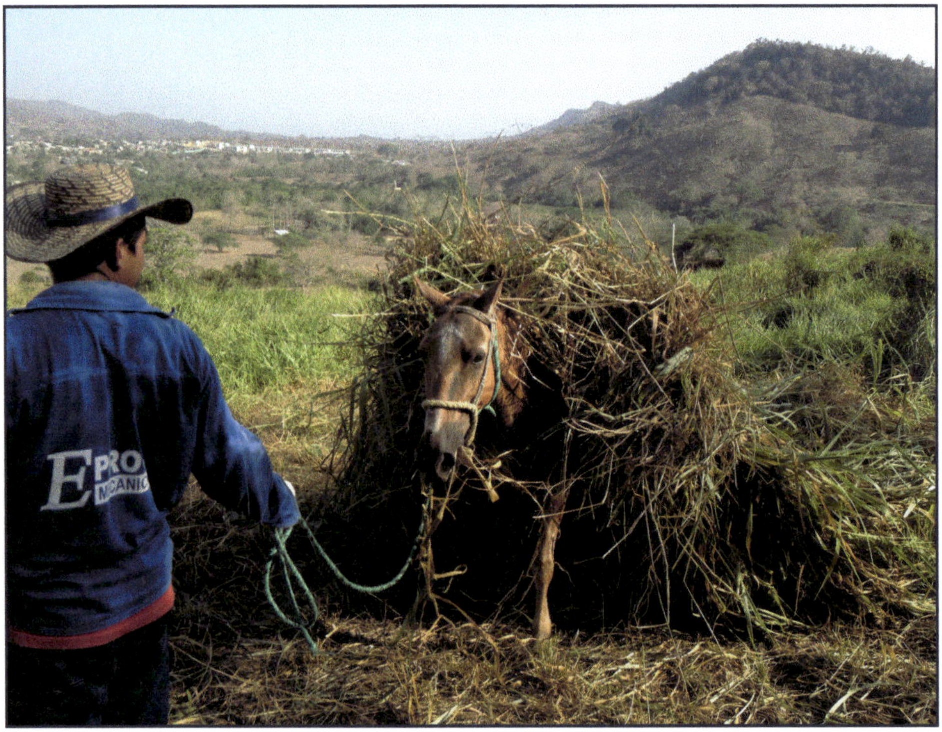

Fig. 8.6. Animal feed production and soil recovery with agroecological practices in tropical dry forest ecosystems in northern Colombia. Picture credit: Authors' own collection (Alexander Navas).

nor men migrated elsewhere, reducing the vulnerability of the family group (Figs 8.6 and 8.7).

Example answer: Points that you may have noted while reading the example include the following:

The social determinants of health in the text include:

- Dignity and wellbeing of people: agroecology aims to create harmonious scenarios where living with dignity is the main motivation for people.
- Social ties and political actions: the approach of agroecology generates bonds of trust and aims to strengthen social ties to provoke political actions for welfare.
- Human wellbeing and quality of life: agroecology recognizes the importance of human wellbeing, quality of life, and participation in decision making for those involved in agricultural systems.
- Gender relations and women's role in agriculture: agroecology promotes **gender equality** and recognizes the significant role of women in agriculture.
- Rural youth prospects: agroecology addresses the challenge of rural youth succession and their prospects as the new generation of family farming professionals.
- Territorial approach to rural development: agroecology seeks to overcome the rural–urban dichotomy and promote rural development with a territorial perspective.

The environmental determinants of health in the text include:

- Protection of the environment: agroecology emphasizes processes of protecting the environment to maintain healthy soils, water and biodiversity.
- Reduction of agrotoxin use: agroecology confronts agrotoxins through diversification, rotation and integration of crops, trees and animals, aiming to minimize climate risks.
- Conservation of native seeds and fight against transgenics: agroecology involves the

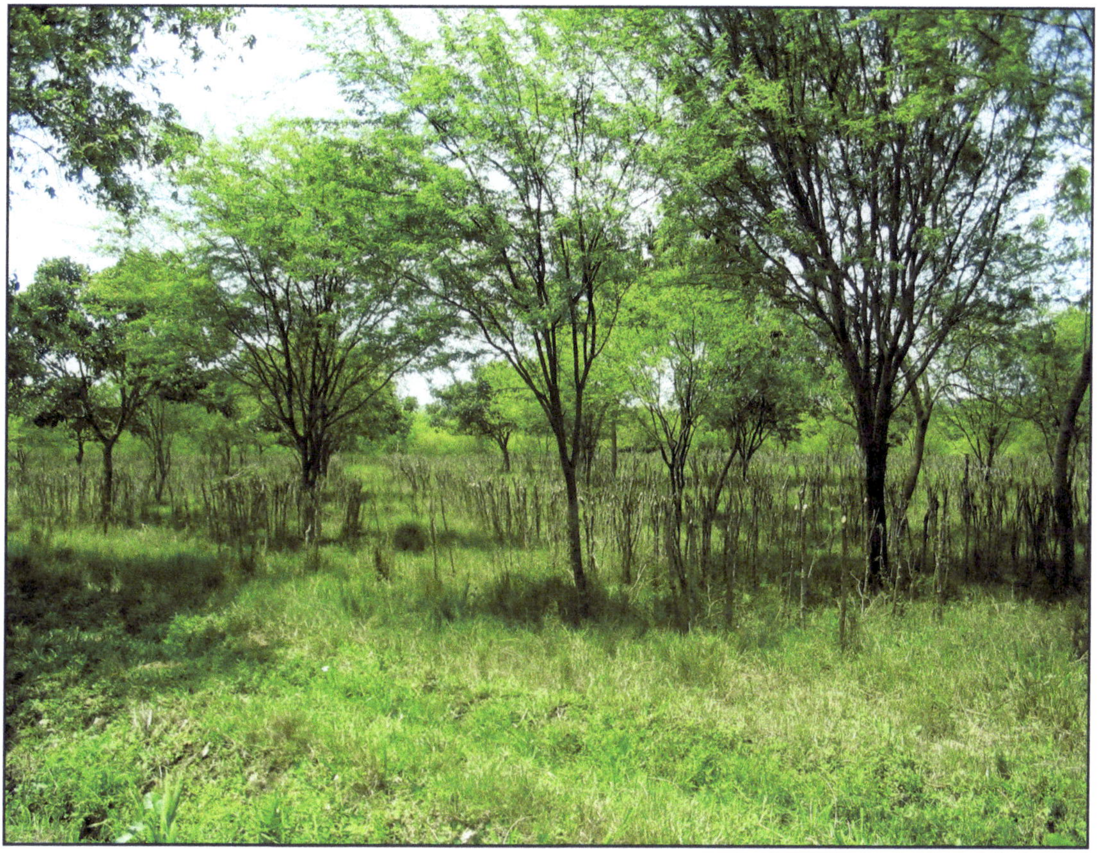

Fig. 8.7. Use of tropical biodiversity in the production of food for animals and people and soil recovery with agroecological practices in Colombia. Picture credit: Authors' own collection (Alexander Navas).

conservation and free exchange of native seeds as a strategy against transgenic crops.

The interconnections among soil, food, animal and human health described in the text include:

- The impact of the food production systems is critical on health conditions, food security and food sovereignty.
- Food systems potentialize harmonious, equitable and sustainable (economic, environmental and social) relationships especially in developing countries where economies are unstable.
- Socio-ecological systems are based on individual actions and choices that create greater transformations around more complex systems. Ethical principles of using 'no harmful' (salutogenic) choices for the soil, earth, animals and humans are political actions made by individuals, but these small actions have the power to generate greater changes within systems.
- Knowledge integration and exchange between the local ancestral knowledge of the communities and the scientific knowledge of different sciences in search of local solutions pertinent to the needs and particularities of the dynamics of the territories.

8.4 Conclusions

- The Alma Mater declaration on Health for All was released in 1978, and the Ottowa Charter on health promotion was promulgated in 1986, stating that the fundamental prerequisities for health are peace, housing, education, food, ecosystem and human health, economic income, stable ecosystems, sustainable resources, social justice and equity. Despite both mandates having existed for over 4 decades, their proclamations are still not yet a reality for many communities worldwide.

- Social Determinants of Health have been useful to explain and understand disease distribution in populations and to advocate for a more equitable society, but they are not sufficient to tackle the challenges posed by the current crises of climate change, biodiversity loss and environmental pollution.
- The profound transformations experienced in recent decades in the social, economic, political and cultural fields, including the pandemic of COVID-19, have generated a landscape of inequality in broad sectors of the population. Consequently, in various parts of the world fundamental human rights, adequate nutrition, decent housing and access to education and healthcare facilities are not available.
- The impacts of environmental degradation and biodiversity loss on health outcomes are most significant among vulnerable populations, especially those most reliant on natural resources and less covered by traditional healthcare such as Indigenous Peoples, rural women, Afro-descendants, etc. The One Health principles of equity, inclusivity and equal access to basic needs, human rights and quality health services at the human–animal–ecosystem interface will serve to implement better, more resilient and more sustainable One Health policies, programmes and plans at global, regional, national and local levels.
- The One Health Agenda is first an equity agenda in many of the low- to middle-income countries, thus all multisectoral endeavours to overthrow the avoidable and unnecessary barriers produced by the unequal distribution of resources and power dynamics in society must be pursued and promoted.

References

Abayineh, A. and Belay, S. (2017) Determinants of smallholder farmers' decision to adopt adaptation options to climate change and variability in the Muger Sub basin of the upper Blue Nile Basin of Ethiopia. *Agriculture and Food Security* 6(64), 1–20. DOI: 10.1186/s40066-017-0144-2.

Altieri, M. and Nicholls, C. (2008) Los impactos del cambio climático sobre las comunidades campesinas y de agricultores tradicionales y sus respuestas adaptativas. *Agroecología* 3, 7–28.

Arcaya, M.C., Arcaya, A.L. and Subramanian, S.V. (2015) Inequalities in health: Definitions, concepts, and theories. *Global Health Action* 8, 27106. DOI: 10.3402/gha.v8.27106.

Arechiga, N., Karunaratna, D. and Aguilar, A. (2014) Control of canine rabies in developing countries: Key features and animal welfare implications. *Scientific and Technical Review* 33(1), 311–321. DOI: 10.20506/rst.33.1.2278.

Balaj, M., York, H.W., Sripada, K., Besnier, E., Vonen, H.D. *et al.* (2021) Parental education and inequalities in child mortality: A global systematic review and meta-analysis. *The Lancet* 398(10300), 608–620. DOI: 10.1016/S0140-6736(21)00534-1.

Barnett, P., Oshinowo, I., Cooper, C., Taylor, C., Smith, S. and Pilling, S. (2023) The association between social class and the impact of treatment for mental health problems: A systematic review and narrative synthesis. *Social Psychiatry and Psychiatric Epidemiology* 58(4), 581–603. DOI: 10.1007/s00127-022-02378-9.

Braveman, P. and Gruskin, S. (2003) Defining equity in health. *Journal of Epidemiology and Community Health* 57(4), 254–258.

Caron, P., Ferrero, G., Loma, O., Nabarro, D., Hainzelin, E. *et al.* (2018) Food systems for sustainable development: Proposals for a profound four-part transformation. *Agronomy for Sustainable Development* 38(4), 41. DOI: 10.1007/s13593-018-0519-1.

Cediel, N.M., Prieto, S., Garzon, A.D.M., Villafañe, M., Rúa, C.V. *et al.* (2022) Woman-sensitive One Health perspective in four tribes of Indigenous People from Latin America: Arhuaco, Wayuú, Nahua, and Kamëntsá. *Frontiers Public Health* 10, 774713. DOI: 10.3389/fpubh.2022.774713.

Centers for Disease Control and Prevention (2021) Zoonotic Diseases. Available at: https://www.cdc.gov/one-health/about/about-zoonotic-diseases.html?CDC_AAref_Val=https://www.cdc.gov/onehealth/basics/zoonotic-diseases.html (accessed 30 July 2024).

Charron, D. (2012) *Ecohealth Research in Practice Innovative Applications of an Ecosystem Approach to Health.* International Development Research Centre, Ottawa. Available at: https://idl-bnc-idrc.dspacedirect.org/bitstream/handle/10625/47809/IDL-47809.pdf?sequence=1 (accessed 8 January 2024).

Cruz, N. (2018) *Co-Colonizing: The Ecological Impacts of Settler Colonialism in the American Supercontinent.* Seattle University. Available at: https://scholarworks.seattleu.edu/cgi/viewcontent.cgi?article=1011&context=ura (accessed 8 January 2024).

Dahlgren, P. and Whitehead, M. (2021) The Dahlgren-Whitehead model of health determinants: 30 years on and still chasing rainbows. *Public Health* 199, 20–24. DOI: 10.1016/j.puhe.2021.08.009.

Del Popolo, F., Jaspers, D. and Cepal, U.N. (2014) Guaranteeing Indigenous People's rights in Latin America. Progress in the past decade and remaining challenges. United Nations, Santiago. Available at: http://hdl.handle.net/11362/37051 (accessed 8 January 2024).

Devakumar, D., Abubakar, I., Achiume, T., Muraaya, K., Paradies, Y. *et al.* (2022) Executive summary. Racism, xenophobia, discrimination, and health. *The Lancet* 400(10368), 2095–2096.

Díaz, A., Pérez, M.V., González, C. and Simon, J. (2004) Conceptos de enfermedad y sanación en la cosmovisión mapuche e impacto de la cultura occidental. *Ciencia y Enfermería* 10(1), 9–16. DOI: 10.4067/S0717-95532004000100002.

Diderichsen, F., Hallqvist, J. and Whitehead, M. (2019) Differential vulnerability and susceptibility: How to make use of recent development in our understanding of mediation and interaction to tackle health inequalities. *International Journal of Epidemiology* 48(1), 268–274.

Field, C.B., Barros, V.R., Dokken, D.J., Mach, K.J., Mastrandrea, M.D. *et al.* (eds) (2014) IPCC: Climate Change 2014: Impacts, adaptation, and vulnerability. Part A: Global and sectoral aspects. *Contribution of Working Group II to the Fifth Assessment Report of the Intergovernmental Panel on Climate Change.* Cambridge University Press, Cambridge, UK and New York.

García, A., Ruiz, D., Colls, C., Mias, M. and Martín, N. (2018) Socioeconomic inequalities in health and the use of healthcare services in Catalonia: Analysis of the individual data of 7.5 million residents. *Journal of Epidemiology and Community Health* 72(10), 871–879. DOI: 10.1136/jech-2018-210817.

Garnier, J., Savić, S., Boriani, E., Bagnol, B., Häsler, B. and Kock, R. (2020) Helping to heal nature and ourselves through human-rights-based and gender-responsive One Health. *One Health Outlook* 1, 1–8.

Gliessman, S.R. (2016) Transforming food systems with agroecology. *Agroecology and Sustainable Food Systems* 40(3), 187–189. DOI: 10.1080/21683565.2015.1130765.

Global Infrastructure Hub (2023) Stakeholder Identification, Engagement and Empowerment. Available at: https://inclusiveinfra.gihub.org/action-areas/stakeholder-identification-engagement-and-empowerment/ (accessed 8 January 2024).

González, J. and Wing Ching, R. (2018) Producción y reproducción de vacas Holstein, Jersey y sus cruces en cinco localidades de Costa Rica. *UNED Research Journal* 10(2), 422–427.

Green, H., Fernandez, R. and MacPhail, C. (2021) The social determinants of health and health outcomes among adults during the COVID-19 pandemic: A systematic review. *Public Health Nursing* 38(6), 942–952. DOI: 10.1111/phn.12959.

Hecht, S. (1999) La evolución del pensamiento agroecológico. In: Altieri, M. (ed.) *Agroecología Bases Para Una Agricultura Sustentable.* Nordan-Comunidad, Montevideo, Uruguay, pp. 15–30.

Kock, R., Queenan, K., Garnier, L., Rosenbaum, S. and Buttigieg, D. (2018) Health solutions: Theoretical foundations of the shift from sectoral to integrated systems. In: Rüegg, S.R., Häsler, B. and Zinsstag, J. (eds) *Integrated Approaches to Health: A Handbook for the Evaluation of One Health.* Wageningen Academic Publishers, Wageningen, p. 22–37.

Marmot, M. (2011) Global action on social determinants of health. *Bulletin of the World Health Organization* 89(10), 702. DOI: 10.2471/BLT.11.094862.

Marmot, M.G. and Wilkinson, R.G. (2006) *Social Determinants of Health* (2nd edn). Oxford University Press, Oxford, UK.

McLeroy, K.R., Bibeau, D., Steckler, A. and Glanz, K. (1988) An ecological perspective on health promotion programs. *Health Education* 15(4), 351–377. DOI: 10.1177/109019818801500401.

Navas, A. (2022) Percepción de pequeños productores sobre cambios en el clima y su efecto en sistemas de producción de leche. *Revista de Investigaciones Veterinarias del Perú* 33(2), e20543. DOI: 10.15381/rivep.v33i2.20543.

One Health High-Level Expert Panel (OHHLEP), Adisasmito, W.B., Almuhairi, S., Behravesh, C.B., Bilivogui, P. *et al.* (2022) One Health: A new definition for a sustainable and healthy future. *PloS Pathogens* 18(6), e1010537. DOI: 10.1371/journal.ppat.1010537.

Palomares Velosa, J.E., Riaño Sánchez, S., Martínez Marín, A. and Cediel Becerra, N.M. (2022) Prevention of exposure to zoonoses in rural Latin America: Social ecological factors in a diverse regional context. *One Health* 15, 100444. DOI: 10.1016/j.onehlt.2022.100444.

Pan American Health Organization (2018) Cuatro países de América Latina y el caribe, los únicos donde la rabia canina sigue actualmente activa. Available at: https://www.paho.org/es/noticias/21-9-2018-cuatro-paises-america-latina-caribe-unicos-donde-rabia-canina-sigue-actualmente#:~:text=La%20rabia%20canina%20solo%20permanece,representan%20el%2010%25%20del%20total (accessed 8 January 2024).

Polanco, N., Cediel, N., Benavides, E. and Villamil, L.C. (2021) Covid-19 como sindemia en la ruralidad colombiana: Brechas y desigualdades. *Equidad y Desarrollo* 37, 53–74. DOI: 10.19052/eq.vol1.iss37.3.

Rabhi, P. (2013) *Vers la sobriété heureuse* [*Towards Happy Sobriety*]. Colibri, Sofia.

Schneider, M.C., Romijn, P.C., Uieda, W., Tamayo, H. and da Silva, D.F. (2009) Rabies transmitted by vampire bats to humans: An emerging zoonotic disease in Latin America? *Pan American Journal of Public Health* 25(3), 260–269.

Solar, O. and Irwin, A. (2010) A conceptual framework for action on the social determinants of health. *Social Determinants of Health Discussion Paper 2 (Policy and Practice)*. Available at: https://iris.who.int/bitstream/handle/10665/44489/9789241500852_eng.pdf?sequence=1 (accessed 8 January 2024).

Stephen, C. and Parmley, J. (2022) *A Transformative One Health Agenda for Livestock Dependent Communities*. ILRI, Nairobi. Available at: https://cgspace.cgiar.org/items/490e61c4-b31a-4e93-8dd5-3e5f5b8df568 (accessed 30 July 2024).

Tulchinsky, T.H. and Lalonde, M. (2018) The health field concept and health promotion. *Case Studies in Public Health*, 523–541. DOI: 10.1016/B978-0-12-804571-8.00028-7.

Villar, M. (2011) Factores determinantes de la salud: Importancia de la prevención. *Acta Médica Peruana* 28(4), 237–241.

Wezel, A., Herren, B.G., Kerr, R.B. *et al.* (2020) Agroecological principles and elements and their implications for transitioning to sustainable food systems. A review. *Agronomy for Sustainable Development* 40, 40. DOI: 10.1007/s13593-020-00646-z.

WHO, Whitehead, M. and Dahlgren, G. (2006) *Concepts and Principles for Tackling Social Inequities in Health: Levelling up Part 1*. World Health Organization, Copenhagen.

Williams, D.R. and Cooper, L.A. (2019) Reducing racial inequities in health: Using what we already know to take action. *International Journal of Environmental Research and Public Health* 16(4), 606. DOI: 10.3390/ijerph16040606.

Williams, J., Allen, L., Wickramasinghe, K., Mikkelsen, B., Roberts, N. and Townsend, N. (2018) A systematic review of associations between non-communicable diseases and socioeconomic status within low- and lower-middle-income countries. *Journal of Global Health* 8(2), 020409. DOI: 10.7189/jogh.08.020409.

World Health Organization (2020) Zoonosis. Available at: https://www.who.int/es/news-room/fact-sheets/detail/zoonoses (accessed 8 January 2024).

World Health Organization (2021) *COVID-19 and the Social Determinants of Health and Health Equity: Evidence Brief*. Available at: https://iris.who.int/bitstream/handle/10665/348333/9789240038387-eng.pdf?sequence=1. (accessed 8 January 2024).

9 Gender Equality in the Context of One Health

Elena Boriani[1,2*], Brigitte Bagnol[2,3*], Sara Savić[2,4], Raffaella Campaner[5], Natalia Cediel Becerra[2,6] and Julie Garnier[2,7]

[1]EB Consult, Hellebæk, Denmark; [2]Network for Ecohealth and One Health (NEOH); [3]Department of Infectious Disease and Global Health, Cummings School of Veterinary Medicine, Tufts University, Boston, USA; [4]Scientific Veterinary Institute 'Novi Sad', Novi Sad, Serbia; [5]Department of Philosophy, University of Bologna, Bologna, Italy; [6]Faculty of Agricultural Sciences, Universidad de La Salle, Bogotá, Colombia; [7]Odyssey Conservation Trust, Bakewell, UK

Reflexivity statement

In this chapter, you may notice that all authors are female, which reflects the composition of our working group, predominantly consisting of female researchers. However, this is not discriminatory; rather, we are actively engaging male researchers to contribute to our collaborative endeavours in promoting gender equity in One Health.

Contents

*The authors have equal contribution

DOI: 10.1079/9781800623002.0010

Chapter Overview

Elevator pitch

Men and women and gender diverse people[1] may have different roles in society, different access to resources and decision making. In consequence they impact their environment and are impacted by it in distinct ways. Other factors such as class, skin colour, cultural, religious, sexual orientation and linguistic origin inform the way people impact and are impacted by their environment. Understanding how those factors intersect and contribute to different layers of vulnerability is important for delivering more impactful work and for contributing to a more equitable and inclusive society.

Book objectives the chapter relates to

- ☐ 1. Understand what One Health and Ecohealth mean
- ☑ 2. Think in a One Health and Ecohealth way
- ☑ 3. Apply One Health and Ecohealth in their professional and personal life
- ☐ 4. Know how to share One Health and Ecohealth knowledge
- ☐ 5. Integrate One Health and Ecohealth knowledge actively
- ☑ 6. Acquire or enhance core One Health competencies

One Health competencies covered

- ☐ 1. Effective communication
- ☑ 2. Collaborative and resilient working
- ☑ 3. Systems understanding
- ☑ 4. Transdisciplinarity
- ☑ 5. Social, cultural and gender equity and inclusiveness
- ☑ 6. Collective learning and reflective practice
- ☐ 7. One Health concepts
- ☐ 8. Theoretical and methodological pluralism
- ☐ 9. Harnessing uncertainty, paradox and limited knowledge

After having worked through this chapter, you will be familiar with key gender concepts and have an understanding of how important they are and how they can be applied to One Health situations.

Learning outcomes

1. Understand a number of key gender concepts (gender roles, equality, equity, discrimination, empowerment, gender-based One Health).
2. Identify the areas where the gender gap is more evident.
3. Use a gender lens in health, agriculture, biodiversity and climate change.

Summary

In this chapter, you will learn about gender and the importance of having a gender sensitive approach when applying One Health. You will also explore the role of gender across disciplines and in various aspects of life. The first part of the chapter presents definitions of gender, sex, gender equality and equity, empowerment and other terms that are increasingly used but not always thoroughly explained. Later in the chapter, examples of a gender equality approach and gender inequalities are illustrated through different One Health topics, including endocrine disruptor chemicals, antimicrobial resistance, COVID-19 and brucellosis. The second part of the chapter includes graphs and pictures to enhance comprehension, with key points highlighted. The primary objective is to identify gender sensitive activities within One Health initiatives and to understand why implementing gender equality or inclusion is crucial, given that the One Health approach should promote equality and inclusion at all levels.

9.1 Gender Equality in the Context of One Health

According to Scott (1988):

> **GENDER** is a 'constitutive element of social relationships based on perceived differences between the sexes, and gender is a primary way of signifying relationships of power'.

At birth, based on the genitalia of a child, a set of values and stereotypes is associated with male and female bodies. Those values and stereotypes often define how people parent, what work people do, what social groups they belong to, who people partner with and how people gain access to resources (FAO, 2014). These differences define roles and access to, control over and benefits of resources such as education, land or decision making.

Gender relations are relations of power. They are not fixed. They are flexible and are affected by other markers of identity such as age, class, skin colour, linguistic group, sexual orientation, religion, and the geographical, economic and political **environment**. Thus, gender takes into consideration relations that are given (colour of skin, age, place of birth, order of birth, etc.) and aspects of people's identity that are acquired (class, education, profession, religion, place of residence, etc.) (Fig. 9.1). Gender relations are not universal, they are specific to a context. Intersectionality is an important approach as it helps us understand how different forms of discrimination interact and exacerbate inequality. For example, an African woman is often discriminated against because she is a woman, because of her skin colour and because of her socio-economic and cultural background.

People facing one or more forms of discrimination are at greater risk of being left behind in accessing disease response services, including testing, treatment, social protection and care.[2] If we fail to integrate intersectionality in our analysis, our understanding of risks and possibilities to prevent diseases is limited.

In Chapters 4 and 5, you learned about the many different forms of **knowledge** and knowledge generation as well as **knowledge integration** and the pathway from **data** to **knowledge** and **wisdom**. Covering all forms of knowledge would go beyond the purpose of this chapter, and we therefore focus here explicitly on scientific knowledge. We acknowledge that people of all genders contribute to various forms of knowledge, and that the intersections of gender with other aspects of identity, such as race, ethnicity and culture, further enrich the diversity of perspectives in knowledge generation. We recognize and value these diverse contributions, as they are essential for fostering holistic and comprehensive understanding in academia, research

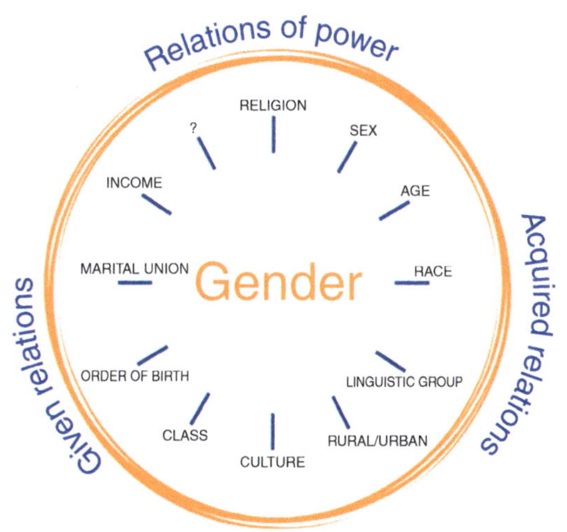

Fig. 9.1. In addition to sex, other markers of identity influence gender relations (figure created by Brigitte Bagnol).

and society as a whole and contribute to transdisciplinarity that is an essential principle of One Health (Chapter 3).

Changes in gender relations often occur over time in response to changing economic, natural or political circumstances, including development efforts. Gender shapes everything we do and all sectors in society. In fact, all institutions, including those related to family, workplaces, politics, arts, sports, culture and development institutions, are gendered. Gender is everywhere in our daily lives, so much so that we usually take many aspects of gender for granted and 'natural'. Development interventions can support or hamper processes of change and reinforce or reduce inequalities between people of different gender (FAO, 2014) including people whose identities do not correspond to established ideas of a gender transformative approach.

Being such a pervasive feature of our lives, gender is clearly intertwined with **health** conditions too. Several authors (Bagnol *et al.*, 2015; FAO *et al.*, 2019; Friedson-Ridenour *et al.*, 2019; Garnier *et al.*, 2020, 2022) have been advocating for the integration of gender and human rights dimensions in the One Health approach. This means to recognize that men and women do not impact the world in the same way and that men and women are impacted differently by the world around them (Bagnol *et al.*, 2015).[3] Roles imposed on people define the ways in which women and men relate with resources and how human disease, animal disease or environmental problems affect women and men and what the impacts are of their activities and behaviours (Garnier *et al.*, 2020). Consequently, this implies differences in perception about risks and solutions and different needs to prevent these. Gender plays an important role in biosafety, as well as in the control, prevention and response to infectious diseases and emerging pandemics.[4] Gender aspects also play a fundamental role in **ecosystem** management,[5] community health management, the effects of climate change,[6] natural disasters and the effects of pollution on health.

Integrating a **gender perspective** in the **One Health approach** allows us to promote a more sustainable world where the health of humans, animals and the environment is balanced and optimized. There cannot be **sustainability** without gender equality; there cannot be a just world without 'the enjoyment of equal rights, opportunities and treatment by men and women and by boys and girls in all spheres of life' (ILO, International Labour Organization) or 'the absence of discrimination on the basis of a person's sex in opportunities, the allocation of resources and benefits, or access to services' (UN Women, 2021).

The integration of gender issues in One Health frameworks and vision has become critical in the 2020 COVID-19 pandemic context, which laid bare social and gender inequities and exposed the need to adopt a gender-responsive One Health approach (Garnier *et al.*, 2020, 2022; UN Women, 2021). WHO (2019) recommended that the health sector takes a gender and equity focus to improve population health in its recent 13th General Program of Work (2019–2023). In fact, women make up 70% of the human health workforce, but only 25% of global health organizations have gender parity at senior management levels (Betron *et al.*, 2019). As a result, women's and gender minorities' voices are barely heard at decision-making tables and gender perspectives are still largely ignored, exacerbating gender and social inequities.

The differences between gender equality and gender equity:

Gender equality refers to women, men and people who identify differently having equal and equally respected rights, and equal access to resources and opportunities. It is equally concerned by the situation of men and of women. However, since it is often women who face greater risks and vulnerabilities in different sectors, it is often associated with a greater focus on women.

Gender equity refers to the process of ensuring fairness for women, men and people who identify differently as part of a gender transformative approach creating a level playing field for them. This goes beyond treating people equally, to actively compensating for the historical processes of discrimination that shape current economic, social and political disadvantages depending on the contexts.

Gender equality is the objective, while gender equity is the process to reach equality.

There are multiple reasons why gender needs to be integrated into One Health in a systematic manner (Garnier *et al.*, 2020):

- Gender equality needs to be recognized as a basic human right.

- Gender equality is critical to address the health, **climate** and **biodiversity** crisis we currently face. These crises impact people differently, often to the detriment of women and people from marginalized groups, and existing gender inequalities are likely to be exacerbated by these crises.
- Gender equity is indispensable for achieving progress in all 17 **Sustainable Development Goals.** Increased gender equity is firmly linked to enhanced productivity, better development outcomes for future generations and improvement in the functioning of institutions.
- Different gender roles and responsibilities in health, food, water and energy management, as well as in the use of other natural resources, contribute to different impacts on the environment and different exposure to risks.
- Men, women and gender-diverse people are impacted differently by human, animal and plant disease, as well as by climate change and environmental disasters, and this impact varies also according to other factors of vulnerability (such as age, skin colour, level of education, class, religion, sexual orientation, etc.).

In 2020, a framework for mainstreaming a gender-responsive One Health approach was proposed by Garnier *et al.* (2020) suggesting (i) 'a change of mindset and paradigm, going from a pursuit of wealth, GDP and overconsumption, towards a goal of well-being of humans and their re-connection to healthy and diverse ecosystems, using a holistic One Health understanding of health and nature' and (ii) 'the integration of gender equity in leadership and the respects of the rights of nature, women and the most vulnerable, including minority ethnic groups and Indigenous People'.

Several One Health networks, such as One Health Central and Eastern Africa (OHCEA), now known as African One Health Network (AFROHUN),[7] and HORN,[8,9] have also recently developed gender modules for their training courses on infectious diseases surveillance, response and control (Bagnol *et al.*, 2015; Amuguni *et al.*, 2018; Friedson-Ridenour *et al.*, 2019). The One Health community now needs to adopt a gender-transformative approach systematically in its **policy** recommendations, research projects and programmes.

SEX refers to biological aspects (chromosomes, genitalia, hormones, reproductive functions). These are the strictly biological, anatomical and physiological characteristics that differentiate individuals. There are fundamental biological differences between men and women at all levels (the body as a whole, the organs and organ systems, and the cells). These biological differences are complex and may confer different advantages on men or women including when it comes to risk of infection (depending on the infectious agent).

9.1.1 How do sex and gender interact?

Sex and gender are interacting variables[10] and may be involved in the transmission and acquisition of diseases and in the success or failure of treatments or interventions. Hence the importance of taking them into account in research, with the aim of reducing inequalities linked to sex and gender in the management of health problems and improving the **wellbeing** of people, whatever their sex and gender. Sex and gender have an impact on exposure to environmental, infectious or other types of risks, and consequently on the susceptibility or resistance to infectious pathologies, and on the type and effectiveness of responses provided, particularly in healthcare interventions.

In 2001, the Institute of Medicine published 'Exploring the Biological Contributions to Human Health: Does Sex Matter?' The Committee on Understanding the Biology of Sex and Gender Differences examined biology from the cellular to the organismal and behavioural levels, and concluded that differences do occur and can have important consequences. They concluded that sex (being male or female) should be recognized as an important variable in research and increased knowledge in this area should be cultivated. The growth of knowledge has become a branch of science known as sex-based biology and has led to the differentiation between the terms 'sex' and 'gender' (Liu and Mager Dipietro, 2016).

Figure 9.2 shows how gender and sex interact. The incidence, duration and severity of disease (shown in the right-hand column) are influenced by both sex and gender in two different ways. On the one hand, sex and gender directly influence vulnerability, exposure to pathogens and response to disease, three key elements of the transmission model. These in turn help to determine incidence, duration and severity. On the other

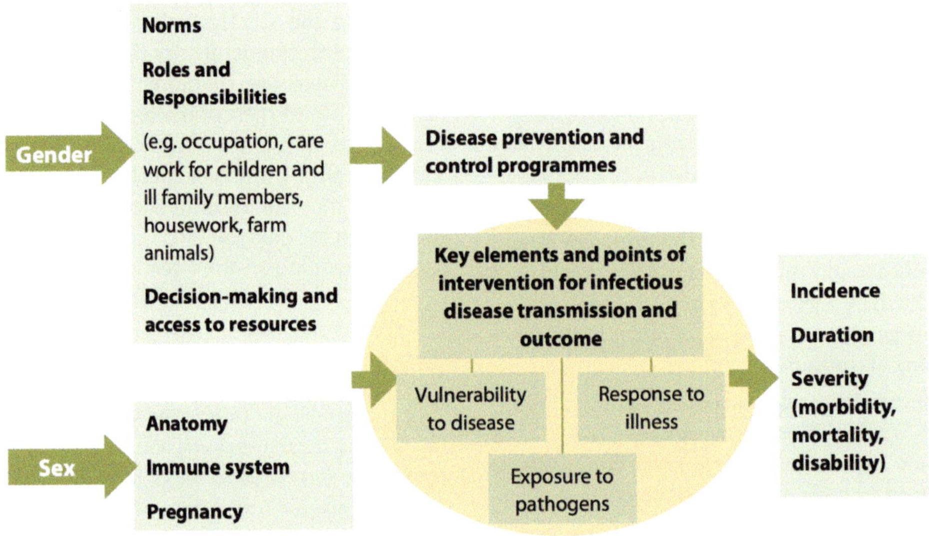

Fig. 9.2. Sex and gender in infectious diseases (WHO, 2013). Reproduced with permission from WHO.

hand, sex and gender indirectly influence incidence, duration and severity through interactions with health interventions that affect vulnerability, exposure and response to disease.

Because of the differences between men and women in many aspects of life in all societies, it is important to understand how they face illness at all stages (prevention, diagnosis, treatment and recovery).

Learning questions: For the context you live in, select an example of gender-typical roles and reflect on how they have evolved over the past decade. Think about the situation of your country and identify the steps, legislation and processes that allowed for the evolution of the situation, if any, in the past few decades.

Example answer 1: Roles in cheese production in the Swiss Alps. Please note that this example may differ substantially from what you will find in your context. What we found interesting about the example below is to see the evolution of the relation between men and women over time. Making cheese evolved from a women's reproductive task to a female productive task with more decision making, reward and recognition for women (Kindstedt, 2012).

Traditional gender roles in alpine livestock farming for cheese production in Switzerland have historically been characterized by distinct divisions of labour based on traditional norms and societal expectations. In this context, men often assumed tasks such as tending to the larger animals, like cattle, and managing the physical demands of farming, such as ploughing fields and managing pastures. Women, on the other hand, typically took on responsibilities related to the household and dairy work, including milking cows, preserving food for the winter and making cheese, a reproductive role as cheese was used mainly for home consumption. Women's role in cheese production was particularly vital, as they were responsible for transforming milk into cheese using traditional methods, a skill that was often passed down through generations. Their expertise was central to maintaining the quality and distinct characteristics of local cheeses.

Advancements in agricultural technology have reduced physical demands, altering traditional gender-based divisions in alpine farming and cheese production. Economic shifts expanded cheese production beyond household consumption and women's roles beyond traditions, enabled by education and career opportunities. Evolving social norms challenged gender roles, fostering greater equality, including in farming. Tourism's fascination with tradition highlights women's roles in cheese production, promoting preservation and recognition. Government policies promoting gender equality bolster balanced labour distribution and acknowledge women's contributions in farming, reshaping gender dynamics in this domain.

As a result of these shifts, there has been a gradual transformation of gender roles in alpine livestock farming for cheese production. Women have gained more visibility and recognition for their contributions beyond traditional domestic roles. They are now taking on leadership positions, participating in decision making, and being recognized as skilled contributors to the entire process of cheese production, from animal care to dairy work. These changes have not only promoted gender equality but have also diversified and strengthened the sustainability of cheese production in the Swiss Alps.

Example answer 2: Government roles in Mozambique. Please note that this example may differ substantially from what you will find in your context. What we found interesting about the example below is how political interventions such as the establishment of gender focal points and a policy on gender issues contributed to changes in the participation of women in the political sphere.

In Mozambique, for example, men used and sometimes still hold most positions of power as politicians, local leaders, businessmen and heads of Ministry, directorate and institutions at all levels (central to local). Gender Units responsible for ensuring the mainstreaming of gender issues in their sector were established in the Ministry of Agriculture in 1992 and in the Ministry of Education in 1994. In 2000, the Ministry of Women and Social Affairs Co-ordination[11] was established and by 2003, most of the Ministries had a Gender Unit and/or Gender focal points in most directorates. In 2001, a National Plan of Action for Women's Advancement (*Plano Nacional de Ação para o Avanço da Mulher 2002–2006*, PNAM) was elaborated including: Women, poverty and employment; Education and training of women and girls; Women, health and HIV/AIDS; Women in power in decision-making location and social communication; Women, environment and agriculture; Institutional mechanisms for the advancement of women. This process led to an increase of the representation of women in the public sphere with the percentage of seats held by women in the parliament reaching 39.6% in 2017[12] and 42% in 2020.[13] However, the percentage of women in **governance** is not the same at provincial and municipality level.

9.1.2 Gender equality and equity and their role in the construction of scientific knowledge

In the past few decades, there has been increasing attention on a number of ways in which science, health professions and academic leadership are gender biased. Who is doing the research and who is participating in the research are important aspects to take into consideration as it can bias the hypothesis, the methodology, the analysis of the results and their presentation. According to Anderson (2012), 'dominant knowledge practices [have] disadvantage[d] women by (1) excluding them from inquiry, (2) denying them epistemic authority, (3) denigrating their "feminine" cognitive styles and modes of knowledge, (4) producing theories of women that represent them as inferior, deviant, or significant only in the ways they serve male interests, (5) producing theories of social phenomena that render women's activities and interests, or gendered power relations, invisible, and (6) producing knowledge (science and technology) that is not useful for people in subordinate positions, or that reinforces gender and other social hierarchies'. In other words, women's standpoints have been regarded as less authoritative in the elaboration of scientific knowledge (Boxes 9.1 and 9.2).

The gender gap in terms of education at secondary and university level as well as in teaching career and position in the university and in research influence the possibility to advocate for more inclusive policy and financing of issues related to inclusion.

Overall, women, poor people, as well as people from minority groups are excluded from educational and academic institutions. Their needs and concerns are not taken into consideration and research related to issues of their interest are less likely to be financed (Figs 9.3 and 9.4).

Box 9.1. Social norms influence academic settings

Latin American women scientists, for example, can face inequity in a society where culturally ingrained masculine pride ('machismo') is normalized and deeply intertwined with the scientific endeavour. Dismissal of women's contributions, patronizing behaviour, and objectification of women's bodies are widely entrenched attitudes in Latin American societies, often extending into academic settings (Bernal *et al.*, 2019).

Box 9.2. Gender distribution in science

Data from UNESCO indicate that women represent 21.7 % of graduates in Africa, 24.3 % in Europe and Central Africa, and 25.6 % in East Asia and the Pacific region in 2015–2020 (UN, 2022). Often, women are at a disadvantage in terms of career path, accessing the position of Principal Investigator, obtaining funding, producing scientific publications because they take a maternity leave which then slows down their career path (Llorens *et al.*, 2021). They might encounter difficulties in returning to their job after the pause and might face difficulties in managing both family responsibilities and their job. Institutional bias in hiring and granting promotion as well as non-**inclusiveness** undermine the retention. In addition, cultural barriers such as gender stereotypes, work environments, and lack of positive female role models still prevent many women and girls from pursuing academic careers. Working closely with academic institutions to identify opportunities for the inclusion of women, especially mid-career, will create a much-needed opportunity or advancement.

Recommendation

All scientific research must be approved by an ethics committee and a selection committee. Ensuring that these committees are gender transformative by providing gender training is crucial. Committee members should be able to evaluate the gender aspects in protocols and to ensure that the research is gender transformative and inclusive. High-quality research protocols integrate gender analysis.

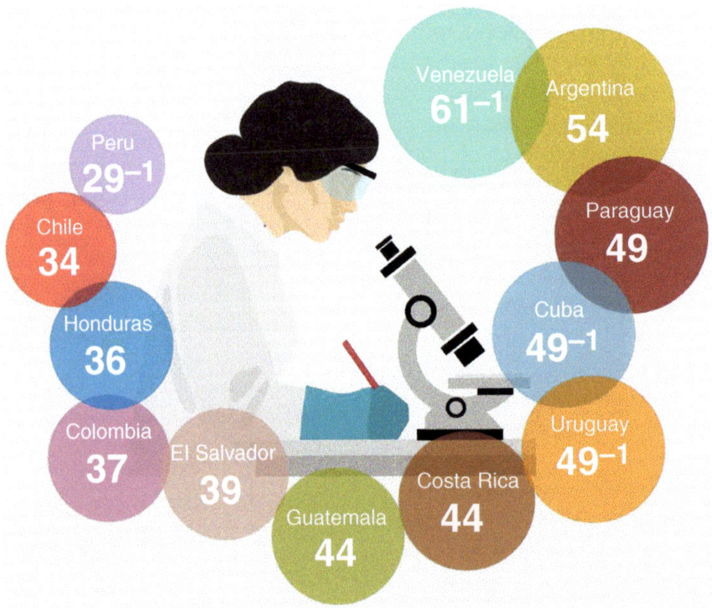

Fig. 9.3. Share (%) of female researchers (Head Count) in Latin America, 2017 or closest year; +n/-n: data refer to n years before or after reference year. From UNESCO (2021), unmodified (CC BY-SA 3.0 IGO: https://creativecommons.org/licenses/by-sa/3.0/igo/).

Knowledge is always situated. This means that researchers are embedded in a social, cultural, ethical, philosophical, religious and political context that defines most of their worldview and their **assumptions** about a specific reality or topic. The question we should ask ourselves is: What is the impact of the fact that most research in science and specifically in Science, Technology, Engineering and Mathematics (STEM) is dominated by men? Is science neutral?

The answer is no. Science is not neutral (Alcoff and Potter, 1993): the question one can ask is how the question is formulated, to whom the question is asked, and how the way the data are analysed will influence the results of the research. In most quantitative research in the past, people interviewed were men, as researchers considered them to be the 'head of the household' and the most appropriate persons to answer questions 'in the name of the household'. This led to a gender bias and to women's knowledge, opinion and needs being dismissed. Similarly, most clinical tests on new drugs were conducted on men, resulting in little knowledge of their impact on women (Fig. 9.5).

Learning questions: An important research question is **how can we develop and use effective vaccines against infectious agents?** Think about the research community as explained in the paragraph above and list at least three points from the perspective of scientific knowledge creators and users that could increase gender balance.

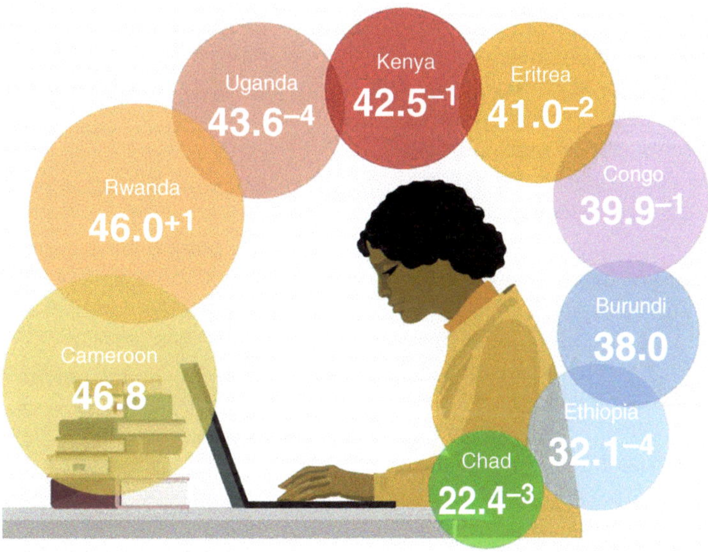

Fig. 9.4. Share (%) of female students enrolled at Central and East African universities, 2018 or closest year; +n/-n: data refer to n years before or after reference year. From UNESCO (2021), unmodified (CC BY-SA 3.0 IGO: https://creativecommons.org/licenses/by-sa/3.0/igo/).

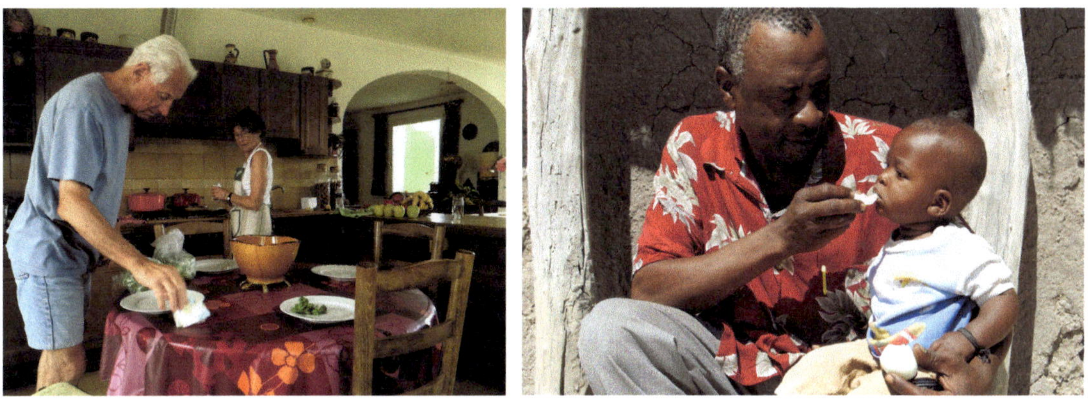

Fig. 9.5. Challenging gender roles (photos by Brigitte Bagnol).

Example answer: You may have come up with similar points to below or addressed different perspectives. The important point here is that you consider aspects relating to both sex and gender.

- **Equitable funding allocation:** Ensure that research funding is distributed among diverse research projects equitably, including those led by individuals from underrepresented gender and minority groups. This supports a broader range of perspectives and research priorities.
- **Mentorship and training:** Establish mentorship and training programmes that specifically target women and marginalized individuals in the field of vaccine research. These programmes can provide support, guidance and opportunities for skill development, fostering a more inclusive pipeline of researchers.
- **Transparent research practices:** Implement transparency in research practices, including data collection, analysis and reporting. Make sure that sex and gender are understood and taken into consideration. Transparent practices help reduce potential biases and ensure that all research contributions are acknowledged and valued, regardless of gender.
- **Public engagement and outreach:** Encourage scientists, including women and underrepresented groups, to engage with the public and communicate their research findings. This promotes visibility, showcases diverse expertise and encourages young individuals from all backgrounds to pursue careers in vaccine research.
- **Collaborative networks:** Establish collaborative networks that bring together researchers, practitioners, policy makers and community members from various backgrounds. These networks can facilitate interdisciplinary and cross-sectoral collaboration, ensuring a holistic approach to vaccine research.
- **Policy advocacy:** Advocate for policies that promote gender equality and diversity in research institutions and funding agencies. These policies can encourage institutional changes that support the recruitment, retention and advancement of women and marginalized groups in vaccine research.
- **Community engagement and participatory research:** Foster meaningful engagement with knowledge users, such as communities that are impacted by infectious diseases. Utilize participatory research approaches that involve community members in the research process, allowing them to contribute their knowledge, experiences and concerns. This ensures that the development and use of vaccines are informed by the needs and priorities of the communities they are intended to benefit.
- **Inclusive research teams:** Ensure that research teams working on vaccine development are diverse and inclusive, including a balanced representation of gender, race and other marginalized groups. This diversity can bring a variety of perspectives, experiences and expertise to the table, leading to more comprehensive and effective research outcomes.
- **Promote equal participation:** Encourage equal participation and engagement of all team members in research discussions, decision making and knowledge exchange. This includes creating an environment where individuals feel valued and comfortable sharing their viewpoints, regardless of their gender or background.
- **Address implicit bias:** Implement strategies to identify and address hidden biases and underlying assumptions in research methodologies and approaches. This involves making these biases explicit and considering how they might influence the research process and outcomes. This can lead to more accurate and unbiased results.

In summary, reflections on gender-related issues strongly point out the impossibility of an 'innocent', 'from nowhere' and detached view of the world. All knowledge has a perspectival component. Therefore, One Health (and other) research initiatives need to include the perspective of the subjugated. On the one hand, the presence of minorities and outsiders is to be acknowledged while revealing specific interests, assumptions and values; on the other hand, the goal is to integrate minorities into scientific communities and in communities who benefit from science and its progress, by promoting equality in knowledge development and knowledge sharing – such as in health-related matters.

9.1.3 Roots of gender inequality

Pervasive gaps persist with the gender transformative approach in order to realize the full spectrum of people's rights, including their access to, control over and benefits from resources, in unpaid work burden, health and safety, and political voice, among other interconnected issues (UNEP, 2021).

Chapter 8 provides an overview of the **social determinants of health**. Many of these determinants are also underlying causes of gender inequality, including:

- Institutional arrangements that create and reinforce gender-based constraints;
- The formal legal system that reinforces customs and practices giving women and minorities groups inferior legal status;
- Sociocultural attitudes as well as ethnic and class-based obligations that determine people's roles, responsibilities and decision-making functions;
- Religious beliefs and practices that limit women's mobility, social contact, access to resources and the types of activities they can pursue;
- Economic factors that limit women's and minorities groups' access to control and benefit from resources, services, activities and knowledge.

All these factors promote gender-based violence that exacerbates inequalities. When these factors are addressed positively and for example transformed into activities that are of value to women and their social networks, multiple benefits can be created, as illustrated in the example of the Tacana women in Bolivia in Fig. 9.6.

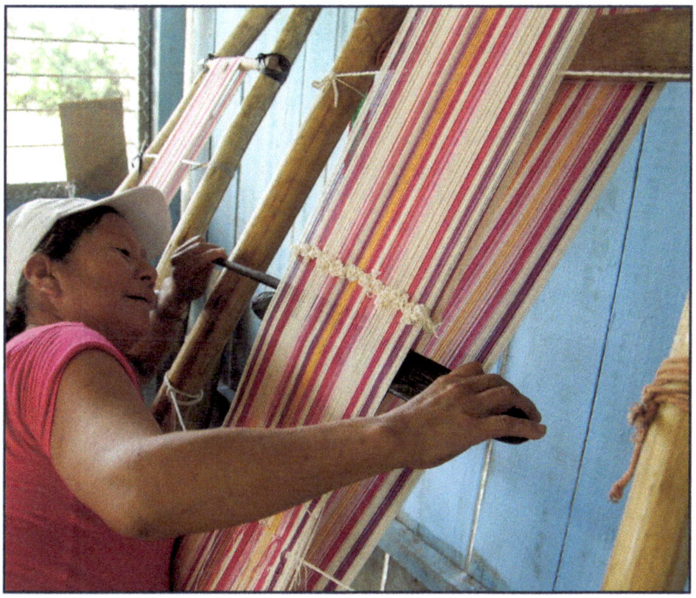

Fig. 9.6. The success of the Tacana women in Bolivia rehabilitating their weaving tradition is multifaceted. It encompasses the revival of cultural heritage, economic empowerment, formation of cooperatives, market access, skill development, community development, empowerment and leadership, and environmental sustainability. This holistic approach has not only improved the economic conditions of the Tacana women but also strengthened their cultural identity and allowed them to have more active roles in their communities. It shows how factors of gender inequality can be transformed into positive change for contemporary benefits, enhancing both individual and community wellbeing (Photo by Julie Garnier).

9.2 Methodology to Assess Gender Issues in the Context of One Health

9.2.1 Gender approaches

In order to analyse the type of (or even absence of) gender approach used in an intervention, an institution, a project and to guide various projects on how to integrate gender, the Interagency Gender Working Group (IGWG) has developed a conceptual framework known as the Gender Integration Continuum[14] (Fig. 9.7).

The notion of a continuum evokes a scale or graduation in the consideration of gender aspects, which goes from a pole where approaches are said to be 'blind' to an opposite pole where approaches are said to be 'transformative'. Among the so-called 'sensitive' interventions, we distinguish 'exploitative', 'accommodating' and finally 'transformative' interventions.

This framework categorizes approaches by how they treat **gender norms** and inequities in the design, implementation and evaluation of a programme or policy. The term **gender blind** refers to policies and programmes that are designed without prior analysis of the culturally defined set of economic, social and political roles, responsibilities, rights, entitlements, obligations and power relations associated with being female and male, and the dynamics between and among men and women, boys and girls. Gender blind programmes or policies ignore gender considerations altogether. In contrast, **gender aware** programmes or policies deliberately examine and address the anticipated gender-related outcomes during both design and implementation. An important prerequisite for all gender-integrated interventions is to be gender aware.

The following definitions of the different gender approaches are adapted from: https://www.igwg.org/wp-content/uploads/2017/05/FG_GendrIntegrContinuum.pdf:

GENDER BLIND policies and programmes do not acknowledge any difference between men and women in any level of the intervention. They develop intervention as if people were facing exactly the same situation without taking into consideration social differences among gender in access, control and benefits over resources, in incidence, duration and severity of disease between men and women.

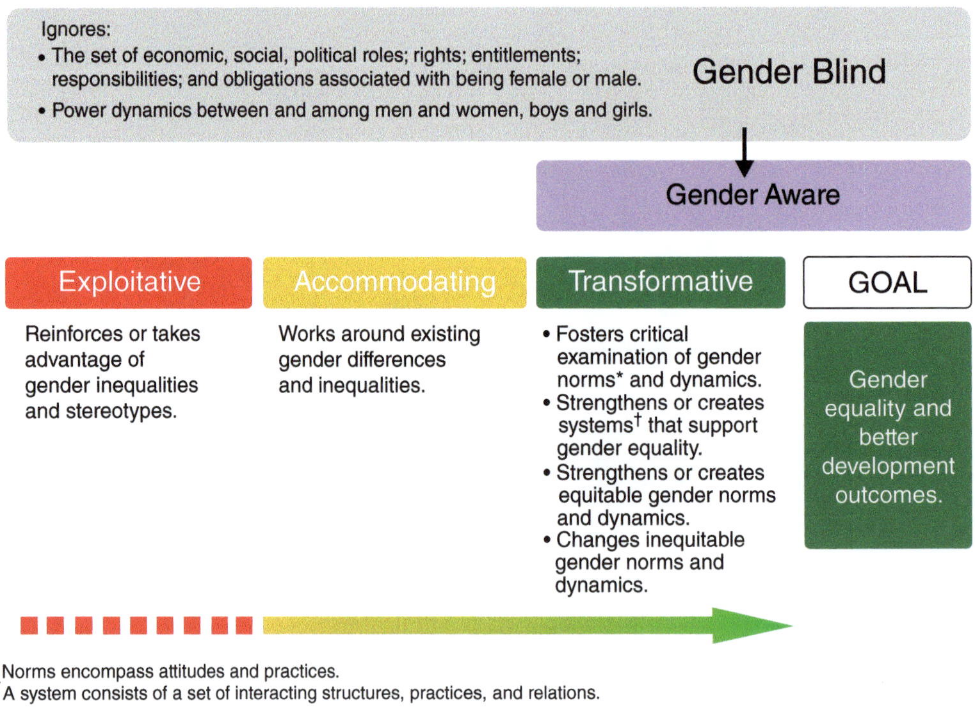

Fig. 9.7. Gender continuum (IGWG, 2017), courtesy of Interagency Gender Working Group (IGWG).

GENDER AWARE policies and programmes take into consideration the set of economic, social and political roles, responsibilities, rights, entitlements, obligations and power relations associated with being female and male and the dynamics between and among genders. They also take into consideration how these factors intersect with other factors.

EXPLOITATIVE GENDER programmes or policies intentionally or unintentionally reinforce or take advantage of gender inequalities and stereotypes in pursuit of project outcomes. This approach is harmful to men, women and for society overall because it reinforces discriminations and inequalities.

ACCOMMODATING GENDER programmes or policies acknowledge gender issues but work around differences and inequalities to achieve project objectives. This approach does not attempt to reduce gender inequalities or address the gender systems that contribute to the differences and inequalities. It reinforces inequalities.

TRANSFORMATIVE GENDER programming includes policies and programmes that seek to transform the power relations between men and women and marginalized groups to promote equality and achieve the programme's objectives. This approach attempts to promote gender equality by: (i) fostering critical examination of inequalities and gender roles, norms and dynamics; (ii) recognizing and strengthening positive norms that support equality and an enabling environment; (iii) promoting the relative position of women, girls and marginalized groups; and (iv) transforming the underlying social structures, policies and broadly held social norms that perpetuate gender inequalities.

9.2.1.1 Empowerment

EMPOWERMENT is the ability to take charge of the course of one's life and to exercise one's 'power to act' on certain events, and implicitly refers to the notion of control. Thus, empowerment is the ability to control one's life through actions that promote change in the factors limiting the individual's ability to take charge of his or her own life. Empowerment refers to people's ability to better understand and exercise their power over the personal, social, economic and political forces that determine the quality of their lives, with the aim of taking action to improve it.

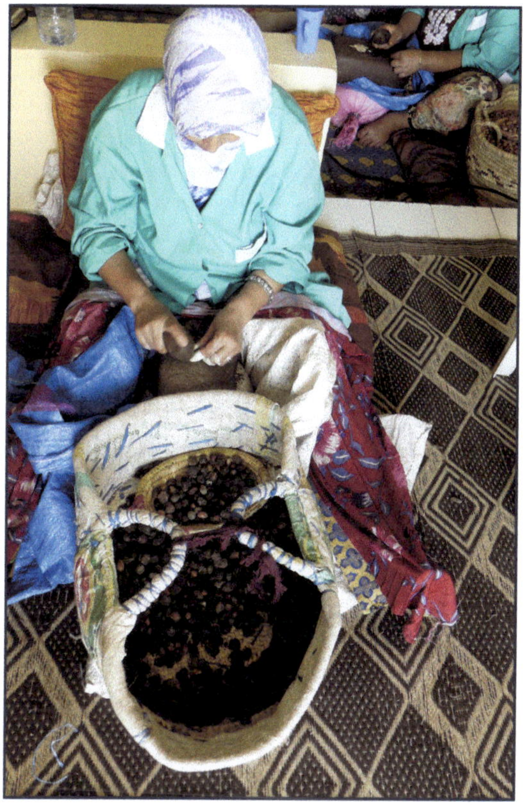

Fig. 9.8. Argan oil's success story in terms of women's empowerment lies in the combination of economic opportunities, cooperative support, skill development, social benefits, sustainable practices, fair trade and external support. These elements together have created a transformative impact on the lives of many women in Morocco (and by extension their children and other family members), making argan oil production a model for women's empowerment and sustainable development. By maintaining control over this sub-sector (often women have been in charge of the care of argan trees and the creation of argan oil), women can continue to benefit from the economic independence, empowerment and social status that they have achieved, while preserving cultural practices and ensuring fair and equitable treatment within their cooperatives (Photo by Julie Garnier).

Empowerment has a relational dimension (family, community, national context) and an individual dimension (age, ethnicity, class, education, etc.). It also occurs at three levels: individuals, organizations and communities. These levels are fundamentally linked. Empowerment is a process similar to a path or a journey, which develops over time. It therefore has a dynamic dimension (Fig. 9.8).

Four definitions of power are now widely used (Munoz Boudet *et al.*, 2007) in gender studies. 'Power within' refers to a transformation of individual consciousness that leads to a new confidence to act. 'Power with' is the power that results from organizing and acting as a group to address common concerns (Gammage *et al.*, 2016). 'Power to' is the power to produce a result or resist change, the power to act. The fourth concept, 'power over', suggests a social relationship of domination or subordination between individuals. It has a negative dimension and is often excluded from areas of analysis.[15]

As defined by the European Institute for Gender Equality (EIGE), 'women's empowerment' comprises five components: women's sense of self-worth; their right to have and determine choices; their right to have access to opportunities and resources; their right to have the power to control their own lives, both inside and outside the home; and their ability to influence the direction of social change to create a more just social and economic order, both nationally and internationally'.[16]

9.2.2 Gender concepts

Gender norms are ideas about how men and women should be and act. These ideas are often learned and internalized as 'rules' early in life and underpin a life cycle of gender socialization and stereotyping. Social inclusion is linked to social exclusion, which refers to when individuals or groups are unable to participate in the economic, social, political and cultural life of their society. They can be economically excluded from or have restricted access to labour markets, land and livelihood opportunities; they can be politically excluded from or have restricted access to citizenship rights, the ability to organize, exercise voice, demand rights and influence decision making that affects their lives; and they can be socially excluded or have restricted access to infrastructure, basic services and amenities, social protection, public safety and social networks. Social inclusion thus refers to improving the ability, opportunity and dignity of people to take part in society.

Gender analysis identifies, analyses and informs action to address inequalities that arise from the different roles of women and men, the distribution of resources, opportunities and power between them, and the consequences of these inequalities on their lives. Gender analysis seeks the perspectives of women and men, and then ensures that these meaningfully inform the development of policies, programmes and projects. It also involves acknowledging the historical and underlying causes of gender inequalities and discrimination in order to inform the setting of relevant and targeted objectives and measures to eliminate gender inequalities. It involves collecting and analysing relevant data to provide a picture of the gender equality situation in a given context; uncovering the underlying causes of gender inequalities; exploring the representation and participation of women and men in different policy sectors and at different levels; and providing evidence-based and credible recommendations for the policies, programmes and projects developed on the basis of it.

Gender planning is a planning that recognizes that because women and men play different roles in society, they often have different needs. Participation of women along with men in project planning enhances project efficiency. It increases project results, cost recovery and improves sustainability. Women's participation serves both practical and strategic needs.

Gender mainstreaming refers to the process of assessing the implications for women and men of any planned action, including legislation, policies or development programmes, in all areas and at all levels. Gender mainstreaming makes women's as well as men's voices, perspectives and expertise central to the design, implementation, monitoring and evaluation of policies and programmes so that women and men benefit equally, and inequality is not perpetuated. The ultimate goal is to achieve gender equality. Gender mainstreaming consists of but is not limited to: analysing gender disaggregated data and qualitative gender analysis data to identify key issues; ensuring the participation of both women and men in determining policy priorities; promoting and modelling gender equal social norms and ways of working as well as positive masculinities; and setting, monitoring and evaluating gender disaggregated policy and programming objectives linked to allocated budgets. Mainstreaming does not necessarily mean that targeted activities to support women are no longer necessary, but the aim is to incorporate the women's and minorities' perspective throughout every policy and programme, even if they are not targeted at women.

Gender roles: Gender planning recognizes that in most societies low-income women have a triple role: women undertake reproductive,

productive and community managing activities, while primarily men undertake productive and community politics activities.

- **Reproductive role:** Child-bearing/rearing responsibilities and domestic tasks often done by women, required to guarantee the maintenance and reproduction of the labour force. It includes not only biological reproduction, but also the care and maintenance of the workforce (male partner and the working children) and the future workforce (infants and school-going children).
- **Productive role:** Work done by both women and men for cash or kind. It includes both market production with an exchange value, and subsistence/home production with actual use-value, and also potential exchange-value. For women in agricultural production, this includes work as independent farmers, peasant wives and wage workers.
- **Community managing role:** Activities undertaken primarily by women at the community level, as an extension of their reproductive role, to ensure the provision and maintenance of scarce resources of collective consumption, such as water, healthcare and education. This is voluntary unpaid work, undertaken in 'free' time.
- **Community political role**: Activities undertaken primarily by men at the community level, organizing at the formal political level, often within the framework of national politics. This is usually paid work, either directly or indirectly, through status and power.

Differential access to and control over resources and benefits: It is important to distinguish between access to resources and control over them when examining how resources (land, labour, credit, income, etc.) are allocated between women and men. How men and women benefit from the resources also should be analysed.

- **Access:** Gives a person the use of a resource, e.g. land to grow crops.
- **Control:** Allows a person to make decisions about who uses the resource or to dispose of the resource, e.g. sell land. Baseline data in a complete gender analysis establish whether there is any differential in men's and women's access to key categories of resources.
- **Benefit**: Allows the person to dispose of the resource in his/her interest.

Condition and position: Development projects generally aim to improve people's living conditions and quality of life. From a gender and development perspective, a distinction is made between the day-to-day condition of women's lives and their position in society. In addition to the specific conditions which women share with men, differential access means that women's position in relation to men must also be assessed when interventions are planned and implemented.

- **Condition:** This refers to the material state in which women and men live, and relates to their responsibilities and work. Improvements in women's and men's condition can be made, for example, by providing safe water, credit and seeds (practical gender needs).
- **Position**: Position refers to women's social and economic standing in society relative to men. This includes, for example, male/female disparities in wages and employment opportunities, unequal representation in the political process, unequal ownership of land and property, and vulnerability to violence (strategic gender needs/interests) (Fig. 9.9).

Gender needs: Women have particular needs that differ from those of men, not only because of their triple role, but also because of their subordinate position in terms of men. It is useful to distinguish two types of needs:

- **Practical gender needs** (PGN) are the needs women identify in their socially accepted roles in society. PGNs do not challenge gender division of labour and women's subordinate position in society. PGNs are a response to immediate perceived necessity. They are practical in nature and tend to concern inadequacies in living conditions such as access to healthcare, education or employment.
- **Strategic gender needs** (SGN) are needs women identify because of their subordinate position in society. They vary according to particular contexts, related to gender divisions of labour, power and control. They may include legal rights, domestic violence, equal wages, and women's control over their bodies. Meeting SGNs assists women to achieve greater equality and contribute to changing existing roles, thereby challenging women's subordinate position.

See also Chapter 13 for information on feminist **economics** that focuses on analysing and addressing gender-based inequalities within economic systems.

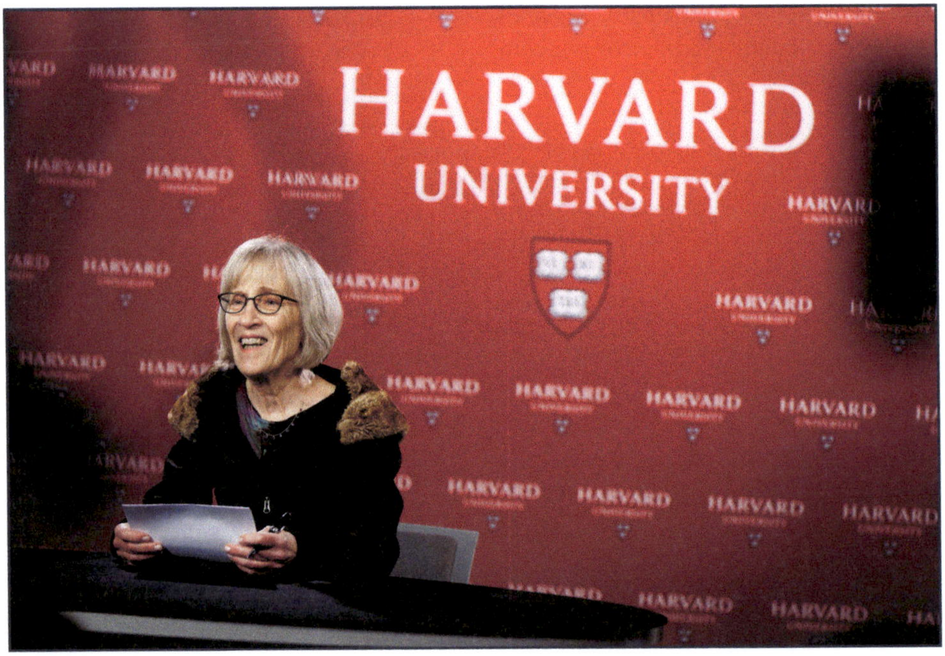

Fig. 9.9. Claudia Goldin won the Nobel Prize for Economics for her groundbreaking work on wage inequality between men and women. She is only the third woman to win the prize (Photo by Stephanie Mitchell / Harvard University with permission from Harvard Public Affairs and Communications).

9.2.3 What is gender analysis?

Gender analysis is the most commonly used tool to integrate a gender perspective into policies, programmes and projects. It is defined by the European Commission as the **'study of differences in the conditions, needs, participation rates, access to resources and development, control of assets, and decision-making powers between men and women in their assigned gender roles'** (EIGE, 2018).

At its simplest, gender analysis is seeing what our eyes have been trained not to see. It is asking about the differences between activities, roles and resources associated with different gender to identify their development needs. Assessing these differences makes it possible to determine gender constraints and opportunities within a sector. Gender analysis can help ensure provision of services that different genders want and that are appropriate to their circumstances. This requires understanding gender roles in the sector by analysing quantitative and qualitative information about their activities, resources and constraints, and benefits and incentives.

The purpose of gender analysis is to identify, understand and explain gaps between individuals with different gender identities that exist in households, communities and countries by:

- Acknowledging differences associated with gender identities based on the unequal distribution of resources, opportunities, constraints and power;
- Ensuring that the different needs of individuals of different gender identities are clearly identified and addressed at all stages of the policy cycle;
- Recognizing that policies, programmes and projects can have different impacts on men and women and people belonging to marginalized/discriminated groups;
- Seeking the viewpoints of men, women, people who identify differently, people facing various forms of discriminations and making their contribution a critical part of developing policies, programmes and projects;
- Promoting all individuals' engagement and participation in community, political and economic life regardless of their gender identity; and
- Promoting better informed, gender-responsive and effective interventions.

When promoting gender-responsive One Health, we need to have interventions and programmes that seek to transform gender relations to promote equality and achieve programmes' objectives (see also Chapter 10 on stakeholder selection and engagement). A good One Health initiative will help to move from an exploitative gender reality to a transformed gender one.

A comprehensive gender analysis will therefore not only provide information to assess and understand gender relations and inequalities in a given context, but it will also explore the causes and effects of gender disparities between groups of people with different power in society. This in turn will allow for developing gender-responsive objectives and measures in order to eliminate gender inequalities in programmes and policies. Ideally, gender analysis is conducted at the design stage, i.e. before a One Health initiative is implemented. Findings of a gender analysis provide the basis for developing gender-responsive indicators, which can be used to monitor trends in gender disparities in One Health decision making, resource control and leadership.

9.2.4 How to undertake a gender analysis

Conducting a gender analysis involves systematically examining how gender roles, norms and power dynamics influence a particular situation, policy, programme or project. The common steps of gender analysis include:

1. Defining the scope and objectives of the gender analysis. Determine in which aspects of a situation or issue you are examining a gender perspective is relevant and why.
2. Collecting relevant data on gender-related aspects, including demographic information, roles, responsibilities, decision-making power, access to resources and societal norms.
3. Identifying data gaps and providing a picture of differences between genders, identifying where further data are needed and what interventions are needed to transform the situation.

Gender-sensitive participatory processes are crucial at all levels, by involving key decision makers along with the groups who will benefit from the policy and projects. Participatory processes will allow for the voices of underrepresented women and men to be heard and to be included in decision-making processes. A number of tools are available to collect relevant data in a participatory manner, such as individual interviews, focus group discussions and resource mapping.

Data collected can be qualitative or quantitative. Qualitative data refer to a broad range of textual or visual information derived from interviews, observations, documents or records. These data are often associated with methods that require 'intensive, often repeated encounters with small numbers of people in their natural environment', often called 'contextual' methods because they attempt to understand human behaviour within the social, cultural, economic and political environment of a locality (FAO, 2014). Quantitative data may derive from official statistics (such as land records or censuses) and surveys. Survey-based methods involve structured interviews of a representative household sample to obtain information on a range of questions, and preformulated, closed-ended and codifiable questions are usually asked to one household member (often the head) during one or two visits, although modifications of the standard interview approach can be used to get more detailed information on gender relations (FAO, 2014).

Data analysis:

- Identify gender roles and norms: identify prevailing gender roles, expectations and norms within the context. Understand how these norms shape the division of labour, decision making and access to resources between genders.
- Assess power dynamics: analyse power dynamics between genders and within different groups. Identify who holds decision-making authority, who has access to resources, and who benefits from existing structures.
- Examine gendered impacts: evaluate how the situation or issue disproportionately affects different genders. Consider both positive and negative impacts, including implications for all genders.
- Analyse access to resources: investigate access to and control over resources such as education, healthcare, land, credit and employment opportunities. Identify whether there are disparities between genders.
- Identify barriers: identify barriers that limit opportunities and participation for specific genders. This could include legal, institutional, cultural and economic barriers.
- Recognize agency: acknowledge the agency and capacities of individuals within different genders. Recognize their contributions, skills and potential for change.

Informing policies, programmes and projects and monitoring, evaluation and learning:

- Develop recommendations: based on the analysis, develop recommendations for promoting gender equality and addressing gender-related disparities. These recommendations can inform policies, programmes and interventions.
- Engage stakeholders: involve stakeholders, including affected communities and gender experts, in the analysis process. Their insights can enhance the accuracy and relevance of the analysis.
- Monitor, evaluate and learn: continuously monitor and evaluate the outcomes of gender-responsive interventions. Adjust strategies based on feedback and evolving gender dynamics.

While these steps will help to ensure that policies, programmes and projects are developed on the basis of sound and accurate information, commitment is needed from all involved to make sure that gender equality and women's empowerment objectives, activities and indicators are embedded systematically into programmes and policies. This also requires ensuring that training programmes on gender and One Health are delivered at all levels, from communities to academic institutions and policy makers.

9.2.5 Gender analysis tools

Most gender analysis frameworks involve collecting quantitative and qualitative information on a set of issues, for which questions must be adapted depending on the project's context and focus areas (Box 9.3).

9.3 Case Studies

In this section, a series of examples are presented for you to work through. They serve the purpose of helping you acquire more awareness of gender domains in One Health. These five examples have been selected to cover different aspects of One Health challenges. For each example, read the description of the issue and the relationship with One Health and think about why it is important to take gender issues into account. Our viewpoints are also given for each example. Please note that these are not exhaustive and that you may have noticed other points that we did not cover.

9.3.1 Endocrine disruptor chemicals

Endocrine disruptor chemicals (EDCs) are substances in the environment (air, soil or water supply), food sources, personal care products and manufactured products that interfere with the normal function of your body's endocrine system.[17] These EDCs have negative consequences for animal health, wildlife health, human health and the environment (Hood, 2005). Some of these compounds are persistent in the environment and can accumulate both in the environment and in the fat of mammalians with subsequent release, for example during pregnancy or lactation, with possible harm to fetal or neonatal susceptible body organs (Lehmann *et al.*, 2018). One such hazard is bisphenol A (BPA), which is used in polycarbonate plastics that are widely used in various everyday items, including food and beverage containers, baby bottles and nipples, or canned food linings. Its use is now banned in several countries worldwide, in particular for baby-related products (Santonicola *et al.*, 2018). Other compounds modify the reproductive organs and avoid normal reproduction in wildlife, such as Atrazine, which is a common herbicide now banned in some countries (Hayes *et al.*, 2011). They can also have consequences in human reproductive organs and present neurotoxicity (Stradtman and Freeman, 2021).

Think about why it is important to take gender issues into account.

Example answer: The most gender- and sex-relevant aspect is that EDCs act on reproductive organs and interfere with hormones (Kumar *et al.*, 2020). Gender should be considered because there are different risks and consequences from being exposed to EDCs[18] (e.g. for human occupational specific exposure, Ribeiro *et al.*, 2017). Furthermore, sex organs in wildlife and humans can have important modifications (e.g. fish and amphibians' feminization; Harris *et al.*, 2011), phase of life (puberty, fertility), pregnancy (in particular along fetus development), menopause, andropause in humans). Recent research also highlights socio-economic status as a relevant factor for exposure and consequences for human health, wildlife and sustainability (Street *et al.*, 2018).

9.3.2 COVID-19

The COVID-19 pandemic started in 2020 was caused by a novel coronavirus, SARS-CoV-2, which has been

Box 9.3. Tools used for gender analysis

Tools	Description	Example
USAID 5 domains of analysis	Laws, policies and regulations Cultural norms and beliefs Access to and control over assets and resources Gender roles, responsibilities and time use Power and decision making	Are women treated equally in legislation related to land rights, employment etc.? Do cultural beliefs hinder women in accessing some opportunities relating to the project? Do men and women have equal access to resources, communication networks, technologies etc.? What are the responsibilities of men and women regarding productive and reproductive activities? Do women hold the power to make decisions and, if so, at what level?
Analysis of 5 forms of capital	Discussing human, social, physical, personal and financial capital, men and women define their access and control over it in the same sex group and give a value between 0 and 10. A comparison between men and women can be done using a radar diagram and discussion on the causes and consequences of the situation can be discussed.	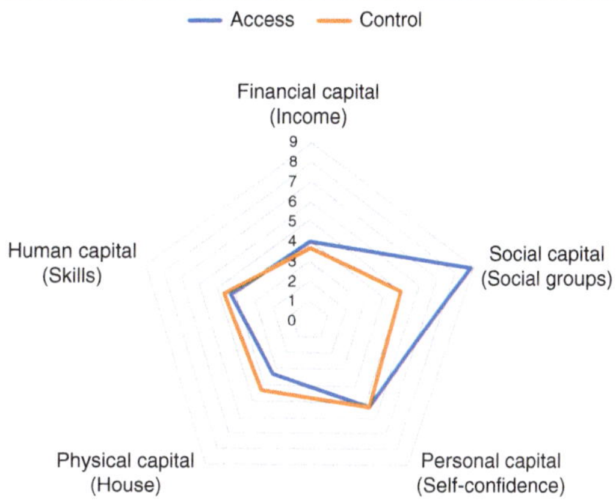 From Opondoh *et al.* (2023) with permission.
Stake-holders analysis	Specific attention to stakeholders demonstrates that different groups have different concerns, capacities and interests, which need to be explicitly understood for problem identification, objective setting and strategy selection.	Stakeholder analysis matrix, SWOT analysis, Venn diagrams or Spider diagrams. 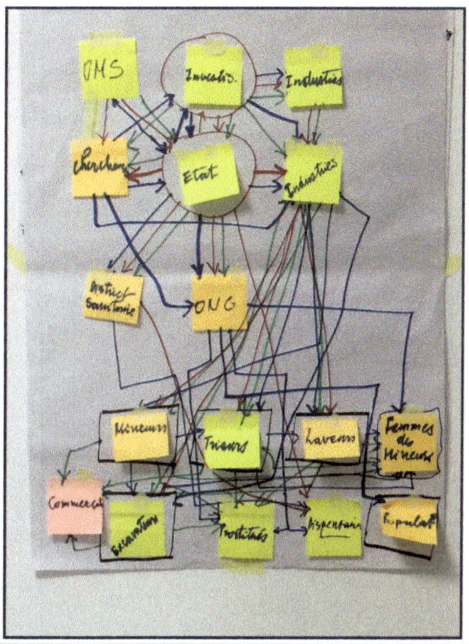

Continued

Box 9.3. Continued.

<table>
<tr><th>Tools</th><th>Description</th><th>Example</th></tr>
<tr>
<td>Harvard tool
Activity profile</td>
<td>Table identifying the different roles that men and women fulfil in the context of your specific work. The example provided here involved rural communities keeping livestock and aimed at identifying the different roles in small livestock production (chickens and goats) during their life cycle.</td>
<td>
<table>
<tr><th>Activities</th><th>Male adults</th><th>Female adults</th><th>Boys</th><th>Girls</th><th>Old men</th><th>Old women</th></tr>
<tr><td>Caring for small species (poultry, goats)</td><td></td><td></td><td></td><td></td><td></td><td></td></tr>
<tr><td>Giving food to these animals</td><td></td><td></td><td></td><td></td><td></td><td></td></tr>
<tr><td>Giving them water</td><td></td><td></td><td></td><td></td><td></td><td></td></tr>
<tr><td>Preparing the chicken house or barn</td><td></td><td></td><td></td><td></td><td></td><td></td></tr>
<tr><td>Preparing where the animal is going to brood or give birth</td><td></td><td></td><td></td><td></td><td></td><td></td></tr>
<tr><td>Cleaning the chicken house or barn</td><td></td><td></td><td></td><td></td><td></td><td></td></tr>
<tr><td>Receiving information on breeding small livestock (poultry, goats)</td><td></td><td></td><td></td><td></td><td></td><td></td></tr>
<tr><td>Caring for sick poultry and goats</td><td></td><td></td><td></td><td></td><td></td><td></td></tr>
<tr><td>Preparing meat from small animals (poultry and goats) for meals</td><td></td><td></td><td></td><td></td><td></td><td></td></tr>
</table>
</td>
</tr>
<tr>
<td>Harvard tool
Access, control and benefits</td>
<td>Table listing resources in relation to the intervention. It also specifies activities carried out by gender and often age. The example provided here involved rural communities engaged in agricultural production.</td>
<td>
<table>
<tr><th>RESOURCES</th><th>WHO HAS ACCESS?</th><th>WHO HAS CONTROL?</th><th>WHO BENEFITS?</th><th>WHAT ARE THE IMPLICATIONS?</th></tr>
<tr><td>LAND (List different land types and status of degradation)
WATER
CROPS (List subsistence and cash crops)
TREES (List important trees)
LIVESTOCK
- Chickens
- Goats and Sheep
- Cows
LABOUR
- Own
- Family
- Hired
INPUTS (Purchased or produced on the farm)
- Fertilizer
- Pesticides
CAPITAL GOODS
- Implements
- Fencing
CASH
- Credit
INFORMATION
MARKET/TRANSPORT
EDUCATION</td><td></td><td></td><td></td><td></td></tr>
</table>
</td>
</tr>
</table>

Continued

Box 9.3. Continued.

<table>
<tr><th>Tools</th><th>Description</th><th>Example</th></tr>
<tr><td>Time use</td><td>This is a 24-hour table where we identify who does what and when. It specifies activities carried out by gender and often age, including sleep, rest, labour, productive, reproductive, community and community politics roles. It shows who works more and who has more resting time.</td><td>
<table>
<tr><td></td><td>1</td><td>2</td><td>3</td><td>4</td><td>5</td><td>6</td><td>7</td><td>8</td><td>9</td><td>10</td><td>11</td><td>12</td><td>13</td><td>14</td><td>15</td><td>16</td><td>17</td><td>18</td><td>19</td><td>20</td><td>21</td><td>22</td><td>23</td><td>24</td></tr>
<tr><td>sleep</td><td></td><td></td><td></td><td></td><td></td><td></td><td></td><td></td><td></td><td></td><td></td><td></td><td></td><td></td><td></td><td></td><td></td><td></td><td></td><td></td><td></td><td></td><td></td><td></td></tr>
<tr><td></td><td></td><td></td><td></td><td></td><td></td><td></td><td></td><td></td><td></td><td></td><td></td><td></td><td></td><td></td><td></td><td></td><td></td><td></td><td></td><td></td><td></td><td></td><td></td><td></td></tr>
<tr><td></td><td></td><td></td><td></td><td></td><td></td><td></td><td></td><td></td><td></td><td></td><td></td><td></td><td></td><td></td><td></td><td></td><td></td><td></td><td></td><td></td><td></td><td></td><td></td><td></td></tr>
<tr><td></td><td></td><td></td><td></td><td></td><td></td><td></td><td></td><td></td><td></td><td></td><td></td><td></td><td></td><td></td><td></td><td></td><td></td><td></td><td></td><td></td><td></td><td></td><td></td><td></td></tr>
</table>
</td></tr>
</table>

designated a **zoonotic disease** by WHO and has an animal origin in an evolutionary sense, being very similar to a coronavirus isolated from bats. However, the exact animal source remains unknown (Haider *et al.*, 2020). The complexity of zoonotic diseases' epidemiology and drivers, including an increasing demand for protein, changing food value chains and biodiversity loss associated with land-use changes, clearly requires an interdisciplinary One Health approach. A survey conducted in four European countries on successful cases of implementing a collaborative, inter-disciplinary and coordinated One Health approach in the context of COVID-19 has been described by Häsler *et al.* (2020). The benefits of nature on people's health, both physical and mental, were also established early in the pandemic by the Gender Working Group of the Network for Ecohealth and One Health who surveyed 345 people in four European countries and found that walking in the countryside was a great help during confinement periods (NEOH Gender WG, unpublished).

Think about why it is important to take gender issues into account.

Example answer: Men and women experience the pandemic differently due to sex and gender differences. In most countries, men have been most affected in terms of fatalities with male to female case fatality ratio ranging up to 3.5 in some cases (Delhingia and Raj, 2021). Sex (biological) factors are likely to be involved because differences in immune systems between men and women are known to contribute to infectious diseases responses (Klein and Flanagan, 2016). Gendered differences associated with risky behaviours (smoking tobacco, drinking alcohol) and co-morbidity including hypertension, cardiovascular disease and some chronic lung diseases might also be associated with adverse outcomes in COVID-19 (Purdie *et al.*, 2020). Nevertheless, women have been disproportionately impacted by COVID-19 (losses of jobs and livelihoods, increase in unpaid care, surge in violence against women and girls) by being at the forefront of the COVID-19 response and through gender roles and responsibilities. As a result, the crisis is threatening to erase decades of progress for women and girls (UN Women, 2021).

9.3.3 Antimicrobial resistance

Antimicrobial drugs, such as antibiotics that are used to treat bacterial infections in humans and animals, allowed improvement in health and survival of animals and humans. But, currently, antimicrobial resistance (AMR) is one of the greatest health threats of our time and is considered a priority challenge for the human and animal health **sectors** (Antimicrobial Resistance Collaborators, 2022). Antibiotics can spill into the soil and the water and resistant strains of bacteria can thus emerge in the environment. These bacteria that are resistant to antibiotics can infect animals including wildlife and humans.

Uncontrolled and irresponsible use in animals and humans, infections from hospital settings, poor monitoring and enforcement, empirical treatment and self-medication are the main causes of AMR. The development of AMR stems in part from the decisions of patients, practitioners, farmers and veterinarians. Identifying who makes decisions about antimicrobial use (antibacterials, antivirals, antiparasitics and antifungals) will allow interventions to be targeted more effectively.

Antimicrobial resistance covers resistance to drugs used for bacterial infections (e.g. urinary tract infections, pneumonia, bloodstream infections) and infections caused by microorganisms, such as parasites (e.g. malaria or helminths), viruses (e.g. HIV) or fungi (e.g. Candida). The direct consequences of human infections with resistant microorganisms are severe and include longer duration of illness, increased mortality, prolonged hospitalization, reduced protection during surgery and other medical procedures, and increased healthcare costs (WHO, 2023). Antimicrobial resistance threatens the successes achieved against tuberculosis, malaria, HIV and other sexually transmitted infections and contributes to the emergence and re-emergence of infectious diseases. By example, the direct consequences of animal infections of antibiotic-resistant diseases such as salmonella, *E. coli* and *Campylobacter* infections in poultry lead to limited growth and a higher level of mortality (Magnusson *et al.*, 2021).

Think about why it is important to take gender issues into account.

Example answer: Those most infected and affected by infectious diseases are most at risk for the consequences of AMR. For example, in 2016, in Senegal, communicable diseases were the cause of death for 35.6 % of men between 15 and 34 years of age and 59.6 % of women in the same age group.[19] In the 15–24 age group, HIV prevalence is twice as high among women (0.02 %) as among men (0.01 %). Therefore, in the age groups mentioned, men and women will not be impacted in the same way by AMR.

Some other points that may be considered:

- **Gendered roles in healthcare and agriculture:** women often play significant roles in healthcare and agriculture, including as caregivers, healthcare workers and farmers. Their responsibilities can influence the use of antimicrobials in both human and animal health sectors.
- **Access to healthcare:** gender disparities in access to healthcare can affect the use of antimicrobials. Women's access to appropriate medical care, diagnostic services and prescription medications may be limited in some regions, which could lead to ineffective treatment practices and contribute to AMR.
- **Self-medication and empirical treatment:** women, especially in regions with limited access to healthcare, may resort to self-medication practices or administer antimicrobials empirically to themselves or their families. This can lead to inappropriate and ineffective use of these medications, contributing to AMR.
- **Gender norms and decision making:** gender norms can influence decision making related to healthcare and livestock management. In some cases, women's voices and knowledge might be excluded from decisions about antimicrobial use, despite their crucial roles in caregiving and animal husbandry.
- **Occupational exposure:** women working in healthcare settings, particularly as nurses or healthcare support staff, may have increased exposure to infections and antimicrobials.
- **Livelihood and economic impact**: in rural communities, where women often manage household livestock and poultry, their decisions about animal health practices can impact the spread of AMR.

9.3.4 Brucellosis

Brucellosis is a zoonotic infectious disease meaning it can be transmitted from animals to humans. The causative agent is a bacteria of *Brucella* spp. Infected female animals most frequently show reproductive problems, including abortions, stillbirths and malformations of the fetus. In male animals, changes in testes can be found. In humans the disease starts with a fever, but after a few weeks it develops into non-specific signs including tiredness, fatigue, headaches and stomach pain which after a few months can evolve into spondylitis, arthritis and endocarditis. In pregnant women there can also be abortions or intrauterine fetal death (Bosilkovski *et al.*, 2020). The most exposed population are people professionally connected with animals like veterinarians, farm workers, breeders and people in the milk or meat industry. People can get infected after direct contact with sick animals or by using milk products from a sick animal, such as raw milk or cheese that is not heat treated (Shakir, 2021).

Think about why it is important to take gender issues into account.

Example answer: Gender needs to be considered because of the gendered nature of work on farms and in the milk industry. Most workers dealing with and manipulating animals in households or small dairy farms in countries where brucellosis is the most prevalent are women. Even in big industrial farms with intensive production women are more often employed for taking care of the animals or milking the animals. This is complicated further by commonly gender-biased access to information, such as livestock management advice and knowledge. The role of the woman in the production and supply chains as well as gender differences in dietary intake of (raw) milk and dairy products is an essential factor. Also, the effects that the infection can have on reproduction is an important element to consider. Pregnant women who contract brucellosis may experience complications, and there can be risks of transmission to the unborn child. Further, women often take on caregiving roles within households, caring for sick family members, including those affected by brucellosis. This can take away their time from other tasks and constitute a burden and potentially loss of income. And yet, gender issues related to brucellosis are commonly addressed in the scientific literature in terms of sex differences. Very rarely is it mentioned that increased presence of women in milking, breeding and caring for the animals can be associated with the transmission of brucellosis and can endanger women more than men (Garnier *et al.*, 2020).

9.3.5 Climate change

Climate change is a global phenomenon that affects natural and managed systems and ecosystems such as water resources, agriculture and food production systems, forestry, coastal-marine areas, and society health in general. Even if rising temperatures can be kept within 1.5°C of pre-industrial levels (and currently we are on course for 2.7°C), the world can expect a future characterized by worsening global food crises, biodiversity loss and more frequent extreme weather events. Fresh water will become scarcer, and disease and malnutrition will rise, contributing to displacement and conflict. Negative impacts will be significant at the local level, especially in those areas or regions where the socio-economic vulnerability is greater (Gonda, 2014). Besides, the global south is not adequately prepared for climate change, mainly due to its high population density in more vulnerable areas, and limited access to resources and poor infrastructure for adequate coping strategies (Roy, 2018). The adverse impacts of climate change are already obvious on agricultural productivity and food security in response to worsening droughts, increasingly vulnerable biodiversity and ecosystems, stressed water resources, human health problems such as infectious diseases spread across newer territories and settlements, migration patterns, energy, transport and industry (Roy, 2018).

Think about why it is important to take gender issues into account.

Example answer: On average, rural women account for nearly half the agricultural workforce in developing countries. Despite their crucial roles in household food security, they face discrimination and limited bargaining power. Patriarchal norms create disadvantages for women farmers, specifically in land rights (small plots, difficulties obtaining ownership, discriminatory inheritance rights), productive resources (no access to credit, extension services or inputs), unpaid work, insecure employment and exclusion from decision making and political representation. Within the household, because of a weaker bargaining position, they frequently eat least, last and least well.

Because gender inequity remains high in the agricultural sector, women farmers who control resources generally have better-quality diets. Women and children bear much of the brunt of climate change, being 14 times more likely than men to die during a disaster. They constitute 70% of people living in poverty in low-income countries who are the most vulnerable to climate change and least able to adapt. Women are also often at greatest risk of displacement: the United Nations Development Program estimates that 80% of climate-displaced people are women, because women are considered to be a weak part of the society and are displaced first in order to be protected (Williamson *et al.*, 2021).

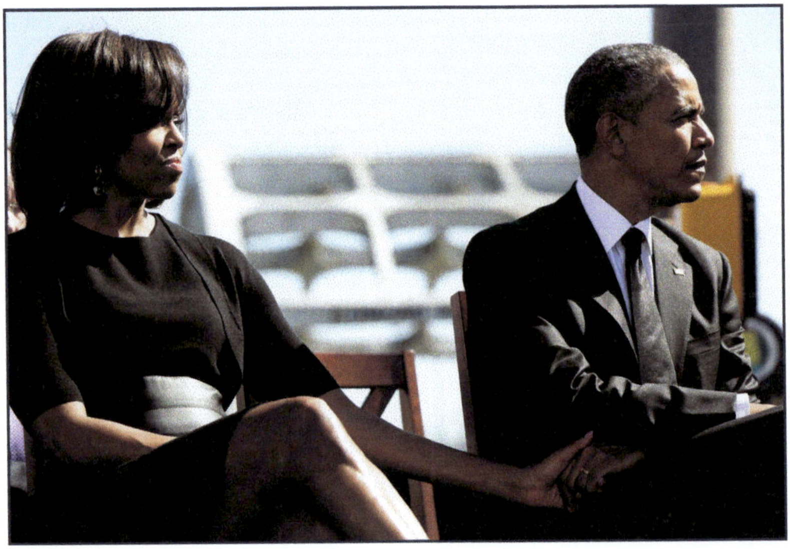

Fig. 9.10. The relationship between Michelle and Barack Obama is widely portrayed and perceived as positive and contributes to promoting respect between men and women (Photo: Courtesy Barack Obama Presidential Library).

9.4 Conclusions

- The gender dimension has started to be acknowledged in the One Health domain but still needs systematic operationalization.
- Integration of gender issues in One Health activities is crucial.
- Elements such as health, equity, environmental and climate crises affect men, women and people who identify differently, most often to the detriment of women.
- Gender analysis provides a tool for allowing the integration of a gender perspective into policies, programmes and projects.
- Presented case studies (endocrine disruptors, COVID-19, AMR, climate change and brucellosis) require a One Health approach with a gender perspective.
- We must move from gender awareness to a gender transformative paradigm to build more resilient and equitable societies (Fig. 9.10).

Notes

[1] We acknowledge that there are gender diverse people who may not identify as men and women and who may be impacted in specific ways by gender issues, but our main focus in this chapter is on the relations between men and women rather than gender identity.

[2] https://www.unfpa.org/sites/default/files/resource-pdf/COVID-19_A_Gender_Lens_Guidance_Note.pdf

[3] We acknowledge that gender identities are not limited to the binary categories of men and women. While our chapter may mention men and women, we recognize and respect the identities of all gender-diverse people who do not identify within these categories.

[4] https://ec.europa.eu/world/avian_influenza/docs/gender_study_0608_en.pdf

[5] https://www.unenvironment.org/news-and-stories/story/why-gender-important-biodiversity-conservation

[6] https://www.iucn.org/resources/issues-briefs/gender-and-climate-change

[7] https://afrohun.org/wp-content/uploads/2021/01/GENDER-ONE-HEALTH-AND-INFECTIOUS-DISEASE-TRAINING-GUIDE-.pdf

[8] https://onehealthhorn.net/

[9] https://www.ecohealthinternational.org/one-health-and-gender-wg/

[10] https://www.inserm.fr/information-en-sante/dossiers-information/genre-et-sante

[11] Ministério da Mulher e Coordenação da Acção Social.

[12] USAID. 2019. Gender Assessment for USAID/Mozambique Country Development Cooperation Strategy. Maputo: USAID. https://pdf.usaid.gov/pdf_docs/PA00WGW3.pdf

[13] https://data.worldbank.org/indicator/SG.GEN.PARL.ZS?locations=MZ

[14] https://www.igwg.org/wp-content/uploads/2017/05/FG_GendrIntegrContinuum.pdf

[15] Such as WEIA and PRO-WEIA, developed by the International Food Policy Research Institute (IFPRI).

[16] https://eige.europa.eu/thesaurus/terms/1102

[17] https://www.endocrine.org/patient-engagement/endocrine-library/edcs

[18] Source of Exposure to EDC : Front. Public Health, 24 September 2020 I https://doi.org/10.3389/fpubh.2020.553850

[19] https://databank.worldbank.org/source/gender-statistics

References

Alcoff, L. and Potter, E. (1993) Introduction. When feminists intersect epistemology. In: Alcoff, L. and Potter, E. (eds) *Feminist Epistemologies*. Routledge, London, pp. 1–14.

Amuguni, J.H., Mugisha, A., Kyewalabye, E., Bagnol, B., Talmage, R. *et al.* (2018) EnGENDERing One Health and addressing gender gaps in infectious disease control and response: Developing a gender, One Health and emerging pandemics threat short course for the public health workforce in Africa. *Advances in Social Sciences Research Journal* 5(5), 467–479. DOI: 10.14738/assrj.55.4640.

Anderson, E. (2012) Feminist epistemology and philosophy of science. In: Zalta, E.N. (ed) *The Stanford Encyclopedia of Philosophy*. Available at: https://plato.stanford.edu/entries/feminism-epistemology/ (accessed 2 August 2024).

Antimicrobial Resistance Collaborators (2022) Global burden of bacterial antimicrobial resistance in 2019: A systematic analysis. *Lancet* 399, 629–655.

Bagnol, B., Alders, R. and McConchie, R. (2015) Gender issues in human, animal and plant health using an ecohealth perspective. *Environment Natural Resources Research* 5(1), 62–76. DOI: 10.5539/enrr.v5n1p62.

Bernal, X.E., Rojas, B., Pinto-E, M.A., Mendoza-Henao, A.M., Herrera-Montes, A. *et al.* (2019) Empowering latina scientists. *Science* 363(6429), 825–826. DOI: 10.1126/science.aaw6.

Betron, M., Bourgeault, I., Manzoor, M., Paulino, E., Steege, R. *et al.* (2019) Time for gender-transformative change in the health workforce. *Lancet* 393(10171): e25–26. DOI: 10.1016/S0140-6736(19)30208-9.

Bosilkovski, M., Arapović, J. and Keramat, F. (2020) Human brucellosis in pregnancy – an overview. *Bosnia Journal Basic Medical Science* 20(4), 415–422. DOI: 10.17305/bjbms.2019.4499.

Delhingia, N. and Raj, A. (2021) Sex differences in COVID-19 case fatality: Do we know enough? *The Lancet Global.*

EIGE (2018) Gender Mainstreaming: Gender Analysis. Available at: https://eige.europa.eu/gender-mainstreaming/methods-tools/gender-analysis (accessed 2 August 2024).

FAO (2014) *Gender in Agriculture. Closing the Knowledge Gap.* Springer, Dordrecht. DOI : 10.1007/978-94-017-8616-4.

FAO, OIE and WHO (2019) A Tripartite Guide to Addressing Zoonotic Diseases in Countries. Available at: https://www.who.int/initiatives/tripartite-zoonosis-guide (accessed 24 August 2024).

Friedson-Ridenour, S., Dutcher, T.V., Calderon, C., Brown, L.D.P. and Olsen, C.W. (2019) Gender analysis for one health: Theoretical perspectives and recommendations for practice. *Ecohealth* 16(2), 306–316. DOI: 10.1007/s10393-019-01410-w.

Gammage, S., Kabeer, N. and van der Meulen Rodgers, Y. (2016) Voice and agency: Where are we now? *Feminist Economics* 22, 1–29. DOI: 10.1080/13545701.2015.1101308.

Garnier, J., Savić, S., Boriani, E., Bagnol, B., Häsler, B. and Kock, R. (2020) Helping to heal nature and ourselves through human-rights-based and gender-responsive One Health. *One Health Outlook* 2(1), 22. DOI: 10.1186/s42522-020-00029-0.

Garnier, J., Savić, S., Cediel, N., Barato, P., Boriani, E., Bagnol, B. and Kock, R.A. (2022) Mainstreaming gender-responsive One Health: Now is the time. *Frontiers in Public Health* 10, 845866. DOI: 10.3389/fpubh.2022.845866.

Gonda, N. (2014) Género y Adaptación al Cambio Climático: Puesta en común y sistematización de experiencias sobre la integración de la perspectiva de género en la adaptación al cambio climático en el ámbito rural en Nicaragua. Agrónomos y Veterinarios sin Fronteras con el apoyo del Programa de Naciones Unidas para el Desarrollo. Available at: https://www.researchgate.net/publication/320799391_Genero_y_Adaptacion_al_Cambio_Climatico_Puesta_en_comun_y_sistematizacion_de_experiencias_sobre_la_integracion_de_la_perspectiva_de_genero_en_la_adaptacion_al_cambio_climatico_en_el_ambito_rural_en_Ni (accessed 24 August 2024).

Haider, N., Rothman-Ostrow, P., Osman, A.Y., Arruda, L.B., Macfarlane-Berry, L. *et al.* (2020) COVID-19: Zoonosis or Emerging Infectious Disease? *Frontiers in Public Health* 8, 596944. DOI: 10.3389/fpubh.2020.596944.

Harris, C.A., Hamilton, P.B., Runnalls, T.J., Vinciotti, V., Henshaw, A. *et al.* (2011) The consequences of feminization in breeding groups of wild fish. *Environmental Health Perspectives* 119(3), 306–311.

Häsler, B., Bazeyo, W., Byrne, A.W., Hernandez-Jover, M., More, S.J. *et al.* (2020) Reflecting on One Health in action during the COVID-19 response. *Frontiers in Veterinary Science* 7, 578649. DOI: 10.3389/fvets.2020.578649.

Hayes, T.B., Anderson, L.L., Beasley, V.R., de Solla, S.R., Iguchi, T. *et al.* (2011) Demasculinization and feminization of male gonads by atrazine: Consistent effects across vertebrate classes. *Journal of Steroid Biochemistry and Molecular Biology* 127(1–2), 64–73. DOI: 10.1016/j.jsbmb.2011.03.015.

Health 9(1), E14–E15. DOI: 10.1016/S2214-109X(20)30464-2.

Hood, E. (2005) Are EDCs blurring issues of gender? *Environmental Health Perspectives* 113(10), A670–A677. DOI: 10.1289/ehp.113-a670.

Interagency Gender Working Group (IGWG) (2017) The Gender Integration Continuum Training Session User's Guide. Population Reference Bureau. Available at: https://www.igwg.org/wp-content/uploads/2017/12/17-418-GenderContTraining-2017-12-12-1633_FINAL.pdf (accessed 5 August 2024).

Kindstedt, P. (2012) *Cheese and Culture: A History of Cheese and its Place in Western Civilization*. Chelsea Green Publishing, Vermont, USA.

Klein, S.L. and Flanagan, K.L. (2016) Sex differences in immune responses. *Nature Reviews Immunology* 16(10), 626–638. DOI: 10.1038/nri.2016.90.

Kumar, M., Sarma, D.K., Shubham, S., Kumawat, M., Verma, V., Prakash, A. and Tiwari, R. (2020) Environmental endocrine-disrupting chemical exposure: Role in non-communicable diseases. *Frontiers in Public Health* 8, 553850. DOI: 10.3389/fpubh.2020.553850.

Lehmann, G.M., LaKind, J.S., Davis, M.H., Hines, E.P., Marchitti, S.A., Alcala, C. and Lorber, M. (2018) Environmental chemicals in breast milk and formula: Exposure and risk assessment implications. *Environmental Health Perspectives* 126(9), 96001. DOI: 10.1289/EHP1953.

Liu, A.K. and Mager Dipietro, A. (2016) Women's involvement in clinical trials: Historical perspective and future implications. *Journal of Pharmacy Practice (Granada)* 14(1), 708.

Llorens, A., Tzovara, A., Bellier, L., Bhaya-Grossman, I., Bidet-Caulet, A. *et al.* (2021) Gender bias in academia: A lifetime problem that needs solutions. *Neuron* 109(13), 2047–2074. DOI: 10.1016/j.neuron.2021.06.002.

Magnusson, U., Moodley, A. and Osbjer, K. (2021) Antimicrobial resistance at the livestock-human interface: Implications for Veterinary Services. *Revue Scientifique et Technique – Office International des Épizooties* 40 (2). Available at: https://www.woah.org/app/uploads/2021/05/402-12-magnusson.pdf (accessed 2 August 2024).

Munoz Boudet, A.M., Petesch, P. and Turk, C. (2007) Power and empowerment. In: VeneKlasen, L. and Miller, V. (eds) *A New Weave of Power, People and Politics*. Practical Action Publishing, Washington DC. Available at: https://justassociates.org/en/resources/new-weave-power-people-politics-action-guide-advocacy-and-citizen-participation (accessed 2 August 2024).

Opondoh, A.A., Muga, G., Kaluwa, C., Oduma, J., Bagnol, B. *et al.* (2023) Women's access to and control over the 5 forms of capital in Machakos Town Sub-County, Kenya. *International Journal of Science and Research* 12, 7. https://www.ijsr.net/archive/v12i7/SR23625065717.pdf (accessed 2 August 2024).

Purdie, A., Hawkes, S., Buse, K. *et al.* (2020) Sex, gender and COVID-19: Disaggregated data and health disparities. Blog *BMJ Global Heath* 2020. Available at: https://blogs.bmj.com/bmjgh/2020/03/24/sex-gender-and-covid-19-disaggregated-data-and-health-disparities/ (accessed 2 August 2024).

Ribeiro, E., Ladeira, C. and Viegas, S. (2017) Occupational exposure to Bisphenol A (BPA): A reality that still needs to be unveiled. *Toxics* 5(3), 22. DOI: 10.3390/toxics5030022.

Roy, S. (ed.) (2018) *Linking Gender to Climate Change Impacts in the Global South*. Springer. ISBN 978-3-319-75776-6 ISBN 978-3-319-75777-3 (eBook) DOI: 10.1007/978-3-319-75777-3.

Santonicola, S., Ferrante, M.C., Leo, G.D., Murru, N., Anastasio, A. and Mercogliano, R. (2018) Study on endocrine disruptors levels in raw milk from cow's farms: Risk assessment. *Italian Journal of Food Safety* 7(3), 7668. DOI: 10.4081/ijfs.2018.7668.

Scott, W.J. (1988) Gender: A useful category of historical gender analysis. In: *Gender and the Politics of History*. Columbia University Press, New York, pp. 28–50.

Shakir, R. (2021) Brucellosis. *Journal of the Neurological Sciences* 420, 117280. DOI: 10.1016/j.jns.2020.117280.

Stradtman, S.C. and Freeman, J.L. (2021) Mechanisms of neurotoxicity associated with exposure to the herbicide atrazine. *Toxics* 9(9), 207. DOI: 10.3390/toxics9090207.

Street, M.E., Angelini, S., Bernasconi, S., Burgio, E., Cassio, A. *et al.* (2018) Current knowledge on endocrine disrupting chemicals (EDCs) from animal biology to humans, from pregnancy to adulthood: Highlights from a national Italian meeting. *International Journal of Molecular Sciences* 19(6), 1647. DOI: 10.3390/ijms19061647.

UN Women (2021) Report on the UN Women Global Response to COVID-19. https://www.unwomen.org/en/digital-library/publications/2021/02/report-on-the-un-women-global-response-to-covid-19 (accessed 2 August 2024).

UN (2022) *Policy Brief STEM Education and Inequalities in Africa*. UN, New York. Available at: https://www.un.org/osaa/sites/www.un.org.osaa/files/un_brand_report_web_august_2020_v36928.pdf (accessed 2 August 2024).

UNEP (2021) Gender and the environment: A preliminary analysis of gaps and opportunities in Latin America and the Caribbean. *United Nations Environment Programme*. PNUMA, Panama City. Available at: https://www.unep.org/events/unep-event/xxii-forum-ministers-environment-latin-america-and-caribbean (accessed 27 August 2024).

UNESCO (2021) Science report 2021. The race against time for smarter development. In: UNESCO, Schneegans, S., Straza, T. and Lewis, J. (eds). UNESCO Publishing, Paris. Available at: https://www.unesco.org/reports/science/2021/en/report-series?TSPD_101_R0=080713870fab2000cdf3904f746e9ac27cccad75921949cc60c76a664f3a26075f2b82bb236bc5a108358dfc3614300073a52731cc4325dac9e0c9ae2be141a7c98faaac9285503b96cadc4f88c597078425c6154e4162c445bcfd6c1f7a7008 (accessed 2 August 2024).

WHO (2013) Taking sex and gender into account in emerging infectious disease programmes. *An Analytical Framework*. WHO Western Pacific. Available at: https://www.who.int/publications/i/item/9789290615323 (accessed 2 August 2024).

WHO (2019) *The Thirteenth General Programme of Work, 2019–2023: Promote Health Keep the World Safe Serve the Vulnerable*. https://iris.who.int/bitstream/handle/10665/324775/WHO-PRP-18.1-eng.pdf?sequence=1

WHO (2023) Antimicrobial resistance. Available at: https://www.who.int/news-room/fact-sheets/detail/antimicrobial-resistance (accessed 2 August 2024).

Williamson, D., Munro, K. and Carlot, M. (2021) Climate Change: A Hunger Crisis in the Making. Available at: https://www.actionagainsthunger.org/sites/default/files/publications/ActionAgainstHunger_Climate_Change_Hunger_Crisis_Report.pdf (accessed 2 August 2024).

10 One Health Implementation Cycle, Stakeholder Analysis and Engagement

Simon R. Rüegg[1,2], Tieble Traore[3], Christina Pettan-Brewer[4], Daniela Figueroa[5,6], Natalia Cediel Becerra[7,2], Verónica Ormea[5,8], Parntep Ratanakorn[9], Tithipong Plangsangmas[10], Kevin Queenan[11], Barbara Häsler[11,2], Catharina B.M. Maassen[12,2] and Séverine Thys[13,2]

[1]Section of Epidemiology, Vetsuisse Faculty, University of Zurich, Zurich, Switzerland; [2]Network for Ecohealth and One Health (NEOH); [3]Emergency Preparedness and Response (EPR) Cluster, World Health Organization, Regional Office for Africa – Dakar Emergency Hub, Dakar, Senegal WHO Regional Office for Africa, Dakkar, Sénégal; [4]School of Medicine and Center for One Health Research, School of Public Health, University of Washington, USA, UNEP Nature for Health (N4H) TAG, International Alliance against Health Risks and Wildlife Trade Steering Committee, CABI One Health Executive Editorial Member and Federal Schools of Minas Gerais (UFMG) and Parana (UFPR), Faculdade Pontificia Catolica (PUC), One Health Brasil (ABRA-SUNI), Brazil, OHLAIC/CYTED Latin America; [5]Red One Health Latinoamerica, Ibero and The Caribbean Network (y El Caribe - OHLAIC); [6]One Health Latin America, Ibero and The Caribbean Network; [7]Faculty of Agricultural Sciences, Universidad de La Salle, Bogotá, Colombia; [8]Faculty of Health Sciences, Universidad Peruana de Ciencias Aplicadas, Lima, Peru; [9]Thailand National Wildlife Health Center, Faculty of Veterinary Science, Mahidol University, Nakhon Pathom, Thailand; [10]Chulabhorn Royal Academy, Bangkok, Thailand; [11]Veterinary Epidemiology Economics and Public Health Group, Department of Pathobiology and Population Sciences, Royal Veterinary College, London, UK; [12]Centre for Infectious Disease Control (CIb), National Institute for Public Health and the Environment (RIVM), Bilthoven, The Netherlands; [13]ASTRE, University Montpellier, CIRAD, INRAE, Montpellier, France

Contents

DOI: 10.1079/9781800623002.0011

Chapter Overview

Elevator pitch

This chapter describes key steps, principles, reflections and recommendations on how One Health can be implemented. It then focuses specifically on how to conduct a stakeholder analysis and provides a set of methods to connect and integrate stakeholders of One Health initiatives. You will learn principles of inclusive stakeholder engagement throughout the One Health implementation cycle. This forms the basis for subsequent chapters that focus on other parts of the cycle and how evaluation (including economic evaluation) can accompany a project.

Book objectives the chapter relates to

☐ 1. Understand what One Health and Ecohealth mean
☐ 2. Think in a One Health and Ecohealth way
☐ 3. Apply One Health and Ecohealth in their professional and personal life
☐ 4. Know how to share One Health and Ecohealth knowledge
☑ 5. Integrate One Health and Ecohealth knowledge actively
☐ 6. Acquire or enhance core One Health competencies

One Health competencies covered

☑ 1. Effective communication
☑ 2. Collaborative and resilient working
☑ 3. Systems understanding
☑ 4. Transdisciplinarity
☑ 5. Social, cultural and gender equity and inclusiveness
☐ 6. Collective learning and reflective practice
☐ 7. One Health concepts
☐ 8. Theoretical and methodological pluralism
☐ 9. Harnessing uncertainty, paradox and limited knowledge

Learning outcomes

1. Know some repertories with tools and methods to engage stakeholders.
2. Be able to articulate a problem statement in an inclusive way.
3. Explain inclusive stakeholder engagement and sketch the development of a stakeholder management plan.
4. Discuss the nature of conflict, reasons for conflicts and their impacts.
5. Know questions and reflections to warrant an equitable and inclusive stakeholder's engagement.
6. Be able to identify indicators of progress in a socio-ecological system.

Summary

The chapter introduces the One Health implementation cycle with all steps that occur during the implementation of a project or policy. We start with an introduction to the implementation of activities in socio-ecological systems (SES), which are, by definition, complex and dynamic. We then explore the kind of challenges we encounter in SES and how these determine the importance of engaging stakeholders in the problem statement, in the understanding of the SES itself and in the co-production of solutions. The cycle starts with stating the problem in an inclusive way and exploring the stakeholders systematically, to leave no one behind. Then, we start a community of practice by co-producing a common understanding of the SES and the challenge. We then reach out and will discover what conflicting perspectives and interests we may encounter and how to deal with them to align behind a common theory of change. This forms the basis for other parts in the implementation cycle, which are covered in Chapters 11, 12 and 13.

10.1 Introduction

IMPLEMENTATION can mean different things depending on the situation. According to the Oxford English Dictionary, it involves beginning, founding, organizing, setting up, developing, placing into action, stabilizing and regulating as examples. Translations in other languages might add more meanings. Some people see implementation as 'starting something new', while others see it as 'developing and regulating existing actions'. The first idea focuses on creating new groups or projects from scratch, while the second looks at turning ideas into real impacts in **socio-ecological systems** (SES), including supporting, funding and further developing what already exists. The problem with the first approach is that it might create competition and division instead of working together as outlined in the One Health vision by experts (Adisasmito *et al.*, 2022; FAO/WHO/WOAH/UNEP, 2022). In this chapter, we are using the second interpretation. This means starting new projects where needed and improving what is already there, like strengthening, coordinating and putting existing ideas into action. In this spirit, it is important to recognize and support initiatives that pioneers have already started. Bringing these efforts together under the One Health approach will help create fair and inclusive ways of doing things.

By **system** we mean a set of elements connected to each other and to the environment with a defined purpose (Anderson and Johnson, 1997). In this case, an SES involves the union between the social system and ecological system, where multiple cultural, political, social, economic, ecological, technological elements and other systems interact (Holling, 2001).

When analysing how a project is put into practice, it is useful to separate different points along the way. As these repeat over time this concept is called the project or policy life cycle. The cycle is quite generic and consistent across many fields of application, but different authors look at the cycle in varying detail and with different numbers of phases. The simplest concept has three phases: (i) conceptualization; (ii) implementation; and (iii) evaluation (Hitziger *et al.*, 2018). To understand better how we move from concept to practice to **evaluation**, however, we will be discussing 14 steps here in what we call the One Health implementation cycle.

Challenges in SES are usually quite messy and intertwined. Studying individuals and organizations involved in a **wicked problem** (or mess) is critical to understand and influence it. This analysis is often guided by two contrasting theories: shareholder theory, focused solely on investors' goals, and **STAKEHOLDER** theory, which acknowledges that value can be expanded to much more than just money (details on **value** are discussed in Chapter 13 on One Health economics). Shareholder theory targets maximizing return on investment (for the shareholders), while stakeholder theory aims to maximize value for stakeholders, emphasizing their diverse qualities (Hester and Adams, 2017, p. 131). Public health, and One Health even more so, is a common good. We therefore use stakeholder theory to guide interventions. According to Hester and Adams:

> Stakeholders exist at the centre of any complex problem-solving effort and holistic consideration of them is a key element of analysing a problem systematically. Stakeholders are the customers, users, clients, suppliers, employees, regulators, and team members of a system. They fund a system, design it, build it, operate it, maintain it, and dispose of it. Each stakeholder contributes their own value-added perspective, as described by the systems principle known as complementarity.
> (Hester and Adams, 2017, p. 132)

A second argument for research- or evidence-based endeavours to engage with stakeholders is their knowledge on local conditions and particularities. This knowledge is held by people that are familiar with the place. This so-called tacit, informal or traditional knowledge is mostly conveyed orally or acquired through observation – and is highly specific to a particular place or situation. To be effective, One Health initiatives must involve the stakeholders in possession of this knowledge during their framing and design phase. The techniques to facilitate this **knowledge integration** are described in detail in Chapter 4 on knowledge integration. This in turn assures that the initiatives are meaningful to the stakeholders and hence facilitates ownership of the challenges and stewardship for their management.

Much of what stakeholders are willing to contribute to a project or programme will depend on the trust they have in it. Hence, trust is paramount for an effective implementation of the

One Health approach. We must acknowledge that the degree of participation and inclusion varies significantly in different contexts. Also, the relationship between governance agents and activities on the ground is very different in different settings. In some instances, citizen engagement may even be absent. However, among participants in a One Health initiative, i.e. those who implement the project or programme, trust in the network of participants will determine how resilient and effective it is. Also, stakes are very different and may give rise to misunderstanding and distrust, simply from the difference in perspective. Bringing together, i.e. coordinating and collaborating, will require overcoming these barriers as a very fundamental practice of One Health. Moreover, political, organizational, economic, ethnic, linguistic, religious and other (mostly human-made) boundaries are generally not respected by wicked problems and will inevitably interfere with a One Health approach. The first effort will thus entail building a trustable ground in which an operation can thrive. This should contain a plan on how to address potential conflicts in the future, even if these seem far off when the endeavour starts.

The transdisciplinary partnership underpinning the **Ecohealth** and **One Health approach** is based on the right of all individuals and social groups to access health; the fundamental need for community development and environmental **sustainability**; the need for an open-minded approach to understand how others see reality; and the importance of social and **gender** considerations to the creation of equal-opportunity societies (Charron, 2012b) (see also Chapter 3 on **transdisciplinarity**). Thus, inclusive stakeholder engagement is one of the best practices for stakeholder management. It requires a deep understanding of how an initiative or project can gain from the inclusion of social groups (attributed to gender, age, ethnicity, employment status and education level, among others), especially those in vulnerable situations. Likewise, mutual learning among participants is a key concept, referring to the process of 'exchange, generation, and integration of existing or newly developing knowledge in different parts of science and society' (Scholz, 2010). A critical component and a goal of transdisciplinary work is to allow for lay persons and experts, researchers and citizens to have equal opportunities to learn from others and to share their knowledge. The practice of equity in a transdisciplinary process is often challenged by power asymmetries between the participating **actors** (Berger-Gonzalez *et al.*, 2022).

Engaging with stakeholders and gaining trust implies that we first recognize ourselves as stakeholders and identify who the others are and understand our and their needs, interests, influence, expectations and concerns in relation to the project or programme. We then should think of a process to involve them in the project or programme and to move forward together. This includes how to communicate, but also sharing input and feedback on how the project or programme is perceived, structure inclusive decision-making processes, and exchange on the progress, changes and challenges. The aim is to create a multi-way communication and interaction to foster trust and collaboration. Acknowledging and respecting the diversity of perspectives is important to make sure all voices are heard and valued. Finally, stakeholder engagement requires continuous monitoring and evaluation of the engagement strategy itself as well as the project or programme to be able to respond and adapt when needed. Inclusive stakeholder engagement will be an important aspect throughout the One Health implementation cycle. There should be a documented process to collect feedback, to present it to technical teams for consideration, to evaluate proposed changes and to feed this back to stakeholders.

There are multiple ways to systematically engage with stakeholders. The aspects of transdisciplinary collaboration, **knowledge** sharing and integration, **data** and **wisdom** as well as **reflexivity** are discussed in more detail in Chapters 2 to 6. All of this contributes to implementation, but it is up to the One Health practitioner or community to choose tools and approaches that are best fit for purpose and correspond to people's preferences. To start exploring, we suggest three repertories of tools, without claim of being comprehensive:

The **TD toolbox for co-production of knowledge**[1] is provided by the Swiss Academies of Arts and Sciences and has three points of entry, depending either on the phases of the project, on the key issue or on alphabetical order. The project phases are: jointly envisage a transdisciplinary project;

jointly frame goals, problems and research; jointly conduct research; or jointly explore ways to impact on science and society. The key issues can be to identify actors, roles and expectations; embrace differences, tensions and conflicts in a transdisciplinary group; strive for societal relevance; navigate through normative goals; integrate different fields of expertise; or review processes and impacts. The methods are often useful for several key issues and phases.

The **Responsible Research and Innovation (RRI) tools**[2] were developed during the European Union's 7th Framework Programme for research by an international consortium. RRI seeks to bring issues related to research and innovation into the open, to anticipate their consequences, and to involve society in discussing how science and technology can help create the kind of world and society we want for generations to come. The site provides resources tailored to policy makers, researchers, educators, business and industry, or civil society organizations. Alternatively, subjects can be selected such as ethics, gender equality, governance, open access, public engagement or science education. Finally, a search engine allows us to filter among the rich variety of resources.

The site of **Integration and Implementation Sciences (i2S)**[3] at the National Centre for Epidemiology and Population Health is part of the College of Health and Medicine at The Australian National University. The page provides a wealth of resources to improve research impact on complex real-world problems among which are tools oriented toward three challenges raised by such problems: knowledge synthesis, unknowns, and policy and practice support. They also maintain a blog on the topics of change, communication, context, decision making, diversity, integration, research, implementation, stakeholder engagement, systems, teamwork and unknowns.

Task: Exploring stakeholder engagement tools

Explore the TD and RRI websites and reflect on the following questions:

1. Who is the audience – who do they address?
2. What are the presented tools used for?
3. Which tools can be used for the different steps in Fig. 10.1?
4. Optional task: From any of the presented tools and methods, choose one and think about how these could work in your context or for your challenge. Do you foresee any difficulties? If yes, what and why?

Further resources that you might find useful: Useful tools on related approaches have been shared by various projects and institutions, e.g. the Companion Modelling collective[4] (ComMod), the STEPS Centre[5] (Social, Technological and Environmental Pathways to Sustainability) at the University of Sussex, and also the Multi-Stakeholder Partnership Guide[6] provided by the University of Wageningen. Further, the United Nations have published a guide for their country teams to link One Health and the UN Sustainable Development Cooperation Framework.[7] In another community of practice, anticipatory approaches use thoughts about the future to make decisions in the present (Poli, 2015). They use a range of instruments from very predictive quantitative models based on data to very exploratory qualitative models based on imagination and creativity, such as causal-layered analysis (Inayatullah, 2008). These approaches are highly related to Post-Normal Science, which is a new understanding of science for situations 'where facts are uncertain, stakes are high, values are in dispute and decisions are urgent' (Funtowicz and Ravetz, 1993). Similar to the methods above, they allow engaging peer communities to define desired objectives, behaviour and attitudes regarding health management within an integrated transdisciplinary approach.

10.2 Steps Along the One Health Implementation Cycle

Figure 10.1 provides an overview of the One Health implementation cycle from the **problem statement** to stakeholder engagement, defining the **theory of change**, implementation and evaluation, which then leads to improvements and closes the circle. In this chapter, we are covering the first seven steps of the cycle, zooming in particularly on stakeholder analysis and engagement. 'Doing One Health' is the focus of Chapter 11, evaluation is covered in Chapter 12 and economic evaluation in Chapter 13.

10.2.1 Problem statement

To orient our activity, we need to state why we are conducting a One Health initiative. We should also reflect on how we can describe the state of affairs with quantitative and qualitative means (both are valid, useful and complementary descriptions). We can retrieve such information from literature, experts and/or local stakeholders. It is important to be aware that problems are perceived very differently by different people who are concerned, e.g. rabies is a different challenge for a dog owner, the mother

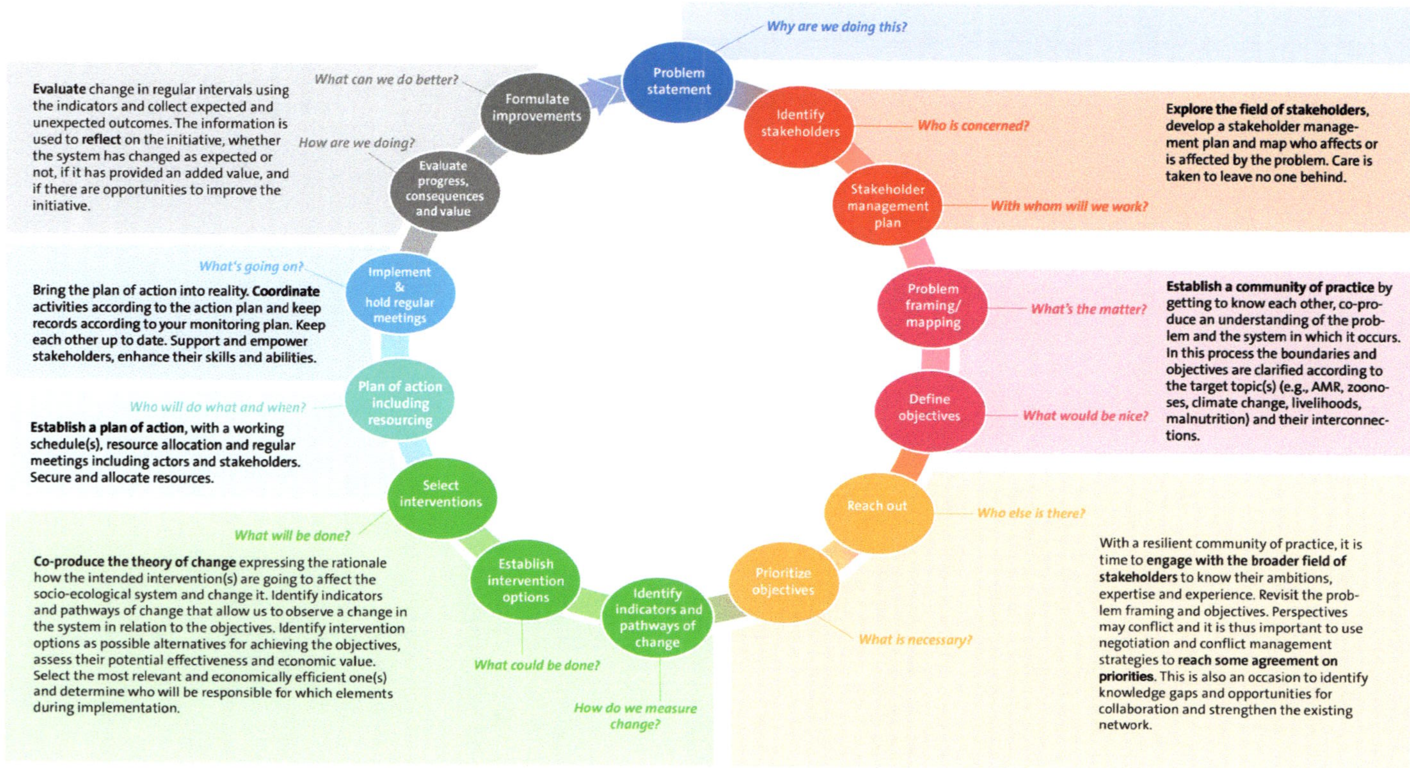

Fig. 10.1. Important stages along the One Health implementation cycle. For sustainability, the cycle repeats regularly. At every point throughout the cycle, attention is needed for inclusive stakeholder engagement.

of a child or a physician. Therefore, the problem statement will have a strong influence if stakeholders feel concerned or not and if they will engage and contribute to the solution. One Health approaches seek to attain equity and leave no one behind, because weak stakeholder engagement decreases the likelihood of an initiative being endorsed by society as a whole (the so-called 'social licence' to proceed) and increases the social risks, leading to delays and cost overruns. We have to understand which stakeholders – people, groups or communities – are at risk of being excluded and what are the specific opportunities and barriers to their inclusion. This begins with the way the problem is stated. We highly recommend reflecting on the stakeholders who may be traditionally marginalized or underrepresented and ensure that the problem statement captures their perspective. Also, the communication must be clear and accessible to all stakeholders, regardless of language and ability. The problem statement explains what the problem is in a way that covers as many perspectives as possible. A first scope of the problem can be established by a project team using methods such as brainstorming or rich picturing (for more details about systems diagrams, see Williams, 2021). Williams distinguishes different approaches depending on the level of knowledge we have about the system; concept mapping requires substantial quantitative knowledge, while rich picturing can be purely qualitative. An overview of concept mapping is provided in Chapter 11.

The sections of the chapter will be accompanied by three examples reflecting different contexts and problems.

Example 1: Vector-borne diseases in the Maasai steppe in Tanzania

The first is a presentation of a case study from Tanzania (Gwakisa *et al.*, 2023).

Problem statement: The effects of zoonotic and vector-borne diseases in the Maasai steppe are likely to increase due to socio-ecological factors, including **climate** variability / change, increased human and livestock populations, agricultural encroachment, competition for land and pastures between humans, livestock and wildlife and water scarcity, which all exacerbate the potential for increased disease burden at the human–animal interface.

Example 2: One Health Networks in Latin America

The second example will present the different steps of the life cycle from an effort to endorse the One Health community in Latin America.

In 2010, the concept of One Health was not well known throughout Latin America. Despite many people working with integrated approaches, few teams knew about each other.

Problem statement (2010): There is a lack of information about One Health in Spanish and Portuguese throughout Latin America. In addition, teams are working in isolation and without communication.

Example 3: Thailand's response to highly pathogenic avian influenza (HPAI)

In the third example, we will discuss how Thailand managed the HPAI outbreak back in 2004.

In 2004, highly pathogenic avian influenza (HPAI) virus of the H5N1 subtype was first confirmed in poultry and humans in Thailand. The public started to lose confidence in poultry products and decreased consumption and import bans started damaging the industry (Tiensin *et al.*, 2005; Retkute *et al.*, 2018).

Problem statement: The lack of information and communication in regard to HPAI has caused panic and questions the credibility of the national authorities.

Learning questions: reflecting inclusiveness of problem statements

Reflect on the problem statement of one of the examples or from your own context or challenge.

The perspective(s) of which stakeholder group(s) is/are represented in the problem statement?

Are there stakeholders at risk of being excluded from the project that have a legitimate interest? If so, how could the statement be formulated to be more inclusive?

Example answer: The problem statement in Example 2 represents the perspective of Latin American researchers who are advocates of One Health. From a strong transdisciplinary stance, citizens are legitimate stakeholders in this process and are excluded. Also, there may be interest groups in other languages that have a legitimate stake in such an approach. However, we must bear in mind that the problem statement implies boundaries and that it may have been a conscious choice to focus on the Spanish- and Portuguese-speaking research community to keep the initiative within reasonable boundaries.

A more inclusive and transdisciplinary statement may be: 'One Health is not well known and rarely applied throughout Central, South America and the Caribbean. There is a need for a regional community of practice around health of people, animals and **ecosystems** and integrated approaches that include researchers and experts from different fields as well as civil society.'

10.2.2 Identify stakeholders and stakeholder management: explore the field and develop a management plan

The next step will be to identify stakeholders, develop a stakeholder management plan and map who is working on integrated approaches to health and topics related to the problem statement in the region / place. We advocate a territorial approach (based on 'place') because this implicitly defines many boundaries from climate to social organizations. Stakeholders exist at the centre of any complex problem-solving effort and a key element of addressing a problem systematically is a comprehensive consideration of them. For the stakeholder management plan, we refer to the recommendations by Hester and Adams (2017) for systemic decision making, because they integrate many aspects of stakeholders that are considered more in isolation with other methods. In Chapter 3 you learn more about empowering stakeholders in transdisciplinary approaches. Of course, these approaches can be combined, modified or complemented by further methods such as social network analysis, power-interest grid, impact-interest grid, engagement scorecards, etc. Our suggested process consists of (i) stakeholder identification; (ii) classification; (iii) attitude evaluation; and (iv) determining the engagement sequence.

During the problem statement you have already thought about who you address and who might be excluded. For a more comprehensive **stakeholder identification**, stakeholders should be listed more systematically. A convenient way to do this is a snowball approach, i.e. ask stakeholders to identify further stakeholders. To maintain a focus on practical aspects of the project, we are guided by the question 'who can affect or is affected by the problem and / or problem solution?' In this process it might be helpful to articulate what stakeholders want from the intervention in the form of a simple sentence. Note that what stakeholders want and what they need may not be the same.

For a problem to be resolved, not everyone gets what they want but the solution hopefully covers everyone's needs, a principle called **SATISFICING**. Thus, the output of the stakeholder identification will be a list of individuals and groups of people with their stake in the problem or its solution, e.g. affected communities, government officials, researchers. It is important at this stage not to restrict the number of stakeholders or to try to limit the list to 'the most important' as this precludes the next steps of our stakeholder analysis.

Stakeholder list for emerging diseases: The implementation of a One Health approach to prevent, detect and respond to emerging infectious diseases requires the engagement of different stakeholders. A starting list at any location would contain the following:

Primary (imminently concerned) stakeholders include citizens of the communities including those practising transhumance, district environment institutions, district department, academic/research institutions, animal health department and human health department.

Secondary (influential) stakeholders include Ministry of Health, Ministry of Environment, Ministry of Education, Ministry of Finance, Ministry of Tourism and national donors and investors.

Tertiary stakeholders may include international organizations, foundations and donors and investors, and neighbouring and other countries.

Conventional stakeholder mapping and engagement will tend to identify those stakeholders with the most influence on the implementation of a project, or those who are most impacted by it. This approach may, however, overlook persons, groups, communities or organizations who are at risk of being under-served or excluded during the development and implementation of the project (G20 Global Infrastructure Hub, 2024). Inclusive stakeholder engagement requires that the project team repeatedly questions the problem statement and verifies which stakeholders are being included; this can be guided by the questions in Table 10.1.

Table 10.1. Ten questions to ask repeatedly throughout the One Health implementation cycle.

Question	Expected reflection
Who are the stakeholders?	Identify diverse groups and individuals, including those from marginalized communities, to ensure a comprehensive representation.
How can we ensure diverse participation?	Explore strategies to actively involve a broad range of voices, considering factors such as gender, ethnicity, socio-economic status, and more.
What barriers might exist?	Identify and address potential obstacles that could hinder the participation of certain groups, ensuring an inclusive process.
Are there specific needs or preferences of stakeholders?	Understand the unique needs and preferences of different stakeholders, especially those related to gender and social considerations.
How can we promote equal decision-making power?	Ensure that decision-making processes are designed to prevent power imbalances and promote equitable contributions from all stakeholders.
What outreach and communication methods are inclusive?	Tailor communication strategies to connect to diverse audiences, considering language, accessibility and cultural relevance.
Are there opportunities for capacity building in different stakeholder groups?	Provide resources and support to empower stakeholders, particularly those who may face systemic barriers to actively participating in the engagement process.
How can feedback mechanisms be inclusive?	Establish feedback channels that accommodate various communication styles and preferences, encouraging open and inclusive dialogue.
Have we conducted impact assessments that consider multiple stakeholders?	Evaluate potential social and gender impacts at different stages of the engagement process and adjust strategies accordingly.
What accountability measures are in place?	Implement mechanisms to hold the engagement process accountable for promoting social and gender equity, ensuring transparency and fairness.

To **classify stakeholders** Hester and Adams (2017) propose to consider three attributes for each stakeholder: power, legitimacy and urgency. The terms are defined as follows:

- Power = A relationship among social actors in which one actor A can get another actor B to do something that B would not usually do.
- Legitimacy = a generalized perception that the actions of an actor are desirable, proper or appropriate.
- Urgency = the degree to which stakeholder claims call for immediate attention.

Each attribute is scored between 0 (none) and 1 (high level). The average of the three scores represents a relative level of importance of the stakeholder to a given problem and is called prominence.

$$Prominence = \frac{Power + Legitimacy + Urgency}{3}$$

We suggest basing the scores on the data collected during the stakeholder identification, but also to review these scores with a panel of diverse stakeholders to ensure a classification that captures multiple perspectives and corresponds to an inclusive stakeholder engagement. Particular attention should be given to power relations among all stakeholders. Understanding power relations is a prerequisite directly affecting the outcomes of a mutual learning process (Mobjörk, 2010) and the direct outcomes in human, animal and ecosystem health.

The way a **stakeholder's attitude** towards the initiative is interpreted also depends on their perspective. To avoid strong bias and misconception, it is advisable to compare this evaluation with the problem statement, and have it reviewed by an inclusive panel. Essentially, we estimate the potential of stakeholders to cooperate with the project or to threaten it. The stakeholder's potential to threaten the project can be either high (score = 1) or low (score = 0), and the same accounts for the potential of this stakeholder to cooperate. We then summarize:

$$Support\ Score = (Potential\ for\ cooperation) - (Potential\ of\ threat)$$

We now combine the Support Score with the Prominence in a table and determine how to manage them:

Support Score \ Prominence	0	1
+1	Collaborate	Involve
0	No action	Monitor
−1	Monitor	Defend

The overall goal is to ensure all active stakeholders are supportive and to successively increase the number of supportive stakeholders, by engaging an ever-increasing diversity. However, since One Health touches on wicked problems, where all stakeholders can rarely reach their ideal outcomes, contradictions and antagonisms will inevitably emerge. The aim is not to avoid these conflicts of goals, but to moderate, negotiate and pacify them. For this conversation, we need to distinguish what stakeholders want and what they need to identify the negotiable space that does not threaten the existential needs of any party. Within this space, **trade-offs** are possible. Still not everyone may agree and it may require quite some effort to lead these negotiations towards a constructive end. We are covering conflict management in more detail in the section on prioritizing objectives, where this issue is the central challenge. Of foremost relevance is development of a trusting collaboration between different stakeholders who (may or may not) share a common interest in the project issues. This is achieved by creating a culture of open dialogue, promoting inclusion of all relevant perspectives (Berger-Gonzalez *et al.*, 2022).

10.2.2.1 Considerations about inclusion and inclusiveness

The One Health principles equity, sociopolitical and multicultural parity and inclusion and engagement of communities and marginalized voices align with inclusive stakeholder engagement (Adisasmito *et al.*, 2022). A systematic approach to ensure inclusiveness is to analyse the **social determinants of health** (SDH) of stakeholders that may cancel or amplify One Health interventions. SDH are underlying, contributing factors of health inequities, i.e. systematic, unfair and avoidable differences in the health status of different population groups (WHO, 2024). They include housing, income, employment, food insecurity, social inclusion (gender, disability, ethnic affiliation) and access to services, among others. They also determine the relationships of people with ecosystems of which they are part, or to which they relate more distantly, their exposure to different health risks and their wellbeing goals (Charron, 2012a), as well as the health and wellbeing of the animals in their care. These differences are generated by policies, social norms and structures that exist at all levels in society. In Chapter 9 you find specific examples of how social categories such as ethnic affiliation and gender can act as gradients that worsen health conditions not only for human populations but also for animal populations and even for the entire ecosystem surrounding those populations.

Inclusive stakeholder engagement ensures that all voices are heard and that decisions are made with the broadest understanding of the impact that they may have. In this regard, some challenging but important concepts should guide our work:

- Treat all people with dignity and respect.
- Give all genders equal opportunities to be heard and engage.
- Show respect for diverse points of view.
- Examine own biases and behaviours.
- Work effectively with people from all backgrounds.
- Do not discriminate against any individual or group.

10.2.2.2 Determine the stakeholder engagement sequence

To determine the sequence in which stakeholders are engaged, the above table allows engagement to be initiated with the most prominent and supportive stakeholders first, building a growing group of supporters of the project step by step. However, in more complex situations, it may be useful to identify the different objectives of stakeholders in relation to the project including identifying to what degree these objectives synergize or are antagonistic. This is an opportunity to revisit the problem statement, perhaps modifying it to attract benevolence from further stakeholders, facilitating their commitment. Generally, engagement works along trusted relationships. These should be used to grow the community and may require involving third parties where direct communication is guarded. With a social network analysis of power relationships or communication links, the driving stakeholders (high out degree) or most important brokers (high betweenness) can then be determined (Hester and Adams, 2017). Drivers are stakeholders who exert power on the SES and can significantly affect the behaviour of others.

If these drivers are not threatening the project, it can be useful to negotiate with them how to modulate (raise or reduce) the use of this influence with the aim of augmenting participation. Alternatively, brokers are highly connected stakeholders in the middle of the SES. Due to this position, they are interesting partners to reach out to new stakeholders, taking a mediation role with stakeholders who are reluctant to engage.

Relationships among stakeholders will change as a project evolves. It is thus important to regularly revisit the stakeholder management plan and adapt it as events unfold.

Example 1: Vector-borne diseases in the Maasai steppe in Tanzania

Maasai communities in the area of Emboret village are the main stakeholders with donors such as WHO, the UN Special Programme for Research and Training in Tropical Diseases (TDR), and the Canadian International Development Research Centre (IDRC) having invested in the region in the past. Actors from diverse **disciplines** were involved from the project inception phase to ensure multi-sectoral representation relevant to the project research problem.

Example 2: One Health Networks in Latin America

The stakeholders were primarily researchers, citizens, groups and institutions at the science–policy interface who were using integrated approaches to health already or had a keen interest in using them in the future.

Throughout South America, and the world, such approaches were applied and implemented prior to the emergence of the term 'One Health', succeeding the various definitions and declarations (see Chapters 1 and 2 for a more detailed account). The aim of this example was to bring everyone together in the Spanish- and Portuguese-speaking realm.

Example 3: Thailand's response to highly pathogenic avian influenza (HPAI)

Initial stakeholders were poultry farmers who were at risk of losing income due to production losses. Their flocks were also at risk of infection, which could lead to death.

Later on, the public poultry product consumers became stakeholders as well as the government authorities responsible for managing the outbreak. International exports were affected, incorporating additional poultry export countries as stakeholders (Tiensin *et al.*, 2005; Retkute *et al.*, 2018).

Task: Reflect on stakeholder engagement.

Read the article about Introducing One Health for brucellosis control in Kazakhstan (Charypkhan and Rüegg, 2022).[8]

1. Identify the stakeholders of brucellosis in Kazakhstan based on the map in Fig. 2 of the paper, which shows the SES as it was perceived by the workshop participants.
2. Compare this with the stakeholders who actually participated in the workshop.
3. Think of possible reasons for this difference.
4. What possible actions could be used to engage a broader diversity of stakeholders?

Example answers:

1. and 2. The map covers animal owners, physicians, veterinarians, slaughterhouse managers, diagnostic laboratories, hospitals, public health and veterinary officials, media, consumers and the wider public. However, at the workshop, 'twenty-one specialists representing veterinary and public health sector, together with researchers, took part'; these are only the governmental and academic stakeholders.

3. No spokespeople for different communities, did not think of them, no inclusiveness policy, no funding to pay for travel and accommodation expenses, misconception of what a stakeholder is …

4. Revisit problem statement, invite other stakeholders. Hold separate workshops to generate a sense of community and successively bring the communities together (it is always easier to voice your opinion when you do not feel alone). Build on the existing map and show the relevance of further stakeholders to better understand the systemic challenges and ways to address them. Sensitize participants for power differentials and explain how they affect the efficacy of mitigation strategies.

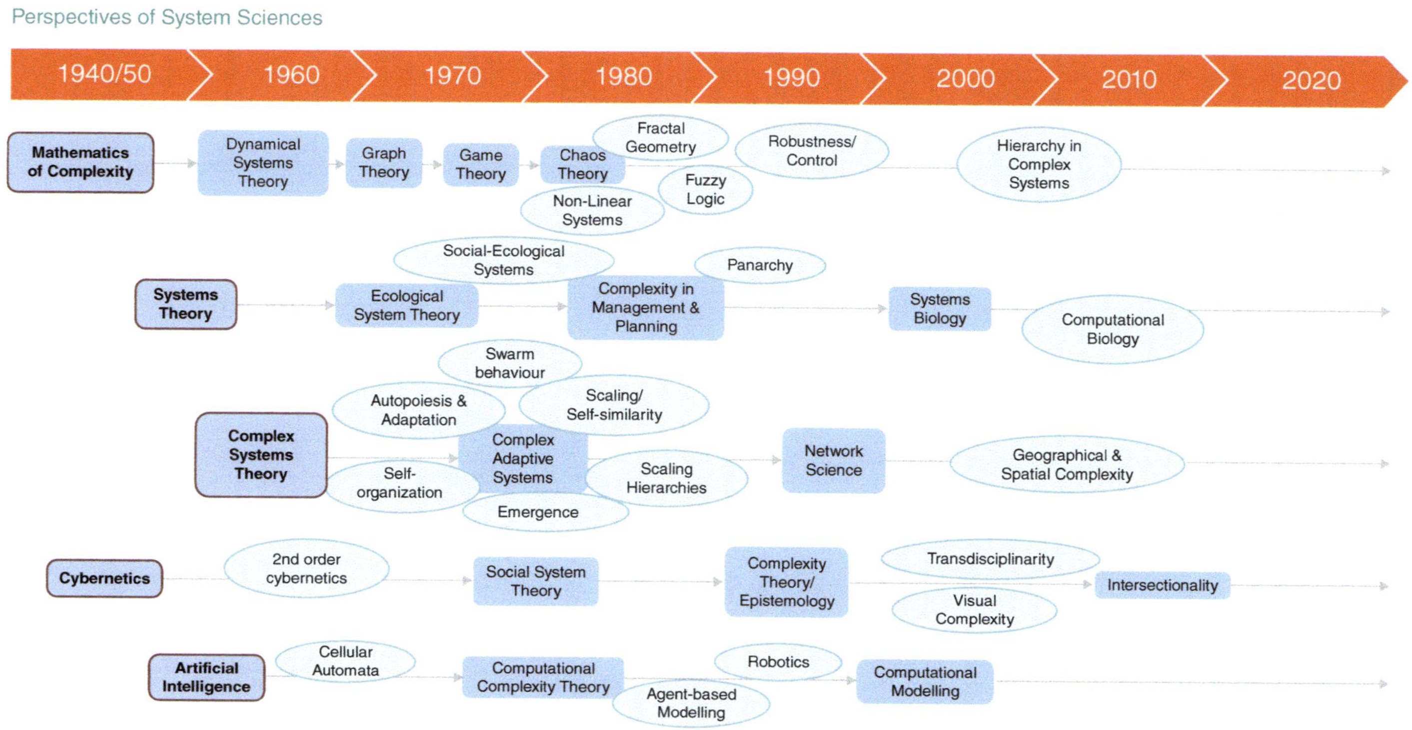

Fig. 10.2. Overview of the evolution of system thinking and complexity since the 1940s. Blue boxes are theories and frameworks, blue circles are methods and fields of application. The evolution is much more intertwined than the linear trajectory may suggest. Figure adapted from Castellani and Gerrits (2021) (https://sacswebsite.blogspot.com/2021/09/q-for-2021-version-of-map-of-complexity.html) (CC BY-SA 4.0 DEED).

10.2.3 Establish a community of practice: problem framing and set objectives

Once it is clear who the stakeholders are, the next step is to engage with them. It may be that in the targeted communities and stakeholders, the concept of One Health is unknown. In these cases, it may be useful to explain the basics with appropriate communication, i.e. digital means, print or mass media, or other ways to reach all stakeholders, whilst paying particular attention to barriers such as digitalization, literacy and access to services. It should also be considered, however, that in the process of co-producing the project with stakeholders, many questions about the significance and meaning of the approach, within the context, will be clarified. Most emphasis should be put on reaching out equally to all stakeholders, including them in the co-production with equitable influence. In many specific cases, the required knowledge and skills to deal with the challenge will then be determined by the challenge itself. However, there is ongoing debate about what One Health literacy would comprise. The concept of 'literacy' in this sense entails the required knowledge, skills and attitudes to take informed decisions about health of people, animals and ecosystems. Due to the breadth of One Health, the distinction to basic education and the more specific health or ecological literacy is fluent. Health literacy and ecological literacy have been studied extensively and for the latter it became apparent that the transdisciplinary process facilitates the development and transmission of the appropriate information and detail (Scholz, 2010).

There are a variety of methods to co-produce knowledge and action with stakeholders, and the field is so vast that we cannot possibly be comprehensive here. Fields of application to explore are identified through keywords such as transdisciplinarity (Chapter 3), knowledge integration (Chapter 4), implementation research, responsible research and innovation (RRI), **citizen science**, systemic leadership, and others. In the Introduction section, we presented some toolboxes that we have found inspiring to explore. It is also advisable to get some support from people with previous experience and/or to test the methods with some colleagues before actually using them. Usually this entails one or more (**physical**) **meetings with the stakeholders** prioritized in the management plan. Some reflection should be done regarding what the initiating/organizing team would like to achieve and how open it is to be guided by co-production. Radical co-production would mean that the objectives of a project will emerge as the stakeholders interact, but in some cases a more prescriptive approach may pre-define or confine the activities and objectives, e.g. because the funder(s) or mandator(s) set conditions. These are the first boundaries that may not be negotiable with the stakeholders, and they should be clearly stated to avoid raising expectations that cannot be met. A second concern may be prevailing conflicts among stakeholders. For pragmatic reasons, it may be wise not to include potentially conflicting parties straight away. The first meetings with stakeholders are sensitive, and it is worth convincing the group to establish a resilient, inclusive community of practice. Later, such a community can deal with tension and conflict much better. It is important to first set the tone and culture of interaction. Then, the methods you use to facilitate the meetings should be culturally appropriate, for example you may not want to use a game in a context in which hierarchies determine how participants interact or hold mixed workshops in a culture where women and men do not interact in public. The reflection on the appropriateness of the meeting facilitation method must be undertaken with persons that are culturally embedded; best practice would be that those also facilitate the meetings (methods for reflection are explained in Chapter 6 on professional reflexivity and **reflective practice**). Note that in a transdisciplinary process everyone evolves, i.e. the facilitators will also gain insights and develop their skills. We do not aim to deliver the perfect product, but to establish an environment that allows everyone to learn. The first meeting aims at:

1. Establishing a trustworthy, inclusive and resilient community of practice.
2. Clarifying the non-negotiable boundaries (financial, political, ecological …).
3. Co-producing the problem statement (again), i.e. identifying the boundaries and objectives set by the stakeholders.
4. Identifying and describing the socio-ecological system in which the project/programme will co-evolve.

Example 1: Vector-borne diseases in the Maasai steppe in Tanzania

The project team conducted a participatory multidisciplinary community-based study targeting sustainable solutions for vector control integration into daily practices.

Example 2: One Health Networks in Latin America

Since the approach is important for essentially anyone, a social media campaign was launched by the project team in Spanish and Portuguese to raise awareness about One Health. Mainly WhatsApp and Facebook[9] were used to share information about the concept of One Health to people who wanted to know about the approach. In parallel, several initiatives promoted networking and exchange among different communities and teams concerned with One Health.

Eventually, the initiating team identified independent researchers from different countries who were concerned about the lack of One Health information in Spanish and Portuguese. With the support of the One Health Commission and the School of Medicine, University of Washington, USA, a 'Who's Who in Latin America webinar'[10] with researchers from Latin America was held in June 2019. This meeting helped exchange on capacities and interests among the participating researchers.

In November the same year, One Health Latin American and Caribbean (OHLAIC) network coleaders met in Monteria, Colombia. Participants came from countries including Colombia, Chile, Brazil, Cuba, Uruguay and Costa Rica with the intention to give the existing informal network of networks a more formal character for the community of practice in Spanish and Portuguese. The OHLAIC group published a manifesto and a memorandum of understanding: https://ciachi.org/es/colaboradores-ohlaic/.

Example 3: Thailand's response to highly pathogenic avian influenza (HPAI)

Public awareness was raised by campaigning about HPAI and that consuming well-cooked poultry products was safe. A 'Big Cleaning Week' was initiated to encourage poultry-related facilities to disinfect their settings, which include but are not limited to poultry houses, farm equipment and vehicles, slaughterhouses and retail markets (Tiensin *et al.*, 2005; Retkute *et al.*, 2018).

10.2.4 System representation and defining objectives

We recommend developing some kind of **system representation** in the form of a map, description or both, as well as a revised textual problem statement as outlined in the step above. Setting the scope of an initiative, i.e. framing the problem, will require knowledge about the SES in which it should be implemented and also technical and scientific knowledge about the challenge or topic itself (Hitziger *et al.*, 2018). First, let us have a look at what we mean by a system.

A **SYSTEM** is an **interacting or interdependent group of items forming a unified whole**. An ecosystem is a good example, describing a biological community of interacting organisms and their physical environment. Ecologists often categorize ecosystems by the type of environment in which they exist: freshwater, oceanic, terrestrial and anthropogenic (artificial – made by humans). A healthcare system is another good example, where a network of people, institutions and resources interact to collectively provide healthcare. A system is NOT just a random collection of things put together without any purpose or coordinated action. For example, a rock collection is interesting and beautiful, but has no collective purpose, function or output.

Regarding the complexity of systems, we can assume that there is a continuum of system 'messiness', from simple to complicated, complex and chaotic:

- A **simple system** is one with a single path to a single output; causalities are clear. It is easy to describe and understand, and is predictable. Consequently, interventions are obvious.
- A **complicated system** is one that has multiple paths leading to an outcome. Complicated systems can be understood. For example, an airplane is a complicated system. It will take much effort to represent and analyse a complicated system, but it

can be done. To govern or steer a complicated system you need to have a good understanding of the influential factors and their positive or negative impacts on the system. This will help you to decide which intervention is the most appropriate to change the system in the right direction.

- A **complex system** has multiple pathways leading to multiple different outcomes. There are no clear causalities. Such a system cannot be grasped in its totality and shows emerging, unpredictable properties. It can be represented in parts, but not comprehensively. Often such systems are adaptive, which means they change based on your interaction with it. In such systems, interventions can have several effects of which many are appropriate, but some may also be unexpected or unwanted. To govern or steer such systems one relies on continuous feedback and adaptability.
- A **chaotic system** has no obvious structure or patterns. Its behaviour lies somewhere between extremely complex patterns and randomness. Therefore, it is also very difficult to describe or analyse it. It is not knowable.

How 'knowable' a system is helps you to understand the predictability of the system and helps to set expectations, plan goals and predict challenges. We can distinguish four types of systems with characteristics that determine 'what we can do': (i) clear is known and familiar; (ii) complicated is knowable and unfamiliar; (iii) complex is unknown; and (iv) chaos is unknowable. These are characteristics that determine 'what we can do'. In chaos, there is nothing to do, while complicated situations require reflection and investigation. In complex questions you first need to think on how to know before investigating. This is why complex problems are addressed differently (co-production) compared to complicated problems (expert teams).

The roots of the OHHLEP definition lie in Ecohealth and the integrated approach to SES, which both assume to operate with complex systems. They consider all the mentioned properties in this paragraph and recognize that any system definition contains an arbitrary boundary, e.g. biological systems are defined by artificial boundaries set by biologists because they are not interested in the social relevance (Holling, 2001). It is important that the boundaries are set, primarily by the stakeholders, and only wherever imperative (e.g. from the funder) by the project team. A nice introduction to methods to represent systems can be found in Anderson and Johnson (1997).

Thus, the next step is to identify the systems involved, and how these interact to understand fully the environment within which to implement your initiative, including the temporal and spatial scale of the problem.

The boundary of a system is a conceptual line that divides the system in which the One Health problem sits from everything else. The environment in which a system sits is anything that can affect the system or be affected by it. For example, when investigating pollution within a freshwater system, the system could be the watershed, but this sits within other systems. Local agricultural production systems could be a source of agrochemical pollution, the watershed sits within a regionally managed water supply, the local town could be influencing the health of the freshwater system as a result of pollution but also riverine management practices in a river (part of the watershed) that goes through the town. There is also a fishery upstream of the town that uses the freshwater supplies.

Therefore, to define your system boundaries you need to:

1. Describe the characteristics of your system.
2. Describe the characteristics of the environment in which the system fits.
3. Describe the influential factors in this environment that impact your system (you can think about a focus question to help with this. This helps to maintain the 'direction' of your later systems thinking).
4. Describe whether the influential factors have positive or negative impacts on your system.
5. Decide which influential factors have the greatest impact, and rank them accordingly so that the interventions developed are most appropriate to the context of the problem.
6. Seek to understand the immediate, underlying and root causes of each positive and negative impact.

Once you understand the boundaries and interactions occurring in your system, you can recognize their interconnectedness so that you can reduce (or compartmentalize) the systems' complexity, conceptualizing and then providing alternative interventions to your One Health problem.

Defining system boundaries and understanding system interactions are important elements of **systems thinking**. Explaining systems thinking in depth would go beyond the scope of this book, but a short overview is provided in Box 10.1.

Box 10.1. Systems thinking

Systems thinking is not a very well-defined theory or method. The term is used in association with complexity sciences or chaos theory and entails a multitude of scientific fields of study between social and natural sciences. Figure 10.2 gives a very simplified overview of the various streams of thought that have contributed to systems thinking. The domains of application have expanded throughout the last century (Sturmberg, 2013; Peters, 2014). More recently, it has become a feature of inter- and transdisciplinary work, such as One Health, given that the latter is increasingly proposed as the approach to resolve several of the complex issues of our times, such as **zoonotic disease** emergence, pandemics, antimicrobial resistance, food safety and security, and climate change (Zexian and Xuhui, 2010).

In contrast to conventional linear analytical (mechanistic and reductionist) approaches, where understanding the whole is based on detailed analysis of component parts, systems thinking posits that due to interrelations of individual elements the whole is more than the sum of its parts. These interrelationships are responsible for the unique (emerging) properties of the whole system that are not evident when the system is separated into its component parts (Laing *et al*., 2023). A further key feature of systems thinking is pluralism, where the different perspectives of numerous individuals operating within the system are considered and appreciated equally, which corresponds well with participatory and transdisciplinary approaches advocated within One Health (Meadows, 2009).

Systems thinking focuses on a system, which can be defined as a collection of interconnected elements that are organized in a coherent manner to fulfil a function or purpose (Laing *et al*., 2023). Systems are responsive, self-organizing, resilient and evolving, and their purpose may only be apparent with observation over time (Laing *et al*., 2023). The structure and contents of systems are determined by their boundaries and are related to the system's purpose or the interests of those who set out to analyse it (Mumford *et al*., 2023). Living systems are self-reproducing and typically subsystems of larger systems. To allow better understanding and feasible analysis, we set boundaries (Laing *et al*., 2023). In such systems, the observing humans inevitably interact with the observed system and influence system behaviour.

Systems thinking has been proposed as a synergistic analytical skillset, used to identify and understand systems, predict their behaviour, and devise modifications to produce desired outcomes (Woodhill and Millican, 2023). When practising systems thinking, certain shifts in mindset are needed, namely: (i) from planning (hard and fast steps) to learning (adaptive and responsive); (ii) from setting targets to establishing a direction of travel; and (iii) from centralized and hierarchical responsibility and blame to a shared and collective accountability (Arnold and Wade, 2015; Mumford *et al*., 2023).

Systems thinking involves identifying the system's structure, including at different scales and levels (both temporal and spatial) and contexts (political, economic, environmental, cultural, religious) through a process of incorporating multiple perspectives and worldviews, whilst accounting for power relationships (Stroh, 2015). Furthermore, it aims to identify and understand the system's dynamics, and infer or estimate the impact of change on the system (Sterman, 2000; Woodhill and Millican, 2023).

Describing the system includes system conceptualization and mapping. This is the qualitative process of generating a visual representation of the system that includes the system's elements and interconnections, which is built based on existing evidence, expert elicitation and participatory methods. The process is typically highly iterative. As knowledge and understanding of the system builds, additional and alternative structural elements and stakeholders' perspectives may be included, boundaries may be broadened or narrowed, and the purpose of the system being considered may change (Duboz *et al*., 2018). System conceptualization forms the foundation of quantitative models that can be parameterized with mathematical equations and is used in scenario simulation analysis and to produce quantitative outputs (DEFRA, 2022).

Systems thinking broadens our understanding of the problem, facilitates communication, encourages shifts in mental models, promotes pluralism and transdisciplinarity, identifies trade-offs, and allows for more informed choices.

Task: Reflect on messiness

Think about the One Health problem of antibiotic resistance in livestock production systems and where it sits in the continuum of messiness. Which aspects of the system are simple and predictable? Can you make aspects more predictable? How does the concept of messiness make you feel? How will it make other stakeholders feel and what may that mean for the implementation of a One Health initiative?

Example answer: Antibiotic resistance is a complex issue that involves interactions between humans, animals and the environment. In this system, some aspects may be relatively simple and predictable. For example, the dosage and frequency of antibiotic use in livestock farming practices can be relatively standardized and follow guidelines. Similarly, the microbial pathways through which antibiotic resistance genes spread in the environment may have some predictable patterns based on factors such as soil composition, water flow and microbial ecology. To make aspects more predictable, interventions can be implemented. For instance, implementing strict antibiotic-use protocols in livestock farming, promoting alternative methods for disease prevention and control, improving waste management to reduce environmental antibiotic contamination, and enhancing surveillance systems to monitor antibiotic resistance trends can all contribute to making the system more predictable in terms of antibiotic resistance dynamics. There are, however, many unpredictable aspects that often relate to human behaviour. The concept of 'messiness' in this context can evoke feelings of complexity and uncertainty, which some people may find paralysing or daunting, whereas others might be inspired by the challenge. It underscores the challenges of implementing interventions that must navigate diverse stakeholders, disciplines and systems. For the implementation of a One Health initiative targeting antibiotic resistance, acknowledging and embracing the messiness is crucial. It means recognizing that solutions must go beyond isolated interventions and involve coordinated efforts across multiple stakeholders. Embracing messiness also calls for adaptive strategies that can evolve as new knowledge emerges and as the system responds to interventions. Applying systems thinking allows us to better understand complex problems by intentionally moving from a smaller focus piece to a broader conceptual perspective. This broader perspective includes attention to overall structures, patterns and system cycles or feedback loops (versus specific system-events alone). It involves consideration of the way system components relate to, and feed back into each other, to help solve specific problems. By analysing the relationships between a system's components, the potential for better decision making and problem solving is increased.

With a system representation in place, stakeholders engaged and a reviewed problem statement available, the group can move to identifying new objectives or reviewing, refining or adapting existing ones. This could for example be facilitated through a collaborative brainstorming session where stakeholders can openly discuss their ideas for project objectives with facilitation that encourages creativity, diversity of viewpoints, and the exploration of potential impact areas in the system that has been defined. Methods to be used here could include round-robin brainstorming, mind mapping, nominal group technique, SWOT analysis, role-storming, storyboarding, brainwriting 6-3-5, fishbone diagram, or similar.

Stakeholders should be given the opportunity to express what their objectives are in relation to the initiative, i.e. what it is that they would like to see change. These objectives can be quantitative and measurable, e.g. reducing the prevalence of a disease, quantitative and non-measurable, e.g. raising public trust in governmental institutions, or qualitative, e.g. establishing a newsletter. Best practice would be if these objectives are operational, i.e. they can be addressed directly and have associated indicators that allow us to observe change, so that they are embedded in the system representation and that at a later point we can use them to articulate the theory of change (see Chapter 12 on evaluation).

10.2.5 Engage more stakeholders: reach out and prioritize objectives

With a resilient community of practice and a set atmosphere of benevolence and inclusiveness, now is the point to **reach out** to further stakeholders who may have conflicting interests, existing conflicts or a lack of interest. Let them share their ambitions, expertise and experience, for example in meetings with oral presentations and discussion groups. This is an occasion to identify knowledge gaps and opportunities for collaboration and to strengthen the community of practice. To include the new participants, it is important to listen to them first, then explain the problem framing and system representation as it has been co-produced in the first steps. The project will demonstrate its inclusiveness through its willingness to embrace and include new perspectives in its problem statement and maybe adopt new objectives. Care should be taken not to gain new participants at the expense of losing others. Knowledge integration implies a process of negotiation and conflict management. Tensions about perspectives, interests and values will rise as the community of practice needs to reach some **agreement on priorities**. Objectives could be prioritized based on their relevance, feasibility, impact potential and alignment with the priorities of the previous and new stakeholders. You could use methods such as voting, ranking or consensus building to reach agreement on key objectives that reflect shared goals and values. Consensus building involves engaging stakeholders in a collaborative process to reach agreement or alignment. Facilitated discussions play a key role, providing a structured platform for stakeholders to express their perspectives and concerns openly. Negotiation strategies help navigate differences and find mutually acceptable solutions, fostering compromise and cooperation. Consensus workshops and voting mechanisms enable stakeholders to prioritize options or proposals based on shared goals and values. Techniques like the Delphi method gather input iteratively, guiding stakeholders towards convergence on complex issues. Continuous engagement and transparent communication throughout the process build trust and sustain momentum towards consensus. This also requires addressing questions of resource allocation, power and leadership and is thus a phase where conflict may easily arise, and engagement may easily be lost. It requires subtlety and diplomacy to navigate in this space, but it is important and inevitable that objectives are prioritized to prepare for the articulation of the theory of change and the definition of the intervention as discussed in the next chapters. Because of potentially diverging views and vested interests, many One Health activities have the potential for conflict and it is therefore important to think about how these can be addressed. Mediation and conflict resolution support constructive dialogue and manage disagreements effectively. See Box 10.2 for more information on conflict and its management.

Box 10.2. Conflict and its management

The effective operationalization of One Health requires not only the technical expertise but also conflict prevention and resolution literacy. As we live in a dynamic interconnected system, with differing values, perceptions, goals, communication styles and emotions, language, economic status, political views and culture among others, it is practically impossible to avoid disagreement that might or might not evolve into conflict. In general, conflict involves at least two or more parties, and it can be derived from disagreement or from issues that threaten stakeholders' interests, values, needs or wellbeing including emotional and /or physical (Weixel Dixon, 2017). Even host–pathogen interactions can be thought of as conflicts possibly requiring medical or veterinary intervention (Schwabe *et al.*, 1977). There are several types of conflict, including structural conflicts and conflict affecting values, relationships and interests. Conflicts can be either hot (aggressive attitude or behaviours, loud emotional expressions) or cold (hidden emotions or invisible stress etc.). Any type of unresolved conflict can lead to inefficiency in our efforts to implement interventions for common good (most One Health initiatives).

One Health practitioners have a central role to engage constructively with various stakeholders, dealing with conflicting opinions and/or knowledge to identify the most appropriate potential outcomes using a variety of tools and approaches, regardless of the nature of the conflict (Stroh, 2015; Dreier *et al.*, 2019). There are several tools and techniques that can be used to deal most effectively with the various types of conflicts, providing optimal outcomes for local as well as for global goods (Waltner-Toews, 2017). Many other tools are available on the web, e.g. on the Coursera platform (Gerzon, 2006). Consequently, effective implementation of One Health requires leadership to turn conflict into opportunities (to minimize or transform potential negative outcomes into positive). Eight mediator's tools identified by Gerzon include: integral vision, systems thinking, presence, inquiry, conscious conversation, dialogue, bridging and innovation. Also, Maslow's theory (triangle) provides a very useful checklist to consider people's basic needs to be addressed to facilitate interest-based negotiation for mitigating conflicts (WHO, 2021).

Example 1: Vector-borne diseases in the Maasai steppe in Tanzania

To address the multiplicity of health issues in the human–animal interface ecosystem, Maasai community members and relevant stakeholders were engaged in consultative meetings to identify and prioritize intervention-researchable areas.

Example 2: One Health Networks in Latin America

Initially the group was called OHLA since it was formed by Latin American country leaders, but later changed its name to OHLAIC as country leaders from Spain, Portugal and the Caribbean countries[11] also joined, and the concept was further disseminated.

When the new countries were included, the statutes of OHLAIC were modified so as not to generate historical conflicts. An objective of the network in the first year was to increase the number of countries involved and to support the consolidation of national networks. Through this expansion, more specialists with resources to carry out research projects also joined the network. The OHLAIC facilitated an environment without competition and without financial means, but with a common ambition to bring the concept of One Health to civil society. With this broad engagement, it was possible to apply for international project funding through the Programa Iberoamericano de Ciencia y Tecnología para el Desarrollo (CYTED),[12] and the network also reached out to social and political scientists.

Example 3: Thailand's response to highly pathogenic avian influenza (HPAI)

Government authorities placed a restriction on movement of all poultry species and surveillance testing was initiated throughout the country. Flocks that tested positive were to be stamped out with compensation to the farmers. Traditional free-ranging duck farming, cockfighting and poultry exhibition were banned to halt the epidemic. The public was encouraged to report any sick or dead avian species as well. Lack of cooperation occurred, however, due to fear of income loss, unawareness of the situation and, in certain cases, pure neglect (Tiensin *et al.*, 2005; Retkute *et al.*, 2018).

Learning questions: Dealing with conflict

Read the project description of the Kedo Diren ('Listen to one another') Project in Mali: https://www.ilri.org/research/projects/local-governance-natural-resources-community-stabilization-central-mali-kedo

1. Who are the parties involved in conflict?
2. What are the causes of the conflict?
3. What conflict mitigation strategies are used?
4. What other conflict mitigation strategies could be suitable here?

Example answer:

1. The conflict involves farmers, militia groups, the government of Mali, the NGO's AMEDD and Sahel Eco and others.
2. The conflict originates through competition for dwindling natural resources fueled by terrorist attacks.
3. The project aims to promote stability through participatory and inclusive management of key land and water resources. It also establishes diversified small ruminant and animal feed businesses operated by women and youth as a strategy to improve community resilience.
4. Co-design new business models to assure livelihoods in changing climate conditions. Establish and promote a solar energy value chain. Establish and promote resilience assistance procedures and services to households. Establish emergency relief infrastructure.

10.3 Conclusions

In this chapter, we covered the different phases of a One Health implementation cycle placing significant emphasis on stakeholder analysis and engagement, recognizing their role in shaping the success of One Health initiatives. We also explored the importance of understanding different perspectives within complex systems, emphasizing the need to incorporate diverse viewpoints for effective problem solving. Additionally, we discussed strategies for identifying and prioritizing objectives, crucial for guiding interventions. In the following chapters, we will continue on the cycle and extend to wider communication, intervention and evaluation aspects. Stakeholder engagement is pivotal in facilitating successful implementation and sustainability of One Health interventions and the aspects and principles covered here apply analogously to the following chapters.

Notes

1 https://naturalsciences.ch/co-producing-knowledge-explained

2 https://rri-tools.eu/

3 https://i2s.anu.edu.au/resources/tools/

4 https://www.commod.org/en

5 https://steps-centre.org/

6 https://mspguide.org/msp-tools

7 https://www.who.int/publications/i/item/WHO-OHI-2023.2

8 https://doi.org/10.1371/journal.pone.0277118

9 https://www.facebook.com/groups/ohlaic/

10 https://www.onehealthcommission.org/index.cfm/37526/96819/quien_es_quien_en_una_salud_en_america_latina___whos_who_in_one_health_in_latin_america_ohla_webinar

11 https://caricom.org/

12 https://cyted.org/USCC

References

Adisasmito, W.B., Almuhairi, S., Behravesh, C.B., Bilivogui, P., Bukachi, S.A. *et al.* (2022) One Health: A new definition for a sustainable and healthy future. *PLoS Pathogens* 18(6), e1010537. DOI: 10.1371/journal.ppat.1010537.

Anderson, V. and Johnson, L. (1997) *Systems Thinking Basics: From Concepts to Causal Loops*. Leverage Networks Inc.

Arnold, R.D. and Wade, J.P. (2015) A definition of systems thinking: A systems approach. *Procedia Computer Science* 44, 669–678.

Berger-Gonzalez, M., Scotti, F., Garcia, A.I., Hesketh, A., Hitziger, M., Thompson, I. and Heinrich, M. (2022) Green Health in Guatemala: How can we build mutual trust and partnerships to develop an evidence-base for local medicines and realize their potential? *Botany* 100(2), 109–126. DOI: 10.1139/cjb-2021-0070.

Buttigieg, S.C., Savić, S., Cauchi, D., Lautier, E., Canali, M. and Aragrande, M. (2018) Brucellosis control in Malta and Serbia: A One Health evaluation. *Frontiers in Veterinary Science* 5, 1–15. DOI: 10.3389/fvets.2018.00147.

Castellani, B. and Gerrits, L. (2021) Map of the complexity sciences. Art and Science Factory, LLC. Available at: https://sacswebsite.blogspot.com/2021/09/q-for-2021-version-of-map-of-complexity.html (accessed 2 August 2024).

Charron, D.F. (2012a) *Ecohealth Research in Practice: Innovative Applications of an Ecosystem Approach to Health*. Springer, New York. DOI: 10.1007/978-1-4614-0517-7.

Charron, D.F. (2012b) Ecosystem approaches to health for a global sustainability agenda. *EcoHealth* 9(3), 256–266. DOI: 10.1007/s10393-012-0791-5.

Charypkhan, D. and Rüegg, S.R. (2022) One Health evaluation of brucellosis control in Kazakhstan. *PLoS One* 17(11), e0277118. DOI: 10.1371/journal.pone.0277118.

de Moura, R.R., Chiba de Castro, W.A., Farinhas, J.H., Pettan-Brewer, C., Kmetiuk, L.B. *et al.* (2022) One Health Index (OHI) applied to Curitiba, the ninth-largest metropolitan area of Brazil, with concomitant assessment of animal, environmental, and human health indicators. *One Health* 14, 100373. DOI: 10.1016/j.onehlt.2022.100373.

DEFRA (2022) Integrating a systems approach into Defra. Department for Environment Food and Rural Affairs, London, UK.

Dreier, L., Nabarro, D. and Nelson, J. (2019) *Systems Leadership for Sustainable Development: Strategies for Achieving Systemic Change*. Harvard Kennedy School, Cambridge, Massachusetts.

Duboz, R., Echaubard, P., Promburom, P., Kilvington, M., Ross, H. *et al.* (2018) Systems thinking in practice: Participatory modeling as a foundation for integrated approaches to health. *Frontiers in Veterinary Science* 5, 303.

FAO/WHO/WOAH/UNEP (2022) *One Health Joint Plan of Action, 2022–2026*. FAO; UNEP; WHO; World Organisation for Animal Health (WOAH) (founded as OIE). DOI: 10.4060/cc2289en.

Funtowicz, S.O. and Ravetz, J.R. (1993) Science for the post-normal age. *Futures* 25(7), 739–755.

Gerzon, M. (2006) *Leading Through Conflict: How Successful Leaders Transform Differences into Opportunities*. Harvard Business School Press, Cambridge, Massachusetts.

G20 Global Infrastructure Hub (2024) *Stakeholder Identification, Engagement and Empowerment*. Available at: https://inclusiveinfra.gihub.org/action-areas/stakeholder-identification-engagement-and-empowerment/ (accessed 2 August 2024).

Gwakisa, P., George, J., Sindato, C., Ngonyoka, A., Nnko, H. *et al.* (2023) Pillars for successful operationalization of one health as an ecosystem approach: Experience from a human-animal interface in the Maasai steppe in Tanzania. *One Health Outlook* 5(1), 11. DOI: 10.1186/s42522-023-00087-0.

Hester, P.T. and Adams, K.M.G. (2017) *Systemic Decision Making* (2nd edn). Springer International Publishing, Cham, Switzerland. DOI: 10.1007/978-3-319-54672-8.

Hitziger, M., Esposito, R., Canali, M., Aragrande, M., Häsler, B. and Rüegg, S.R. (2018) Knowledge integration in One Health policy formulation, implementation and evaluation. *Bulletin of the World Health Organization* 96(3), 211–218. DOI: 10.2471/BLT.17.202705.

Holling, C.S. (2001) Understanding the complexity of economic, ecological, and social systems. *Ecosystems* 4(5), 390–405. DOI: 10.1007/s10021-001-0101-5.

Inayatullah, S. (2008) Six pillars: Futures thinking for transforming. *Foresight* 10(1), 4–21. DOI: 10.1108/14636680810855991.

Laing, G., Duffy, E., Anderson, N., Antoine-Moussiaux, N., Aragrande, M. *et al.* (2023) Advancing One Health: Updated core competencies. *CABI One Health* 1–13.

Meadows, D.H. (2009) *Thinking in Systems: A Primer*. Wright, D. (ed.) The Sustainability Institute. Earthscan, London.

Mobjörk, M. (2010) Consulting versus participatory transdisciplinarity: A refined classification of transdisciplinary research. *Futures* 42(8), 866–873. DOI: 10.1016/j.futures.2010.03.003.

Mumford, E.L., Martinez, D.J., Tyance-Hassell, K., Cook, A., Hansen, G.R. *et al.* (2023) Evolution and expansion of the One Health approach to promote sustainable and resilient health and well-being: A call to action. *Frontiers in Public Health* 10, 1056459. DOI: 10.3389/fpubh.2022.1056459.

Peters, D.H. (2014) The application of systems thinking in health: Why use systems thinking? *Health Research Policy and Systems* 12(1), 1–6.

Poli, R. (2015) The implicit future orientation of the capability approach. *Futures* 71, 105–113. DOI: 10.1016/j.futures.2015.03.002.

Retkute, R., Jewell, C.P., Van Boeckel, T.P., Zhang, G., Xiao, X. *et al.* (2018) Dynamics of the 2004 avian influenza H5N1 outbreak in Thailand: The role of duck farming, sequential model fitting and control. *Preventive Veterinary Medicine* 159, 171–181. DOI: 10.1016/j.prevetmed.2018.09.014.

Scholz, R.W. (2010) *Environmental Literacy in Science and Society: From Knowledge to Decisions.* Cambridge University Press, Cambridge, UK.

Schwabe, C.W., Riemann, H.P. and Franti, C.E. (1977) *Epidemiology in Veterinary Practice.* Lea and Febiger, Philadelphia, Pennsylvania.

Sterman, J.D. (2000) *Business Dynamics: Systems Thinking and Modeling for a Complex World.* Irwin/McGraw-Hill, Boston.

Stroh, D.P. (2015) *Systems Thinking for Social Change: A Practical Guide to Solving Complex Problems, Avoiding Unintended Consequences, and Achieving Lasting Results.* Chelsea Green, Hartford, Vermont.

Sturmberg, J. (2013) *The Handbook of Systems and Complexity in Health.* Springer, New York.

Tiensin, T., Chaitaweesub, P., Songserm, T., Chaisingh, A., Hoonsuwan, W. *et al.* (2005) Highly pathogenic avian influenza H5N1, Thailand, 2004. *Emerging Infectious Diseases* 11(11), 1664–1672. DOI: 10.3201/eid1111.050608.

Waltner-Toews, D. (2017) Zoonoses, One Health and complexity: Wicked problems and constructive conflict. *Philosophical Transactions of the Royal Society B: Biological Sciences* 372(1725), 20160171. DOI: 10.1098/rstb.2016.0171.

Weixel Dixon, K. (2017) *Interpersonal Conflict: An Existential Psychotherapeutic and Practical Model.* Routledge, Abingdon, UK. DOI: 10.4324/9781315626437.

WHO (2021) Leadership in Emergencies: Building Competencies for Effective Leadership in All-Hazards Emergency Response. Available at: https://www.who.int/news/item/16-11-2021-leadership-in-emergencies-building-competencies-for-effective-leadership-in-all-hazards-emergency-response (accessed 14 March 2024).

WHO (2024) WHO Social Determinants of Health. Available at: https://www.who.int/health-topics/social-determinants-of-health (accessed 2 August 2024).

Williams, B. (2021) *Systems Diagrams* (1st edn). Available at: https://gum.co/systemdiagrams (accessed 2 August 2024).

Woodhill, J. and Millican, J. (2023) *Systems Thinking and Practice: A Guide to Concepts, Principles and Tools for FCDO and Partners. K4D.* Institute of Development Studies, Brighton, UK.

Zexian, Y. and Xuhui, Y. (2010) A revolution in the field of systems thinking: A review of Checkland's system thinking. *Systems Research and Behavioral Science* 27(2), 140–155.

11 Doing One Health! Using Participatory and Systems-Thinking Steps to Develop and Implement a One Health Intervention

K. Marie McIntyre[1,2], Deborah J. Thomson[2,3], Dominic Travis[4], Elena Boriani[2,5], Ana Glória Fonseca[2,6] and Steve Unwin[7]

[1]Modelling, Evidence and Policy Group, School of Natural and Environmental Sciences, Newcastle University, Newcastle, UK; [2]Network for Ecohealth and One Health (NEOH); [3]One Health Lessons, Arlington, Virginia, USA; [4]The Marine Mammal Center, Fort Cronkhite, Sausalito, USA; [5]EB Consult, Hellebæk, Denmark; [6]NOVA Medical School, Campo Mártires da Pátria, Lisbon, and Department of Medicine, Hospital Garcia de Orta, Almada, Portugal; [7]Wildlife Health Australia, Canberra, Australia, and School of Biosciences, University of Birmingham, Edgbaston, UK

Contents

 Principles of One Health for a better planet (eds B. Häsler, A. Tvarijonaviciute and S. Savić)
DOI: 10.1079/9781800623002.0012

Chapter Overview

Elevator pitch

To develop acceptable and feasible actions and interventions against a health outcome needing a One Health solution, you can use a series of steps to guide you through the participatory and systems thinking that are useful when working with your stakeholders. Vital to all of this is efficient and effective communication. Following up from the previous chapter, we focus on how to create a One Health intervention and implement it, including relevant challenges and solutions.

Book objectives the chapter relates to

☑ 1. Understand what One Health and Ecohealth mean
☑ 2. Think in a One Health and Ecohealth way
☑ 3. Apply One Health and Ecohealth in their professional and personal life
☑ 4. Know how to share One Health and Ecohealth knowledge
☑ 5. Integrate One Health and Ecohealth knowledge actively
☑ 6. Acquire or enhance core One Health competencies

One Health competencies covered

☑ 1. Effective communication
☑ 2. Collaborative and resilient working
☑ 3. Systems understanding
☑ 4. Transdisciplinarity
☑ 5. Social, cultural and gender equity and inclusiveness
☑ 6. Collective learning and reflective practice
☑ 7. One Health concepts
☑ 8. Theoretical and methodological pluralism
☑ 9. Harnessing uncertainty, paradox and limited knowledge

Learning outcomes

Be able to:

1. Identify acceptable and feasible intervention(s) to address (a) One Health problem(s).
2. Describe the challenges and solutions to participatory working for One Health outcome interventions.
3. Have awareness of available One Health educational and networking opportunities and how these will help you to improve your One Health working practices.

Summary

This chapter describes the necessary thought processes to develop interventions to improve a health outcome using One Health approaches, considering how you will share and disseminate knowledge learned by communicating with colleagues and collaborators. Whilst developing acceptable and feasible interventions against problems needing a One Health solution, you work with your stakeholders, mapping out the systems' complexities including identifying feedback loops and exploring alternative dynamics to mitigate system instability. Then, you develop a potential intervention(s) whilst considering mechanisms to balance the dynamics of stakeholders within the system, as well as the temporal and spatial scales at which your intervention(s) will operate. Effectively communicating will facilitate the collaborative process. Finally, dissemination of your findings is vital to create appropriate impact for your work. Having worked through this chapter, you will understand how to share and synthesize ideas using systems thinking, and efficient and effective communication, to best disseminate the knowledge learned.

11.1 Introduction

The **One Health approach** involves overcoming social barriers developed within and between societal structures, e.g. governing bodies including governments. Academic **disciplines** also create barriers; silos in methods and ideas, when many are shared between disciplines and complex health problems, and their solutions can benefit from integration across disciplines and participation of **stakeholders** (see **multi-, inter-** and **transdisciplinarity** in Chapter 3). To make One Health approaches sustainable and effective we need: evidence that spending time and money using One Health approaches provides **value** (Chapter 13); sufficient connections and close working – cohesion between the different stakeholders in projects (Chapter 10); and effective communication by One Health advocates so that its concept, approach and importance are understood, knowledge can be synthesized, stakeholders remain engaged, and projects are co-produced with society (Gibbs, 2018).

One Health recognizes links between disciplines, **sectors** and other bodies of knowledge (see Chapter 4 on **knowledge integration**), which are vital to properly address human, animal and environment health problems. As outlined in Chapter 10, the development of One Health initiatives describes a sequence of planning, from thinking in abstract isolation, to forming a cohesive planning group that recognizes the steps needed to implement the initiative. The One Health initiative could, for example, be a development project, education programme, research project or intergovernmental strategy, such as to improve the surveillance of a disease and develop interventions to reduce a complex health problem (Rüegg *et al.*, 2017). The One Health approach necessitates developing a common vocabulary, systems thinking, shared conceptualizations, inclusion of multiple perspectives and knowledge systems, and forming good working relationships and trust between those involved, to develop efficient, effective interventions.

Some organizations are not aligned to facilitate working using One Health approaches, e.g. they may include departments and working groups which reflect academic disciplines, or which focus on aspects of health such as for livestock, humans, the environment or wildlife. The departments and groups may themselves be physically separated, and if they include clinical services, their main foci may be separately financed and managed. In addition, funding is often developed into siloed funding streams which are not necessarily comparative in size; it can be difficult to develop mechanisms in which physical resources and funding can be shared, but also where the importance and contributions of different disciplines are both properly described and appreciated, e.g. human clinical medicine historically tends to receive greater funding than public health and veterinary medicine, and this can sometimes create conflicts related to access to resources due to territorialism.

Planning using One Health approaches requires that aims, understanding of the health problem and its health outcomes, the responsibilities and any financing consciously deal with different organizations' structures and hierarchies, to sectors and disciplines; the roles, tasks, responsibilities and competencies (including leadership, power and authority) of those involved must be firmly established, carefully balancing relationships to attain equitable outcomes. This highlights the necessity for excellent knowledge sharing, communication and dissemination to improve One Health working practices (Rüegg *et al.*, 2017). Knowledge on topics can be understood by thinking about interactions between actors (including stakeholders) with a **gender** perspective (see Chapter 9 on **gender equity**) and processes involved in different systems of knowledge that describe human, animal and environment health.

Systems thinking (see Box 10.1 on systems thinking in Chapter 10) promotes One Health values, helping to: (i) explore problems from a systems perspective; (ii) show the potential of solutions that work across subsystems and that anticipate and mitigate against destabilizing causes and effects within the system; (iii) promote dynamic networks of diverse stakeholders; (iv) inspire learning; (v) foster more system-wide planning, evaluation and research; and (vi) embrace dynamics, uncertainty and emergence in real world systems (Savigny and Adam, 2009). **Socio-ecological systems** rely on societies with cultural and community understanding to provide balance in the social, economic and environmental policies around **ecosystems** so that they can support all human, animal and plant species (Whitmee *et al.*, 2015). Without this understanding, the systems become unstable; this is demonstrated, for example, by the **impacts** of changing weather patterns and **climate** shocks and stresses on food systems (Falloon *et al.*, 2022). Thus, interventions need to be cognizant of the dynamics of these systems to achieve sustainable and effective outcomes.

11.1.1 What is an intervention?

Developing appropriate working practices is important for different sorts of One Health actions and initiatives. To remain within the scope of one chapter, we have focused on examples centred around developing interventions to improve health outcomes through healthcare, as illustrations of One Health problems.

But what do we mean by an **INTERVENTION**? In healthcare, an intervention is defined as any activity undertaken to improve a health outcome by preventing, curing or reducing the duration or severity of (infectious or non-infectious) disease, by restoring function that was lost because of injury or disease. Interventions to improve outcomes can be to prevent disease or reduce the incidence of new cases, or they can be to provide therapeutic solutions by treating, mitigating or postponing the effects of disease that is already present. Interventions can be both preventive and therapeutic (Anonymous, 2015). When extending One Health approaches to think about the health outcomes of the environment, health outcomes can include the resilience of ecosystems in terms of their ecosystem services; restoring ecosystem functioning because of damage to the physical and biological properties of the ecosystem (see Chapter 7 on **biodiversity** and ecosystems for more understanding on this). Interventions can also be focused on adjustments to **policy** to change outcomes.

Recently, the characteristics of a One Health intervention have been suggested. This includes: an intervention being a multisectoral and multidisciplinary initiative where this benefits the health outcome; equal partnership in activities across the project; shared technical, personnel and financial resources; and the joint defining of measurable outcome deliverables to help evaluate the social and economic contributions and benefits of the activities associated with the intervention across each sector and discipline (Nzietchueng *et al.*, 2023). In response to this definition, we argue that One Health must take an interdisciplinary or transdisciplinary approach, rather than being multidisciplinary.

Challenges of finding suitable interventions for different One Health problems: The following examples highlight the importance of understanding interconnections among diverse populations and factors, which enables a comprehensive approach and facilitates the planning of interventions with broader, more impactful outcomes.

- Mariki *et al.* (2015) carefully showed the complex web of relations that contributes to the One Health problem of human–elephant conflict and how it can affect the effectiveness of interventions. The study authors acknowledge a missed opportunity in relation to human–elephant conflict, where the poisoning of wildlife and contamination of the environment have caused major impacts in Tanzania. However, their drivers are land use and local community perceptions of the problem. Interventions to lessen conflicts should have involved supporting local communities as key stakeholders for environmental health, and reducing their marginalization and disempowerment, which have created resistance to conservation efforts.
- The way a problem is framed will determine its boundaries. This in turn will determine whether a One Health approach is needed or not. It may not be advisable to articulate every problem as a One Health problem and care should be taken to reflect if One Health is appropriate or not. One Health approaches should consider human, animal and environment dimensions, as necessary, but One Health interventions do not always happen, perhaps because appropriate approaches have not yet emerged. Forest fires are an example of when a One Health approach has not necessarily been used. Either managed or left to run wild, they impact wildlife populations (e.g. Kinnaird and O'Brien, 1998; Tiedemann *et al.*, 2000; Harper *et al.*, 2016; Andrus *et al.*, 2021). Interventions to lessen fire impacts often focus on ecosystem health, not just the health of local wildlife species and public health (e.g. Mott *et al.*, 2002; Schweizer and Cisneros, 2017). So far, however, an integrated

systems-level One Health approach remains elusive, though this may be changing, because general forest health now considers changes in global human activity as having an important influence upon forest health (e.g. see Trumbore *et al.*, 2015).

- Toxic events and the poor state of UK waterways have been widely reported in the general media (Ashworth, 2021), and are under constant governmental review (Anonymous, 2022a). Impacts on ecosystem health, public health, biodiversity and livestock production make this a One Health issue; however, current management continues to compartmentalize aspects of the problem, leading to fractured solutions, e.g. feminized fish populations resulting from steroid oestrogen contamination (Gross-Sorokin *et al.*, 2006), and recreational river users' health impacted by contaminated sediments (Scholes *et al.*, 2008). Systems understanding is vital to aid sustainable development of interventions to ameliorate all impacts, because solutions to these problems involve examining clinical impacts (in fish and humans) as well as environmental contamination by artificial hormones and potentially chemicals including heavy metal sources.

When more than one sub-system is involved, you have multiple interacting units, meaning that the system is inherently complex because you will have different sets of system structures, hierarchies and linear and non-linear processes operating for each sub-system, potentially at different (and at multi-) scales (San Miguel, 2023). Interventions need to account for this by adopting a holistic approach that considers the interactions and interdependencies among the various sub-systems. This involves understanding the diverse system structures, hierarchies and processes at play within each sub-system and across different scales. By acknowledging the inherent complexity and interconnectedness, interventions can be designed to address not only the immediate issues but also the underlying systemic factors that contribute to the complexity. Supported by a strong consortium of stakeholders that is willing to solve problems together and encourage collective change, existing structures, knowledge and behaviours can be leveraged to lead to more impactful solutions.

11.2 Intervention Steps and Communication along the One Health Implementation Cycle

Figure 11.1, first introduced in Chapter 10 (Fig. 10.1), provides an overview of the One Health implementation cycle from the problem statement to stakeholder engagement, defining the **theory of change**, implementation and evaluation, which then leads to improvements and closes the circle. In this chapter, we are focusing on the intervention aspects of the cycle with explicit emphasis on 'doing One Health' and communication that can facilitate effective and impactful interventions (Fig. 11.1). The co-production of the theory of change is covered in more detail in the **evaluation** chapter (Chapter 12) together with wider evaluation aspects.

As we have already seen, teamwork is essential in the One Health approach. Many higher education institutes have developed One Health-focused programmes at undergraduate, graduate and professional levels, and these involve many shared topics, e.g. management, communication and informatics, values and ethics, leadership, team and collaboration, roles and responsibilities, and systems thinking (Togami *et al.*, 2018; Amuguni *et al.*, 2019). It is not necessary to undertake formal training; however, when this has been completed, One Health graduates are often trained in a specific discipline (e.g. veterinary medicine, public health, ecology) but have had additional training including in communication skills and entrepreneurship. Entrepreneurship involves adapting quickly to a changing situation whilst being open-minded, thinking broadly about current challenges, whilst respectfully listening to others, including external stakeholders' needs and contributions; this also describes a good chairperson. A One Health leader can communicate across their team, maintaining the well-functioning of the team, both morally and financially, even when unforeseen complications arise.

When identifying the group of stakeholders involved in or affected by a One Health problem, and from within this group, forming a team to formulate the problem and prioritize objectives with the view to develop interventions (as described in Chapter 10), it is important to consider who should guide the stakeholders in discussions around interventions (e.g. a group of leaders or coordinators, a facilitator or a single

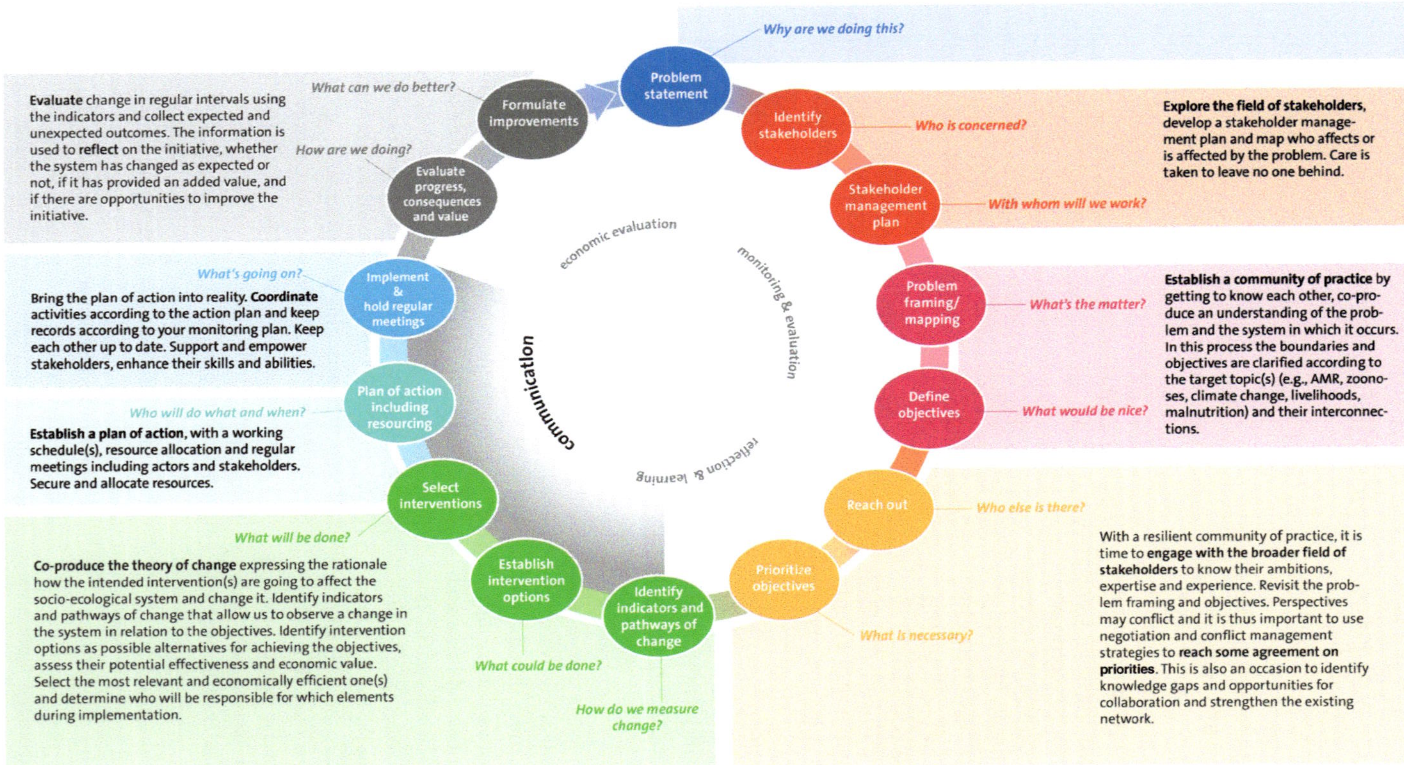

Fig. 11.1. Important stages along the One Health implementation cycle. After engaging your stakeholders, agreeing on the problem(s) and objectives, describing your system, conceptualizing the relevant system(s) boundaries, and expanding to reach a wider group, you then proceed to the elaboration of an intervention or set of interventions and theory of change. The theory of change outlines the causal pathways between inputs, activities, outputs, outcomes and impacts of an intervention or programme. It helps you to develop conceptual understanding for how your intervention (or a combination of interventions) will change your One Health problem, creating pathways describing possible solutions. A conceptual pathway is therefore a theoretical construct that describes the sequence of steps or events that lead to a particular outcome. You work through the systems' sub-systems including causal (feedback) loops using your previously developed planning coalition of key actors; systems dynamic modelling can help with this, combined with concept mapping or fuzzy cognitive mapping. This helps you to identify different intervention options that will help you achieve your objectives. There are always trade-offs within complex systems so that when we are improving one aspect of the system there are negative changes to another aspect; these trade-offs must be dealt with by strategically prioritizing the most important system components using joint decision making, whilst considering equity and social justice, and adaptation and flexibility in intervention design. Following this, you assess their potential effectiveness and economic value, and select the most efficient ones. Having a solid plan of action and a good communication plan underpinning this will help you to most effectively implement your intervention(s). You need to develop strong, active engagement with stakeholders throughout development, to ensure effective communication and coordination that will facilitate your transdisciplinary working. Knowledge sharing should be appropriate to different audiences to ensure greater mobilization of knowledge.

chairperson). Whomever is chosen, they do not need to be the most highly educated, and nor do they need to have the best understanding of the problem or have a specific opinion on interventions. They do need to have moral authority and the trust of group members so that they can speak openly, facilitate discussions, and offer guidance and support to the group.

When tackling One Health problems in a transdisciplinary way (Chapter 3), there are challenges when it comes to achieving a common understanding through language (including technical language) shared because of different backgrounds, ways of life, knowledge and expertise. Thus, One Health interventions need to be planned with attention not only to systems and science, but also to cultural inclusiveness. Cultural inclusiveness is essential in fostering collaboration and engagement across diverse communities. It involves respecting and recognizing the value of different cultural backgrounds, actively listening to diverse perspectives, and promoting open dialogue without judgement. Inclusive intervention planning ensures that all relevant voices are heard. Learning and using, for example, a local language shows respect for the community's heritage and facilitates more meaningful interactions. Engaging with someone else's art, traditions and cultural practices demonstrates not only an interest, but facilitates access to understanding each other's worldviews and values. Providing cultural sensitivity training, language support and adapting practices to align with cultural values can further help in communication. Involving stakeholders broadly in decision-making processes empowers them to shape initiatives according to their needs and aspirations to foster trust, promote mutual respect, and potentially generate ownership for interventions.

Before delving into the details of how interventions can be developed and prioritized, let us spend some time thinking about an applied example and how to generate a good foundation for intervention planning. This is an opportunity for you to bring in what you learned in Chapter 10.

The photogenic keystone sea otter: Considered endangered, the omnivorous sea otter (*Enhydra lutris*) draws tourists to your community. Populations are, however, becoming fatally infected with the protozoan parasite *Toxoplasma*, which leaches into the sea otter's ecosystem via contaminated water run-off from terrestrial stray cat populations. When sea otter numbers decrease, sea urchin numbers (their favourite meal) conversely increase, leading to smaller kelp (brown seaweed) forests resulting from sea urchin overgrazing.

Reduced kelp forests no longer hold back strong ocean currents, causing coastal erosion, endangering expensive houses bordering beaches and risking human lives. What must change? Many variables contribute to the problem and will influence interventions (e.g. human lives at risk, property and community-led ecotourism loss). The original cause of coastal erosion is decreased sea otter populations. Engineers will stabilize the land, and politicians will redirect local funds to shore-up beach integrity, houses and ecotourism, adjusting policies to manage *Toxoplasma* contamination. Marine biologists focus on the kelp forest and sea otters, and wildlife veterinarians care for the sea otters. Animal welfare groups manage the stray cats. Every group will probably have different interventions to this complex problem; sustainable interventions will develop a coalition of key actors and larger stakeholder groups to fully and appropriately represent all concerned, ensuring the problem is properly defined, conceptualized and iteratively adapted to optimize interventions.

Learning questions: For this example, each group of stakeholders will approach the situation with their own expertise in mind. You are given the role of acting as the One Health chairperson. How would you address the following points?

1. Determine who (what groups) should be involved.
2. Ensure everybody understands the entire situation (between stray cats, *Toxoplasma*, sea otters, sea urchins, kelp forest, erosion, homes at risk, loss of ecotourism meaning that less money is coming into the community).
3. Ensure everybody feels respected.
4. Ensure deadlines are met.

Once you have concluded the activity, compare your answers with the example answer below and reflect on how they differ and why. Note that there are multiple ways of answering this question and there is not one single correct solution.

Example answer:

1. Possible groups to involve include: spay/neuter veterinary group(s), policy makers, tourism board, wildlife veterinarians, parasitologists, ecologists, marine biologists, water specialists, engineers, architects, construction workers and the media.
2. Host early and frequent meetings to ensure people from the different groups start to trust and respect each other for their skills and knowledge. Explain early the entire situation while staying humble and asking for feedback and points of collaboration.
3. A way to ensure everybody feels respected is to set expectations very early when gathering people together and create a plan where each group presents their ideas to solve the problem. Create an atmosphere where everybody feels heard and it is safe to speak and brainstorm ideas.
4. The deadlines must be made clear at the first meeting. The multiple teams that you are managing as the chairperson must be held accountable or else the entire project would be delayed. Make this clear from the start.

11.3 Developing Intervention(s)

Intervention design in the context of addressing One Health problems requires a comprehensive and integrated approach that considers the interconnectedness of human, animal and environment health. This involves considering not only the immediate health outcomes but also the underlying causes, social determinants and environmental factors contributing to the problem.

So far, in Chapters 10 and 11, we have spent time defining and understanding the problem and its causes; identifying and engaging stakeholders in a community of practice; clarifying the characteristics of the system, its environment and boundaries; and deciding which influential factors have greatest scope for change.

Now we move on to identify how we can bring about change and how to deliver the change via an intervention or group of interventions. To do so, we need to pay attention to:

- The full spectrum of intervention options: often, in One Health interventions, preventive strategies are emphasized such as vaccination programmes, disease surveillance systems, biosecurity measures, biodiversity loss or pollution prevention. Given the complexity of health problems, One Health interventions often involve some form of attitude or behaviour change among communities, healthcare providers, farmers and other stakeholders. Environmental management strategies are often needed to protect ecosystems; these may include sustainable land-use practices, pollution control measures, habitat conservation and ecosystem restoration efforts.
- Dealing with trade-offs: while there are multiple opportunities for co-benefits (see Chapter 13 on economic evaluation), One Health interventions often need to deal with trade-offs, because resources are probably limited and decisions must be made about competing needs or goals; improving one aspect may come at the expense of another. Dealing with trade-offs in interventions requires strategic prioritization, systems-based planning, stakeholder engagement, joint decision making, flexibility and adaptability supported by robust monitoring and effective collaboration and coordination.
- Importance of equity and social justice: One Health interventions are commonly expected to promote equity, inclusivity and social justice. Consequently, the needs of marginalized communities, vulnerable populations and underserved areas need to be considered and underlying **social determinants of health** (see Chapter 8 for more information on these determinants) need to be addressed.
- Adaptation and flexibility: given the dynamic nature of One Health problems and the associated systems, there is a need to be adaptable and flexible in intervention design to respond to changing contexts, emerging challenges and lessons learned from implementation. Thus, the monitoring of progress and evaluation of effectiveness throughout (as explained in Chapter 12) can lead to iterative adaptations based on feedback and evolving needs.

11.4 Conceptualizing Pathways to Particular Outcomes

11.4.1 Elaborating change pathways and interventions in a collaborative approach

After engaging your stakeholders, agreeing on the problem(s) and the objectives, describing your system, conceptualizing the relevant system(s) boundaries, and expanding to reach a wider group, you then proceed to the elaboration of an intervention / set of interventions and theory of change. The details of that including the selection of indicators are explained in Chapter 12 on evaluation, but a brief overview is provided here:

A **theory of change** is a comprehensive and systematic approach that outlines the causal pathways between inputs, activities, **outputs**, outcomes and impacts of an intervention or programme. It is a visual or narrative representation that helps to explain how and why the desired changes are expected to occur as a result of the intervention. It begins with identifying the inputs, which encompass the resources and assets required for the intervention, such as funding, personnel, equipment and expertise. These inputs are then utilized through a series of planned activities, which are the specific actions or strategies undertaken as part of the programme. The outputs of these activities are the immediate and tangible products, services, or deliverables produced by the intervention. Moving beyond outputs, the theory of change delves into outcomes, which represent the changes or results expected as a direct consequence of the outputs. These outcomes can vary in timing and scope, encompassing short-term, medium-term and long-term changes in behaviour, attitudes, conditions or systems. Central to the theory of change are the underlying **assumptions** and logic that connect inputs, activities, outputs and outcomes. These assumptions form the theoretical basis for how the intervention is expected to bring about the desired changes. Finally, the theory of change includes indicators and measurement tools that allow for tracking progress, evaluating effectiveness and assessing whether the intervention is achieving its intended objectives. This process of theory of change elaboration can help greatly to develop conceptual pathways describing how the intervention (or a combination of interventions) will change your One Health problem, working through its sub-systems including causal (feedback) loops using your previously developed planning coalition of key actors (Chapter 10); systems dynamic modelling can help with this (Trochim *et al.*, 2006), combined with concept mapping (Box 11.1) or fuzzy cognitive mapping (Voinov *et al.*, 2018).

A **conceptual pathway** is a theoretical construct that describes the sequence of steps or events that lead to a particular outcome. It may include visual representations of relationships between concepts, variables and factors, and can be used to describe complex ideas (e.g. Fig. 11.2).

Another way to organize knowledge is concept mapping, which is a visual and analytical tool used to organize and represent knowledge or ideas in a structured format creating graphical representations of concepts, ideas or information, along with the relationships between them. Concept maps are typically hierarchical diagrams that consist of nodes (representing concepts or ideas) and labelled lines or arrows (indicating the relationships or connections between the concepts). They help to provide understanding of negative and positive effects of interventions on different system components. Iterative adaptations are then used to redesign the intervention, optimizing synergies and positive impacts whilst avoiding (or minimizing) negative impacts (Savigny and Adam, 2009). See Box 11.1 for more detail on concept mapping using the example of intervention.

The design for optimized intervention(s) should then be shared for input with the larger stakeholder group/community of practice, to ascertain that the needs of different stakeholders are met in the planned intervention(s) (Table 11.1), and to clarify that issues are framed and prioritized appropriately by different groups (see the applied example) at appropriate temporal and spatial scales.

All stakeholder groups work to their strengths as much as they are able, but they all also have limitations. These can be, for example, in relation to niche knowledge, community networks and technology availability. Consider applying the strengths of one stakeholder group to fill the limitations of another, to fill these gaps and to be gender equitable (see Chapter 9 on gender). This must include examining whether interventions are or can be made acceptable, affordable, sustainable and equitable for all groups and whether they might not exacerbate some existing gender imbalances. Iterative changes to intervention(s) need to be explored at the planning stage until this balance is achieved across the organizations and groups of people impacted by the intervention.

Box 11.1. Concept mapping for an intervention

Systems-thinking methods can be applied using specific tools to organize ideas and concepts. Systems diagrams can be used to describe and visualize complex situations, helping to address any identified problems, with approaches including Rich Picturing, Influence diagrams, Causal diagrams, Cynefin, Viable System Models and Cultural Historical Activity System Models (Williams, 2021). While systems diagrams can use purely qualitative information, concept mapping uses more quantitative understanding, and is explained here in more detail. It uses a structured process that is amenable to many health professionals, and is focused on a topic or construct of interest with the aim to produce an interpretable pictorial view of the ideas and concepts, and how these are interrelated, of inputs from multiple (a group of) participants (Trochim, 1989). The six-step model of concept mapping (Trochim *et al.*, 2006; Kane and Trochim, 2007; Trochim and McLinden, 2017) includes:

1. Preparation: (a) selecting the participants – your One Health consortium (e.g. the community of practice set up following the steps in Chapter 10) identifies the strengths and weaknesses of different groups of actors to be included in the mapping process. Once selected, the concept mapping team plans the logistics for mapping, including materials preparation and participants' contacting timelines. (b) Developing the focus to frame your problem, including defining the focus for the brainstorming, and defining the human, animal and environment dimension(s) on which each of the brainstormed elements will be rated. If problem and system (including boundaries) descriptions are available already, these can be included at this step. Otherwise, time should be spent on these aspects. Together these form a short summary of your One Health problem including describing the system boundaries and environment.
2. Generation: the concept mapping team brainstorm to generate statements or concepts for mapping, including key facets of the conceptual domain. Key facets of the intervention domain are explored, ranked based on importance and feasibility, and then conceptually linked to form an intervention framework. They explore the relative importance of concepts (or statements describing these concepts), and then rank them using Likert-like scales. A diagram depicting relationships between statements or concepts is created, with overarching concepts broken down into smaller components using arrows and linking words demonstrating connections between ideas and demonstrating how interventions interact and contribute to desired outcomes. Concepts are perceived regularities or patterns in events or objects, designated using a label and shapes in the diagram. For example, they might be drivers of an issue such as arrows depicting El Niño patterns causing flooding, which then creates run-off from agricultural land, which causes *Vibrio* species pathogens to be flushed into an estuary, creating infectivity in mariculture blue mussel farms, which then causes potential food contamination when the mussels are harvested. Linking words and lines describes relationships between concepts, and feedback loops in diagrams explain the behaviour of the system, describing cause and effect relationships between components. Feedback loops are where part of the output of a system returns to its input, creating a loop. In the *Vibrio* example above, otters might search for food along the shore front and eat *Vibrio*-affected mussels; in foraging on the cropped farmland above the shore, they then defecate on the crops, exacerbating the prevalence of *Vibrio* in the environment. Anonymous brainstorming (or an alternative method) ensures that minority views are included. The final statement or concept set describing the operationalized conceptual domain is edited and synthesized from a wider number of statements or concepts (e.g. using structured editing processes and content analysis).
3. Structuring: the structuring step includes collecting demographic variables describing participants, sorting data (e.g. based on their similarity, to help organize complexity), and collating statement or concept ratings information. The sorting and collating of data focus on organizing intervention ideas based on their relevance and potential impact. Demographic information classifies participants into sub-groups. Statements or concepts are arranged into logical participant group sets (often using software to help). Participants then rate each intervention idea statement or concept based upon their perception of an item's

Continued

Box 11.1. Continued.

importance or another relevant value qualifier, e.g. feasibility, priority, effort involved and expected outcomes. The ratings are usually Likert-like scales (e.g. 1–5, 1–7) based on some kind of continuum. For ratings to be representative of the population, it is useful to first scan the list of statements to gain an idea of the highest and lowest priorities within the set; you can then make sure that these are included in the full range of rating values. The overall structuring process can be implemented using proprietary software, e.g. (Anonymous, n.d. a; Anonymous, 2022b).

4. Representation: the data collected from the intervention generation and structuring steps during the data generation step are represented as results clustering intervention ideas based on their alignment with intervention goals and strategies. An NxN binary symmetric matrix of similarities Xij is first developed for each participant, and then a total NxN similarity matrix Tij is created. The total NxN similarity matrix Tij is then analysed using nonmetric multidimensional scaling with a two-dimensional solution. This leads to the development of a two-dimensional (x,y) configuration of the set of statements or concepts based on the idea that statements piled together more often are located more closely than those piled together less (these are further apart). The x,y configuration that is created is thereafter used as the basis for defining a cluster in a cluster analysis in which a final number of clusters is selected that is a balance of preserving the most detail but also simplifying the results so that they can be interpreted. The multidimensional scaling results are graphed in two dimensions providing a point map which shows the brainstormed statements which are most similar being closer to each other. A cluster map can also be developed based on the multidimensional scaling results which uses the outermost points for the final clusters as cluster boundaries. Generally, the larger the cluster in the final cluster set then the broader are the meanings around the statements or concepts within that cluster. The rating data are averaged across participants for each item statement or concept and each cluster; they are shown in a point rating map including the original point map with third dimension vertical columns describing the average rating per item and in a cluster rating map showing the clusters in three dimensions. Additional representations can be made of the data collected; for full details see Trochim and McLinden (2017).

5. Interpretation: normally undertaken using a structured joint participatory collaboration (Trochim, 1989), during interpretation, after reminders describing the brainstorming, scoring and rating processes, participants are shown the listing of clustered statements or concepts. They then describe each using short phrases or words, and a facilitator helps find consensus for each statement. Cluster labels are thereafter appended to the cluster map and examined for: representativeness; to identify interpretable cluster groups; and pattern-matching for degree of consensus to statement or concept ratings. Go-zone plots provide drilled-down results information.

6. Utilization: the final outputs provide a framework of intervention statements derived from the concept mapping process. This map serves as a guide to identify, prioritize and plan appropriate interventions for addressing the One Health problem effectively.

When developing a transdisciplinary, cross-cultural and inter-sectoral team for interventions, expectations must be agreed on early in intervention development. Considering spatial scale ensures that the project can be applied at a certain targeted scale, e.g. local community versus entire country. Spatial and temporal scales will only be fully considered within interventions if the design focuses on their coverage, and it can be easier to reduce project scale and resolution than to increase these. For example, if managing a disease outbreak, the sooner data are understood at the local level, the easier it will be to explain national trends. There are, however, often issues of equitable data access and sharing that need to be considered (Box 11.2 on factual and data sharing constraints). The understanding of the appropriate spatial and temporal scales for the One Health problem starts when considering your systems' boundaries during initial brainstorming (Chapter 10).

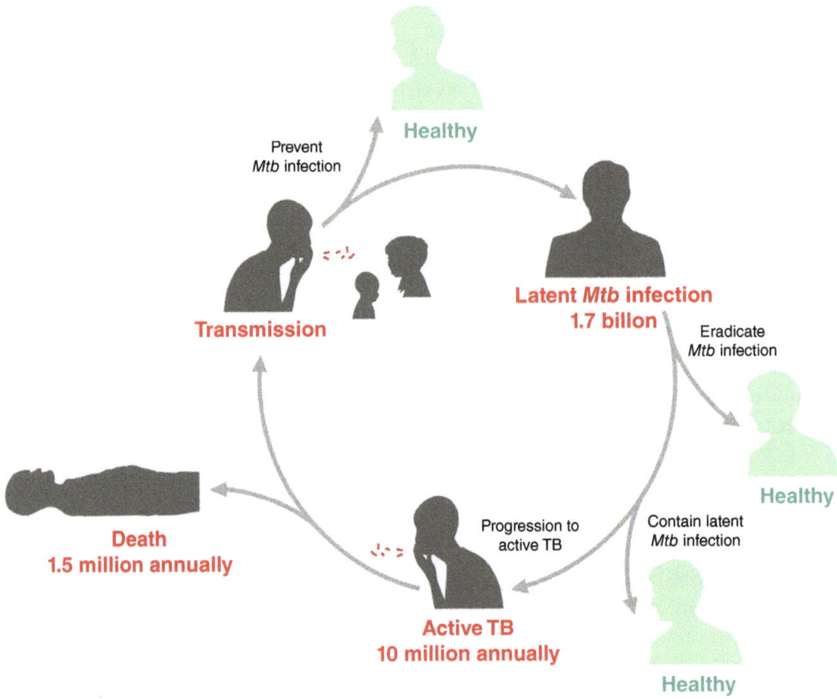

Fig. 11.2. The clinical cycle of human tuberculosis (TB) and health status during different stages of the disease. The simple links and loops describe the chronological flow of this disease process. This conceptual pathway diagram depicts a complex system (partially knowable and predictable, and adaptive) in a single visualization. Taken from Kaufmann (2020), unmodified (CC BY 4.0 DEED: https://creativecommons.org/licenses/by/4.0).

Table 11.1. Summary of potential power imbalances in stakeholder groups, and how these might be redressed within planned interventions.

<table>
<tr><th>Stakeholder group</th><th>How might the group influence or be ignored in the planned intervention?</th><th>How might these influences or incapacities be redressed within the planned intervention?</th></tr>
<tr><td>Principal stakeholders</td><td>Could have greater power within decision making than less-empowered groups. Their perspective on ideal interventions may contrast with less-empowered groups.</td><td rowspan="2">By including representation from less-empowered groups in the coalition of key actors and respecting a gender balance, and in the larger stakeholder group during planning of interventions (and/or the structuring stage in concept mapping).
By ensuring that all groups have a single 'vote' (no weighting on opinions during decision making).</td></tr>
<tr><td>Certain genders, ethnic and/or resource-poor groups, or groups indirectly impacted by the planned intervention (for more information see Bagnol *et al.*, 2016; Friedson-Ridenour and Pierotti, 2019; Garnier *et al.*, 2020; Garnier *et al.*, 2022)</td><td>Particular groups have differing access to education, land, healthcare etc.
Particular groups have differing abilities to make decisions causing power imbalances.
Particular groups are treated differently, meaning that they are impacted differently by the world around them.
Differences in resources and power can lead to different perceptions about risks and interventions in One Health.</td></tr>
</table>

Box 11.2. Factual and data sharing constraints

Knowledge sharing involves volunteering information, data and understanding between different agents and organizations. This enables learning, collaborative problem solving and capacity building, promoting innovation, creating new theories or ideas, and establishing new research principles. It also creates a common repository of reusable knowledge. Within One Health, it can refer to general information or awareness sharing, data and information sharing, methods and results sharing, and institutional memory and resilience within system change. Knowledge sharing promotes progress, enables knowledge production and integration to collaboratively tackle complex health problems at the human, animal and environment interface.

Information and data sharing within One Health approaches involves transparency of data, with greater, holistic analysis and discussion that considers perspectives greater than those of data owners. This strengthens analysis and research methods, fosters collaboration and builds trust, minimizing bias and duplication of data collection, ensuring optimization of resources.

Barriers to sharing are common, including data accessibility and ownership issues. Despite growing enthusiasm for public, open-access datasets, gaining data and information access can be burdensome, involving complex bureaucratic processes, time delays, high costs, technical constraints and mistrust issues. Confidentiality issues associated with sharing sensitive data, such as Personally Identifiable Information, are particularly difficult, requiring obtaining ethical permissions for data gathering and use. Frequently, such data are collected for specific purposes, and cannot be used for new or alternative studies without securing additional permissions. Secure data storage and sharing mechanisms within specific data centres are often necessary to guarantee anonymized storage, maintenance and data access, regardless of individual or institutional changes. Anonymization, however, can hamper interoperability when trying to merge databases, reducing potential data reuse. As the culture of knowledge sharing evolves, sharing between institutions and collaborators should be defined and conceptualized at institution (or project) set-up, to positively influence how data are collected, stored and shared. Memorandums of understanding that are often signed between collaborating organizations can help with data sharing issues, as can recent Open Data initiatives, whereby data from projects are made accessible using Digital Object Identifiers (DOIs).

11.4.2 Checking the impact of feedback loops on system stability, for new scenarios

Most systems are self-organizing, non-linear and counter-intuitive, history dependent, constantly changing, tightly linked, governed by feedback and resistant to change. The use of systems thinking (see Box 10.1 on systems thinking in Chapter 10) to create One Health interventions for health outcomes involves focusing on the nature of key facets within the conceptual domain (relationships between building blocks), relationships between statements or concepts (space between blocks and understanding of what happens there), and synergies between concepts or components (synergies emerging from interactions among blocks). Causal (feedback) loops describing cause and effect relationships between system components make the system more complex, potentially destabilizing interventions. This highlights the need in systems thinking for thought, clarity, and efficient and effective communication during the development and application of system-level interventions, which target multiple system building blocks directly or generically. For example, weak stewardship (leadership and **governance**) can lead to system instability, as interventions are not appropriately situated in policy and practice if governance and knowledge sharing are inadequate (Savigny and Adam, 2009). The systems-thinking approach explores alternative dynamics within the system to mitigate system instability, such as in the following applied example.

Disease risk communication and mitigation: In 2021, stakeholders interested in reducing risk of African Swine Fever (ASF) in the Philippines were brought together by the IUCN Species Survival Commission wild suid specialist group. It had been acknowledged that disease mitigation focusing on domestic pig health and human food security was insufficient; there was a need to consider biodiversity and ecosystem health. A disease risk analysis (DRA) workshop (utilizing Jakob-Hoff *et al.*, 2014) identified that including wild pigs in ASF control and prevention measures and risk communication would reduce the disease's economic and food security impacts by improving surveillance and transmission pathway identification, providing improved containment understanding for decision makers. The system's communication pathways were mapped during the DRA process, and this identified parallel reporting systems including different participants, and risk of failure as not all disease pathways were highlighted for control. A combined communications network was therefore developed, based on enhanced understanding of feedback loops in the system, to improve ASF disease risk communication and mitigation efforts.

11.4.3 Deciding which intervention(s) is/are most appropriate and finalizing using an 'ecological' perspective

Hawe *et al.* (2009) defined an intervention as 'a series of inter-related events occurring within a system where the change in outcome (attenuated or amplified) is not proportional to the change in input'. This means that interventions can also be interpreted as an ongoing social process in an ongoing context, which seems pertinent to One Health. Whilst an intervention in a **simple system** can potentially also be simple, because the context of the system is well understood, in a more complex and therefore less predictable system, the process of identifying potential interventions is more onerous. So how can this be done? Rather than focusing on simplifying a problem to identify interventions, in a **complex system** it is appropriate to take an 'ecological' systems-based perspective and focus on dynamic processes that occur in the context of the system in which you are going to introduce the intervention, and with which your intervention will interact (see the applied example on orangutan conservation). In doing this, you might improve understanding on how to expand the effectiveness of your intervention because you harness the intervention to the system's dynamics. This is also particularly important when doing evaluations of One Health interventions because these will need to stay open to both intended and unintended effects, as described in Chapter 12. As you are assuming that the changes in the system because of the intervention are not going to be uniform, this means that the input of the intervention will not be identical across sub-systems within the greater system; it will instead adapt to different initial conditions. As described within the structure of the implementation cycle, the initial steps to rationalize the most appropriate intervention include: defining your One Health problem (Gibbs, 2018); identifying and gathering the actors involved (Rüegg *et al.*, 2017); and describing your system (Savigny and Adam, 2009).

To assess system-level changes that will occur because of potential interventions, you need to:

1. **Explore how each potential intervention (or combination of these) is linked to the context of your system** – think about how far across the system it would have impact, and how intensive the impact would be relative to what occurs now. What key activities, settings or events would the intervention impact if introduced, and how much would it change the status quo for each?
2. **Track changes in the relationships in your system that would occur because of each potential intervention (or combination)** – your system is described by a network; a social structure within which you can track changes in structural relationships across time. These changes might be in the interactions between network actors (people or organizations running activities), or links between settings or events. Are changes in the network such as new relationships occurring because of new technologies being introduced in the intervention(s), meaning that the importance of some network actors is changing? You might see the network becoming sparser, which means that there are fewer interactions, or it might become denser and more cohesive, meaning that there are more interactions.
3. **Focus on the distribution and transformation of resources in your system that would occur because of your potential intervention(s)** – what is going to change in terms of your key activities, settings or events, and in what way? Will the outcome you are interested in change in place and time, and by how much?

4. **Assess the activities which are displaced in your system by the potential intervention** – you need to clarify that it really is the effects of the intervention(s) that are changing the system. It might be that the activities that are displaced truly account for the changes in your outcome.

By understanding these different facets, you will be able to capture the full benefits, as well as an understanding of potential negative impacts on some stakeholders, of potential interventions. For example, assuming that capacity building is the intervention objective, you can more completely assess its effect, such as enablement, improving the structural position of network actors, settings or events so that more can be achieved. By focusing on dynamic processes that occur in your system because of your potential intervention(s) you will also be able to maximize your strategic investment by best harnessing the system's complexity, due to focusing on specific sub-systems and processes within them. You will be able to prospectively track changes in the network actor's relationships, using your improved knowledge to steer the strategic direction when choosing the most appropriate intervention(s), e.g. capitalizing on positive feedback loops and counteracting negative feedback loops (Hawe *et al.*, 2009). This dynamic intervention effect poses challenges for evaluation and economic evaluation, as discussed in Chapters 12 and 13, respectively.

Orangutan conservation: Now that we have worked through the steps of agreeing on a problem, engaging stakeholders, identifying objectives and elaborating the intervention(s), we are going to look at an applied example that chronicles a risk-based approach to highlight concerns about continued orangutan translocations in Indonesia during the COVID-19 pandemic (Sherman *et al.*, 2021) (Fig. 11.3).

This applied example allows you to practise how to identify and bring together the actors involved in this problem (this example covers a multidisciplinary set), to identify acceptable and feasible intervention(s) against this problem(s), and to describe the challenges and solutions to participatory working for One Health interventions. This example highlights how decisions can be assessed for effectiveness and feasibility via a properly analysed rationale to improve decision making and the need for systems thinking, including challenges of understanding decision-maker motivation, knowledge and politics.

The target audience was not only practitioners, but government-level decision makers who had been advocating relocating the entire *Pongo tapanuliensis* orangutan species into captivity (see the highlighted section, surrounded in bold, in Fig. 11.4). *P. tapanuliensis* was only described as a distinct species in 2017 and is critically endangered, according to the International Union for Conservation of Nature (IUCN) Red List of Threatened Species (Anonymous, 2017). The rationale for relocation was to avoid the transmission and spread of COVID-19 to wild populations through the relocation / keeping in capacity with biosecurity measures. A study team was pulled together to elaborate a problem statement and conduct a disease risk assessment related to orangutan releases based on data from Indonesia.

Task: Have a look at Fig. 11.3 and think about how you would engage stakeholders, and organize factors and information to create a foundation for interventions. Summarize some key points in writing and then continue reading.

You will see that the study team used a One Health approach by following a wildlife disease risk analysis (DRA) process (an effective One Health tool) that allowed them to map out causal pathways of risk factors to health, with a focus on environmental health, wildlife health and human health, emphasizing that a healthy system is not just absence of disease – a fundamental One Health tenet.

To test the validity of the systems approach, the authors considered the risk of COVID-19 in orangutan translocations. However, they did not only focus on that, but utilized the qualitative risk analysis process to assess the relative risk of translocation decision-making options on species survival and ecosystem impact. A qualitative risk assessment matrix can be used by practitioners to consider overall threats associated with orangutan translocations (see Fig. 11.4).

The study team described the potential consequences of translocation, highlighting that a One Health approach was needed to provide:

- health surveillance of wild, captive and released orangutans, and information sharing among stakeholders;

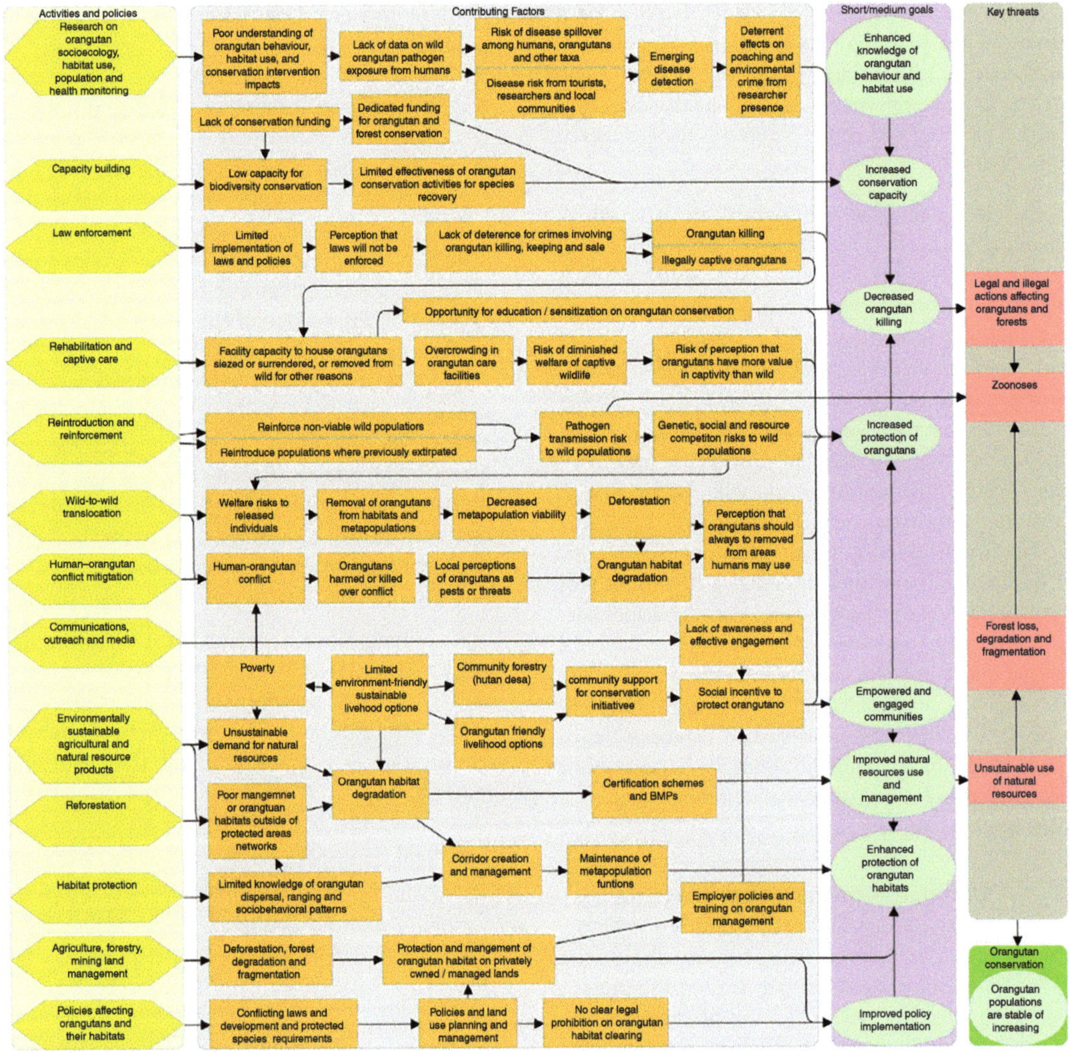

Fig. 11.3 Orangutan conservation complexity. Cells in the far-left column are activities and policies affecting orangutans. Central section cells describe positive and negative factors that affect orangutan conservation outcomes. The second column from the right shows the interim goals of activities and policies. Key threats that activities and policies aim to address are in the far-right column. Arrows indicate relationships between cells. From Sherman *et al.* (2021), unmodified (CC BY 4.0 DEED: https://creativecommons.org/licenses/by/4.0/).

- collaboration among government, local communities and non-governmental organizations (NGOs) to address health and biodiversity conservation;
- a disease risk assessment conducted with orangutan conservation and translocation stakeholders and wildlife health experts;
- investment in education and policy that recognizes the direct dependence of human health on functional ecosystems and biodiversity; and
- improved law enforcement to address orangutan killing, trade and clearance of orangutan habitats in agricultural concessions, addressing negative human interactions with orangutans, and protecting large intact forests and forest fragments that have been identified as orangutan conservation priorities.

The necessary interventions were developed to minimize human–orangutan interactions so that:

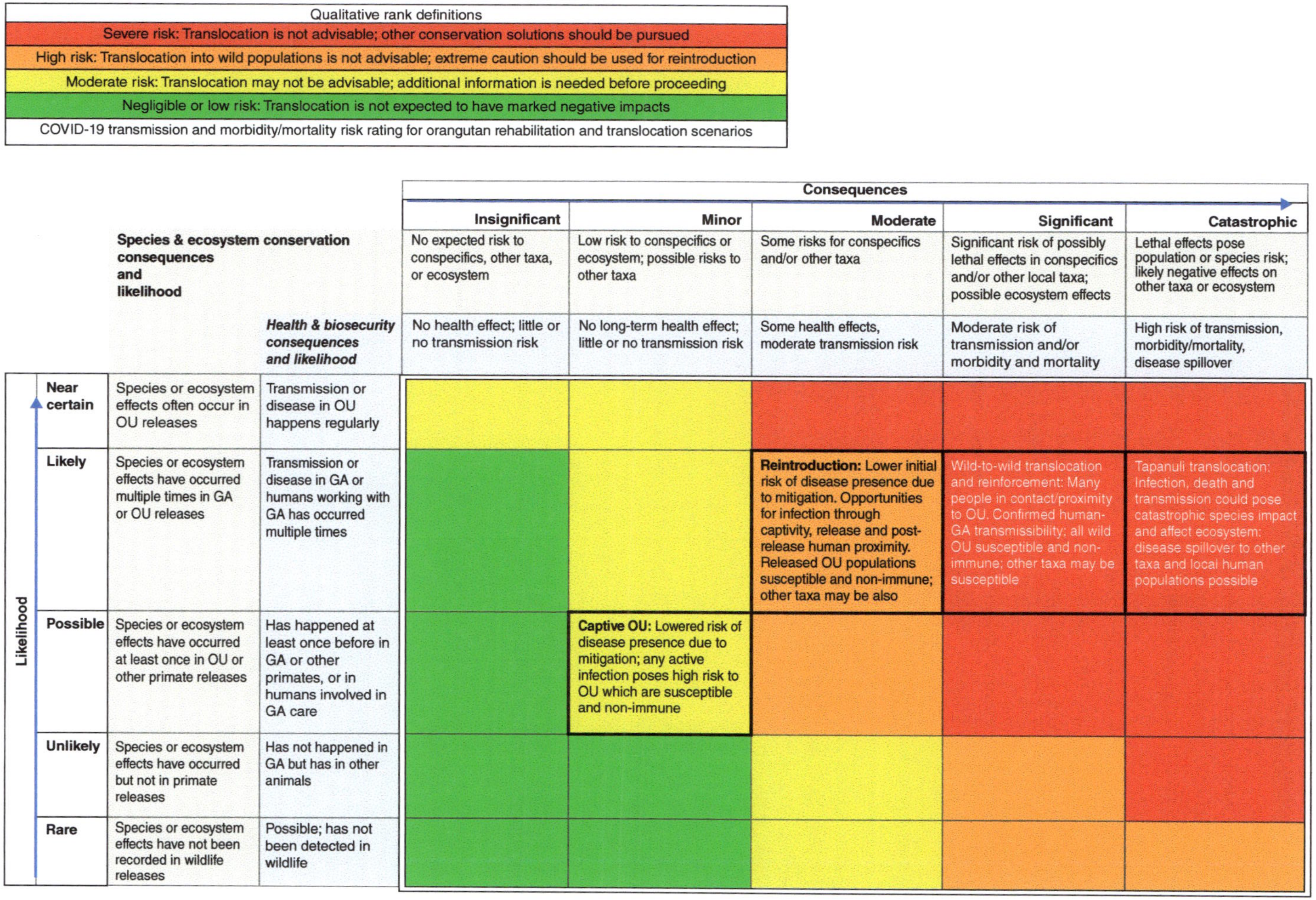

Fig. 11.4 Qualitative risk matrix for orangutan translocation using a COVID-19 example. OU = orangutans; GA = great apes. Coloured cells inside double lines denote overall qualitative rank. Consequence definitions are presented in the two cells beneath each category name, with species and ecosystems in the top cell and health and biosecurity in the cell below. Likelihood category definitions are presented in the two cells to the right of each category name, for species and ecosystems, and then for health and biosecurity from left to right. Cells relevant to OU translocation scenarios have a thick border and list factors considered in risk ranking. From Sherman *et al.* (2021), unmodified (CC BY 4.0 DEED: https://creativecommons.org/licenses/by/4.0/).

- Wild-to-wild translocations should be the only option in extraordinary circumstances, such as when orangutans cannot escape forest fires, or people are likely to kill them and cannot be swayed by legal consequences or alternative interventions. Otherwise, outreach measures should be pursued to protect orangutans *in situ*.
- Interventions should be determined in collaboration with local communities, to address their specific needs, including providing financial benefits, employment opportunities, or improved livelihoods.
- Effective strategies to provide positive impacts of interventions for the local population could be demonstrated, e.g. healthcare services tied to illegal logging reductions and community forest management initiatives.
- When orangutans needed to be moved between forest blocks within agricultural landscapes, unpalatable crops such as shade-grown coffee can be used, as they would discourage orangutans from returning to the area.
- Potentially negative interactions could be forestalled by engaging local community members to serve as 'orangutan guardians' by providing indirect incentives such as enhancing infrastructure and civic facilities, or direct financial incentives.
- Long-standing positive relationships with surrounding communities could be used to maximize crucial local support when developing interventions, because rescue and research centres, and NGOs are often significant sources of local employment.

Problem descriptions such as the applied example on orangutan conservation can be useful tools to help communicate and forge agreement among stakeholders. This is vital for successful risk communication and advancing the DRA process (Jakob-Hoff *et al.*, 2014; Wolf *et al.*, 2019). Anecdotally, the lack of a problem statement is where a lot of DRA processes fail: when stakeholders cannot agree on the problem, it is more challenging to convince decision makers to follow the DRA recommendations for risk management (Unwin, unpublished data). The context and drivers of orangutan translocations further complicate potential disease and conservation risks by creating pressure for translocation as an ostensibly rapid, short-term solution to protect orangutans.

The study (Sherman *et al.*, 2021) linked NGOs with government decision makers by communicating the role of locally based NGOs being crucial to developing solutions, as they have long-standing relationships with surrounding communities, and often serve as significant sources of local employment. At the time of writing, the Indonesian Government had paused its original requirement to bring the species into captivity as indicated in the paper, based on the evidence of risk presented. This provides evidence of increased leverage on events by transmitting a message (in this case a scientific journal article) that was received by decision makers in a manner that allowed for change in a decision that improved, however slightly, the One Health problem.

11.5 Implementation

For implementation, stakeholders use their role and competence within the socio-ecological system to bring the plan of action into reality. During the scheduled meetings, information about activities is fed back to the community of practice to see if the project is on track and the actions are coordinated. Stakeholders may be encouraged to support each other and synergize towards achieving the objectives, and there should be space for mutual learning. Some changes may have to be made to adapt the action plan to the realities in the field or respond to unexpected events.

The time required to achieve impacts depends largely on the size of the project, where larger initiatives with many stakeholders and changes in infrastructure may take decades, and small-scale projects may have imminent effects. This is due to the characteristic time of systems, which designates the time that a system requires to respond to a stimulation and depends on its size, e.g. a cell responds within minutes to adapt to a change of acidity in its environment, while an ecosystem may take decades to recover from a landslide.

The implementation of a One Health intervention generally follows the same basic steps as other interventions, namely:

1. Development of a detailed implementation plan based on all the steps conducted above and an assessment of the resources needed in alignment with the change mechanisms, pathways and theory of change.

2. Gathering of necessary resources, including personnel, funding or financing, equipment and materials. Training and orientation of staff or stakeholders involved in the intervention.

3. Conducting small-scale pilot tests of the intervention to identify any potential issues, refine procedures, and confirm expected feasibility.

4. Rolling out of the intervention on a larger scale according to the finalized plan including close monitoring of progress to address any challenges that arise and enable adaptive implementation.

5. Documenting and communicating aspects of the intervention, including processes, outcomes, lessons learned and best practices. Disseminating findings to relevant stakeholders and the broader community.

However, One Health interventions commonly add a layer of difficulty owing to the problems that are being tackled and the complexity of working with diverse disciplines, stakeholders and perspectives. These added layers of difficulty need to be considered and addressed through effective communication, collaboration and adaptive management strategies.

With the overview of activities, a plan of action is established, with working schedule(s), resource allocation and regular meetings. The activities are delegated to the competent stakeholders. Care should be taken to match tasks, resources, competencies and responsibilities appropriately. The plan of action should also foresee coordination and collaborations, either formally through memorandum(s) of understanding, or less formally with oral agreements. Monitoring plans can support the implementation of the intervention as described in Chapter 12. It is important that all actors are clear about their roles and the expectations towards them.

Thus, it is important to have effective communication plans for the implementation of the intervention.

11.5.1 Communication plans to support effective implementation of the intervention

We have highlighted the importance of the 'human factor' in One Health practice. It follows that effective communication is vital to build knowledge, influence attitudes, raise awareness and build perceptual associations between recommendations and stakeholders' or audiences' values, customs and beliefs. Furthermore, effective communication focuses on outcomes for the audience or stakeholder, rather than activities of an organization or its partners. During the communication process, it is important to find the right time to act, engage with the real world, and not bombard people with evidence; effective communication is vital to successful management of an intervention. A communications plan should be inclusive and respectful of the needs of different stakeholders.

A communication plan for a transdisciplinary intervention must address the unique challenges posed by diverse stakeholders and interdisciplinary collaboration. The plan should reflect the stakeholder analysis conducted including the respective roles, interests and communication preferences of each group involved. The project objectives elaborated and agreed on and the community of practice established will be helpful in tailoring communication pathways for the intervention.

Timely and regular updates are essential to keep stakeholders informed about project progress, milestones, challenges and outcomes. Two-way communication channels should be established to encourage feedback, questions and contributions from stakeholders. It is important to create an environment where stakeholders feel heard and valued, fostering open dialogue and participation. Communication channels may encompass a mix reflecting the project including a combination of regular meetings, email updates, project newsletters, social media platforms and collaboration tools. Engagement strategies could involve workshops, training sessions, feedback mechanisms, and opportunities for co-creation and collaboration.

Conflict resolution mechanisms should be in place to address any disagreements or misunderstandings that may arise among stakeholders during the implementation of the intervention (see Chapter 10 for more information on conflict resolution). Finally, the communication plan should include mechanisms for evaluation and feedback to assess the effectiveness of communication strategies and make necessary adjustments. Documentation and knowledge sharing are also crucial for maintaining continuity, facilitating learning, and ensuring that project information is accessible to all relevant stakeholders.

Risk communication: Risk communication is a specialized form of communication that focuses on conveying information about risks, hazards and uncertainties to stakeholders, decision makers and the public. It involves explaining potential dangers, uncertainties and potential consequences associated with certain actions, events or situations. Risk communication aims to facilitate understanding, promote informed decision making, and mitigate negative impacts by providing relevant and timely information.

An example of how efficient and effective communication prevented both panic and the spread of misinformation was the identification of COVID-19 in captive wildlife in American zoos (Daly, 2021). The zoos managed to communicate successfully to the media at multiple points (e.g. Fig. 11.5) about the risk of zoonotic transmission of COVID-19, having identified disease in apes, tigers, snow leopards and other animals. They controlled the risk message by being transparent, honest and open to scrutiny (Anonymous, 2021).

A map of transmission routes for tuberculosis at the human–animal interface is shown in Fig. 11.6. The One Health problem depicted is transmission of tuberculosis in free-living and semi-captive chimpanzees, and in humans living locally. This is categorized as a One Health problem, because interventions are needed in the human, semi-captive and free-living chimpanzee populations in order for disease transmission to be reduced; this will involve actors from all three dimensions, as otherwise the disease will re-emerge in the different sets of hosts due to the complex transmission cycle. Expected primary causes and transmission routes in sanctuary-housed chimpanzees are displayed with a pink outline. Unknown or not proven transmission routes have a blue question mark. In the five bubbles with different colours, we see transmission within the sub-populations involved. The

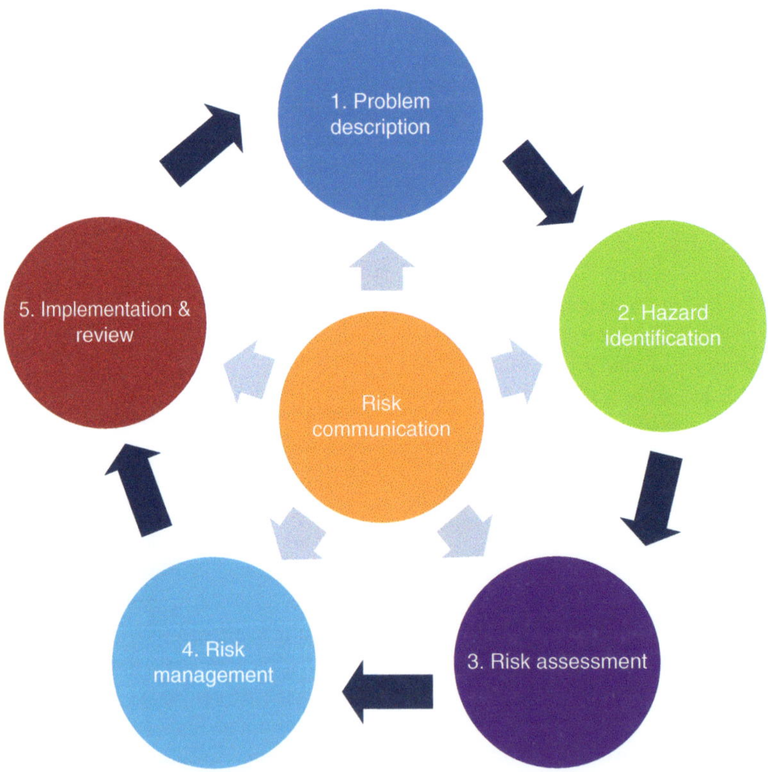
1. Problem description
2. Hazard identification
3. Risk assessment
4. Risk management
5. Implementation & review
Risk communication

Fig. 11.5. Risk communication within effective management of a health issue. Taken from the IUCN's wildlife disease risk analysis (DRA) programme (Jakob-Hoff *et al.*, 2014), with permission.

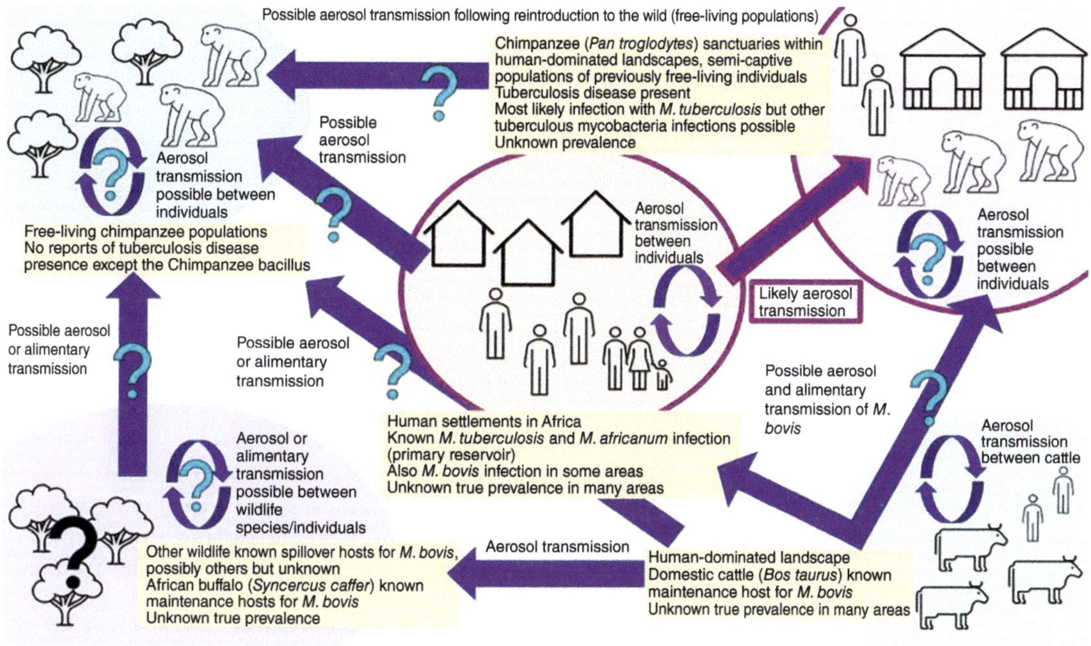

Fig. 11.6. Possible transmission routes for free-living and semi-captive sanctuary chimpanzee (*Pan troglodytes*) populations impacted by *Mycobacterium tuberculosis* and *M. bovis*. This figure was developed by J. Quinlan and used with permission, with information adapted from Coscolla *et al.* (2013); Fitzgerald and Kaneene (2013); Law and Floyd (2020); Sanchez and Hidalgo-Hermoso (2022).

boxes explain the main host and pathogens impacting them, where known. A possible target audience for this map is the Department of Environment and Forestry, as the department responsible for protecting the environment that this map represents. The advantages of using this figure are that it provides a visualization of where there is uncertainty in the system (question marks), and so helps decision makers to understand where to focus limited resources, to close data gaps. A disadvantage is that it could include misinterpretation without context, such as seeing chimpanzees as the disease threat, which would potentially lead to unintended consequences on the chimpanzee population, for example, less support for their conservation.

11.6 Strong Engagement and Effective Communication Facilitate Transdisciplinary Working

When developing transdisciplinary project work and findings, it is important to engage in an active, meaningful manner with relevant collaborators including scientific, other research community members, government and stakeholder groups. By holding prolonged discussions when progressing the One Health project, a common vocabulary, trust and respect will be established, leading to the most sustainable interventions. Also, as described in Chapter 10, a meaningful problem statement and framing and a participatory approach to intervention planning (see above) can promote engagement, ownership and agency. Throughout Chapters 10 and 11, the importance of communication is highlighted in multiple forms, which is also greatly supported by **reflexivity** as described in Chapter 6. Here, we want to reiterate the communication focus of the various steps in the One Health implementation cycle and emphasize critical messages.

11.6.1 Remember the importance of active, meaningful stakeholder engagement throughout, while considering communication challenges

Multidisciplinary, interdisciplinary and transdisciplinary teams present many challenges, including each team member having different strengths (and weaknesses). It is therefore important to maintain active, meaningful stakeholder engagement throughout, while considering communication challenges. Counter-productive interactions can be transformed into productive ones, including aspects of conflict (see Chapter 10), adherence, compliance, stewardship etc. used with advantage to improve participatory interactions in the team during participatory activities such as identifying and gathering your stakeholders, describing your system, and when exploring and developing potential interventions, as well as during dissemination of your work and overall findings.

11.6.2 Enable knowledge sharing among different audiences

Knowledge sharing between scientific and non-scientific collaborators is essential to ensure sound interventions that can help to produce positive health outcomes while minimizing eventual collateral damage. One Health practice implies reaching out and engaging with researchers, academics, practitioners and policy makers from multiple disciplines and fields as well as the local community. To share knowledge effectively, it is important that those sharing information understand their audience, and which aspects of knowledge need sharing and in what form. Thus, there are a variety of audiences, and they may have very different needs. For example, communities affected by the problem may need to know how an intervention can be done and how it will affect them, and not necessarily the minutiae of a situation.

To best learn about your stakeholders, listen to them to gain understanding of their perspective and interests; this will help you create the best sound bite for your work. Your messages must be clear, using plain, accessible language, and avoiding disciplinary or field-specific jargon and terminology; they must also present a positive tone. Your language needs to be gender-sensitive, meaning that your language reflects your consideration of gender equality (Anonymous, 2024). Gender equality in language is attained when any genders are addressed through language as persons of equal value, dignity, integrity and respect. Knowledge can be shared using (amongst other methods) storytelling, writing textbooks, teaching classes, designing games, experiencing arts, performing rituals, meditating together or conducting podcasts.

Any information shared must be cognizant of ethical considerations (e.g. personal identifiable information), intellectual property laws, invention patents and trade-marking concerns, particularly if working with non-academic partners who may not want others to use their ideas. Understanding data and making them understandable is critical to create trust and collaboration amongst all involved in solving complex health problems and advocating One Health. Methods such as using multiple data-sharing strategies, visual representation or visual elements like infographics, videos or illustrations can help make data more understandable. To help with understanding, it is recommended that you tell stories to capture attention and illustrate data relevance (so that data are compelling to the audience). Data sharing and presenting strategies are based on delivery by writing, speaking and using information technologies. Writing could be in peer-reviewed research publications, technical reports, book chapters and books, newsletters, and media advisories or press releases. Speaking in-person or online could be at conferences or congresses, giving lectures, presentations, webinars, workshops and training sessions, holding meetings or conversation sessions. Using information technologies includes via websites, online discussion forums, social media platforms (X, Facebook, Instagram, WhatsApp), podcasts and blogs or email listservs. This information sharing is an essential activity in One Health collaborations and an important, albeit insufficient, element for the knowledge integration that is described in Chapter 4.

Efficient and effective communication outputs can always be repurposed, with One Health groups not always having to start from scratch. For example, CDC's 13 steps to outbreak investigation, which includes media at multiple points (Anonymous, n.d. b), were incorporated with good impacts into a continuing professional development programme including a tuberculosis hierarchy of controls at the human–wildlife interface in Africa. Social media can also be a powerful tool for One Health in general (e.g. see Mekaru and Brownstein, 2014). It can be used to target specific problems, such as to detect and locate wildfires (Boulton *et al.*, 2016), identify **zoonotic disease** risk in human–wildlife interactions (McLean *et al.*, 2022), and monitor environmental observations (e.g. Mosites *et al.*, 2018). There is, however, also a risk to using social media. This was exemplified for COVID-19 in India, where social media had a major negative impact, spreading misinformation and creating fear around transmission of the virus via chickens. This led to a collapse in demand for chickens, which then had wide-reaching consequences for farmers and the birds (in terms of animal welfare), as well as other parts of the economy (Kolluri *et al.*, 2021).

11.6.3 Promote continuous learning in an iterative One Health process

One Health requires teamwork between people of different backgrounds, disciplines and strengths to prevent and solve health problems (Thomson, 2021). The One Health definition and approaches are increasingly appreciated, and gaining momentum in research, government and policy-maker environments, as well as in industry. At time of publication, there is a significant lack of specifically badged One Health education in primary and secondary schools, particularly in low- and middle-income countries. By teaching One Health in primary and secondary schools, communities are empowered, and future One Health interventions are more likely to be accepted by community members and leaders. At tertiary level, network organizations and postgraduate training in One Health approaches are increasingly available around the world and tailored to country requirements, e.g. Africa One Health University Network (AFROHUN), the USAID-funded Predict programme One Health Workforce, the UKRI GCRF HORN programme, the Network for Ecohealth and One Health (NEOH), One Health Commission, South East Asia One Health University Network (SEAOHUN) and SETAC. The Quadripartite Organizations (FAO, UNEP, WHO and WOAH) have also published their One Health Joint Plan of Action which includes an action track to enhance One Health capacities to strengthen health systems (World Health Organization *et al.*, 2022).

A noteworthy example of a One Health team is One Health Lessons. This global educational organization inspires children and adults to value One Health, with a vision to help societies create a more sustainable planet by delivering high-quality learning materials. Intern teams within the first two years of One Health Lessons have included professionals from: dentistry, public health, law, global health, medicine, economics, veterinary medicine, American Sign Language, environmental health and international relations, and nations including: Basque Country, Brazil, Canada, Ecuador, Guatemala, Indonesia, Hong Kong, Hungary, Japan, Malawi, Mexico, Nepal, Nigeria, North Macedonia, Taiwan, Turkey, Ukraine, UK, USA and Uganda. In the first two years, more than 25,000 students have been educated, creating over 25 partnerships of like-minded organizations, 11 age-appropriate lessons have been taught in over 25 languages (e.g. One Health Lessons, 2021), and 200 volunteers have been trained to teach lessons on One Health to children in their own communities through the Lesson Leaders Programme. One Health Lessons aims to snowball global networks of connected and trained people, by training volunteers to become Lesson Leaders who then deliver teaching. By facilitating global education on One Health, the programme will increase global understanding of health problems from a One Health perspective, facilitating the development of the most appropriate future solutions, including interventions.

Continuous learning is facilitated also through monitoring and evaluation by creating dynamic feedback loops that inform decision making. Monitoring and evaluation systems track progress, identify successes and challenges, and provide valuable insights into the effectiveness of a project or programme. It promotes a culture of adaptive management, where strategies are flexible and responsive to changing circumstances. By engaging in continuous learning through monitoring and evaluation activities, stakeholders can enhance their understanding of what works, what does not and why, leading to more impactful and sustainable outcomes. This is the focus of the next chapter.

References

Amuguni, H., Bikaako, W., Naigaga, I. and Bazeyo, W. (2019) Building a framework for the design and implementation of One Health curricula in East and Central Africa: OHCEAs One Health training modules development process. *One Health* 7, 002–2.

Andrus, R.A., Martinez, A.J., Jones, G.M. and Meddens, A.J.H. (2021) Assessing the quality of fire refugia for wildlife habitat. *Forest Ecology and Management* 482, 118868.

Anonymous (2015) Types of intervention and their development. In: Smith, P.G., Morrow, R.H. and Ross, D.A. (eds) *Field Trials of Health Interventions: A Toolbox.* (3rd edn). OUP Oxford, Oxford, UK.

Anonymous (2017) International Union for Conservation of Nature and Natural Resources. Available at: https://www.

iucnredlist.org/species/120588639/247632253 (accessed 5 August 2024).

Anonymous (2021) Snow Leopard at the San Diego Zoo Suspected Positive for COVID-19. Available at: https://sandiegozoowildlifealliance.org/pr/SnowLeopardatSanDiegoZooSuspectedPositiveforCOVID-19 (accessed 5 August 2024).

Anonymous (2022a) Water Quality in Rivers. Fourth Report of Session 2021–22. House of Commons Environmental Audit Committee: Parliamentary Copyright House of Commons.

Anonymous (2022b) Concept System1 Global MAX. Available at: https://www.conceptsystems.com/home (accessed 5 August 2024).

Anonymous (2024) Gender-sensitive communication. Available at: https://eige.europa.eu/publications-resources/toolkits-guides/gender-sensitive-communication?language_content_entity=en (accessed 5 August 2024).

Anonymous (n.d. a) groupwisdom™. Available at: https://groupwisdom.com/ (accessed 5 August 2024).

Anonymous (n.d. b) Section 2: Steps of an Outbreak Investigation: Centers for Disease Control. Available at: https://archive.cdc.gov/#/details?url=https://www.cdc.gov/csels/dsepd/ss1978/lesson6/section2.html (accessed 5 August 2024).

Ashworth, J. (2021) The Deadly Effects of Sewage Pollution on Nature Natural History Museum. Available at: https://www.nhm.ac.uk/discover/news/2021/november/the-deadly-effects-of-sewage-pollution-on-nature.html (accessed 5 August 2024).

Bagnol, B., Clarke, E., Li, M., Maulaga, W., Lumbwe, H., McConchie, R. *et al.* (2016) Transdisciplinary project communication and knowledge sharing experiences in Tanzania and Zambia through a One Health lens. *Frontiers in Public Health* 4, 10. DOI: 10.3389/fpubh.2016.00010.

Boulton, C., Shotton, H. and Williams, H. (2016) Using Social Media to Detect and Locate Wildfires. *Proceedings of the International AAAI Conference on Web and Social Media* 10(2), 178–186.

Coscolla, M., Lewin, A., Metzger, S., Maetz-Rennsing, K., Calvignac-Spencer, S. *et al.* (2013) Novel mycobacterium tuberculosis complex isolate from a wild chimpanzee. *Emerging Infectious Diseases* 19(6), 969–976.

Daly, N. (2021) More Species are Found to be Susceptible to the Coronavirus, with Most Cases Detected in Zoos. Available at: https://www.nationalgeographic.com/animals/article/more-animal-species-are-getting-covid-19-for-the-first-time (accessed 10 December 2021).

Falloon, P., Bebber, D.P., Dalin, C., Ingram, J., Mitchell, D.M., Hartley, T. *et al.* (2022) What do changing weather and climate shocks and stresses mean for the UK food system? *Environmental Research Letters* 17, 051001.

Fitzgerald, S.D. and Kaneene, J.B. (2013) Wildlife reservoirs of bovine tuberculosis worldwide: Hosts, pathology, surveillance, and control. *Veterinary Pathology* 50(3), 488–499.

Friedson-Ridenour, S. and Pierotti, R.S. (2019) Competing priorities: Women's microenterprises and household relationships. *World Development* 121, 53–62.

Garnier, J., Savić, S., Boriani, E., Bagnol, B., Häsler, B. and Kock, R. (2020) Helping to heal nature and ourselves through human-rights-based and gender-responsive One Health. *One Health Outlook* 2.

Garnier, J., Savić, S., Cediel, N., Barato, P., Boriani, E. *et al.* (2022) Mainstreaming gender-responsive One Health: Now is the time. *Frontiers in Public Health* 10, 845866.

Gibbs, E.P.J. (2018) Musings on the future direction of One Health, William Hunting and tuberculosis, while listening to blackbirds sing. *Veterinary Record* 183(2), 57–62.

Gross-Sorokin, M.Y., Roast, S.D. and Brighty, G.C. (2006) Assessment of feminization of male fish in English rivers by the environment agency of England and Wales. *Environment Health Perspective* 114(Suppl 1), 147–151.

Harper, C.A., Ford, W.M., Lashley, M.A., Moorman, C.E. and Stambaugh, M.C. (2016) Fire effects on wildlife in the central hardwoods and Appalachian regions, USA. *Fire Ecology* 12(2), 127–159.

Hawe, P., Shiell, A. and Riley, T. (2009) Theorising interventions as events in systems. *American Journal of Community Psychology* 43(3–4), 267–276.

Jakob-Hoff, R.M., MacDiarmid, S.C., Lees, C., Miller, P.S., Travis, D. *et al.* (2014) *Manual of Procedures for Wildlife Disease Risk Analysis.* World Organisation for Animal Health, Paris.

Kane, M. and Trochim, W.M.K. (2007) *Concept Mapping for Planning and Evaluation.* Sage Publications, Thousand Oaks, California.

Kaufmann, S.H.E. (2020) Vaccination against tuberculosis: Revamping BCG by molecular genetics guided by immunology. *Frontiers in Immunology* 11, 316.

Kinnaird, M.F. and O'Brien, T.G. (1998) Ecological effects of wildfire on lowland rainforest in Sumatra. *Conservation Biology* 12(5), 954–956.

Kolluri, G., Tyagi, J.S. and Sasidhar, P.V.K. (2021) Research note: Indian poultry industry vis-à-vis coronavirus disease 2019: A situation analysis report. *Poultry Science* 100(3), 100828.

Law, I. and Floyd, K. (2020) Group tATPS. National tuberculosis prevalence surveys in Africa, 2008–2016: An overview of results and lessons learned. *Tropical Medicine and International Health* 25(11), 1308–1327.

Mariki, S.B., Svarstad, H. and Benjaminsen, T.A. (2015) Elephants over the cliff: Explaining wildlife killings in Tanzania. *Land Use Policy* 44, 19–30.

McLean, H.E., Jaebker, L.M., Anderson, A.M., Teel, T.L., Bright, A.D. *et al.* (2022) Social media as a window into human-wildlife interactions and zoonotic disease risk: An examination of wild pig hunting videos on YouTube. *Human Dimensions of Wildlife* 27(4), 307–320.

Mekaru, S.R. and Brownstein, J.S. (2014) One Health in social networks and social media. *Revue Scientifique et Technique* 33(2), 629–637.

Mosites, E., Lujan, E., Brook, M., Brubaker, M., Roehl, D., Tcheripanoff, M. *et al.* (2018) Environmental observation, social media, and One Health action: A description of the Local Environmental Observer (LEO) network. *One Health* 6, 29–33.

Mott, J.A., Meyer, P., Mannino, D., Redd, S.C., Smith, E.M. *et al.* (2002) Wildland forest fire smoke: Health effects and intervention evaluation, Hoopa, California, 1999. *The Western Journal of Medicine* 176(3), 157–162.

Nzietchueng, S., Kitua, A., Nyatanyi, T. and Rwego, I.B. (2023) Facilitating implementation of the one health approach: A definition of a one health intervention. *One Health* 16, 100491.

One Health Lessons (2021) The Story Behind the COVID-19 Vaccine. Available at: https://onehealthlessons.org/covid19_vaccine (accessed 5 August 2024).

Rüegg, S.R., McMahon, B.J., Häsler, B., Esposito, R., Nielsen, L.R., Ifejika Speranza, C. *et al.* (2017) A blueprint to evaluate One Health. *Frontier Public Health* 5, 20.

San Miguel, M. (2023) Frontiers in complex systems. *Frontiers in Complex Systems* 1, 1080801.

Sanchez, C.R. and Hidalgo-Hermoso, E. (2022) *Mycobacterium tuberculosis* sensu stricto in African apes, what is its true health impact? *Pathogens* 11(5), 484.

Savigny, D.D. and Adam, T. (2009) *Systems Thinking for Health Systems Strengthening Alliance for Health Policy and Systems Research.* WHO, Geneva.

Scholes, L., Faulkner, H., Tapsell, S. and Downward, S. (2008) Urban rivers as pollutant sinks and sources: A public health concern for recreational river users? *Water, Air, and Soil Pollution: Focus* 8(5), 543–553.

Schweizer, D.W. and Cisneros, R. (2017) Forest fire policy: Change conventional thinking of smoke management to prioritize long-term air quality and public health. *Air Quality, Atmosphere and Health* 10(1), 33–36.

Sherman, J., Unwin, S., Travis, D.A., Oram, F., Wich, S.A. *et al.* (2021) Disease risk and conservation implications of orangutan translocations. *Frontiers in Veterinary Science* 8.

Thomson, D. (2021) *The Art of Science Communication: Sharing Knowledge with Students, the Public, and Policymakers.* Thomson Publishing, USA.

Tiedemann, A.R., Klemmedson, J.O. and Bull, E.L. (2000) Solution of forest health problems with prescribed fire: Are forest productivity and wildlife at risk? *Forest Ecology and Management* 127(1), 1–18.

Togami, E., Gardy, J.L., Hansen, G.R., Poste, G.H., Rizzo, D.M., Wilson, M.E. *et al.* (2018) Core Competencies in One Health Education: What are we Missing? NAM Perspectives Discussion Paper, National Academy of Medicine, Washington, DC.

Trochim, W.M.K. (1989) An introduction to concept mapping for planning and evaluation. *Evaluation and Program Planning* 12(1), 1–16.

Trochim, W.M., Cabrera, D.A., Milstein, B., Gallagher, R.S. and Leischow, S.J. (2006) Practical challenges of systems thinking and modeling in public health. *American Journal of Public Health* 96(3), 538–546.

Trochim, W.M. and McLinden, D. (2017) Introduction to a special issue on concept mapping. *Evaluation and Program Planning* 60, 166–175.

Trumbore, S., Brando, P. and Hartmann, H. (2015) Forest health and global change. *Science* 349(6250), 814–818.

Voinov, A., Jenni, K., Gray, S., Kolagani, N., Glynn, P., Bommel, P. *et al.* (2018) Tools and methods in participatory modeling: Selecting the right tool for the job. *Environmental Modelling and Software* 109.

Whitmee, S., Haines, A., Beyrer, C., Boltz, F., Capon, A.G. *et al.* (2015) Safeguarding human health in the Anthropocene epoch: Report of The Rockefeller Foundation-Lancet Commission on planetary health. *Lancet* 386(10007), 1973–2028.

Williams, B. (2021) *Systems Diagrams* (1st edn). Available at: https://gum.co/systemdiagrams (accessed 5 August 2024).

Wolf, T.M., Miller, P., Primus, A. and Travis, D.A. (2019) Aquatic disease risk analysis: Applications for the conservation and management of freshwater mollusks. *Freshwater Mollusk Biology and Conservation* 22, 90–97.

World Health Organization, Food, Agriculture Organization of the United Nations, World Organisation for Animal Health, United Nations Environment Programme (2022) *One Health Joint Plan of Action (2022–2026): Working Together for the Health of Humans, Animals, Plants and the Environment.* World Health Organization, Geneva.

12 Evaluation of One Health Initiatives

Ilias Chantziaras[1,2], Joana Pessoa[3], Daniele de Meneghi[2,4], Maurizio Aragrande[2,5], Ana Glória Fonseca[2,6] and Barbara Häsler[2,7]

[1]Faculty of Veterinary Medicine, Ghent University, Merelbeke, Belgium; [2]Network for Ecohealth and One Health (NEOH); [3]Technical University of Denmark, National Food Institute, Kongens Lyngby, Denmark; [4]Department of Veterinary Sciences, University of Turin, Turin, Italy; [5]Department of Agricultural and Food Sciences, University of Bologna, Bologna, Italy; [6]NOVA Medical School, Campo Mártires da Patria, Lisbon, and Department of Medicine, Hospital Garcia de Orta, Almada, Portugal; [7]Veterinary Epidemiology Economics and Public Health Group, Department of Pathobiology and Population Sciences, Royal Veterinary College, London, UK

Contents

DOI: 10.1079/9781800623002.0013

Chapter Overview

Elevator pitch

This chapter will help you to familiarize yourself with the use of standardized methodologies to evaluate One Health initiatives. It helps you to understand how you can assess the effect your initiative is having and provide evidence on the added effect of integrated and transdisciplinary approaches. This is of great importance when communicating with governments, researchers, funding bodies and other stakeholders.

Book objectives the chapter relates to

☐ 1. Understand what One Health and Ecohealth mean
☑ 2. Think in a One Health and Ecohealth way
☐ 3. Apply One Health and Ecohealth in their professional and personal life
☐ 4. Know how to share One Health and Ecohealth knowledge
☐ 5. Integrate One Health and Ecohealth knowledge actively
☑ 6. Acquire or enhance core One Health competencies

One Health competencies covered

☐ 1. Effective communication
☐ 2. Collaborative and resilient working
☑ 3. Systems understanding
☐ 4. Transdisciplinarity
☐ 5. Social, cultural and gender equity and inclusiveness
☑ 6. Collective learning and reflective practice
☑ 7. One Health concepts
☐ 8. Theoretical and methodological pluralism
☐ 9. Harnessing uncertainty, paradox and limited knowledge

After working through this chapter, you will understand the methodologies available to evaluate One Health initiatives and their strengths and weaknesses and know what to consider when planning an evaluation of One Health.

Learning outcomes

1. Understand and use standardized methodologies to evaluate One Health initiatives.
2. Know different existing tools and frameworks that are used to evaluate different One Health initiatives and their strengths and weaknesses.
3. Be able to make an informed choice of a suitable evaluation tool according to the context, intended use and/or discipline.

Summary

This chapter equips you with the tools to evaluate One Health initiatives that address health issues at the intersection of humans, animals and the environment. It emphasizes the importance of a systematic approach to assess these initiatives' effectiveness and impact. The chapter uses the Theory of Change (ToC) as a framework for outlining how the initiative will achieve its goals. Stakeholder involvement is a key theme, as you will learn how to collaborate with them to define the evaluation approach and select measurable indicators based on the ToC. The chapter also dives into data collection methods for both quantitative (surveys) and qualitative (interviews) data. Ultimately, it equips you to use evaluation results to inform decisions, improve programme design and strengthen future One Health efforts, ensuring a lasting positive influence on interconnected One Health topics across various sectors.

12.1 Introduction

By definition, a One Health initiative spans collaboration across various **sectors**, and it is expected that effects are seen in more than one sector and that social **impacts** are generated (Rüegg *et al.*, 2018a). Capturing these effects is an important aspect in the monitoring and **evaluation** of One Health.

Evaluating One Health initiatives is essential to ensure **effectiveness** and **efficiency**, and facilitate the generation of impacts on human, animal, plant and environment **health** while contributing to the overall **wellbeing** of communities and **ecosystems**. It allows a holistic assessment of the effectiveness of addressing interconnected health issues and their impacts. The evaluation results inform decision making and can be combined with economic analyses to provide evidence on the return on investment (Narrod *et al.*, 2012). Moreover, the evaluation fosters continuous learning, adaptation and **sustainability**, ensuring that actions are efficient, successful and capable of safeguarding wellbeing in the face of emerging health challenges. Because of the interconnected and cross-sectoral nature of One Health, it is important to think about how to capture the different integrated activities and effects.

One Health activities are expected to be beneficial to multiple **STAKEHOLDERS**. Among them, one main group of beneficiaries of One Health activities are usually social **ACTORS**, who may be a source of information to understand the complexity of the system and, at the same time, be actors in specific activities. They are defined as a subgroup of stakeholders such as 'any individual, group or organisation who acts, or takes part' in the context of a One Health initiative (Anonymous, 1999). Collectively they are referred to as stakeholders in Chapter 10, where we explore in detail the importance of wide engagement and community of practice building to include and integrate diverse **knowledge** (including social knowledge) in the design of the One Health project in a transdisciplinary process (see Chapter 3 for **transdisciplinarity**). This transdisciplinary engagement of stakeholders in all parts of the project implementation is a critical aspect of One Health and is expected to increase the likelihood that One Health initiatives will lead to successful **outcomes**.

One Health commonly aims to achieve distinct outcomes including sustainability, health and **welfare**, **interspecies equity** and stewardship, effectiveness and efficiency (Rüegg *et al.*, 2017). When referring to cross-sector impacts, it means that the activities conducted in one sector generate effects not just in the same sector, but also in other sectors (Fig. 12.1). They also include the diverse causal relationships such as direct or indirect causations, feedback loops and other interactions that mutually influence these sectors.

Sectoral activities are routed in the structures that were built over time in our societies and span people, institutions and organizations with social, political and anthropological dimensions. They are embedded in society and may impact it in different ways depending on the social organization (Speranza *et al.*, 2018). Social organization is a complex and dynamic concept, largely varying across cultures and time, in close mutual influence with the economic and political organization (Blane *et al.*, 1996). Social groups (i.e. parts or groups of the society that show a relative homogeneity according to one or more variables such as revenue, lifestyle, workers of certain sectors, religion, age) may be affected in different ways by One Health initiatives. For example, a programme against rabies may have a bigger impact on low-income people working or living in close contact with potentially infectious animals. **Gender** is a widely recognized factor that may differentiate the impacts of health programmes because of the different characteristics and roles of genders in society also in relation to health (for example because of specific health problems, access to services, degree of economic or moral independence). Any society is subjected to rules and laws, decided and administered by public institutions that play an important role in the implementation of One Health initiatives (Burris *et al.*, 2010). Consumers (i.e. people who spend their revenue to purchase goods or services in a market context) may also be impacted by a One Health initiative.

Importantly, an evaluation should not only consider the positive outcomes of a One Health initiative but consider both the negative and positive changes that are generated by a One Health initiative to gain a full picture. This includes consideration of **emergent properties**, i.e. new characteristics or behaviours that arise from the interactions within a system that often go beyond what was initially anticipated. For example, a rabies control activity focusing on awareness raising may cause increased reporting of cases (Hasanov *et al.*, 2018), but also stimulate undesired behaviours. Promotional

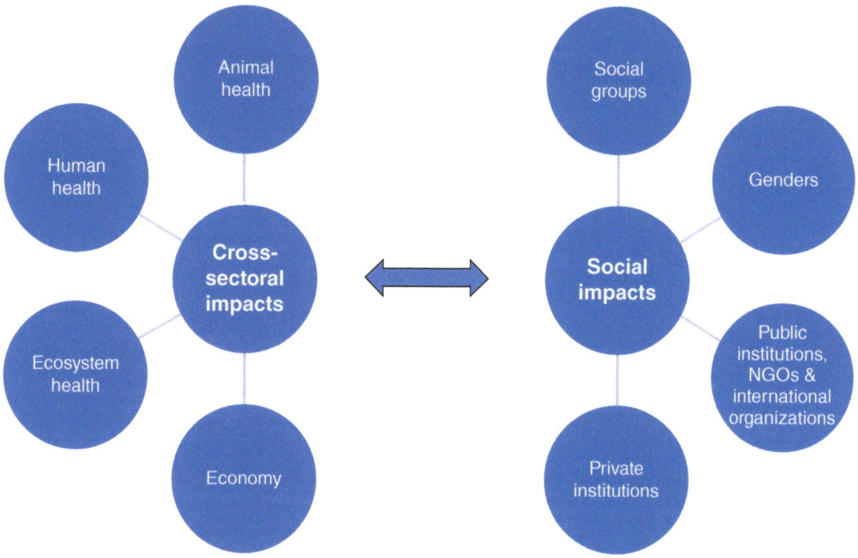

Fig. 12.1. Cross-sectoral and social impacts of One Health. Developed by the authors.

materials depicting aggressive-looking dogs and severe bites may unintentionally reinforce misconceptions about rabies risk and bite severity, potentially discouraging people from seeking care for a seemingly minor bite or scratch (Castillo-Neyra *et al.*, 2020).

12.1.1 The importance of monitoring and evaluation in the One Health implementation cycle

Evaluation of One Health initiatives (e.g. an intervention) provides evidence-based insights into its effectiveness, informs decision making, enhances accountability, facilitates learning and adaptation, and ensures **value** for money (Speranza *et al.*, 2018). By systematically assessing how well an initiative is working, decision makers can optimize their efforts to address complex challenges. It involves gathering and analysing **data** to understand how well an initiative is achieving its intended objectives and outcomes and provide evidence-based insights into the success, strengths, weaknesses, and areas for improvement of the subject under review.

Although we highlight evaluation as a particular section in the One Health implementation cycle (Fig. 12.2), monitoring and evaluation should be more of a fundamental attitude throughout the project than a single activity at its end. Evaluations can occur before, during and/or after a project implementation. However, at this last stage at the end of the cycle, we take more time and effort to check how it went and what has been achieved. Depending on how a One Health initiative was evaluated and what was found, we might change it, rethink it, or keep it the same, before we start the cycle again. This is particularly important when continuing through multiple cycles and over longer periods.

In One Health initiatives, the above focus on the improvement of the initiative and ensuring that it is fit for purpose is very important, as the ultimate objective is to achieve or improve One Health **OUTCOMES** (Zinsstag *et al.*, 2009). The One Health evaluation community is, however, also interested in understanding whether more or less One Health or weaker or stronger One Health allows the achievement of better outcomes (Rüegg *et al.*, 2018b). One of the underlying tenets of One Health claims that improved coordination, collaboration, capacity building and communication (the 4 Cs) in One Health allows achieving improved outcomes (Mettenleiter *et al.*, 2023). To be able to answer this question in full, it is necessary to understand both the strength of a One Health initiative (or its 'One Healthness') and compare it to the resulting outcomes (Rüegg *et al.*, 2018a). A growing number of evaluations of this kind will allow building an evidence base that can be used in future **meta-analyses** (i.e. the combination and

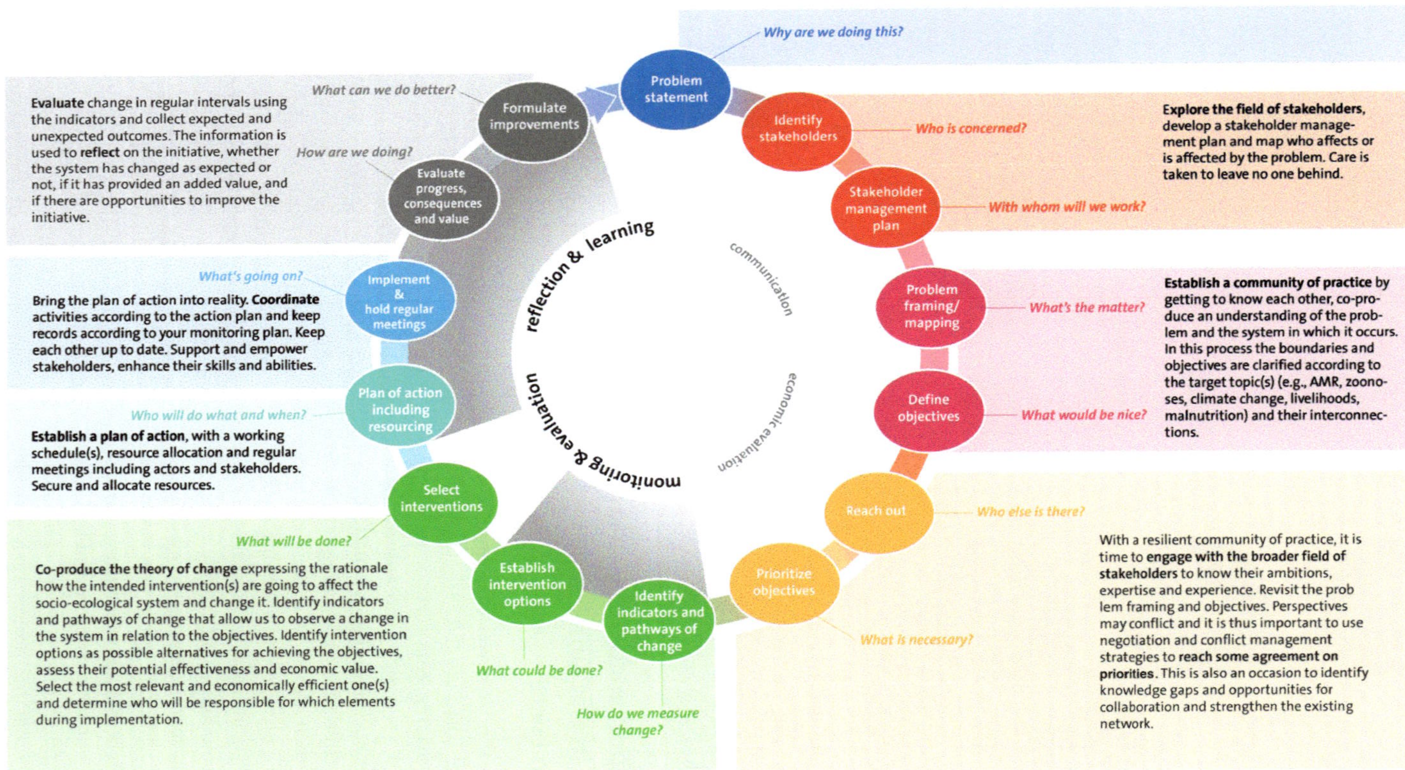

Fig. 12.2. Important stages along the One Health implementation cycle. The areas covered in this chapter in relation to the evaluation of One Health are highlighted in the centre. Developed by the authors.

analysis of results from multiple independent studies on a particular topic or research question) to establish the relationship between One Healthness and outcomes. Moreover, an individual evaluation allows generating useful insights for decision makers on the strengths and weaknesses of the 4 Cs in their initiatives.

12.2 Evaluating One Health

12.2.1 General overview

Evaluation is the process of systematically and objectively determining the relevance, effectiveness and impact of organized initiatives in the light of their objectives. To produce accurate findings it should be practical, realistic (context-based) and feasible, and conducted ethically according to a set of guidelines or principles. Constraints and limitations related to resources, time and political context also need to be considered.

Defining the goal of the evaluation is an important first step to establishing an evaluation plan and is crucial to understand the scope, and expectations, and to allocate time and budget to this task.

Because of the complexity and multitude of relationships within a system, when evaluating One Health initiatives, it is essential to focus on the aspects outlined in Fig. 12.3.

In the Network for Evaluation of One Health (NEOH) evaluation handbook *Integrated Approaches to Health: a Handbook for the Evaluation of One Health* (Rüegg *et al.*, 2018a), detailed guidance is provided on these general steps including the description of an overarching evaluation framework, three chapters on key outcomes and their meaning, and measurement and **knowledge integration** in relation to the policy cycle.

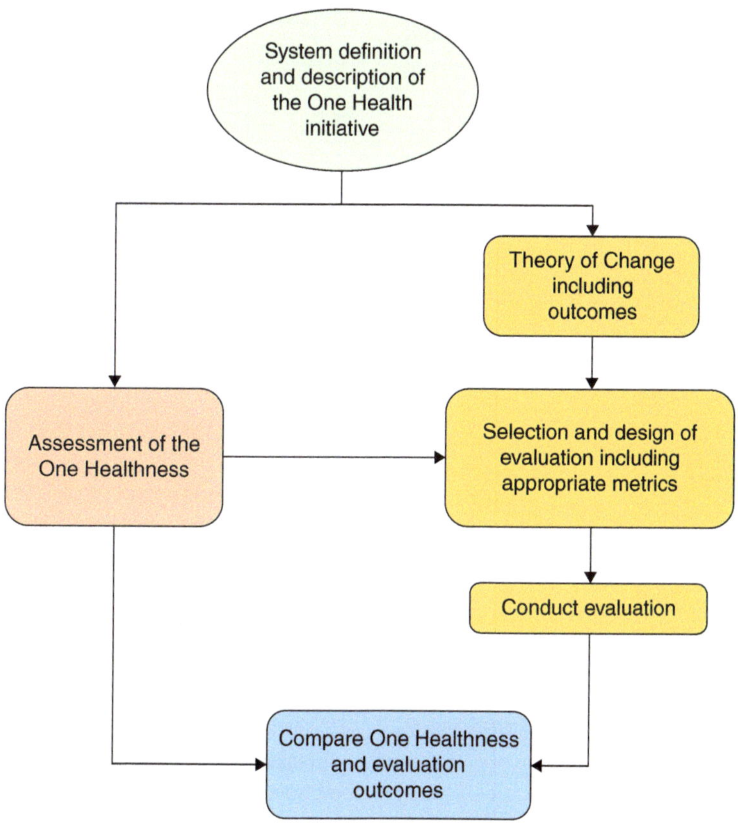

Fig. 12.3. Simplified overview of the evaluation framework elaborated by the Network for Evaluation of One Health (adapted based on Rüegg *et al.*, 2018a).

The evaluation framework suggests as a first element the system definition and the description of the One Health initiative, which has been covered in Chapters 10 and 11. Next, it suggests a **THEORY OF CHANGE** (ToC) to identify expected outcomes and create the foundation for unexpected outcomes. The One Healthness assessment focuses on the operations and infrastructure contributing to the One Health initiative. The selection and design of the evaluation including appropriate metrics is an essential part to determine outcomes achieved. Finally, the One Healthness and the outcomes can be compared to gain information on whether the strength of One Health influences the outcomes.

In this chapter, we are emphasizing the elaboration of the ToC as a critical method to understand the expected pathways to change, the assessment of the One Health aspects of the initiative, the selection of the evaluation design and the measurement of indicators to support the implementation cycle. We are also looking at some tools that may be helpful when conducting evaluations of One Health initiatives.

12.2.2 Assess the One Health aspects of the initiative

An important aspect in One Health evaluation is to assess the One Health aspects of an initiative. This helps us to see how initiatives grow, their structures, and the activities they involve, such as communication and advocacy. One Health initiatives focus on sharing, collaborating and learning across different fields and sectors, which affects how these initiatives are delivered, how they cause change, and how external factors shape them.

In the NEOH evaluation framework (Rüegg *et al.*, 2018a), we used process evaluation to understand how initiatives are carried out (like the methods and resources used), how they cause change (like how people interact with them), and how external factors affect them. We identified six aspects that collectively reflect the 'OH-ness' of an initiative, namely: (i) One Health thinking; (ii) One Health planning; (iii) One Health working; (iv) sharing; (v) learning; and (vi) systemic organization. We further created assessment tools like the OH index (OHI) and OH ratio (OHR) to evaluate these aspects in a holistic way. These tools use questions and scoring systems to measure how well an initiative meets these One Health characteristics. The goal is to ensure that our evaluation methods capture the unique aspects of One Health initiatives effectively. This includes the assessment of the extent and quality of collaboration and coordination among experts from different fields and groups in society to address the complex health issues at the human–animal–plant–environment interface as well as the quality and extent of community involvement, participation and ownership including the alignment with community needs, priorities, and social and cultural practices. Moreover, it includes looking at the extent and quality of communication and sharing (including data, resources, knowledge) between the different groups involved and the learning that is occurring at the individual, group and institutional level. Finally, it looks at how effective leadership helps to navigate **complex systems** by leveraging key points of influence to drive change. You will find an applied example later in the chapter.

12.2.3 Co-produce a ToC, select evaluation design and indicators of change

12.2.3.1 Definition and overview

A ToC is a comprehensive and systematic description of how and why a desired change is expected to occur. It explains all the different pathways that might lead to the desired effect of an initiative showing the activities, **outputs**, outcomes and impact of an initiative as well as outlining (and explaining) the causal linkages, assumptions and barriers. Each effect is shown in a logical relationship to the other elements. The ToC describes how an initiative is meant to change the current situation toward the desired objectives. In Chapter 10, we have seen the multiple steps needed from problem statement to the analysis and engagement of stakeholders and a process of agreeing on prioritized objectives. In Chapter 11, we have built on this to elaborate interventions; the ToC fits into that process.

A ToC is a dynamic and adaptable concept utilized throughout an implementation cycle to guide actions and measure progress. Initially, a ToC outlines the logic behind how and why a desired change is expected to occur. It identifies the key interventions, activities and outcomes that lead to the desired impact. As the implementation progresses and data and information are collected, however, the ToC requires revisiting at regular intervals. The initial ToC serves as a roadmap, providing a structured framework for understanding the expected cause-and-effect relationships between activities and outcomes. As data are collected and analysed during implementation, the ToC may need adjustments based on real-world insights, emerging challenges or unexpected outcomes. This iterative process allows stakeholders to assess whether the planned interventions are effective, identify areas needing improvement, and make informed decisions to optimize the intervention strategy.

In essence, the ToC evolves alongside the implementation process, reflecting a continuous learning and adaptive approach to achieve meaningful and sustainable change.

Task: Figure 12.4 shows a ToC from a project in Northern Botswana to tackle illegal bushmeat hunting (Heermans *et al.*, 2021), as this is an important contributor to the decline of wildlife populations. Bushmeat refers to the meat of wild animals from forests or other natural habitats encompassing a wide variety of wildlife species, including mammals, birds, reptiles and amphibians, that are hunted (often illegally) for subsistence or trade (Cawthorn and Hoffman, 2015). The ToC was developed to facilitate the elaboration of a novel community-based approach focusing on husbandry and livestock production. Have a look at the ToC and think about what it tells you and what the different boxes and arrows illustrate.

Example answer: The ToC shows a common structure using activities, outputs, outcomes and impact and identifies three main pathways. The impact encompasses the intended positive, primary and secondary long-term effects produced by the initiative; it is commonly outside the control of the people implementing the initiative (OECD, 2023). We then see three levels of outcomes. Outcomes are the likely or achieved short-term and medium-term effects of a One Health initiative's outputs or deliverables. They usually occur along a wider time horizon and with an amplification effect that is outside of our control, but still within our sphere of influence. Here, we are looking at pathway-specific outcomes, as well as cross-cutting outcomes, which may be intermediate outcomes towards achievement of the overall outcome. In the red boxes we see the results, also called outputs or deliverables. They usually constitute the products, capital goods and services that result from a One Health initiative; they are commonly within the control of the people implementing the initiative. An activity in a ToC refers to a specific action or intervention designed to bring about a desired change or outcome. Next down come the actions or activities or, in other words, the practical steps or strategies implemented within an initiative to achieve the intended goals. Here, both implementation-specific activities are given as well as activities to generate an enabling environment. Finally, we see the pathways that involve enhancing local enforcement institutions, creating incentives for responsible ecosystem management, and reducing the challenges associated with coexisting with wildlife. Pathways are the sequences or routes to outcomes or impacts; they describe the logical connections between inputs, activities, outputs, outcomes and impacts. Here, the effectiveness of these pathways relies on foundational enabling actions, such as establishing robust institutional frameworks, empowering communities to adopt sustainable farming practices, and fostering commitments to manage resources responsibly, enhancing resilience to environmental and economic challenges. What is missing in this ToC are the barriers to change and the assumptions supporting it.

12.2.3.2 Intended and unintended outcomes

In One Health, sustainability, health and welfare, interspecies equity and stewardship, effectiveness and efficiency are key intended outcomes (Rüegg *et al.*, 2017):

- **Health outcomes:** Assess the initiative's impact on improving health outcomes, including reductions in disease transmission, morbidity and mortality in humans, animals and plants.
- **Environmental outcomes:** Examine how the initiative addresses ecosystem health concerns, such as the preservation of biodiversity, ecosystem balance and reduction of pollution (see Chapter 7 for more details).
- **Social outcomes:** Evaluate the initiative's social impact by assessing changes in community awareness, behaviour and engagement, such as community participation, empowerment and equity in

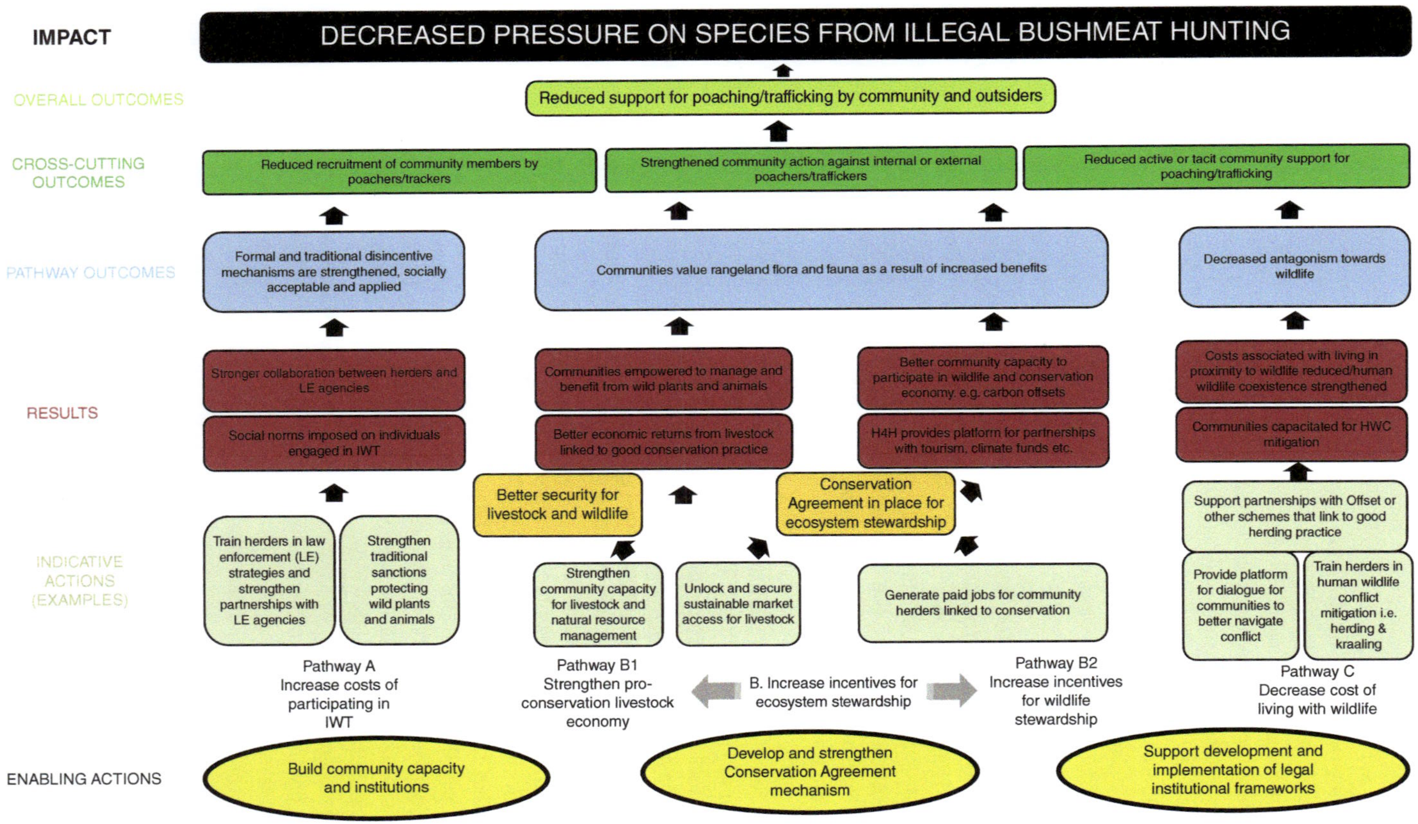

Fig. 12.4. A Theory of Change (ToC) of identifying the roles agropastoral communities can have in decreasing the pressures from illegal bushmeat hunting. IWT, illegal wildlife trade; LE, law enforcement. Figure from Heermans *et al.* (2021), unmodified (license CC4.0: https://creativecommons.org/licenses/by/4.0/).

decision-making processes (see Chapter 8 and Chapter 9 for more details).

- **Economic outcomes:** Analyse the economic value of the initiative, including its economic impact on communities, healthcare systems, and the different sectors involved or affected (see Chapter 13 for more details).

While these are the outcomes that we are commonly striving for in One Health, there are also unintended effects and we need to be prepared to capture those when implementing the initiative. Emerging properties refer to new characteristics or behaviours that arise from the interactions within a system, often beyond what was initially anticipated. These properties can lead to non-linear impacts, where small changes in one part of the system can result in significant, unexpected effects elsewhere. Therefore, a systematic approach based on the ToC, while essential for standardizing evaluation, must also remain open to capturing potentially emerging systemic effects through non-linear impact evaluation methods.

Non-linear impact evaluation is a methodology that recognizes the complex and interconnected nature of interventions, such as those in One Health systems, and aims to capture the non-linear relationships and emergent properties that can arise within these systems. Unlike traditional linear evaluation methods that assume cause-and-effect relationships follow a straightforward path, non-linear impact evaluation acknowledges that outcomes can be influenced by multiple factors interacting in dynamic and often unpredictable ways.

By incorporating non-linear impact evaluation approaches, we can better capture the complexity and dynamism of systems like we see in One Health initiatives. This approach acknowledges that initiatives are embedded in dynamic and interconnected systems where feedback loops, unintended consequences and emergent properties are common. It allows us to not only assess intended outcomes but also detect and understand unforeseen effects, contributing to more comprehensive and insightful evaluations.

12.2.3.3 Systems thinking and participation

Systems thinking is based on **interdisciplinarity** and transdisciplinarity, meaning that the combination of academic and social knowledge in a transdisciplinary, multi-actor approach allows for the understanding of a system's complexity and for the variety of relationships (see Chapter 3 on transdisciplinarity and Chapter 10 for information on systems thinking). Thus, stakeholder engagement is crucial in this process, as it allows for a comprehensive understanding of the problem context, diverse stakeholder roles and expectations for change. The steps in Chapter 10 and Chapter 11 have led to a situation where workshops, focus groups, interviews and surveys can be employed to gather inputs and co-create the ToC collaboratively and in a participatory way. As seen previously, using systems mapping techniques is essential to visualize the interconnectedness and dynamics within the system. This includes identifying key actors, resources, causal links, feedback loops and system structures that influence the problem and potential solutions. Problem analysis tools such as problem trees and causal loop diagrams help to uncover root causes, drivers and underlying issues contributing to the problem. A practical approach (Belcher and Claus, 2020) is provided with useful preparatory documents. More recently, Claus *et al.* (2023) provide guidance on how to build further ToC for transdisciplinary research.

The elaboration of a visual representation of the ToC is an essential aspect, defining clear long-term and intermediate outcomes aligned with the desired change and a structured framework depicting the pathways that connect activities, outputs, outcomes and impacts. **Assumptions**, underlying beliefs about necessary conditions for outcomes, must be identified, evaluated for plausibility and challenged. Stakeholders' diverse perspectives aid in this process. Testing key assumptions during implementation, documenting rationales, and regularly reviewing and updating assumptions based on new information are vital. Risk and uncertainty associated with assumptions should be considered, and contingency plans developed.

Regular iterative reviews and adaptations of the ToC are necessary to respond to changing contexts, emerging insights and new data gathered during implementation. This iterative and participatory approach fosters a dynamic ToC that guides effective decision making and course corrections, leading to impactful interventions in complex settings.

One Health initiatives, with their inherent complexity and far-reaching impacts, demand a comprehensive evaluation process to ensure their success and maximize their benefits across human, animal, and environment health. Including an evaluation process is a crucial step to not only validate the initiative but also to improve its effectiveness (Sandberg *et al.*, 2021); to inform decision making; to generate science-based evidence and build knowledge on efficacy, effectiveness and efficiency. Evaluation results are valuable for all those involved in project management and decision making, such as project administrators, funding partners, and policy and decision makers.

An example focusing on health more closely may be found in the vaccination of an animal population. The output of a vaccination plan is the number of vaccinated humans or animals as the result of a vaccination campaign (the process) (Fig. 12.5).

Outcomes are the consequences of the inputs. Vaccination is meant to protect individuals against a disease: the greater the number of vaccinated individuals, the lower the diffusion of the disease in the society. The improvement of the health status of the population can be considered an outcome of the vaccination campaign. In turn, improved population health allows for a series of secondary outcomes or impacts: a healthier population has greater productivity, spends less money for healthcare, shows a stronger sense of confidence and trust in societal institutions; if animals are vaccinated, producers may have greater access to domestic and foreign markets; net public health expenses may lower because of vaccination. Conversely, unexpected outcomes may appear (i.e. negative reaction to vaccination), which result in negative outcomes lowering the social benefits of vaccination. All of these effects contribute to defining the ToC of a vaccination campaign.

12.2.3.4 Determining the evaluation approach

With the ToC elaborated and the evaluation purpose determined in line with the implementation cycle and the stakeholder needs, priorities and expectations, the evaluation approach can be determined. In One Health, it will often include a combination of linear impact evaluation, non-linear impact evaluation and economic evaluation for the reasons explained earlier. Once the evaluation approach is chosen, it is time to develop a detailed evaluation plan. The plan should outline the evaluation design, methods, data collection instruments, analysis techniques, reporting mechanisms and timeline. It should be well documented, transparent and communicated to relevant stakeholders to ensure alignment and understanding of the evaluation process. Regular communication and feedback loops with stakeholders throughout the evaluation process are essential to address emerging aspects, adjust the approach if necessary, and ensure the evaluation remains relevant and useful.

12.2.3.5 Selecting indicators

The ToC builds on the steps described in Chapter 10 and Chapter 11. Once the ToC has been elaborated and

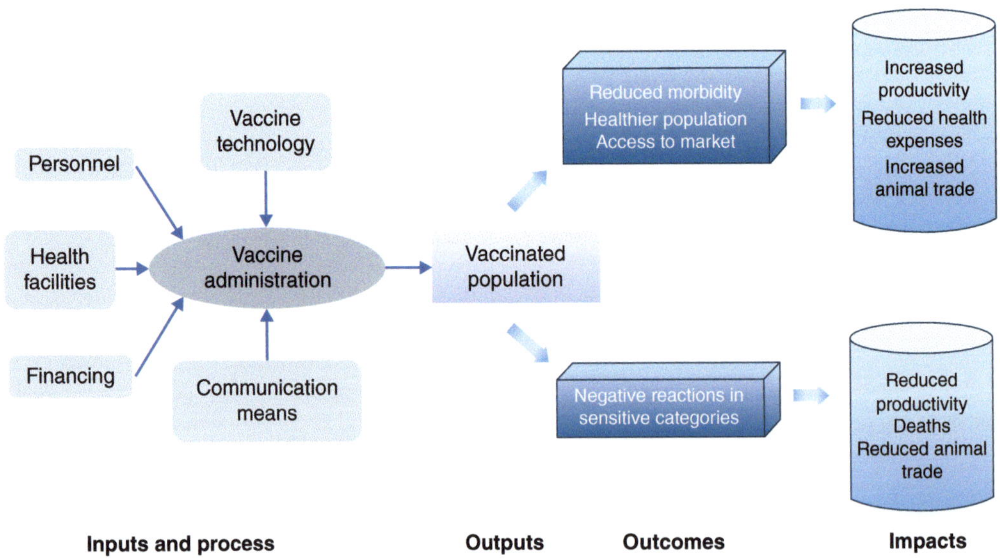

Fig. 12.5. Basic elements of a Theory of Change of a vaccination strategy in an animal population. Developed by the authors.

the evaluation approach determined, it is necessary to identify indicators of change. These are elements of the **socio-ecological system** (SES) that can be observed or assessed with qualitative or quantitative means. It is expected that the actions implemented manifest in a change of the outcomes and the associated indicators. Such actions can be very different depending on the need of the initiative: for example, vaccination campaigns, applying for (research) funding, conducting research, teaching or capacity building, networking, etc. (Rüegg *et al.*, 2018, Chapter 3; Cassetti and Paredes-Carbonell, 2020; de Moura *et al.*, 2023a; Mettenleiter *et al.*, 2023).

It is important that the stakeholders agree on these indicators because they will serve to evaluate the evolution of the SES, i.e. they are the feedback from the SES towards the stakeholders. This requires careful facilitation and exchange to generate a list of potential indicators based on the defined objectives, stakeholder input and criteria developed. Given the nature of One Health initiatives and the expected outcomes, both quantitative and qualitative indicators should be considered that capture different aspects of the initiative's impact and progress. The following points should be considered.

- **Clarity and specificity:** ensure that indicators proposed focus on a well-delineated aspect to avoid ambiguity and facilitate data collection and analysis.
- **Relevance:** the indicators should be directly related to the goals and objectives of the One Health initiative as elaborated in the ToC.
- **Feasibility:** consider the practicality of collecting information on the indicators within the available resources, time and data. Choose indicators that can be measured in a realistic and achievable way, given the evaluation context.
- **Measurability:** ensure that the indicators can be quantitatively or qualitatively assessed and that data sources for their assessment exist or can be generated.
- **Importance:** prioritize indicators that are most relevant to stakeholders and decision makers. Choose indicators that will provide valuable insights to inform programme improvements and decision making.
- **Context sensitivity:** make sure that the indicators are specific to the context of the One Health initiative considering its unique characteristics, challenges and opportunities of the target population and setting.
- **Consider multiple perspectives:** make sure that indicators reflect the different parts of the ToC and achieve a balance in terms of the priorities of the various stakeholders involved.

After generating a list of potential indicators, first they need to be prioritized based on relevance, measurability and alignment with project goals. This prioritization ensures that resources are allocated efficiently, and focus is placed on key metrics that drive project success. Second, pilot testing the selected indicators in a real-world setting allows for practical assessment of their validity, reliability and **feasibility** of measurement. This phase helps refine the indicators and address any challenges or limitations discovered during testing. Finally, developing a comprehensive monitoring and evaluation plan is crucial, outlining how each indicator will be measured, data collection methods, frequency of measurement, responsible parties and data analysis procedures. An example of what such a template can look like is given in Table 12.1. This plan ensures consistent and systematic monitoring of project progress and impact, enabling informed decision making and adaptive management throughout the project life cycle.

Task: Quantitative and qualitative indicators in a socio-ecological system.
Think about the socio-ecological system of a coral reef ecosystem and the human communities that depend on it for various resources and services. In this system, both ecological and social components interact and influence each other, creating a complex and interconnected network of relationships. Coral reefs are under heat stress from **climate** change with coral bleaching becoming more common. One intervention to protect them is to improve water quality by reducing pollution and runoff from land-based sources, which can help mitigate stress on coral reefs. Implementing best management practices in agriculture, reducing sedimentation and controlling nutrient inputs can improve overall water quality and reduce stress on coral reefs. What indicators can you think of that would allow us to measure if the intervention is achieving its objectives and progressing?

Example answer: Indicators to measure the effectiveness of interventions aimed at improving water quality and reducing stress on coral reefs include monitoring water quality parameters like nutrient levels and sedimentation rates, assessing

Table 12.1. Example template for the monitoring of the indicators selected.

Indicator name	Definition of indicator	Baseline value	Target value	Data source for measurement	Who is responsible for measurement	Comments

coral health and bleaching events, tracking changes in biodiversity and ecosystem services, evaluating community engagement and compliance with conservation measures, quantifying reductions in land-based pollution, and conducting long-term trend analysis to gauge overall ecosystem resilience. For instance, reduced nutrient concentrations, healthy coral populations, increased fish diversity, active community involvement and downward trends in pollution levels would indicate successful progress toward intervention objectives and the protection of coral reef ecosystems.

In addition to ecological indicators, assessing the effects of interventions on humans and wildlife will be important here. Indicators such as changes in human health indicators (e.g. reduced waterborne diseases), livelihood impacts (e.g. increased fish catch volumes, tourism revenue), social wellbeing (e.g. community satisfaction levels), wildlife health (e.g. disease prevalence among marine species), provision of ecosystem services to wildlife, and community resilience and adaptation capacities can provide a holistic understanding of intervention impacts. For instance, improvements in human health, economic benefits to local communities, healthy wildlife populations, and enhanced community resilience would indicate positive outcomes and sustainability of intervention strategies in protecting coral reefs and promoting water quality.

12.2.4 Monitor, evaluate and reflect

12.2.4.1 Monitoring and measurement of the activities, outputs, outcomes and impacts of One Health initiatives

The selected indicators can be measured and monitored using various methods depending on the nature of the indicator and the project's context. Common methods include quantitative data collection through surveys, interviews, observations or existing databases. Qualitative data collection methods such as focus group discussions or case studies can also be valuable for capturing nuanced information related to indicators.

The measurement and monitoring of indicators should be done systematically and planned well to ensure that it is not overly cumbersome. It requires careful consideration of data collection tools, frequency of measurement, data quality assurance processes, and data analysis methods. Utilizing technology such as data management software, mobile data collection apps and statistical analysis tools can support the process.

Key resources needed for measuring and monitoring indicators include trained personnel for data collection and analysis, appropriate data collection tools and instruments, access to relevant stakeholders or target populations, and sufficient financial resources to support data collection efforts and technology if necessary. Effective planning, stakeholder engagement and clear protocols for data collection and analysis are crucial to ensure the measurement and monitoring process is efficient and yields reliable data for decision making. See Box 12.1 for a discussion of selected indicators and their measurements. The provision of a full overview of all possible indicators is beyond the scope of this chapter, but relevant resources are provided for those interested in gaining more information.

A particular set of indicators in One Health relates to the One Health nature of the initiative (see the applied examples below), the One Health outcomes and the economic value of an initiative. For the latter, relevant economic analyses allow determining whether it is economically efficient or viable. Investors will be interested in the return on investment and the careful planning of financing and resourcing is a crucial step in the implementation cycle. These aspects are covered in detail in Chapter 13.

12.2.4.2 Analysis (including attribution analysis)

Analysing monitoring and evaluation data in complex and interdisciplinary One Health projects requires a

Box 12.1 The challenge of identifying and measuring suitable indicators

Here, we are looking at three indicators to illustrate key points that need to be considered when measuring the outcomes of One Health initiatives. The first example looks at the burden of disease in the human health sector; the second one at the impact of animal disease; and the third one at social outcomes.

Measuring the burden of disease in humans: In the human health sector, the impact of a disease can be measured by its incidence and/or the number of deaths (mortality) caused by it in a population (Devleesschauwer *et al.*, 2018). However, using only these two population health measures, the impact of a disease on human health is not depicted accurately (Devleesschauwer *et al.*, 2018). In fact, a disease might have a very high incidence but cause a very low burden due to its mild symptoms, or because it is mostly asymptomatic. How can we compare a disease with an incidence of 300,000 cases, low severity and 0% mortality with a disease causing three cases with high severity and 33% mortality? Furthermore, ignoring the age at which people die from a specific disease can also be problematic. What if two diseases have the same incidence and the same mortality rate, but the deaths in one occur in younger people? Likewise, if those population health measures are the same, but one disease only causes acute symptoms (i.e. have a short duration) and the other chronic lifelong sequelae? To overcome these limitations, the Disability-Adjusted Life-Year (DALY) metric was developed (Murray and Lopez, 1996) and is currently the most used metric to estimate the burden of disease in humans (Gao *et al.*, 2015). The concept of the DALY metric is simple: it represents the years lived with disability (YLD), i.e. years lived with decreased quality of life, and the years of life lost (YLL) due to premature death as a consequence of a given disease or condition, at the individual or population level (Pires *et al.*, 2024). By incorporating morbidity, mortality and disability in one metric, the DALY enables the comparison and ranking between diseases for all regions of the world (Murray and Lopez, 1996).

Let us have a look at how this works using the example of iron deficiency: iron deficiency is a common health issue that can affect individuals across different age groups, including young women. First, DALYs account for the years of life lost (YLL) due to premature mortality caused by severe iron deficiency-related conditions such as anaemia (Vos *et al.*, 2020). For instance, if a young woman dies prematurely due to severe anaemia resulting from iron deficiency, the YLL component of DALYs captures the impact of this premature death on population health. Second, DALYs also consider the years lived with disability (YLD) due to iron deficiency-related health issues. This includes factors such as fatigue, weakness, impaired cognitive function and reduced work productivity experienced by individuals affected by iron deficiency. An example of the burden of iron deficiency is provided by Wang *et al.* (2022), where a longitudinal, comparative burden-of-disease study was set to examine regional and sex inequalities in global iron deficiency from 1990 to 2017. A downward trend was observed globally but an uptrend was observed in its inequalities (higher in men).

For more details, see the following resources:

- The **Global Burden of Disease (GBD)** (https://www.healthdata.org/research-analysis/gbd) is a comprehensive study that quantifies the impact of diseases, injuries and risk factors on populations worldwide using the DALY. It provides crucial data on mortality, morbidity and disability, guiding public health policies and interventions to address major health challenges and improve population health outcomes globally.
- The **COST Action CA18218, European Burden of Disease Network** (https://www.burden-eu.net) focuses on assessing the health burden caused by diseases, injuries and risk factors across Europe. It aims to improve methodologies, data collection and analysis related to disease burden estimation, facilitating evidence-based decision making and healthcare resource allocation within the region.
- **WHO's Estimating the burden of foodborne diseases** (https://www.who.int/activities/estimating-the-burden-of-foodborne-diseases) quantifies the impact of foodborne illnesses globally. It gathers data on disease incidence, mortality and disability caused by unsafe food consumption, informing

Continued

Box 12.1 Continued.

policies and strategies to reduce foodborne disease burden, improve food safety and protect public health worldwide.

Another important health metric is the Quality-Adjusted Life-Year (QALY) that quantifies the impact of a health condition by considering both the duration and quality of life gained from a medical intervention, incorporating preferences for health states. It is often used to evaluate the effectiveness of specific healthcare interventions (Weinstein *et al.*, 2009).

Measuring the impact of disease in animals: For the animal health sector, a recent project – the Global Burden of Animal Diseases Programme (GBADs) – was developed to improve the human relationship with animal production and to build a more sustainable world. Its aim is to quantify the global burden of animal diseases considering not only animal production losses and expenditures, but also effects on animal welfare, human health, and the environment. To achieve this, GBADs brings together an international network of experts who combine methodological progress with data and tool integration from a variety of sources and contexts. The burden estimates are expected to improve decision making and support strategic investments. Consistent and transparent attribution of economic costs to various diseases and conditions provides a comprehensive overview of what causes the burden and enables comparisons between different animal species, production systems, and geographies.

For more information see: https://animalhealthmetrics.org/ and https://gbads.woah.org/

Measuring social cohesion: Social cohesion can be measured using various quantitative and qualitative indicators that reflect the degree of connectedness, trust, cooperation and solidarity within a community or society. Surveys and questionnaires play a crucial role by gathering data on trust levels, social networks, community engagement and feelings of belonging. These tools delve into perceptions of safety, willingness to help others and participation in communal activities, providing valuable insights into interpersonal relationships. Additionally, social network analysis (SNA) techniques offer a deeper understanding of social structures, identifying key individuals, connections and interaction patterns. Qualitative methods such as interviews and focus groups complement these quantitative approaches by exploring individuals' experiences, values and perspectives related to social cohesion and community identity. Here, we are looking at social network analysis as a possible method and metric for social cohesion. The SNA can also be useful for project planning as described in Chapter 10.

SNA is a method used to study relationships and interactions between individuals, groups or organizations within a social system. It involves mapping and analysing connections to uncover patterns, structures and dynamics within networks. SNA focuses on nodes (entities like people or organizations) and edges (connections or relationships between nodes), examining factors such as centrality (importance of nodes), clustering (groups of interconnected nodes) and information flow. By visualizing and quantifying these elements, SNA provides insights into social behaviours, information diffusion, influence and overall network health, helping us understand how social structures function and evolve. Using an example from the social science domain, SNA was used to investigate how individual and group-level features in the school class are related to prosocial behaviour and social capital (generalized trust) (Van den Bos *et al.*, 2018). In detail, the social networks within 22 classrooms of adolescents were mapped and data on social behaviours towards peers were collected. Through the use of SNA, it was shown that individuals with high centrality show both higher levels of prosocial behaviour and relational aggression. Also, greater social cohesion in the classroom was associated with: (i) reduced levels of antisocial behaviour towards peers; and (ii) increased generalized trust. Using this line of research provides novel insights and opens possibilities to connect with various behavioural dimensions.

To address the multifaceted health/One Health networks, various references exist for further reading (Leppin *et al.*, 2018; Albery *et al.*, 2021; Mwatondo *et al.*, 2023). The benefits of using SNA to address One Health have been addressed in a national context (Hoe *et al.*, 2019; Larkins *et al.*, 2024) and more broadly (Vink *et al.*, 2022).

thoughtful approach to derive meaningful insights and assess project outcomes effectively (Rüegg *et al.*, 2022). The process begins with data cleaning and preparation, ensuring that the datasets are accurate, complete and structured appropriately for analysis. Descriptive analysis plays a crucial role in summarizing key indicators and variables using measures such as means, frequencies, percentages and standard deviations where appropriate to provide a foundational understanding of the data's central tendencies and distributions. Moving forward, comparative analysis techniques may be employed to compare outcomes across different groups or time periods for quantitative data (e.g. t-tests, ANOVA, chi-square tests, regression analyses for quantitative data) or thematic analysis, content analysis or coding frameworks to extract themes and patterns from qualitative data.

In addition, impact evaluation methods are crucial for assessing causal impacts and attributions in One Health interventions (Rüegg *et al.*, 2018b; Aenishaenslin *et al.*, 2021). Techniques like difference-in-differences (DID), propensity score matching (PSM) or regression discontinuity design (RDD) help in estimating causal effects by comparing outcomes between intervention and control groups while accounting for confounding factors. Counterfactual analysis is also employed to estimate what would have happened in the absence of the intervention, providing a clearer picture of the intervention's actual impact.

Spatial and temporal analysis techniques further enhance the data analysis process, especially when dealing with geographic or time-series data. GIS mapping, spatial clustering and temporal trend analysis are utilized to visualize geographic patterns, spatial relationships and trends over time. Data visualization tools such as charts, graphs, maps and dashboards are employed to present findings effectively and communicate key insights to stakeholders and decision makers.

Once such information is available, an important aspect is to gauge to what extent observed changes or outcomes can be attributed to the One Health initiative. Attribution analysis aims to isolate and quantify the contribution of the intervention itself versus other external factors or influences that may also affect the outcomes. Attribution analysis can be complex and challenging, especially in situations where multiple interventions or external factors are at play, making it difficult to establish direct causal links. For example, a statistical model within a Bayesian estimation framework was developed to combine attribution estimates from expert elicitations with estimates from microbial subtyping and case-control studies of sporadic infection with zoonotic pathogens to reach consensus estimates reflecting the available empirical evidence (Mughini-Gras *et al.*, 2022). For further reading, you may want to refer to Mäesaar *et al.* (2020) and Cento *et al.* (2024).

12.2.4.3 Reflection, learning and adaptation

Ultimately, stakeholder engagement throughout the data analysis process is critical. Involving stakeholders in data validation, interpretation and insights gathering ensures that the analysis remains relevant, actionable and aligned with stakeholders' needs and perspectives. By combining these analytical approaches and engaging stakeholders effectively, One Health projects can derive actionable insights, assess impact and effectiveness, and inform evidence-based decision making for improved health and environmental outcomes.

Evaluation should be an attitude of vigilance throughout the project life cycle to adhere to inclusive principles and observe the co-evolution of the project in its environment. Because we are dealing with a complex adaptive system, new behaviours or structures may emerge due to our actions. Hence it is imperative to collect unexpected outcomes using qualitative methods such as Most Significant Change technique (Davies and Dart, 2005), outcome harvesting (Wilson-Grau and Britt, 2012) or other methods described by the Better Evaluation network (https://www.betterevaluation.org).

The information generated through the evaluation is used to reflect on the initiative, whether the system has changed as expected or not and if there are opportunities to improve the initiative. It also provides accountability to the stakeholders more generally. The deeper reflection can be guided by questions and practices as explained in Chapter 6. With the conclusions drawn from the evaluation and the reflection, the project cycle can be reiterated by revisiting the problem statement.

12.3 Evaluation Tools

Within the myriad existing tools to assess One Health initiatives, it is important to understand what distinct frameworks and tools have to offer. Identifying the correct tool for a specific One Health problem depends on the evaluation goals and objectives. When selecting an evaluation tool, it is important that you think carefully about what you want to achieve with your evaluation and support a tool that can facilitate your process. It is recommended that you document well your full process and thereby achieve a good understanding of what you are doing and why. This will be helpful when you look at suitable tools that can be applied during the evaluation. Please note that it is not necessary to use an existing tool and that you can define your own evaluation design; however, the application of existing tools helps with standardization and comparison across countries (Moura *et al.*, 2023a).

The One Health High-Level Expert Panel (OHHLEP) is a Quadripartite (FAO, UNEP, WHO, WOAH) advisory panel that is used to provide guidance to the four partner organizations (Mettenleiter *et al.*, 2023). Together with the Quadripartite's guide for implementing their One Health Joint Plan of Action (WHO *et al.*, 2023a), OHHLEP provided an inventory with 50 tools relevant to the implementation (including evaluation) of One Health initiatives (WHO *et al.*, 2023b, Barthon Behravesh *et al.*, 2024).

Because antimicrobial use and resistance (AMU and AMR, respectively) are global threats requiring urgent multisectoral action, several of these One Health evaluation tools were developed specifically to evaluate AMU and AMR surveillance systems. Indeed, within the activities of the project 'Convergence in evaluation frameworks for integrated surveillance of AMU and AMR' (CoEvalAMR), a guide was created to provide support towards the evaluation of surveillance systems for AMU and/or AMR and was made available online (https://guidance.fp7-risksur.eu). This guidance includes a comprehensive list of different valuation tools and frameworks, views their characteristics, and helps the reader in the selection of the most useful and appropriate tool to use for the evaluation of AMU/AMR surveillance systems. Because AMU and AMR are by definition One Health problems, this guidance also includes tools that can be used for general One Health initiatives that do not focus on this particular topic.

Table 12.2 shows a compilation of selected existing tools for the evaluation of One Health initiatives and provides an overview of their aims and a brief description. For each tool, an example or a case study is provided where applications and user experiences of each tool can be found.

In this applied example, we are using the NEOH evaluation approach using the example of the Cysticercosis Surveillance design in Portugal (Fonseca *et al.*, 2018).

In Portugal, an Observatory of Taeniasis and Cysticercosis (OTC) was created to establish a One Health-based national disease surveillance system, aiming to detect and treat tapeworm carriers to reduce the risk of infection in humans and pigs. The rationale and background is that: (i) emerging *Taenia solium* taeniasis and cysticercosis in urban areas of different European countries challenge the traditional view of the disease as only affecting low-middle-income countries; (ii) it is a preventable parasitic infection transmitted through contaminated food and water; (iii) it impacts human, animal and environmental health and welfare.

1. Define the evaluation question

The evaluation question was: is the OTC designed according to One Health characteristics and requirements? All phases of the OTC (design and implementation) were evaluated.

2. Define the system and elaborate the ToC

This One Health initiative is a subsystem aimed at the surveillance of Taeniasis and Cysticercosis, impacting human, animal and environmental health. The system's boundaries are determined by geographical, life, knowledge, legislative, networking and economic dimensions. The actors and stakeholders include human and animal health directorates, human and animal health academic institutions, public health and healthcare providers, practitioners in human and animal health, and laboratories. Stakeholders also include the community, patients and political decision makers.

The theory of change for this study is to increase awareness and knowledge of the epidemiology of cysticercosis in Portugal through an integrated human and animal health surveillance system (Fig. 12.6). This system will combine passive and active surveillance activities, consider ecological and environmental variables, and result in the efficient identification and treatment of human tapeworm carriers. The expected outcomes include disease awareness, identification of carriers, effective treatments and the development of guidelines. The interdisciplinary outcomes involve the creation of

Table 12.2. A compilation of tools used for the evaluation of One Health initiatives.

Tool	Aim and brief description	Case studies/examples
Network for the Evaluation of One Health Framework (**NEOH**)	Assessment of the added value of One Health and other integrated approaches to health: 'One Healthness'. This tool assesses One Health initiatives based on six aspects: systemic thinking, planning, transdisciplinary working, sharing, learning and systemic organization. Provides a qualitative assessment and semi-quantitative scorings to determine the degree of 'One Healthness'.	Selected case studies and examples can be found in Frontiers' research topic: '*Concepts and experiences in framing, integration and evaluation of One Health and EcoHealth*' (https://www.frontiersin.org/research-topics/5479/concepts-and-experiences-in-framing-integration-and-evaluation-of-one-health-and-ecohealth) and in the case studies provided by the Co-Eval-AMR: https://guidance.fp7-risksur.eu/welcome/case-studies/
Evaluating knOwLedge Integration Capacity (**EVOLvINC**)	This tool derives from NEOH and also assesses 'One Healthness'. It arranges the same six aspects used in the NEOH tool along the three stages of the project life cycle (formulation, implementation and evaluation). Qualitative assessment and semi-quantitative scorings to determine the level of knowledge integration capacity (median criteria scores) at each of the three stages of project life cycle.	An example can be found in: Hitziger *et al.* (2019) and in the case studies provided by the Co-Eval-AMR: https://guidance.fp7-risksur.eu/welcome/case-studies/
Evaluation tool for One Health epidemiological surveillance capacities and capabilities (**OH-EpiCap**)	Developed to assess, characterize and monitor surveillance capacities and capabilities in order to identify opportunities to improve the One Healthness of collaborations in the surveillance of any specific hazard. It encompasses three thematic domains, each with four different targets assessed by four different questions in a total of 48 standardized indicators. The level of One Healthness is shown by a semi-quantitative scale.	Access to the user guide and the tool can be found at: https://freddietafreeth.shinyapps.io/OH-EpiCap/

new data sources, networks and projects, as well as increased collaboration and transparency. Additionally, the initiative brings innovation by introducing a new model for disease control in European settings.

3. Select the evaluation tool

Considering the intention to assess the One Health aspects of the initiative, the OTC was evaluated using the Network for Evaluation of One Health framework.

The NEOH framework uses a systems approach and a mix of qualitative and quantitative assessments to evaluate the degree and structural balance of One Healthness, which includes operational aspects and supporting infrastructure aspects. The six different aspects of a perfect OH approach were scored using standardized assessment tools: namely, One Health thinking, One Health planning, One Health working, sharing, learning and systemic organization. Each one consisted of a series of up to 17 questions and an associated scoring system with values between 0 and 1, with a score of 1 an ideal scenario.

- One Health **thinking** evaluates how actors and stakeholders think about the One Health initiative and its operating system (context), with scoring criteria that include coverage and balance of dimensions, a match between the initiative and the environment, integrative health approach, the system features and targets, sustainability, socio-ecological considerations, perspectives and Theory of Change factors.
- One Health **planning** evaluates planning and resource allocations in the initiative. The scoring criteria are common aims; stakeholder and actor engagement; self-assessment and plan revisions; and individual objectives.

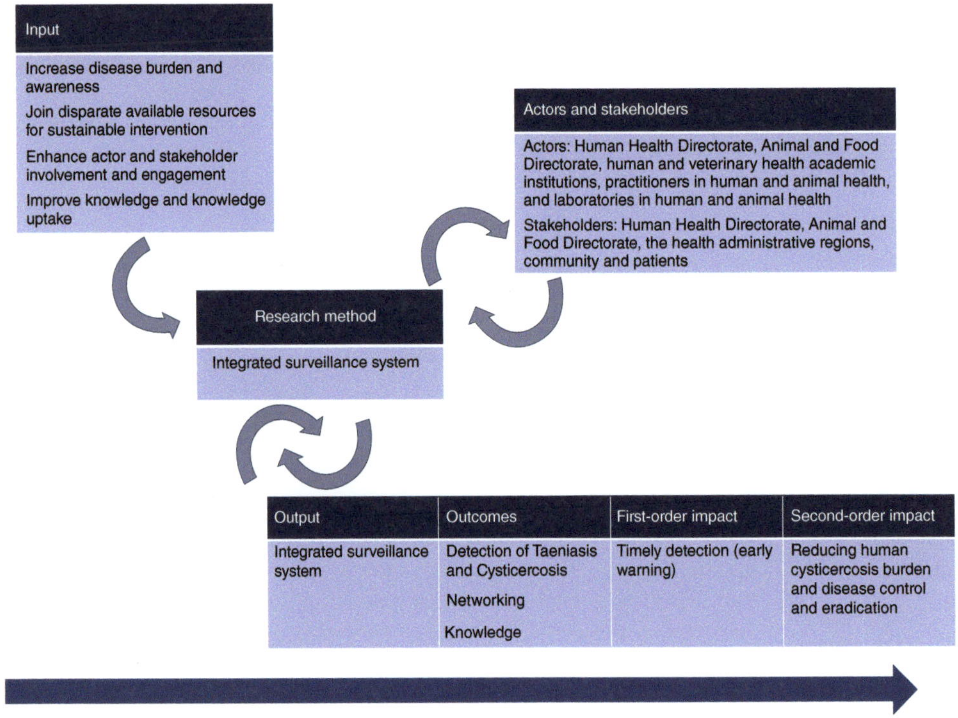

Fig. 12.6. Theory of Change applied for awareness and knowledge on the epidemiology of cysticercosis in Portugal. Unmodified from Fonseca *et al.* (2018) (CC BY 4.0 DEED: https://creativecommons.org/licenses/by/4.0/).

- One Health **working** is performed using specific scoring criteria to evaluate the interdisciplinary and participatory engagement in One Health initiatives. These criteria include broadness, collaboration, transdisciplinary balance, cultural and social balance, flexibility and adaptation.
- **Sharing** evaluates the extent and methods of information and data sharing infrastructures in One Health initiatives. It uses the following scoring criteria: general information and awareness sharing; data and information sharing; methods and results sharing; institutional memory and resilience to change.
- **Learning** evaluates the learning infrastructure of the initiative (scoring criteria: focus on adaptive and generative individual learning; focus on adaptive and generative team learning; adaptive and generative organizational learning; direct learning environment supportive of adaptive and generative learning; general learning environment supportive of adaptive and generative learning).
- **System organization** evaluates the systemic organization of the initiative, focusing on leadership skills and criteria for effective teamwork. The scoring criteria are team structure; social and leadership structures and skills; competence; focus on innovation.

The **OH index** (OHI) and **OH ratio** (OHR) were calculated to reflect the degree of integration of operational aspects and infrastructure and the balance between them. In this case, the evaluation aimed to ensure that a newly started initiative would achieve One Health characteristics in the longer term by correcting its design on the way.

4. Interpret the results

The OH index and OH ratio were calculated (0.31 and 1.98 respectively) and illustrated with a spider diagram (Fig. 12.7). The diagram's shape and surface area indicated the extent of One Health implementation and the balance between operational and supporting means. The initiative's main strengths were in the operational levels, specifically One Health thinking and One Health working, which showed a multidimensional approach and transdisciplinary nature. However, there were weaknesses in the supporting infrastructure, such as sharing, team structure and organizational learning. This evaluation

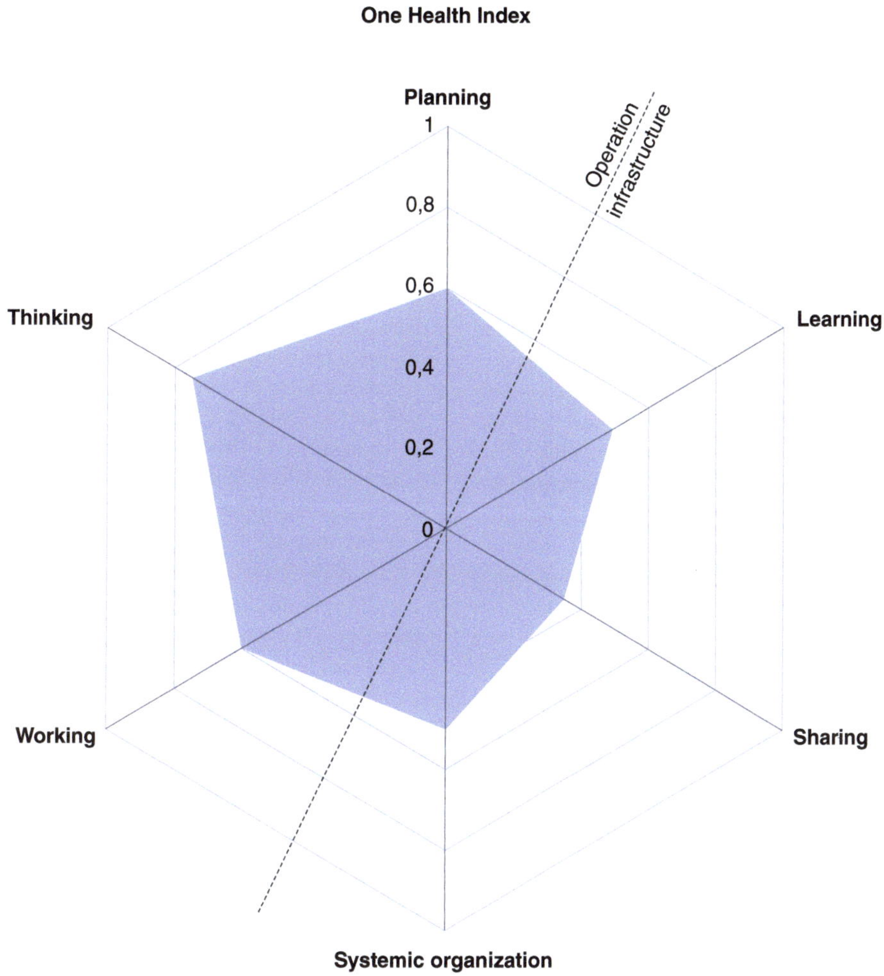

Fig. 12.7. Spider diagram illustrating the degree of One Health implementation and the balance between the operational and the supporting means of the Observatory of Taeniasis and Cysticercosis in Portugal. Unmodified from Fonseca *et al.* (2018) (CC BY 4.0 DEED: https://creativecommons.org/licenses/by/4.0/).

only looked at the strength of One Health and not at any of the outputs and outcomes it produces.

Evaluating the 'One Healthness' of DANMAP: The Danish Integrated Antimicrobial Resistance Monitoring and Research Programme (DANMAP) has been evaluated using the OH-EpiCap tool to identify areas for improvement. DANMAP is a One Health programme that aims to prevent potential risks related to antimicrobial resistance (AMR) in humans and animals. The evaluation focused on surveillance components of the programme related to the spread of AMR monitored in clinical isolates from humans and indicator bacteria from food-producing animals. The OH-EpiCap tool is developed by the MATRIX consortium, funded by the One Health European Joint Programme (https://onehealthejp.eu/).

The purpose of the OH-EpiCap is to help identify opportunities to enhance collaboration in the surveillance of a hazard in a One Health context (Tegegne *et al.*, 2023). It consists of three thematic domains with four targets each, totalling 48 standardized indicators, presented in Table 12.3. These indicators are answered using a semi-quantitative scale ranging from 1 to 4, with 4 being the ideal scenario in most cases.

Figure 12.8 provides a visual representation of the results of the OH-EpiCap evaluation of DANMAP, which scored well in every dimension, with an average score above 3 in all target areas, indicating a high level of One Health collaboration (Moura *et al.*, 2023b).

The evaluation identified the following points as relevant for discussion. Regarding Dimension 1 (Organization), three areas for improvement were identified. First, all supporting documentation related to DANMAP should be compiled and shared in a common digital location to improve accessibility. Second, the steering committee should include representatives from all sectors relevant to One Health surveillance, including the environment. Third, while all actively engaged sectors are represented in the programme's coordination group, more representatives from the livestock industry and environmental sector could strengthen the One Health approach. The exclusion of environmental data from the surveillance programme was based on previous research but is now being reconsidered due to increased animal production and hospital activity. However, including these data would require additional resources. While the programme has evolved and undergone regular internal evaluations, a more standardized methodology could improve the implementation of corrective measures. The current resources are sufficient for the programme's objectives, but an additional budget would be required for emerging issues and new components, such as environmental aspects.

Dimension 2, which focuses on operational activities, suggests that improving the harmonization of indicators and methodology for sampling animals for AMR surveillance may be challenging due to budget constraints. Additionally, a joint multisectoral analysis could potentially be enhanced in the future, and transparency, communication and accessibility of data should be regularly assessed as changes in methodology or programme objectives may impact these factors. Furthermore, investing in additional training for professionals responsible for prescribing and using antimicrobials could also be considered.

Lastly, for Dimension 3, since One Health surveillance has always been a fundamental component of DANMAP, the tool did not specifically assess the added value of adopting a One Health approach. None the less, the programme's

Table 12.3. Dimensions, targets and indicators evaluate by the OH-EPICap tool – based on Henaux *et al.* (2022).

Dimension 1: Organization			
Target 1.1 Formalization: common aim, support documentations, shared leadership, and the definition of roles/composition of coordination committees.	Target 1.2 Coverage: inclusion of all relevant actors, disciplines, sectors, geography, populations, and related hazards.	Target 1.3 Resources: budget and human resources, programme training, and sharing of resources.	Target 1.4 Evaluation and resilience: internal and external evaluations, development/ implementation of corrective measures, and adaptability to change.
Dimension 2: Operational activities			
Target 2.1 Data collection and methods sharing: multisectoral collaboration in the design of surveillance protocols and data collection, harmonization of laboratory techniques and data warehousing.	Target 2.2 Data sharing: data sharing agreements, assessment of data quality, the usefulness of shared data, and the compliance of data with the FAIR (findability, accessibility, interoperability, reusability) principle.	Target 2.3 Data analysis and interpretation: multisectoral integration for data analysis, sharing of analysis techniques, sharing of scientific expertise, and harmonization of indicators.	Target 2.4 Communication: internal and external communication, dissemination to decision makers, and information sharing in case of suspicion / particular events.
Dimension 3: Impact			
Target 3.1 Technical outputs: timely detection of emergence, epidemiological knowledge improvement, increased effectiveness of surveillance, and reduction of operational costs.	Target 3.2 Collaborative added value: strengthening of the One Health team and network, international collaboration, and common strategy (roadmap) design.	Target 3.3 Immediate and intermediate outcomes: advocacy, awareness, preparedness, and interventions based on the information generated.	Target 3.4 Ultimate outcomes: research opportunities, policy changes and behavioural changes and better health outcomes.

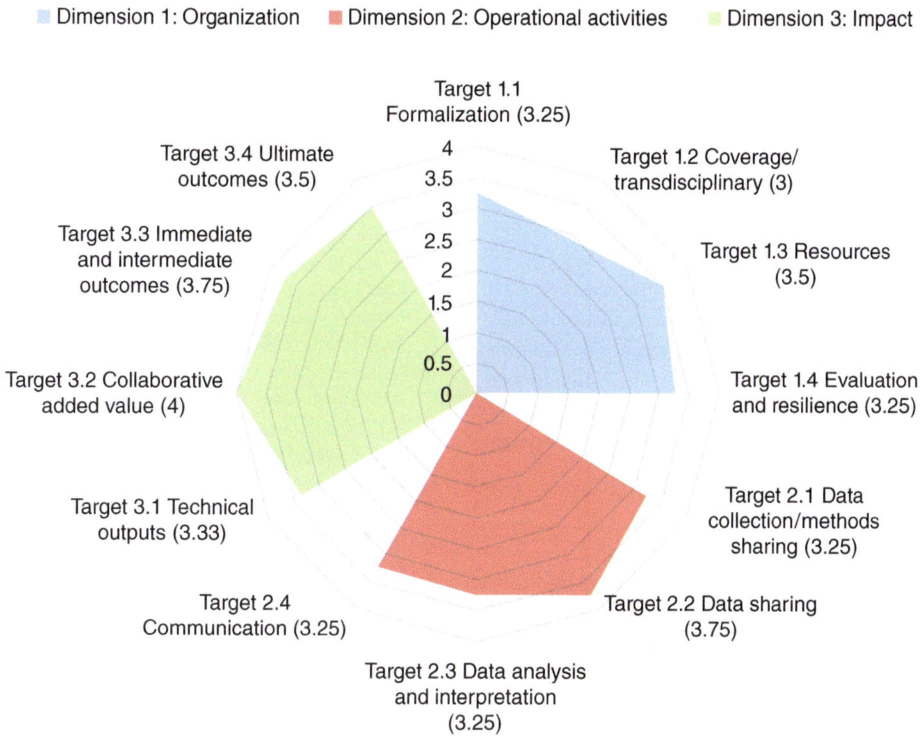

Fig. 12.8. Average scores of DANMAP for the target areas covered by the OH-EpiCap tool, segmented into three dimensions. The average scores for each of the target areas are indicated in brackets. Unmodified from Moura *et al.* (2023b) (CC BY 4.0 DEED: https://creativecommons.org/licenses/by/4.0/).

impact on epidemiological knowledge over its 25+ years of operation is significant and has influenced sector interventions and policy changes. In Denmark, there is a strong commitment to collaborative work, and the level of awareness among stakeholders is high, although there is room for improvement in translating this into action.

12.4 Conclusions

In this chapter, you have learned about basic principles of evaluation of One Health initiatives as they are embedded in the One Health project life cycle. This knowledge should help you to conceptualize, understand or make use of One Health evaluations. It should help you also to know how evaluation can be used, what questions can be answered and how evaluation can support the effectiveness of One Health initiatives, thus allowing you to gain deeper insights about:

- How to assess if the One Health initiative improved health or other One Health outcomes of interest, e.g. to what extent did the integrated One Health approach reduce the incidence of **zoonotic diseases** in the target population?
- Collaboration effect: how effective were the collaborative efforts between sectors, partners and/or groups in society, e.g. human and veterinary health sectors in preventing disease outbreaks at the human–animal interface?
- Process evaluation: is the One Health initiative being implemented as planned?
- Capacity assessment: what is the One Health capacity and how is it evolving over time? To what extent did the capacity-building programmes enhance the knowledge and skills of healthcare professionals, veterinarians and environmental experts in applying One Health principles?
- Governance: how effective were the collaborative mechanisms and governance structures in promoting intersectoral coordination and information sharing among relevant agencies and stakeholders? Did the establishment of joint task forces or

committees lead to more efficient and timely responses to One Health challenges?

- Communication: did public awareness campaigns and advocacy efforts increase understanding and support for One Health approaches among target audiences? How did effective communication strategies impact behaviours related to human–animal–environment interactions?

In the next chapter, we look at how we can use economic evaluation to gain insights into the economic value of One Health and how economic analyses can help us to inform resource allocation. This will allow us to understand what the socio-economic benefits are of One Health interventions for communities and what that means for One Health investments.

References

Aenishaenslin, C., Häsler, B., Ravel, A., Parmley, E.J., Mediouni, S. *et al.* (2021) Evaluating the integration of One Health in surveillance systems for antimicrobial use and resistance: A conceptual framework. *Frontiers in Veterinary Science* 8, 611931.

Albery, G.F., Kirkpatrick, L., Firth, J.A. and Bansal, S. (2021) Unifying spatial and social network analysis in disease ecology. *Journal of Animal Ecology* 90(1), 45–61.

Anonymous (1999) Interactive Terminology for Europe. Available at: http://iate.europa.eu (accessed 1 March 2024).

Barton Behravesh, C., Charron, D.F., Liew, A., Cediel Becerra, N., Machalaba, C. *et al.* (2024) An integrated inventory of One Health tools: Mapping and analysis of globally available tools to advance One Health. *CABI One Health* 3(1). DOI: 10.1079/cabionehealth.2024.0017.

Belcher, B. and Claus, R. (2020) Theory of Change. td-net toolbox Profile (5). Swiss Academies of Arts and Sciences: td-net toolbox for co-Producing Knowledge. Available at: www.transdisciplinarity.ch/toolbox (accessed 7 August 2024).

Blane, D., Brunner, E. and Wilkinson, R.G. (eds) (1996) *Health and Social Organization: Towards a Health Policy for the Twenty-First Century.* Psychology Press, London.

Burris, S., Wagenaar, A.C., Swanson, J., Ibrahim, J.K., Wood, J. and Mello, M.M. (2010) Making the case for laws that improve health: A framework for public health law research. *The Milbank Quarterly* 88(2), 169–210.

Cassetti, V. and Paredes-Carbonell, J.J. (2020) Theory of change: A tool for participatory planning and evaluation in community health. *Gaceta Sanitaria* 34(3), 305–307.

Castillo-Neyra, R., Buttenheim, A.M., Brown, J., Ferrara, J.F., Arevalo-Nieto, C. *et al.* (2020) Behavioral and structural barriers to accessing human post-exposure prophylaxis and other preventive practices in Arequipa, Peru, during a canine rabies epidemic. *PLoS Neglected Tropical Diseases* 14(7), e0008478.

Cawthorn, D.M. and Hoffman, L.C. (2015) The bushmeat and food security nexus: A global account of the contributions, conundrums and ethical collisions. *Food Research International* 76, 906–925.

Cento, G., Mancin, M., Cibin, V., Villa, L., Ricci, A. *et al.* (2024) Application of the EFSA Source Attribution Model (SAM) to compare the main sources of human salmonellosis in Italy related to the national production over the period 2018–2020. *Food Control* 160, 110315.

Claus, R., Davel, R., Heykoop, C., Pinto, D. and Belcher, B.M. (2023) How to build Theories of Change for transdisciplinary research: Guidance and considerations. *GAIA-Ecological Perspectives for Science and Society* 32(1), 186–196.

Davies, R. and Dart, J. (2005) The 'Most Significant Change' (MSC) Technique. A Guide to its Use, p. 10. Available at: https://www.mande.co.uk/wp-content/uploads/2005/MSCGuide.pdf (accessed 7 August 2024).

Devleesschauwer, B., Haagsma, J.A., Mangen, M.J.J., Lake, R.J. and Havelaar, A.H. (2018) The global burden of foodborne disease. In: *Food Safety Economics: Incentives for a Safer Food Supply.* Springer, Cham, pp. 107–122.

Fonseca, A.G., Torgal, J., De Meneghi, D., Coelho, A.C. and Vilhena, M. (2018) One Health-ness evaluation of cysticercosis surveillance design in Portugal. *Frontiers in Public Health* 6, 315166.

Gao, T., Wang, X.C., Chen, R., Ngo, H.H. and Guo, W. (2015) Disability adjusted life year (DALY): A useful tool for quantitative assessment of environmental pollution. *Science of the Total Environment* 511, 268–287.

Hasanov, E., Zeynalova, S., Geleishvili, M., Maes, E., Tongren, E. *et al.* (2018) Assessing the impact of public education on a preventable zoonotic disease: Rabies. *Epidemiology and Infection* 146(2), 227–235.

Heermans, B., Van Rooyen, J., Fynn, R., Biggs, D., Lewis, M. and McNutt, J. (2021) Husbandry and herding: A community-based approach to addressing illegal wildlife trade in northern Botswana. *Frontiers in Conservation Science* 2, 675493.

Henaux, V., Tegegne, H., Bogaardt, C., Lailler, R., Collineau, L. and Prada, J. (2022) Deliverable D-JIP-MATRIX-WP4.2 OH-EpiCap tool and tutorial. Available at: https://zenodo.org/record/7006654.

Hitziger, M., Aragrande, M., Berezowski, J.A., Canali, M., Del Rio Vilas, V. *et al.* (2019) EVOLvINC: EValuating knOwLedge INtegration Capacity in Multistakeholder Governance. *Ecology and Society* 24(2). https://www.jstor.org/stable/26796961.

Hoe, C., Adhikari, B., Glandon, D., Das, A., Kaur, N. and Gupta, S. (2019) Using social network analysis to plan, promote and monitor intersectoral collaboration for health in rural India. *PLoS One* 14(7), e0219786.

Larkins, A., Vannamahaxay, S., Puttana, V., Chittavong, M., Southammavong, F. *et al.* (2024) Scaling up One Health: A network analysis in Lao PDR. *One Health* 18, 100661.

Leppin, A.L., Okamoto, J.M., Organick, P.W., Thota, A.D., Barrera-Flores, F.J. *et al.* (2018) Applying social network analysis to evaluate implementation of a multisector population health collaborative that uses a bridging hub organization. *Frontiers in Public Health* 6, 315.

Mäesaar, M., Tedersoo, T., Meremäe, K. and Roasto, M. (2020) The source attribution analysis revealed the prevalent role of poultry over cattle and wild birds in human campylobacteriosis cases in the Baltic States. *PLoS One* 15(7), e0235841.

Mettenleiter, T.C., Markotter, W., Charron, D.F., Adisasmito, W.B., Almuhairi, S. *et al.* (2023) The one health high-level expert panel (OHHLEP). *One Health Outlook* 5(1), 18.

Moura, P., Collineau, L., Sandberg, M., Tomassone, L., De Meneghi, D. *et al.* (2023a) Users' perception of the OH-EpiCap evaluation tool based on its application to nine national antimicrobial resistance surveillance systems. *Frontiers in Public Health* 11, 1138645.

Moura, P., Borck Høg, B., Alban, L., Sönksen, U.W., Ribeiro Duarte, A.S. and Sandberg, M. (2023b) Evaluating the OH-EpiCap tool using the Danish integrated surveillance program for AMU and AMR as a case study. *Frontiers in Public Health* 11, 1127701.

Mughini-Gras, L., Benincà, E., McDonald, S.A., de Jong, A., Chardon, J., Evers, E. and Bonačić Marinović, A.A. (2022) A statistical modelling approach for source attribution meta-analysis of sporadic infection with foodborne pathogens. *Zoonoses and Public Health* 69(5), 475–486.

Murray, C.J. and Lopez, A.D. (1996) Evidence-based health policy: Lessons from the global burden of disease study. *Science* 274(5288), 740–743.

Mwatondo, A., Rahman-Shepherd, A., Hollmann, L., Chiossi, S., Maina, J. *et al.* (2023) A global analysis of One Health networks and the proliferation of One Health collaborations. *The Lancet* 401(10376), 605–616.

Narrod, C., Zinsstag, J. and Tiongco, M. (2012) A one health framework for estimating the economic costs of zoonotic diseases on society. *EcoHealth* 9, 150–162.

OECD (2023) *Glossary of Key Terms in Evaluation and Results-based Management for Sustainable Development* (2nd edn). OECD Publishing, Paris. DOI: 10.1787/632da462-en-fr-es.

Pires, S.M., Redondo, H.G., Pessoa, J., Jakobsen, L.S. and Thomsen, S.T. (2024) Risk ranking of foodborne diseases in Denmark: Reflections on a national burden of disease study. *Food Control* 158, 110199.

Rüegg, S.R., McMahon, B.J., Häsler, B., Esposito, R., Nielsen, L.R. *et al.* (2017) A blueprint to evaluate One Health. *Frontiers in Public Health* 5, 20.

Rüegg, S.R., Häsler, B. and Zinsstag, J. (eds) (2018a) *Integrated Approaches to Health: A Handbook for the Evaluation of One Health.* Wageningen Academic Publishers, Wageningen, The Netherlands.

Rüegg, S.R., Nielsen, L.R., Buttigieg, S.C., Santa, M., Aragrande, M. *et al.* (2018b) A systems approach to evaluate One Health initiatives. *Frontiers in Veterinary Science* 5, 23.

Rüegg, S.R., Antoine-Moussiaux, N., Aenishaenslin, C., Alban, L., Bordier, M. *et al.* (2022) Guidance for evaluating integrated surveillance of antimicrobial use and resistance. *CABI One Health* 2022, p.ohcs20220007.

Sandberg, M., Hesp, A., Aenishaenslin, C., Bordier, M., Bennani, H. *et al.* (2021) Assessment of evaluation tools for integrated surveillance of antimicrobial use and resistance based on selected case studies. *Frontiers in Veterinary Science* 8, 620998. DOI: 10.3389/fvets.2021.620998.

Speranza, C.I., Wüthrich, T., Rüegg, S., Zinsstag, J., Keune, H. *et al.* (2018) Evaluating the contributions of One Health initiatives to social sustainability. In: *Integrated Approaches to Health.* Wageningen Academic, Wageningen, The Netherlands, pp. 86–125.

Tegegne, H.A., Bogaardt, C., Collineau, L., Cazeau, G., Lailler, R. *et al.* (2023) OH-EpiCap: A semi-quantitative tool for the evaluation of One Health epidemiological surveillance capacities and capabilities. *Frontiers in Public Health* 11, 1053986.

Van den Bos, W., Crone, E.A., Meuwese, R. and Güroğlu, B. (2018) Social network cohesion in school classes promotes prosocial behavior. *PLoS One* 13(4), e0194656.

Vink, D., Haesler, B., Peyre, M.I., Tomley, F., Apgar, M. and Fournié, G. (2022) The role of Social Network Analysis (SNA) as an evaluation tool in complex One Health partnership networks. In: *16th International Symposium of Veterinary Epidemiology and Economics – Connecting Animals, People, and their Shared Environments: Abstract book.* ISVEE. Halifax: ISVEE, Résumé. International Symposium of Veterinary Epidemiology and Economics (ISVEE 16). 16, Halifax, Canada, p. 627.

Vos, T., Lim, S.S., Abbafati, C., Abbas, K.M., Abbasi, M. *et al.* (2020) Global burden of 369 diseases and injuries in 204 countries and territories, 1990–2019: A systematic analysis for the Global Burden of Disease Study 2019. *The Lancet* 396(10258), 1204–1222.

Wang, M., Gao, H., Wang, J., Cao, C., Ying, X. *et al.* (2022) Global burden and inequality of iron deficiency: Findings from the Global Burden of Disease datasets 1990–2017. *Nutrition Journal* 21(1), 16.

Weinstein, M.C., Torrance, G. and McGuire, A. (2009) QALYs: The basics. *Value in Health* 12(1), S5–S9.

Wilson-Grau, R. and Britt, H. (2012) *Outcome Harvesting.* Ford Foundation, Cairo.

World Health Organization, Food and Agriculture Organization of the United Nations, United Nations Environment Programme and World Organisation for Animal Health (2023a) *A Guide to Implementing the One Health Joint Plan of Action at National Level.* Geneva. Available at: https://openknowledge.fao.org/handle/20.500.14283/cc7916en (accessed 7 August 2024).

World Health Organization, UNEP United Nations Environment Programme and World Organisation for Animal Health (2023b) *Implementing the Global Action Plan on Antimicrobial Resistance: First Quadripartite Biennial Report.* World Health Organization, Geneva. Available at: https://iris.who.int/handle/10665/375008 (accessed 7 August 2024).

Zinsstag, J., Schelling, E., Bonfoh, B., Fooks, A.R., Kasymbekov, J., Waltner-Toews, D. and Tanner, M. (2009) Towards a 'One Health' research and application tool box. *Veterinaria Italiana* 45(1), 121–133.

13 The Economic Evaluation of One Health Interventions

Massimo Canali[1,3], Valentina Suprani[1], Maurizio Aragrande[1,3], Martin Hitziger[3,4] and Barbara Häsler[2,3]

[1]Department of Agricultural and Food Sciences, University of Bologna, Bologna, Italy; [2]Veterinary Epidemiology Economics and Public Health Group, Department of Pathobiology and Population Sciences, Royal Veterinary College, London, UK; [3]Network for Ecohealth and One Health (NEOH); [4]Section of Epidemiology, Vetsuisse Faculty, University of Zurich, Zurich, Switzerland

Contents

DOI: 10.1079/9781800623002.0014

Chapter Overview

Elevator pitch

Understanding the economic value of One Health is crucial for making decisions on One Health investments. In this chapter, you will learn about the basic principles of economic evaluations of One Health. You will discover what is needed to design these evaluations using a One Health lens and how the information can be used to prioritize resource allocation and justify investments in One Health. This will equip you with skills to help make a compelling case for sustainable and impactful One Health implementation.

Book objectives the chapter relates to

☐ 1. Understand what One Health and Ecohealth mean
☑ 2. Think in a One Health and Ecohealth way
☐ 3. Apply One Health and Ecohealth in their professional and personal life
☐ 4. Know how to share One Health and Ecohealth knowledge
☐ 5. Integrate One Health and Ecohealth knowledge actively
☑ 6. Acquire or enhance core One Health competencies

One Health competencies covered

☐ 1. Effective communication
☐ 2. Collaborative and resilient working
☑ 3. Systems understanding
☐ 4. Transdisciplinarity
☐ 5. Social, cultural and gender equity and inclusiveness
☐ 6. Collective learning and reflective practice
☑ 7. One Health concepts
☐ 8. Theoretical and methodological pluralism
☑ 9. Harnessing uncertainty, paradox and limited knowledge

After working through this chapter, you will understand what to consider when planning a One Health economic evaluation and how this information can be used in decision making for One Health implementation.

Learning outcomes

1. Understand the basic principles of economic evaluation of One Health initiatives.
2. Know what to consider when conceptualizing a One Health economic evaluation.
3. Discuss the economic evaluation results and how to use them for decision making on One Health investments.

Summary

In this chapter, you explore the basics of economic assessments in One Health initiatives addressing key questions such as why these assessments are important for One Health implementation and what they entail. You learn about how to conceptualize economic evaluations of One Health and delve into the costs and benefits associated with One Health interventions, covering tangible and intangible costs, market prices of resources, and the evaluation of benefits over time. You get to know various economic evaluation methods that can help to provide insights into how these methods quantify the economic value of interventions. Furthermore, you engage with different metrics and valuation approaches and how to address the challenge of uncertainty through sensitivity analyses, ensuring robustness in your conclusions for decision making. Finally, you learn about wider dimensions including different economic paradigms, financing and funding.

13.1 Introduction

One Health has gained significant momentum in recent years as a holistic approach to address complex **health** challenges spanning humans, animals, plants and the **environment**, emphasizing the narrative that the interconnectedness of these domains causes cascading effects of benefits or problems in other **sectors**. Numerous proof-of-concept studies showcase the **effectiveness** and added **value** of One Health initiatives (Pitt and Gunn, 2024). While much of the initial focus of economic evidence of the **One Health approach** was on **zoonotic diseases** and food safety, there is now growing evidence of the benefits of applying One Health to tackle global development concerns such as antimicrobial resistance (AMR) and environmental pollution (Destoumieux-Garzón *et al.*, 2018). For instance, there is a strong, documented investment case that shows that the value of reducing air pollution is substantial, as it not only benefits human health but also has positive implications for animal health and overall environmental **sustainability** (Manisalidis *et al.*, 2020; Pansini and Shi, 2022).

After the COVID-19 pandemic, with the increasing recognition of One Health's potential, there has been a corresponding rise in funding and financing opportunities for such initiatives. Governments, international organizations, philanthropic foundations and private sector entities are showing greater interest in supporting One Health initiatives. This trend reflects a broader acknowledgment of the interconnected nature of health challenges and the need for collaborative, multisectoral solutions (FAO *et al.*, 2022; Lefrançois *et al.*, 2023; The World Bank Group, 2023).

Despite the progress made, however, challenges remain in fully realizing the potential of One Health through sustainable, long-term and dedicated investments. While there is ample evidence supporting certain aspects of One Health initiatives, gaps exist in demonstrating the added value and return on investment across One Health domains more broadly. Addressing financing and funding challenges is essential for the long-term sustainability of One Health activities. Efforts to strengthen economic arguments, expand evidence across diverse One Health domains, and secure sustainable financing mechanisms are key to advance the One Health agenda and achieve meaningful **impact** on global health and **wellbeing**.

Thus, economic **evaluations** are critical in the One Health implementation cycle as a tool for decision making (Drummond *et al.*, 2015). As resources are limited, they help us to make the best use of them to satisfy our needs. For instance, a government decision maker may wonder what projects or programmes to invest in when they have a budget available for One Health initiatives and a particular epidemiological situation; should they opt for a rabies eradication programme, a blue-tongue vaccination programme, a brucellosis surveillance programme, or maybe a programme to decrease **biodiversity** loss or non-communicable diseases? A mixed group of **stakeholders** working in a wider programme may wonder about investments through private–public partnerships. A private industry actor, such as a vaccine producer, might be interested in the potential financial return on the vaccine development. An NGO involved in conservation might be interested in knowing what the value is of preserving a certain species.

Knowing that the economic value of what we decide to do is given by what we give up – in economics, this is called '**opportunity cost**' (Palmer and Raftery, 1999) – economic evaluations should, therefore, help us to obtain from One Health initiatives an added value when comparing the benefits to the costs.

13.1.1 Economic evaluations in the One Health implementation cycle

When looking at our One Health implementation cycle, we are interested in two big questions. The first question revolves around assessing whether our One Health initiative is economically acceptable and offers sufficient benefits (both monetary and non-monetary) to justify the resources invested. This requires robust economic evaluations tailored to different One Health contexts and interventions. The second question pertains to the financing mechanisms for One Health initiatives. Identifying sustainable funding sources, fostering partnerships among stakeholders, and exploring innovative financing models should help to ensure the long-term success of a One Health initiative.

While the principles outlined are applicable to any type of One Health initiative, we are focusing on One Health interventions here, as a wider coverage of different types of One Health initiatives would go beyond the scope of this chapter.

In the implementation cycle (Fig. 13.1), the economic evaluation links to establishing intervention options where we identify the possible alternatives for achieving the objectives defined. Sometimes, this might just be a

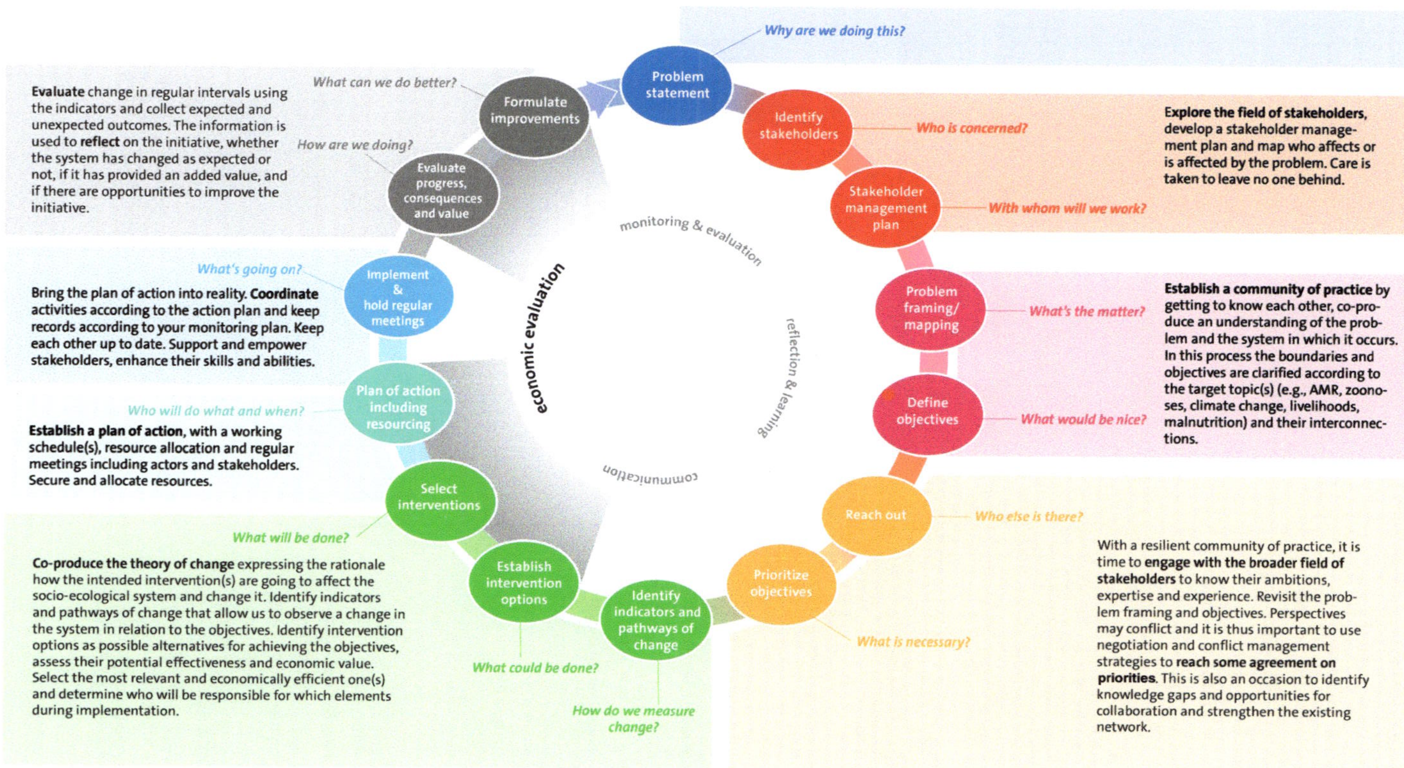

Fig. 13.1. Economic evaluation comes in at various steps of the One Health implementation cycle including the assessment of intervention options, when planning the implementation, and during and after implementation with the aim to find out if the initiative is likely to or has generated economic value.

single intervention, but we might often find a package of interventions (e.g. rabies awareness campaign combined with vaccination of dogs and people). The economic evaluation can be structured based on the participatory approach taking place to define the problem, objectives and possible interventions, and the associated **Theory of Change** (ToC). The selection of the intervention to be implemented should be informed not only by technical considerations, but also by the economic value of these interventions. From an economic point of view, an intervention is acceptable when the resulting benefits outweigh the costs. This can be established in an *ex-ante* (or prospective) analysis to inform the selection of interventions and ensure that sufficient funds are allocated to it. The latter may necessitate the generation of funds through various investment channels and partnerships. Once the intervention is implemented, economic evaluation *ad interim* (while the intervention is ongoing) can be used to determine whether we are on track or need to implement corrective measures. Furthermore, economic evaluation may take place after an intervention has gone through a first phase of this cycle in a process of *ex-post* (retrospective) evaluation that allows us to capture both the progress and unintended consequences (both positive and negative) and determine the value achieved for the investment made. This information then helps to think about a new phase or cycle, reflect on lessons learned, explain variations from the original planning and formulate improvements (Pearce *et al.*, 2006).

The focus of this chapter is on explaining the basic steps of an economic evaluation in alignment with the One Health implementation cycle. It refers to the problem statement, stakeholder engagement, prioritization, systems mapping, implementation and monitoring and evaluation steps discussed in Chapters 10, 11 and 12, and makes use of these foundations to explain what we need to consider in the economic evaluation. Emphasis is also placed on valuation approaches and the challenges of measuring certain One Health outcomes. Finally, we spend some time thinking about how these analyses link to funding and financing and what more complex analyses will look like.

13.2 Economic Evaluations of One Health Interventions

Economic evaluations assess alternative One Health interventions by comparing their respective costs and consequences across the different sectors involved.

Figure 13.2 shows the main characteristics of two alternative surveillance programmes and associated interventions to mitigate bovine brucellosis in the dairy farms of a given area. Bovine brucellosis is a One Health challenge due to its multi-species impact, zoonotic potential, economic ramifications and the necessity for a collaborative approach (Pal *et al.*, 2017; Buttigieg *et al.*, 2018; Franc *et al.*, 2018; Ghanbari *et al.*, 2020). It affects various animals, including cattle, sheep and wildlife, while posing risks of transmission to humans through direct contact or consumption of contaminated products. Its economic consequences can be far-reaching

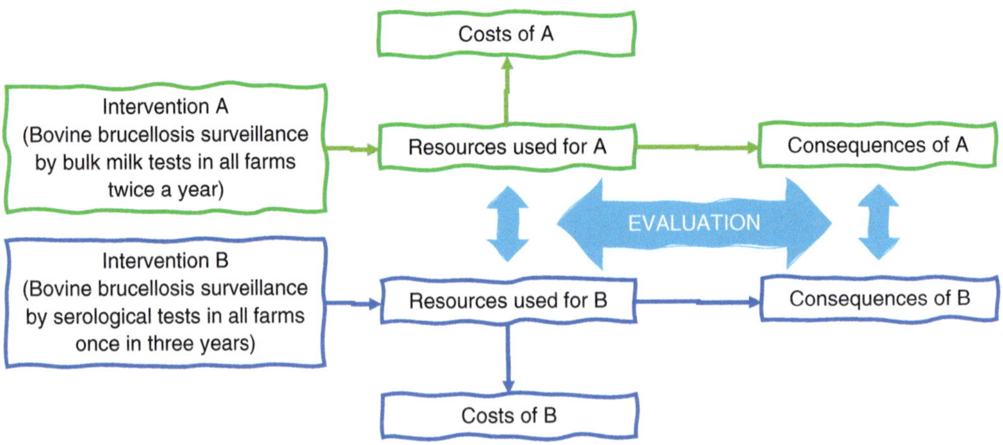

Fig. 13.2. Main characteristics of two surveillance and intervention options against bovine brucellosis in the dairy farms of an area and elements subject to economic evaluation.

and span reduced productivity in livestock, trade limitations and human health impacts. Addressing brucellosis requires coordinated efforts between veterinary or agriculture, public health and wildlife management sectors, emphasizing the interconnectedness of health across species and the importance of a holistic One Health approach (Buttigieg *et al.*, 2018; Moriyón *et al.*, 2023). We will use the example of this disease throughout the chapter to illustrate the principles covered.

One of the alternative surveillance options of Fig. 13.2 involves indirect testing of bulk milk samples from all the farms in the area twice a year, followed by serological testing of suspected herds and animals. The alternative surveillance option tests serological samples from all dairy cows every three years. Positive animals are culled, and positive farms are isolated to avoid infection of other animals and to reduce the risk to people and wildlife. The identification of the aetiological agent in the organs of culled animals triggers a sanitization protocol for the farm.

Both programmes require resources, such as skilled personnel, transportation, laboratory infrastructure and materials, which have associated costs. Each programme also has consequences in terms of reduced risks of infections in animal and human populations. The economic evaluation process involves comparing the costs and the consequences of the two alternative programmes to determine which gives the most benefits at the lowest cost.

What economists consider a 'full' economic evaluation requires two conditions: the first is that there must be at least two alternative interventions to be examined (knowing that a situation with no intervention can be one of the alternatives); the second condition is that both the costs and the consequences of all the alternatives are analysed (Pearce *et al.*, 2006; Drummond *et al.*, 2015). From this point of view, if the analysis is limited to one intervention, it is not an economic evaluation in the conventional sense but merely a description of costs, results, or both costs and results (Table 13.1). An analysis considering multiple alternatives but only evaluating their consequences is an evaluation of effectiveness, which allows the identification of the intervention that produces the best effects for the intended objective (see Chapters 10–12). Alternatively, if only costs are examined, we have a cost analysis (CA), which identifies the intervention implementable at the lowest costs compared to the alternatives. Descriptions of cost and results, evaluations of effectiveness, and CAs are partial evaluations. When we examine two or more alternative interventions, assessing the costs

Table 13.1. Partial and full economic evaluations (authors' own elaboration based on Drummond *et al.*, 2015).

Alternatives examined	Analysis of costs and/or consequences and type of evaluation	Partial or full evaluation
One intervention only	Only the consequences are examined: • Description of the results produced	Partial evaluations
	Only the costs are examined: • Description of costs	
	Costs and consequences are examined: • Description of costs and results	
Two or more alternative interventions	Only the consequences are examined: • Evaluation of effectiveness	
	Only the costs are examined: • Cost analysis (CA)	
	Costs and consequences are examined: • Cost-minimization analysis (CMA) • Cost-effectiveness analysis (CEA) • Cost-utility analysis (CUA) • Cost–benefit analysis (CBA)	Full economic evaluations

and the consequences of each, we conduct a full economic evaluation.

There are several types of full economic evaluations. When the effects of the alternatives under consideration are the same, the best solution is the one entailing the lowest costs and is identified through a cost-minimization analysis (CMA) (Rai and Goyal, 2018). When the effects of the alternative interventions are different and can be compared through a physical parameter (e.g. gains in terms of fewer infections or deaths in the human population, fewer days of hospitalization, less livestock culling, fewer animals dying, reduction in air pollution, etc.), the cost-effectiveness analysis (CEA) indicates the solution that provides the best result at the lowest cost or at a higher cost deemed acceptable. For example, a more expensive solution that guarantees fewer infections than the alternative one may be preferable if the additional costs do not exceed what the decision makers consider spendable for that outcome (Briggs *et al.*, 2006; Diamond and Kaul, 2009; Glick, 2015a).

In evaluations related to human health, when the alternatives are compared in terms of the quality of human life provided over time through specific indicators such as the Disability-Adjusted Life-Years (DALYs) and the Quality-Adjusted Life-Years (QALYs), we have a cost-utility analysis (CUA), which prefers the solutions achieving the best quality of life for the longest time at the minimum cost or with costs deemed affordable (Robinson, 1993; Coons and Kaplan, 1996; Nuijten and Dubois, 2011). For animal lives, new metrics are becoming available that are similar to the DALYs and QALYs, such as Welfare-Adjusted Life-Years (WALYs) (Teng *et al.*, 2018). A cost–benefit analysis (CBA) evaluates all the costs and outcomes of the examined alternatives in monetary terms. In this case, the best solution is the one that generates the highest net present value (NPV), i.e. the highest difference between all the benefits and the costs produced over time expressed in terms of present values[1] (Sunstein, 2005; Pearce *et al.*, 2006; Glick, 2015b; Guerriero and Pacelli, 2020).

In our brucellosis example, we are focusing on a full economic evaluation using a One Health lens where we are looking at two interventions in the animal sector, but with consequences in other sectors. We could of course expand this to have, for example, a package of interventions (with integration points) in both the human and animal sectors with consequences in both. However, for the sake of simplicity and covering basic principles, we are starting with the animal sector example and later show you how to expand this to add more complexity and One Health aspects. The underlying concepts of One Health evaluations and the use of CMA, CEA, CUA and CBA are described in detail in Canali *et al.* (2018) and Häsler *et al.* (2021); we suggest that you refer to these chapters for more information on how to conduct these analyses. Here, we provide a basic coverage of the main steps involved in these analyses and spend some time discussing valuation approaches.

But before doing so, we want to discuss how to conceptualize economic evaluations given the complexity of One Health problems and their solutions. Note that economic evaluations, particularly in the context of healthcare and public health interventions, are often associated with neo-classical economic theory due to their emphasis on efficiency, rational decision making, and resource allocation based on CEA or CBA. **Neo-classical economics** is a school of economic thought that emphasizes the role of individual rational behaviour, market mechanisms and the efficient allocation of resources to maximize societal **welfare** (Pigou, 1920; Kelman, 1981; Hansson, 2007; Glick, 2015b). There are other schools of economic thought that can be relevant to One Health; a short overview of three selected ones is provided in Box 13.1.

13.3 The Challenges of Designing and Conducting Economic Evaluations of One Health Initiatives

Economic evaluations of complex One Health initiatives pose significant challenges due to the inherent complexity and dynamic nature of these initiatives. One of the primary difficulties arises from the diverse and dynamic outcomes that we often see associated with One Health interventions. Unlike traditional healthcare interventions with relatively clearly delineated outcomes, such as reduced mortality or improved quality of life, One Health initiatives often target multifaceted problems involving human, animal, plant and environment dimensions and it is not uncommon that we face **trade-offs**. Thus, economic evaluations of One Health need to deal with a wide range of outcomes across various sectors, making it

Box 13.1. Three selected alternative schools of economic thought with relevance for One Health

Ecological economics: Ecological economics emphasizes the interconnectedness of human economies with the natural environment. It highlights that economic activities are embedded within and dependent on our planet's **ecosystems**, which provide essential resources and services that sustain life and economic activities. It acknowledges the finite nature of natural resources and the ecological limits of the planet. It advocates for meeting present human needs without compromising the ability of future generations to meet their own needs. This involves adopting practices and policies that promote resource conservation, reduce pollution and waste, and promote regenerative approaches to economic activities, such as de-growth, green growth and circular economies. It focuses on the importance of clean air and water, biodiversity, soil fertility, climate regulation, and other ecosystem functions that directly or indirectly contribute to human wellbeing and economic prosperity. Furthermore, ecological economics challenges traditional measures of economic progress, such as Gross Domestic Product (GDP), by advocating for alternative indicators that reflect broader wellbeing and the health of the environment. This includes metrics like Genuine Progress Indicator (GPI), Ecological Footprint, and measures of social and environmental resilience (Martinez-Alier and Schlupmann, 1987; van den Bergh, 2001; Baumgärtner *et al.*, 2008).

Doughnut economics: Doughnut economics is a concept developed by Kate Raworth that proposes a new economic model centred around social and planetary boundaries (Raworth, 2017a, b). It can be seen as a sub-set within the wider framework of ecological economics. The essence of doughnut economics lies in creating a balance between meeting the needs of people without overshooting the Earth's ecological limits. The 'doughnut' represents two concentric rings: the inner ring represents the minimum social standards that everyone should have access to (such as food, water, healthcare, education), while the outer ring represents the ecological ceiling beyond which human activity risks damaging the planet (such as **climate** change, biodiversity loss, pollution). The goal is to operate within this 'safe and just space for humanity', ensuring social **equity** and environmental sustainability. Doughnut economics encourages rethinking traditional growth-focused models and emphasizes sustainable development that respects planetary boundaries and promotes wellbeing for all. The goal of downscaling is met with several challenges related to the behaviour of **complex systems**, dealing with trade-offs and difficult questions in decision making and agreeing on goals when considering different scales (Turner and Wills, 2022) – all aspects that the One Health approach can help us address.

Feminist economics: Provides a critical lens that examines economic theories and practices through the prism of **gender equality** (see Chapter 9) and **social justice**. At its core, it challenges the traditional economic model's **assumptions** and methodologies (Nelson, 1995), which often overlook or undervalue the contributions and experiences of women and marginalized groups. One key aspect of feminist economics is its emphasis on recognizing and valuing unpaid labour, such as caregiving, household work and community support, which are predominantly shouldered by women (Antonopoulos and Hirway, 2010; Benería *et al.*, 2015; Winders and Smith, 2019; Stevano *et al.*, 2021). This perspective sheds light on the hidden economic contributions that sustain societies but are often ignored in conventional economic analyses (Mair, 2020). Feminist economists also highlight the intersectionality of gender with other axes of identity like race, class and sexuality, acknowledging that individuals experience economic systems differently based on their unique social positions (Antonopoulos and Hirway, 2010). Moreover, feminist economics advocates for policies and interventions that promote gender equality, economic empowerment, and inclusivity in decision making. This includes initiatives to address pay gaps, enhance access to education and employment opportunities for women, and challenge discriminatory practices within economic institutions. By centring social justice, equity and diversity in economic discourse and policy making, feminist economics aims to create more inclusive and sustainable economies that prioritize the wellbeing and agency of all individuals, irrespective of their gender or social identities (Razavi *et al.*, 2012; Braunstein, 2015; Bachelet, 2022).

challenging (but not impossible!) to capture and quantify their full impacts comprehensively.

Furthermore, the multisectoral nature of One Health adds layers of complexity to economic evaluations. One Health initiatives typically involve collaboration and coordination among diverse stakeholders from public health, veterinary medicine, environmental science, agriculture and other sectors. Each sector may have distinct priorities, metrics and methods of assessment, making it difficult to integrate economic data and analyses across sectors. This multiplicity of perspectives and outcomes complicates the task of assigning economic values to different aspects of One Health interventions. It is important to consider explicitly the One Health elements and structures of an evaluation if we want to determine the added value of One Health (Auplish *et al.*, 2024).

Economic evaluations often use monetary terms, and these may not adequately capture the full spectrum of outcomes and impacts associated with One Health interventions. The potential intangible benefits of such interventions, such as **ecosystem services**, social equity improvements or resilience enhancement, are challenging to quantify in monetary terms despite knowing that these benefits have value to communities and society. Additionally, **data** availability and quality for economic evaluations in One Health can vary widely, especially when dealing with interconnected systems and long-term effects. For example, when effects on the environment are considered, the benefits often reach far into the future and questions of intergenerational values and equity must be considered.

Addressing these challenges involves developing and adapting the evaluation frameworks and methods that can accommodate the diverse outcomes, perspectives and uncertainties inherent in One Health initiatives. Collaborative efforts among economists, public health experts, environmental scientists and other stakeholders are crucial for advancing methodological tools, data collection strategies and analytical techniques tailored to the complexities of One Health. By improving the capacity for economic evaluations in One Health, decision makers can better understand the value proposition of these initiatives and make informed investment choices for promoting global health, sustainability and resilience. We will revisit these challenges later, but for now look at the different steps of capturing the costs and benefits of One Health interventions.

Task: Thinking about the brucellosis intervention from Fig. 13.2, list any consequences that you can think of resulting from these two interventions covering livestock health, agriculture, wildlife and public health sectors.

Example answer 1: For a context, where brucellosis is endemic and transmission to people directly through animals or milk is a common occurrence, we might think about the following:

- Livestock health: Reduction in brucellosis prevalence among dairy cows due to removal of infected animals would be a positive aspect and contribute to improved overall health of dairy herds with fewer disease outbreaks.
- Agriculture: A positive effect would be increased productivity in dairy farming as infected cows are removed, preventing further spread, thereby contributing to more economic resilience of the sector. On the negative side, there could be economic losses for small-scale farmers due to culling of infected cows.
- Wildlife: A positive effect could be the reduced risk of transmission to wildlife species sharing habitats with infected cattle.
- Public health: A positive effect could be the decreased transmission of brucellosis to humans through consumption of contaminated milk or direct contact with infected animals and improved public health outcomes with fewer brucellosis cases among the population.

Example answer 2: For a context, where brucellosis has been eliminated and the intervention focuses on maintaining the situation of freedom from disease, the consequences may include the following:

- Livestock health: The testing might lead to the detection of some rare cases of brucellosis in dairy cows that may lead to slaughter of some animals. On the positive side, there might be a good reputation of the sector for having eliminated the disease and keeping it away.
- Agriculture: With the detection and removal of (few) positive animals if a reintroduction occurs, there can be some economic losses to the animal owners. On the positive side, the wider sector benefits from the disease absence.

- Wildlife: A positive effect is the limited risk of transmission to wildlife as brucellosis is largely absent in livestock.
- Public health: A positive effect is the very low risk of human brucellosis cases due to effective control measures and eradication efforts. Improved confidence in food safety and reduced public health concerns related to brucellosis transmission.

From this and the previous sections you know the main challenges of performing economic evaluations by comparing costs and consequences of alternative One Health initiatives. In the next section, we are going to discuss how we can put values on these elements and compare them.

13.4 What are the Costs and Benefits of One Health Interventions and How Do We Evaluate Them?

When individuals experience a decrease in their wellbeing, they incur a cost. The resources, skills and time used to fulfil given needs cannot be used to satisfy other needs. This trade-off or sacrifice is the cost incurred by pursuing a particular activity. Additionally, any suffering, discomfort, pain or reduction in wellbeing experienced by an individual is also considered a cost. When the wellbeing improves (e.g. less human disease, better livestock welfare, more biodiversity), the reduction of the negative effect transforms into a benefit. The magnitude of the benefit that we can achieve through an intervention gives us an upper limit of how much we can invest to achieve these benefits and break even (a break-even point is a term commonly used in economics and business to describe the point at which total revenue equals total costs, resulting in neither profit nor loss). In other words, an investment is economically worthwhile if the investment costs are recovered by the resulting benefits.

In One Health, the costs may be borne by different **actors** and the benefits may include both private and public goods. A **PRIVATE GOOD** is both excludable and rivalrous in consumption and includes most consumer products, such as food or clothing typically bought and sold in markets. A **PUBLIC GOOD** is non-excludable and non-rivalrous in consumption, i.e. consumption is open to all and if one individual consumes it, there is still availability or benefits for others, e.g. public parks or clean air. Public goods often have positive EXTERNALITIES, i.e. the impact of an economic activity that affects third parties who are not directly involved in the activity and whose interests are not taken into account in the market price, meaning their benefits spill over to society as a whole beyond those directly consuming or paying for goods or services.

13.4.1 Market prices of resources

How do we value what we have defined as costs? The materials, work time, and skills we use for One Health interventions are generally available on the market. **MARKET PRICES** are indicators of the availability of these resources and the competition for their use among economic operators in their activities. Then, market prices show how much the resources in a One Health intervention are worth. This cost reflects what we give up by not using those resources for other possible purposes.

13.4.2 Tangible and intangible costs

When implementing an activity, the costs related to resource use for which market prices can be identified, such as fuels, energy and other utilities, raw materials, consumable and durable goods, facilities, personnel and professional services, are defined as **TANGIBLE COSTS** (measurable costs that can be quantified in monetary terms). Their assessment is based on information on technical parameters (how much energy, how many materials, how much labour, what kind of facilities, etc.) and price data.

We have also seen that the occurrence in individuals of suffering, discomfort, pain or reduced wellbeing is a cost. To estimate these costs, we cannot refer directly to market prices. For this reason, costs originating from non-market goods are defined as **INTANGIBLE COSTS** and are estimated by analysing the behaviour of individuals through a range of methods. In the context of the evaluation of One Health initiatives, we often also consider the intangible costs related to animal welfare losses in farms (Bozzo *et al.*, 2019; Alonso *et al.*, 2020) and those related to losses in the 'non-use' values of environmental goods. The latter refers to the value individuals attribute to keeping in existence an environmental good even though there is no actual, planned or possible use of it (see also Section 13.7 on valuation later in the chapter). People's value could stem from the concern for the good itself (e.g. a threatened landscape or animal species), a feeling of responsibility for it (existence values), or a sentiment that the good should be available to others (altruistic value) or future generations (bequest value) (Pearce *et al.*, 2006).

Methods for estimating intangible costs are based on the assessment of individuals' willingness to pay[2] (WTP) to avoid the associated welfare losses. They include revealed and stated preference methods, which derive values based on observed behaviours or stated opinions of individuals respectively (Whitehead *et al.*, 2008). This makes it possible to attribute monetary values to intangible costs: an example is the social cost of carbon used specifically for environmental intangible costs (Nordhaus, 2017). The concept of the 'intrinsic' value affirms that environmental goods have value in themselves independently of human preferences and WTP (Attfield, 1998; Batavia and Nelson, 2017). However, this notion cannot be incorporated into evaluation procedures that attribute values to assets based on objective criteria and people's WTP (Pearce *et al.*, 2006). In other words, when we assume that the value of an environmental good is not related to individual preferences, we do not know how to quantify this 'intrinsic' value objectively in monetary terms.

13.4.3 Direct and indirect costs of an intervention

Direct costs are those directly related to the implementation of an intervention, for example:

- employment of health and administrative personnel;
- use of medicines, vaccines, supplements, medical instruments, personal protective equipment, etc.;
- use of health facilities, laboratories, health equipment, vehicles, etc.;
- third-party services (insurance, rental of vehicles and equipment, banking services, consultancy, etc.);
- monitoring and evaluation to track the progress and effectiveness of the intervention; and
- activities and processes in the environment, such as construction, planting, or habitat restoration efforts.

Indirect costs are those that arise as a consequence of the implementation of the intervention; typical indirect costs are the so-called productivity losses when people and animals are affected, but there are also other types of indirect costs:

- time spent by workers or community members participating in or supporting the intervention instead of their regular activities or jobs;
- temporary declines in animal health and productivity or welfare due to side effects of the intervention;
- trade disruptions in the agricultural or animal production sector caused by the intervention; and
- impact on local businesses or industries due to changes in environmental regulations or interventions, such as restrictions on fishing or logging.

13.4.4 Resources that do not exhaust their functionality with use

There are resources that exhaust their utility with use, such as medicines, electricity, fuel for vehicles, disinfectants, detergents, hours of work, which once used cannot be reused at other times. Therefore, their value in use corresponds to the price we pay to buy them.

For resources such as buildings, medical and laboratory instruments, health equipment, vehicles, furniture and hardware, which do not exhaust their functionality with use and can also be used beyond the specific intervention we are evaluating, it is necessary to estimate the COST OF DEPRECIATION in the context of the intervention considered. For example, the depreciation cost of a vehicle used by the public veterinary service to collect samples for the alternative surveillance options, outlined in Fig. 13.2, can be calculated with the formula:

$$C_{int} = \frac{NV}{TT} * T_{int}$$

Where:

NV = price of purchasing the vehicle as new (e.g. a minivan, price: US\$40,000);

TT = estimated total time of use of the vehicle by the public veterinary service until its decommissioning (e.g. 10 years);

T_{int} = estimated time of use of the vehicle for the interventions:

6 months per year in the case of intervention A (bulk milk testing in all farms twice a year);

1 month per year in the case of intervention B (serological testing in all farms once in three years).

C_{int} = cost of depreciation of the vehicle for its use in the interventions:

for intervention A (bulk milk testing in all farms twice a year) = (\$40,000/10 years) * 6/12 = \$2000 per year;

for intervention B (serological testing in all farms once in three years) = (\$40,000/10 years) * 1/12 = \$333 per year.

Task: Assuming the vehicle of the above example is used for an average annual distance travelled of 30,000 km, estimate the depreciation cost per km travelled.

Answer: The annual depreciation cost of the vehicle is calculated by dividing the NV (\$40,000) by the estimated total time of using the vehicle (10 years), which results in an annual depreciation cost of \$4000 per year. Next, we calculate the depreciation cost per kilometre travelled. We know the vehicle travels an average annual distance of 30,000 km. We calculate the depreciation cost per kilometre by dividing the annual depreciation cost by the average annual distance travelled, i.e. \$4000/30,000km = \$ 0.1333/km.

13.4.5 Benefits

Contrary to costs, anything that causes an increase in an individual's or population's state of wellbeing determines a benefit, for example:

- a decrease in the state of suffering, discomfort, pain, or the induction of a state of greater pleasure or satisfaction in an individual;
- improved water quality, increasing biodiversity, and providing recreational opportunities enhancing the overall wellbeing of the community and ecosystem;
- increasing crop and animal yields to ensure a stable food supply, reducing hunger and malnutrition;
- generating more equitable education opportunities promoting empowerment of disadvantaged groups; and
- saving resources in satisfying a need so that they can be allocated to meet other needs as well as productivity improvements.

Benefits assessment generally follows the same logic and classifications seen for costs regarding tangibility, direct and indirect correlation to the implementation of the intervention, distribution over time (see below), and application of methods to determine their value.

13.4.6 The evaluation timeframe, values over time and discounting

The timeframe of an evaluation is the period over which the costs and consequences of an intervention are assessed. It should cover the time needed for the intervention to develop all its relevant impacts regarding the use of resources and wellbeing creation. Typically, this goes through a first phase in which most of the investments necessary for intervention implementation are deployed, with dominance of costs over benefits. In the second phase, the intervention runs at its ordinary capacity with operating costs being incurred, and benefits often prevailing.

Therefore, resource consumption and effects of a One Health intervention develop over time, and the same happens for the costs and benefits that the intervention produces, which is a problem for economic evaluations because values generated at different moments are not directly comparable.

Getting a benefit of \$1000 today is better than getting a benefit of \$1000 in one year's time and supporting a cost of \$1000 in one year's time is better than disbursing such an amount today, because money available now is worth more than the same amount in the future due to its potential earning capacity. Therefore, to compare benefits and costs occurring at different moments, it is necessary to convert them to present-day values, a process called **discounting**:

$$PV = \frac{FV}{(1+r)^t}$$

Where:

PV = present value;

FV = future value;

r = discount rate;

t = time

Discounting gives account of time preference of individuals. A classical problem is that a future value discounted at present appears to us smaller the later in time it occurs, and the higher the discount rate is. Figure 13.3 illustrates the distribution over time of the net values created by a One Health intervention that extends its relevant impacts over 20 years. Net investments of

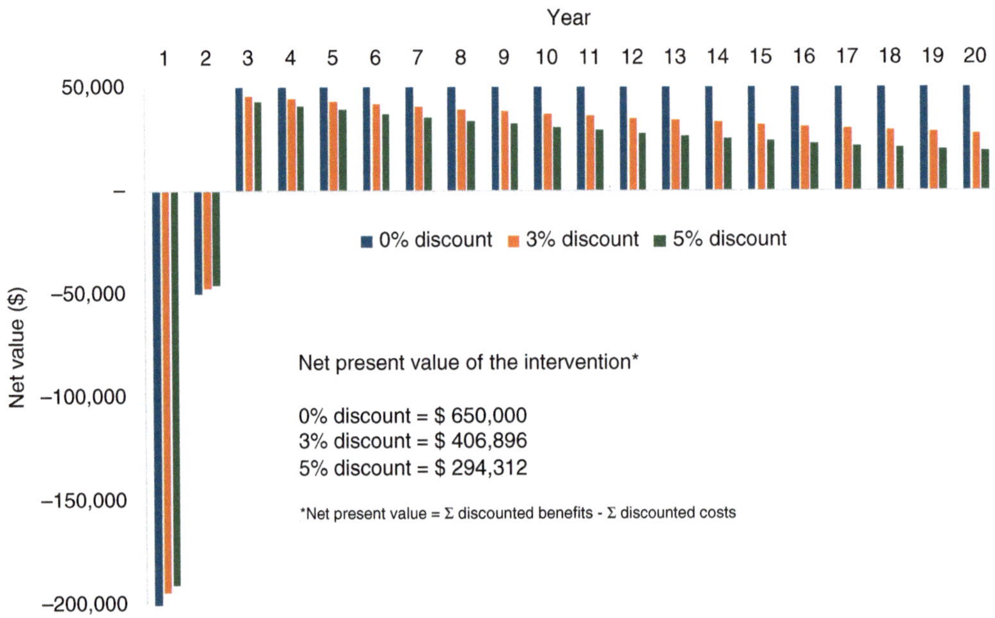

Fig. 13.3. Distribution over time of the net values created by a One Health intervention over a 20-year timeframe calculated at different discount rates (0%, 3% and 5%), and respective net present values (see details in the text).

\$200,000 and \$50,000 are planned in the first two years. The intervention brings an annual net benefit of \$25,000 between the third and the twentieth year.

These values have been discounted at different rates:

- 0%, i.e. no discount applied (blue bars in the graph);
- 3% discount (orange bars in the graph);
- 5% discount (green bars in the graph).

The graph highlights the difference between the annual values when discounted at different rates and the further away from the start of the project in time. Figure 13.3 also shows the intervention's net present value (NPV), i.e. the difference between the sum of all the discounted benefits and the discounted costs accumulated over time. Not applying discounting, the intervention achieves a net present value of \$650,000. With a discount rate of 3%, the attractiveness of the intervention decreases considerably to an NPV of \$406,896. If we apply a discount rate of 5%, the NPV is \$294,312.

The choice of the discount rate can, therefore, significantly influence the final economic judgement on an intervention:

- In the case of health interventions, reference is made to the so-called 'social time preference rate' or 'social discount rate', generally indicated by government authorities for projects that have public utility implications (Zhuang *et al.*, 2007). They can be lower than market rates to reflect societal preferences for intergenerational equity. The WHO suggests applying in health assessments a discount rate of 3% (Tan-Torres Edejer *et al.*, 2003). The European Commission often uses a range of 3% to 5% for CBAs related to public investments, including environmental projects.[3]
- Financial discount rates are used in financial analysis to evaluate investments, projects or assets from the perspective of investors or businesses. For interventions operated with private financing (for example, in the agriculture sector), a reference can be the rate of return of alternative investments in the private sector.

The social discount rate emphasizes societal values and intergenerational equity, while the financial discount rate focuses on maximizing financial returns and investment decisions.

Discount rates proposed by governments for public interest initiatives vary significantly across countries and over time for the same country. Zhuang *et al.* (2007) analysed the different approaches public authorities adopted in different countries. Following the mentioned WHO suggestion, as well as the advice of the US Panels on Cost-Effectiveness in Health and Medicine, the 3% discount rate is often used for evaluations concerned with global health (Basu and Ganiats, 2016; Haacker et al., 2020).

Discounting future values related to environmental assets is deemed to underestimate the potential damage to future generations from the current use of natural resources; this is called the 'Tyranny of Discounting'. Many environmental interventions, such as conservation projects or pollution reduction efforts, generate benefits that accrue over extended time periods, sometimes spanning generations. Discounting these benefits at standard rates can diminish their perceived value in present terms. Another argument is that some environmental changes, such as species extinction or habitat destruction, are irreversible or have long-lasting consequences and that discounting may not adequately capture the irreversible nature of these losses. Proposed alternatives to the supposed unfairness of discounting towards future generations are the adoption of zero discounting or discount rates that diminish in the far future for economic evaluations involving the environment (Broome, 1992; Pearce *et al.*, 2003; Polasky and Dampha, 2021). These approaches want to induce incremental savings of natural resources by the current generation to safeguard the prosperity of future generations. However, zero discounting implies that future values are accounted the same as current values by neglecting individuals' time preference, which does not fit with human behaviour. Moreover, the zero-discounting perspective entails that there are no limits on how many future generations are entitled to benefit from current savings, creating relevant paradoxes, including inequity regarding the possibilities of improving the conditions of the most disadvantaged populations within the current generation (Pearce *et al.*, 2003, 2006).

Over the last decades, researchers have found that time-declining discount rates align better with the behaviour of individuals compared to the conventional practice of discounting at a constant rate over time (Hansen, 2006). The human attitude of discounting future values has been attributed to **uncertainty** about the future or the economy. In contrast, the application of time-declining discount rates addressing intergenerational equity is rooted in a prescriptive approach stemming from environmental ethics and climate-change policies. Despite this considerable difference – and other shortcomings related to the logic consistency of time-declining discounting when concretely applied (Hansen, 2006) – the two approaches could opportunistically find some convergence (Pearce *et al.*, 2003; Hansen, 2006; Polasky and Dampha, 2021).

13.4.7 The evaluation point of view

What is a cost for the government is often not a cost for an individual patient or farmer. Moreover, the interest of the entire national community is not necessarily the same for a specific region, territory or health facility.

The 'point of view' or 'perspective' considered in economic evaluation is relevant. For example, two alternative viewpoints are adopted in the economic assessment of health interventions that have public interest implications (Hurley, 2000; Brouwer *et al.*, 2008; Drummond *et al.*, 2015), namely:

- Given the available resources, the 'societal' point of view pursues the maximum interest for the whole community of reference; this is the 'welfarist' approach.[4] One solution is better than another if it increases someone's wellbeing without damaging anyone else (or providing compensations for those supporting damages);
- The point of view of the health structure that provides the service is the position of an institution that, with the budget assigned, must optimize the services to which it is committed in quantitative and qualitative terms, under the hypothesis that the institution's decision makers act in the interest of the community: this is the 'extra-welfarist' approach.

In the first case, the judgement on the convenience of an intervention should also consider the possible alternative uses of resources in society's sectors other than the One Health sectors. In the second case, the choices about the intervention directly concern the management of the specific institution or service.

In the context of One Health, the costs and benefits associated with interventions can vary depending on the perspective adopted. Unlike traditional health evaluations, where costs for the public health service may not directly impact individual patients or farmers, One Health interventions often involve interconnected systems where costs and benefits extend beyond the health sector alone.

Consider, for example, a vaccination programme targeting **zoonotic diseases** in both human and animal populations. From a societal perspective, the 'welfarist' approach seeks to maximize overall wellbeing across all sectors of the community. This perspective considers not only the health benefits but also the broader societal impacts, such as economic productivity, environmental sustainability and social equity. In this view, an intervention is deemed favourable if it increases overall wellbeing without causing harm to any sector and considers potential trade-offs between One Health sectors and other societal needs.

Task: Using the brucellosis example with interventions to be applied in an endemic context, work through the different steps as outlined in this section and for each step write down what you would consider in your analysis.

Example answer:

- Market price of resources: Consider the cost of resources such as vaccines, diagnostic tests, personnel and medical equipment based on market prices. This will allow you to estimate the costs of the intervention accurately.
- Tangible and intangible costs: By analysing both tangible and intangible costs, direct and indirect costs, we can get a more complete picture of the economic burden associated with the two options. Evaluate tangible costs like extra labour needed or labour lost when people are sick, medicines and facilities used, and costs for the culling of animals as well as the costs incurred for personnel (veterinarians, technicians) involved in testing of the animals. Both programmes might lead to productivity losses for farmers owing to time spent handling testing procedures and culling. Restrictions on animal movement due to positive tests could also lead to indirect costs. The tangible costs can be estimated using market prices for personnel, testing materials and equipment. Moreover, consider intangible costs such as animal welfare losses when livestock get ill, environmental non-use values (see Section 13.7 on valuation), and societal wellbeing impacts. Both interventions involve culling infected animals, which can be a source of stress and suffering for the animals. This can be considered an intangible cost. Estimating the intangible cost of animal welfare is challenging. We cannot directly use market prices, but we can consider studies that assess people's WTP to reduce animal suffering in farm settings.
- Resources that do not exhaust their functionality with use: Estimate costs related to resources that retain functionality over time, such as buildings and medical equipment, considering their use beyond the specific intervention.
- Benefits: Assess benefits in terms of reduced disease burden, increased productivity, societal wellbeing, improved animal welfare and environmental benefits.
- The timeframe of the evaluation: Define the time over which the One Health intervention deploys its relevant consequences in terms of the use of resources and impacts on humans, animals and health of the environment. Note that the timeframe for proposed interventions affects the inclusion of benefits. Longer timeframes can be more useful to see environment health benefits, but if timeframes are too long, the results become much less certain.
- The values over time and discounting: Apply discounting to compare costs and benefits over time, considering the present value of the intervention and the choice of discount rate based on public or private financing perspectives.
- The point of view of evaluation: Consider the evaluation perspective, whether it is from a social viewpoint aiming for maximum community or sector benefit or if it is an intervention that benefits society more widely. In some cases, it may also be of interest to include the perspective of a specific health facility managing its resources optimally (e.g. a chain of veterinary practices involved in brucellosis control).
- Applying the framework: This information, along with the potential benefits (improved animal health, reduced public health risk), can be used to conduct a CBA and determine the most cost-effective programme for controlling brucellosis in the specific context.

13.5 Combining Different Metrics and Decision Parameters

The main methods of economic evaluation do not substantially differ in considering costs, which are always expressed in terms of monetary values, but rather in the ways in which the consequences of the interventions examined are compared. Even when the comparison is made with reference to non-monetary effects, such as in the CEA and CUA, these effects should be discounted. Table 13.2 provides an overview of how the different

Table 13.2. Types of economic evaluations for One Health interventions, parameters for the evaluation of costs and consequences, and published examples on brucellosis.

Type of evaluation	Costs	Consequences	Description and decision parameters	Examples on brucellosis
Cost-minimization analysis (CMA)	Monetary values	The examined alternatives have identical health effects expressed with the same indicator	Compares the costs in monetary terms of alternative interventions that have equivalent outcomes. Aims to identify the least costly option among equally effective alternatives.	Cost comparison of two surveillance strategies on cattle with the same diagnostic accuracy in a brucellosis officially free area in Northern Italy (Aragrande *et al.*, 2020).
Cost-effectiveness analysis (CEA)	Monetary values	The examined alternatives have different health effects expressed with the same indicator in natural (physical) units	Compares the costs and health outcomes of alternative interventions calculating the cost per unit of outcome achieved to identify the most cost-effective solution. The alternatives are compared through the incremental cost-effectiveness ratio (ICER, see in the main text).	The sensitivity in detecting brucellosis and the costs of the French surveillance system for the disease are compared to those of 19 alternative surveillance scenarios (Hénaux and Calavas, 2017).
Cost-utility analysis (CUA)	Monetary values	Different effects expressed in terms of better health status of individuals over time	As in CEA (often CUA is also considered to be a type of CEA), except for the outcomes that are always expressed as individuals' quality of life over time with specific indicators, e.g. disability-adjusted life-year (DALY) or quality-adjusted life-year (QALY).	Cost-utility comparison in terms of cost per DALY averted between two testing methods, namely the Febrile Antigen Brucella Agglutination Test (FBAT) and the Rose Bengal Test (RBT) in Kenyan hospitals (Alumasa *et al.*, 2021). Comparison of different test-and-slaughter strategies for brucellosis control achieving different levels of livestock culling for cattle and sheep in Armenia (Anyanwu *et al.*, 2024).
Cost–benefit analysis (CBA)	Monetary values	Effects expressed in monetary values	Considers the monetary values generated over time by alternative interventions in terms of both costs and the benefits to identify the solution that generates the highest net present value (NPV, see Section 13.4.6). Other parameters for decision in CBA are the benefit–cost ratio (BCR) and the internal rate of return (IRR). There are also parameters that do not use discounted values, such as the pay-back period (PBP).	Cost–benefit evaluation of a proposed improved annual mass vaccination programme for sheep and goats targeting all animals older than 3 months with the Rev. 1 vaccine, compared to a current annual programme vaccinating only female animals between 3 and 6 months of age in Northern Iraq (Al Hamada *et al.*, 2021). Comparison of different test-and-slaughter strategies for brucellosis control achieving different levels of livestock culling for cattle and sheep in Armenia (Anyanwu *et al.*, 2024).

Continued

Table 13.2. Continued.

Type of evaluation	Costs	Consequences	Description and decision parameters	Examples on brucellosis
Mixed analysis	Monetary values	Effects expressed in monetary and non-monetary values	A mixed One Health analysis that combines both cost-effectiveness analysis and cost–benefit analysis and looks at effects in multiple sectors.	For the human population, an incremental cost-effectiveness analysis to compare the cost and health effects of a vaccination programme with current practice. Combined with a cost–benefit analysis for different vaccination strategies in livestock. Consideration of reduced transmission from livestock to people (Roth *et al.*, 2003). From a societal perspective, the value of reduced disease in humans, households and animal production outweighed the total intervention costs and the $ per DALY averted became negative.[5]

types of economic evaluations can be applied using different brucellosis examples.

For the CBA, an important parameter informing decisions between the examined interventions is the NPV described in Section 13.4.6. Other parameters used in CBA are the benefit–cost ratio (BCR) and the internal rate of return (IRR). The BCR of an intervention is calculated by dividing the sum of its discounted benefits by the sum of its discounted costs, as follows:

$$BCR = \frac{\sum discounted\ benefits}{\sum discounted\ costs}$$

An intervention creates a positive value (i.e. NPV > 0) when the BCR > 1. Between alternative interventions, we should prefer the one with the highest BCR. If two alternatives have the same NPV, the one that implies the lower costs is better, and this can be detected with the BCR.

The IRR is the discount rate that results in an NPV equal to zero. It can be calculated based on the equation:

$$\sum discounted\ benefits = \sum discounted\ costs$$

Between alternative interventions we should prefer the one with the highest IRR.

All three decision criteria are ideally considered in decision making. The IRR has the advantage of avoiding the choice of the discount rate to be adopted in the valuation. However, the literature advises against its use as the main evaluation parameter of an intervention, as it is influenced by the distribution of costs and benefits over time and has several accounting drawbacks: e.g. it is possible for an intervention to have more than one IRR or even no IRR at all (Pearce *et al.*, 2006).

There are also decision parameters for CBA that do not make use of discounted values. One is the pay-back period (PBP), which is the time needed to recover the initial investment of the intervention with the generated net benefits. For example, if an intervention requires an initial investment of \$1 million, and generates net benefits of \$100,000 per year, its PBP is ten years. Between alternative interventions, we should choose the one with the shorter PBP.

Regarding CEA and CUA, the cost-effectiveness of alternative interventions is compared through the incremental cost-effectiveness ratio (ICER), which expresses the difference in costs related to the difference in effectiveness between the alternatives:

$$ICER = \frac{C_N - C_O}{E_N - E_O}$$

Where C_N and C_O are the costs of the new intervention and the old (existing) alternative, and E_N and E_O are the respective effects.

The ICER expresses the cost-effectiveness of N compared to O. If N is less expensive and more effective than O, it should be preferred. If it results in being more costly and less effective, it should be rejected. If it is more costly but also more effective than O, the decision maker should establish if the incremental effect of N justifies its incremental cost, according to a cost-effectiveness threshold that, in a societal perspective, sets the maximum willingness to pay of society for such an improvement.

For details on how to conduct the different analyses summarized in Table 13.2, please refer to Canali *et al.* (2018) and look at the references provided with illustrative examples. Here, we are now moving on to think about how to combine different effects in these economic evaluations.

Learning questions: Building on the example above and the different effects that you identified, think about how these outcomes could be measured and how they would be included in an economic evaluation. Would they all have the same metric? Would they all have the same weight? Why?

Example answer:

- Improved animal health productivity can be measured through indicators such as disease incidence rates, animal mortality rates, reproductive success and livestock productivity metrics (e.g. milk yield, weight gain). In the economic evaluation, improved animal health productivity would involve assessing the costs of veterinary services, disease prevention measures, animal husbandry practices, and access to quality feed and healthcare. The benefits can be assessed in terms of increased income from livestock products, reduced healthcare expenses and overall economic gains for farmers.
- Improved human health resulting from the interventions can be measured through various indicators such as changes in disease incidence and prevalence, morbidity and mortality rates, healthcare utilization patterns including hospital admissions and primary care visits. Also, qualitative assessments can be used such as quality of life surveys and patient feedback to determine metrics such as QALYs and DALYs. The interventions also come with healthcare associated costs that need to be considered.
- Biodiversity gain can be measured using ecological metrics such as species richness, habitat diversity, ecosystem stability and presence of indicator species. In the economic evaluation, biodiversity gain would involve assessing the costs associated with conservation efforts, habitat restoration and biodiversity monitoring. The benefits can be assessed in terms of ecosystem services provided, such as pollination services, soil fertility, water purification and carbon sequestration.
- Social **empowerment** can be measured through indicators such as increased participation in decision-making processes, enhanced **knowledge** and skills among community members, and improved access to resources and opportunities. The economic evaluation can assess the cost of **capacity-building** programmes, community training sessions, and infrastructure development aimed at empowering individuals. The benefits can be measured through factors like increased community resilience, reduced social inequalities and improved overall wellbeing.
- Each outcome would require different metrics for measurement due to their unique nature (social, ecological and economic). For example, social empowerment may use qualitative and participatory methods, while biodiversity gain may rely on ecological surveys.
- The weights assigned to each outcome in the economic evaluation would depend on various factors such as the project goals, stakeholder priorities and societal values. For instance, in an area with high biodiversity importance, biodiversity gain may be given more weight, whereas in a community facing social challenges, social empowerment may be prioritized. These weights would reflect the relative importance and impact of each outcome on the overall success and sustainability of the One Health intervention. They can be determined with the community of practice and stakeholders set up during the implementation cycle.

You will see from the activity above that there are important considerations and decisions to be made when it comes to the combination of diverse outcomes. Using our example of two interventions for brucellosis in dairy farms, we now present the hypothetical results of their application in a region recording 100 human cases annually.

Task: Given the two interventions summarized in Table 13.3, considering a period of 10 years, and a discount rate of 3%, calculate:

- The NPV of the two interventions from a societal perspective and from the viewpoint of the national health service, and indicate the best solution; and
- The ICER per averted human case of the two interventions with respect to the current situation from a societal perspective and from the viewpoint of the national health service and indicate the best solution.

Answer:

The subscripts A and B indicate interventions A and B, respectively, and the figures highlighted in bold indicate the preferred intervention from an economic point of view.

Net present value:

- Societal perspective: **NPV_A $29,378,019**; NPV_B $26,968,236.
- Health service perspective: **NPV_A $20,165,400**; NPV_B $18,101,090.

Incremental cost-effectiveness ratio:

- Societal perspective: **$ICER_A$ $-43,050** per DALY; $ICER_B$ $-41,058 per DALY (for both solutions the ICER is negative, which in this case means that both generate a benefit per DALY averted).
- Health service perspective: **$ICER_A$ $-29,550** per DALY; $ICER_B$ $-27,558 per DALY (for both solutions the ICER is negative, which in this case means that both generate a benefit per DALY averted).

Table 13.4 shows the costs and benefits for the two interventions A and B as compared to the current situation. Note that the benefits (both monetary and non-monetary) can be estimated directly using the averted costs, i.e. no comparison with the current situation (i.e. the baseline) is needed.

Table 13.5 shows the calculated net present value and the ICER for both options A and B. Here, the total monetary value calculated was compared to the DALYs averted. Because the NPV is already positive, the DALYs averted are an additional benefit, adding to the monetary benefit that is created in the livestock sector. One DALY equates to a year of healthy life lost, i.e. averted DALYs constitute a benefit. Here, we are now facing a situation where we are seeing a benefit for each DALY averted. As explained in the note cited previously (note 5), this can be difficult for decision makers to understand and it may make sense to present this outcome in a different way.

We often see situations where there is a net cost and the averted DALYs are used to decide whether an intervention is economically worthwhile. Hence, we might

Table 13.3. Results stemming from a hypothetical *ex-ante* economic analysis of two new intervention options (to replace the current one) for brucellosis in dairy farms in an endemic region where 100 human cases are annually recorded, with resulting benefits in human and animal populations. One of the two options will substitute the current farm control strategy of the public veterinary service.

Item	Intervention A	Intervention B
Total cost of the current farm control strategy of the public veterinary service ($/year)	20,000	20,000
Transportation costs of public veterinary service staff with the new farm surveillance system ($/year)	25,000	7,000
Costs of sample collection in dairy farms by the public veterinary service with the new farm surveillance system ($/year)	23,000	145,000
Laboratory testing costs by the public veterinary service with the new farm surveillance system ($/year)	8,000	56,000
Averted farm costs for suspected animal culling and farm sanitation protocols with the new farm surveillance system ($/year)	800,000	770,000
Averted costs for human healthcare and hospitalizations by the public health service with the new farm surveillance system ($/year)	2,400,000	2,310,000
Averted costs of productivity losses for human cases with the new farm surveillance system ($/year)	280,000	269,500
Number of averted DALYs with the new farm surveillance system (DALYs/year)	80	77

Table 13.4. Overview of the different costs and benefits, both monetary and non-monetary, over a time period of 10 years, discounted and undiscounted.

Years	1	2	3	4	5	6	7	8	9	10
COSTS										
Current control strategy cost ($)	20,000	20,000	20,000	20,000	20,000	20,000	20,000	20,000	20,000	20,000
Transportation costs + sample collection + laboratory testing for A ($)	56,000	56,000	56,000	56,000	56,000	56,000	56,000	56,000	56,000	56,000
Difference in costs current and A (i.e. the extra costs of A compared to current) ($)	36,000	36,000	36,000	36,000	36,000	36,000	36,000	36,000	36,000	36,000
Discounted difference in costs (i.e. the extra costs of A compared to current in present value terms) ($)	**34,951**	**33,933**	**32,945**	**31,986**	**31,054**	**30,149**	**29,271**	**28,419**	**27,591**	**26,787**
Transportation costs + sample collection + laboratory testing for B ($)	208,000	208,000	208,000	208,000	208,000	208,000	208,000	208,000	208,000	208,000
Difference in costs current and B (i.e. the extra costs of B compared to current) ($)	188,000	188,000	188,000	188,000	188,000	188,000	188,000	188,000	188,000	188,000
Discounted difference in costs (i.e. the extra costs of B compared to current in present value terms) ($)	**182,524**	**177,208**	**172,047**	**167,036**	**162,170**	**157,447**	**152,861**	**148,409**	**144,086**	**139,890**
BENEFITS										
Societal perspective A										
Averted farm costs + averted human health costs + averted productivity losses ($)	3,480,000	3,480,000	3,480,000	3,480,000	3,480,000	3,480,000	3,480,000	3,480,000	3,480,000	3,480,000
Discounted benefits societal perspective ($)	**3,378,641**	**3,280,234**	**3,184,693**	**3,091,935**	**3,001,879**	**2,914,445**	**2,829,558**	**2,747,144**	**2,667,130**	**2,589,447**
Health service perspective A										
Public health perspective: Averted costs for human healthcare and hospitalization ($)	2,400,000	2,400,000	2,400,000	2,400,000	2,400,000	2,400,000	2,400,000	2,400,000	2,400,000	2,400,000
Discounted benefits health service perspective ($)	**2,330,097**	**2,262,230**	**2,196,340**	**2,132,369**	**2,070,261**	**2,009,962**	**1,951,420**	**1,894,582**	**1,839,400**	**1,785,825**
Societal perspective B										
Averted farm costs + averted human health costs + averted productivity losses ($)	3,349,500	3,349,500	3,349,500	3,349,500	3,349,500	3,349,500	3,349,500	3,349,500	3,349,500	3,349,500

Continued

Table 13.4. Continued

Years	1	2	3	4	5	6	7	8	9	10
Discounted benefits societal perspective ($)	3,251,942	3,157,225	3,065,267	2,975,987	2,889,308	2,805,154	2,723,450	2,644,126	2,567,113	2,492,343
Health service perspective B										
Public health perspective: Averted costs for human healthcare and hospitalization ($)	2,310,000	2,310,000	2,310,000	2,310,000	2,310,000	2,310,000	2,310,000	2,310,000	2,310,000	2,310,000
Discounted benefits health service perspective ($)	2,242,718	2,177,397	2,113,977	2,052,405	1,992,626	1,934,589	1,878,241	1,823,535	1,770,423	1,718,857
Human cases averted										
Intervention A (DALYs)	80	80	80	80	80	80	80	80	80	80
Discounted values (DALYs)	78	75	73	71	69	67	65	63	61	60
Intervention B (DALYs)	77	77	77	77	77	77	77	77	77	77
Discounted values (DALYs)	75	73	70	68	66	64	63	61	59	57

Table 13.5. Net present value and ICER for options A and B calculated for a ten-year time period using the values shown in Tables 13.3 and 13.4. The preferred option using economic criteria is highlighted.

Net Present Value (NPV)	Across 10 years	
Societal perspective	A	B
Total discounted costs (Sum Years 1 to 10) ($)	307,087	1,603,678
Total discounted benefits (Sum Years 1 to 10) ($)	29,685,106	28,571,914
NPV societal perspective ($)	**29,378,019**	**26,968,236**
Health service perspective		
Total discounted costs (Sum Years 1 to 10) ($)	307,087	1,603,678
Total discounted benefits (Sum Years 1 to 10) ($)	20,472,487	19,704,769
NPV health service perspective ($)	**20,165,400**	**18,101,090**
INCREMENTAL COST-EFFECTIVENESS RATIO (ICER)		
Societal perspective		
Difference in costs (intervention option compared to the baseline) ($)	−29,378,019	−26,968,236
Total discounted effects (Sum Years 1 to 10) (DALYs)	682	657
Cost per averted DALY ($/DALY)	**−43,050**	**−41,058**
Health service perspective		
Difference in costs (intervention option compared to the baseline) ($)	−20,165,400	−18,101,090
Total discounted effects (Sum Years 1 to 10) (DALYs)	682	657
Cost per averted DALY ($/DALY)	**−29,550**	**−27,558**

see a situation where the benefits from the livestock sector are not sufficient to recoup the investment and the benefits in humans decide if the investment is worthwhile. Let us look at this with an illustrated (hypothetical) example: if intervention B produced a net cost of say $–1,034,566 and we compared that to the DALYs averted, then the cost per DALY averted would be $1576. To know if this is good value for money, we could aim to find a cost-effectiveness threshold. Many health economic evaluations use specific thresholds to determine whether an intervention is cost-effective. These thresholds can vary by country and health system but are often benchmarked against a country's GDP per capita or specific policy targets. For instance, the World Health Organization (WHO) has suggested that interventions costing less than three times the GDP per capita per DALY averted are considered cost-effective, while those costing less than the GDP per capita per DALY averted are considered highly cost-effective.

13.6 The Problem of Uncertainty and Sensitivity Analyses

Economic evaluations of One Health interventions are based on assumptions about the accuracy of the information, reference data and the occurrence of certain events in the future (e.g. incidence of diseases, availability of resources, prices of materials to be used, etc.). The concrete usefulness of an evaluation depends on the correctness and the occurrence of these assumptions. Each evaluation is therefore affected by uncertainty: it represents a probable, but not certain, situation.

13.6.1 Sensitivity analysis

Economic evaluations are subject to **sensitivity analyses** to address uncertainty that make it possible to assess the extent to which an evaluation outcome is sensitive to variations in the parameters used for calculations (e.g. epidemiological indicators, quantity of resources to be used, reference prices, etc.). In other words, it is a question of seeing if the outcome of the evaluation is confirmed in the presence of possible changes in the values of the parameters adopted, especially those that appear more uncertain.

Deterministic and probabilistic sensitivity analyses:

1. Deterministic sensitivity analyses, on the one hand, consist in varying a specific parameter (univariate) or a set of relevant parameters (multivariate) of the evaluation, then the results are examined to verify the impact of these changes on the initial evaluation.
2. Probabilistic sensitivity analyses, on the other hand, tend to incorporate uncertainty within the evaluation process.

In a probabilistic analysis, first, we define the statistics (i.e. type of distribution, mean, standard error) of the relevant parameters of the evaluation model. On this basis, a new value is randomly extracted for all the model parameters to calculate a new evaluation outcome for the intervention that will be different from the result of the baseline evaluation. Available software can easily repeat this process thousands of times and randomly produce thousands of possible outcomes, of which one part will indicate the achievement of the intervention goal and the other will not. This allows estimating the probability of a successful intervention outcome by integrating uncertainty into the evaluation procedure.

By way of example, Fig. 13.4A shows the result of a probabilistic sensitivity analysis of a hypothetic CUA comparing the cost utility of a One Health intervention to a no-intervention scenario in a societal perspective. The scattered orange points on cost-effectiveness represent the ICER of the intervention resulting from 1000 random iterations. Most points fall in the first quadrant of the cost-effectiveness plan, denoting a high probability that the intervention is more effective for gained QALYs but costlier than no intervention. A consistent number of points also fall in the fourth quadrant, which indicates the favourable occurrence that the intervention is more effective and less costly than no intervention. Few iterations give an outcome where the intervention is costlier and less effective (second quadrant) or less costly and less effective (third quadrant) than no intervention.

Figure 13.4B shows the cost-effectiveness acceptability curve (CEAC) of the intervention. The intersection of the curve with the vertical axis indicates that the

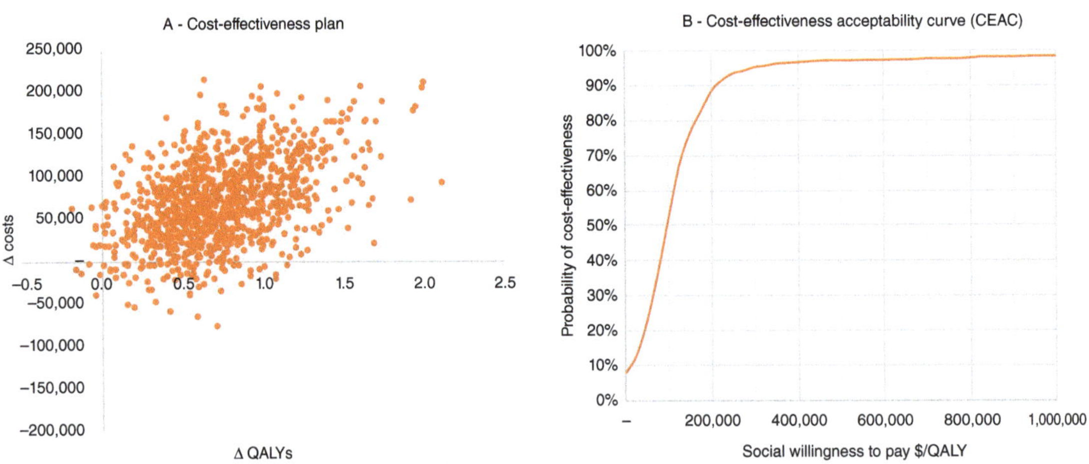

Fig. 13.4. (A) Representation of the probabilistic sensitivity analysis of a hypothetic CUA in the cost-effectiveness plan and (B) the resulting cost-effectiveness acceptability curve (see explanations in the text).

intervention has a 7.8% probability of being more cost-effective than the no-intervention scenario without any additional cost to society. The probability of cost-effectiveness of the intervention increases with the increase of the social willingness to pay for QALY gains. Within a social willingness to pay threshold of $100,000 per QALY, the cost-effectiveness probability of the intervention rises to 52.8% and 88.5% if the threshold is $200,000.

13.7 The Valuation Problem and Approaches to Address it

The previous sections demonstrated the variety of outcomes we may consider and the importance of measuring them for inclusion in economic evaluations. A big topic in One Health nowadays is the value of nature and other outcomes that do not have a market price. The intimate links between biodiversity, various kinds of ecosystem services and One Health have been illustrated in Chapter 7 on biodiversity. This section adds a conceptual reflection on value and valuations, which is particularly relevant for decision making in One Health; for example, when planning development projects or exploiting natural resources or creating projects that affect the social fabric of communities.

13.7.1 Valuation

VALUATION plays a crucial role in various fields of economics (e.g. health economics or environmental economics), but each field approaches it from distinct perspectives and focuses on different aspects. In simple terms, it refers to the process of assigning a quantifiable monetary value to various entities, outcomes or impacts. Valuations play a crucial role in evidence-based decision making, allowing the incorporation of intangible values into economic analyses and thereby ensuring that policies and interventions are aligned with societal values and goals.

Learning questions: What is value? Take a few minutes to think about what 'value' means to you. What has value to you and why? How do you know that something has value? Will this be similar to the value other people attribute to this?

Example answer: Here are two examples – yours may be similar or completely different; there is no right or wrong!

1. *I perceive value based on my personal beliefs and life experiences. To me, value encompasses various aspects depending on my priorities and what brings meaning to my life. For me, wealth, finance and success are important, and provide value in the form of material possessions, financial stability and economic opportunities. Investments, business ventures and financial assets hold significant value in my eyes as they contribute to my financial security, status and ability to achieve my desired lifestyle.*

2. *For me, there is only one thing that really has value, namely nature. My perception of value is deeply rooted in spiritual and environmental considerations. I find immense joy in the interconnectedness of all living beings, the tranquillity of nature, and the harmony of ecosystems. If a tree is unwell, I feel physically sick and I cannot witness the felling of trees, as it breaks my heart.*

Reading these statements and having thought about your own values, you will appreciate that there are many different forms of value and many different value systems. For some people, personal relationships and moments of joy hold great value as they contribute to emotional wellbeing and happiness. Similarly, knowledge and personal growth are valuable as they enrich life experiences and enable continuous learning. Value can also be attributed to tangible items like time, health and financial security, which are essential for overall wellbeing and quality of life. These aspects have value because they contribute to a sense of security, stability and fulfilment.

The perception of value is subjective and influenced by various factors such as cultural background, personal beliefs and life experiences. What holds value for one person may not hold the same value for another. For instance, a painting may hold significant emotional value for an art enthusiast because of its aesthetic appeal and artistic meaning, while others may not find the same level of value in it.

Understanding that value is subjective and can vary among individuals is crucial in appreciating diverse perspectives. It highlights the importance of empathy, open-mindedness and respect for different values and beliefs in interpersonal interactions and decision-making processes.

Given the multitude of perspectives, interests and value systems encountered in transdisciplinary processes, it is difficult to come up with valuations for inclusion in economic evaluations that do justice to the diversity encountered. Also, there are disciplinary silos that contribute to the challenge. In human health economics, valuation primarily revolves around health-related measures and outcomes, such as improvements in health status, life expectancy or quality of life. On the other hand, environmental economics focuses on valuing natural resources, ecosystem services and environmental impacts. This includes assigning monetary values to aspects such as clean air and water, biodiversity conservation, climate change mitigation and land-use changes. Valuation also extends to social aspects, encompassing factors such as social equity, community wellbeing, cultural heritage and human rights. Next, we are going to look at these diverse valuation challenges and then reflect on how to bring everything together and what this means for our implementation cycle.

13.7.2 Ecosystem valuation

Ecosystem services are gains or benefits to humankind derived from surrounding ecosystems. The primary challenge associated with this definition is the concept of 'gains'. A gain, benefit or ecosystem service is more than an objective description of the state, components or processes relating to an ecosystem: it entails an **anthropocentric** valuation of this very state, components or processes. This valuation determines whether a certain ecosystem state, component or process is seen as a benefit, or service that provides some gain. This valuation problem is the normative dimension which is inherent to any effort to identify or quantify ecosystem services. It is also related to the concept of '**environmental health**', which likewise contains an element of anthropocentric judgement about what is considered a 'healthy' environment.

This valuation problem can be broken down into two key aspects:

- How do we assess the value of the ecosystem service? This question becomes particularly relevant when we intend to compare several ecosystem services, or to account for the benefits and losses incurred by different actions.
- From whose perspective is an ecosystem service identified? That is, which stakeholders determine what is to be considered an ecosystem service?

Many standardized approaches to measuring subjectively perceived values have been developed by economists, psychologists and decision-making scientists that are relevant to valuing ecosystem services. Most such approaches are based on the concept of '**utility**'. Utility was first introduced by moral philosophers (Bentham, 1879; Mill, 1863) to designate pleasure or happiness. In this context, utility represents general qualities that apply in similar ways to different people. From the perspective of ecosystem services, this concept of utility thus comes closest to the concept of environmental health as a measure of 'optimal' state of ecosystems.

Modern economics and game theory defined utility as personal and subjective preference order over a set of choices (Pareto, 1923). Importantly, any such preference order is considered subjective, even if it refers to material goods, commodities or natural resources (Baron, 2008). From the perspective of ecosystem services, this definition emphasizes the subjective nature of gains and services that can be derived from ecosystems. By implication, different states of ecosystems could be considered desirable, depending on the utilities attached to them by different individuals. The question of which state of an ecosystem was to be considered 'healthy' would thus become a matter of negotiation or selection between different perspectives.

The concept of utilities was further refined by mathematicians (Von Neumann and Morgenstern, 1953), who developed it into 'expected utilities', which describe the relative preference of choices, the outcomes of which are not known for certain, but are uncertain. The overwhelming complexity of virtually any ecosystem will always make it impossible to base one's choices regarding the environment on full knowledge of the outcomes of different actions. Expected utilities that consider uncertain outcomes are thus a key concept for valuing ecosystem services in One Health initiatives.

The mathematician Herbert Simon and psychologists Tversky and Kahneman reconsidered the valuation concept (Simon, 1957; Kahneman and Tversky, 1979; Kahneman, 2011). Their key insight is humans' limited capability to amalgamate large bodies of information, and uncertain outcomes of extended sets of choices, into clear and consistent preference rankings. Instead, they tend to use incomplete information to make 'heuristic' choices, which can be described as establishing one's preference orders by rules of thumb. This approach may be a good approximation as to how humans and societies tend to value and decide about choices that impact on the ecosystem services that they profit from.

The school of 'bounded rationality' focuses on how to help people making better choices, by considering more available information and reflecting about potential inconsistencies in their preferences (Sent, 2018). One key tool relevant to the valuation of ecosystem services is multi-criteria decision methods, which are promoted and used in various One Health contexts (Hitziger *et al.*, 2018). These decision-making support procedures enable the elicitation of values and preferences between several alternative choices through a variety of criteria. In a case study by Aenishaenslin *et al.* (2013) on Lyme disease in Canada, multi-criteria methods are used to analyse stakeholder preferences and impact of disease management interventions along 16 criteria, which include public, animal and environmental health, as well as social, economic and surveillance criteria.

Multi-criteria analysis can incorporate valuations from stakeholders with differing perspectives and objectives. It is the responsibility of the analyst to ensure that all relevant stakeholders are included in the analysis and that the voices of underrepresented and marginalized groups or populations are considered. Valuing ecosystem services using economic models has been criticized as inadequate for incorporating non-utilitarian, cultural or sacred values regarding the environment that are held by many groups of Indigenous Peoples. Some assessment processes for ecosystem services, in particular the IPBES[7] (Pascual *et al.*, 2017), have therefore developed an alternative framework for integrating complementary valuations into their assessments. In this framework, the conceptual approach to measuring ecosystem services is used in addition to a holistic valuation of 'nature's gifts'.

13.7.3 Social outcome valuation

Social impact assessment (Freudenburg, 1986; Esteves *et al.*, 2012; Vanclay *et al.*, 2015) and social cost–benefit analysis (Chawla, 1987; Kumar, 2017) are methodologies used to quantify and evaluate social values, addressing issues such as income distribution, access to essential services, social cohesion and inclusivity. Valuation in the social realm aims to highlight the broader impacts of policies, projects or interventions on society, beyond purely economic or environmental metrics, to ensure holistic decision making and sustainable development.

The social aspects are also an important part of what is called the Social Return on Investment (SROI), which is a framework for measuring and accounting for a broader concept of value by incorporating social, environment and economic costs and benefits. It can be seen as an expansion of the CBA described above because it includes environmental and social outcomes more comprehensively, but requires careful consideration of the use of counterfactuals (baselines) and study time horizons (Banke-Thomas *et al.*, 2015). Social impacts may, for example, consider improvements in quality of life or social cohesion, enhanced skills and knowledge, or increased access to services and opportunities for marginalized groups. Environmental impacts may be a reduction in environmental degradation or conservation of natural resources and the economic effects may be health service costs saved in animal and human health sectors. Thus, this approach lends itself to One Health, but has not yet been used widely in the One Health community.

13.7.4 Health valuation

Health valuation refers to the process of assigning a quantitative value or monetary value to health outcomes or health-related interventions. It involves assessing and measuring the benefits or improvements in health resulting from specific healthcare interventions, policies or programmes. The most common metrics are QALYs and DALYs to measure the impact on quality of life and overall health status. This valuation helps decision makers prioritize healthcare resources, allocate funding efficiently, and make informed choices regarding healthcare investments based on the expected health benefits and their associated costs.

In animals, many of the effects can be a combination of physical coefficients and market price information. It can include, for example, measuring parameters such as disease incidence and prevalence, mortality rates, physiological indicators of health (e.g. body condition scores) and output (e.g. litres of milk, number of eggs produced per unit of livestock). Multiplying these by the market prices of the animals or the products can give us the magnitude of a certain effect. Like for human health, there are also efforts to come up with behavioural assessments and overall quality of life indicators that allow capturing the welfare of an animal. For example, the Welfare-Adjusted Life-Years (WALYs) for animals reproduce the QALYs used in humans. WALYs aim to measure the overall wellbeing or quality of life of animals, based on both the duration and the quality of their lives (Teng *et al.*, 2018). It involves assessing various aspects of animal welfare, such as physical health, behaviour, social interactions, environment and mental wellbeing, and then assigning a quantitative value to these factors. WALYs consider the impact of different health conditions, treatments or interventions on an animal's welfare over time. For example, an animal experiencing chronic pain or suffering from a disease may have a lower WALY score compared to a healthy, well-cared-for animal. By combining measures of welfare with time, WALYs provide a way to evaluate and compare the overall impact of different management practices, treatments or interventions on animal wellbeing, helping inform decisions related to animal welfare policies, veterinary care and ethical considerations.

In terms of integrated metrics, the zDALY provides a metric for zoonotic diseases that spans people and livestock (Torgerson *et al.*, 2018). In the zDALY, the losses from animal disease are converted to a metric using the local gross national income per capita to be able to compare them to human life-years. This allows estimating the time required to earn the income needed to make up for the loss incurred. Based on this, a so-called animal loss equivalent (ALE) is estimated and added to the DALY associated with human disease to give the zDALY (Torgerson *et al.*, 2018).

13.8 Dealing with Additional Levels of Analysis and Complexity

So far, we have looked at how to conceptualize the cross-sectoral interventions and effects when it comes to an example like a zoonotic disease intervention where we may see multiple activities and multiple effects in different populations. We looked at how we can identify and compare the different inputs and the consequences in common types of economic evaluations. These are analyses often used to determine the value of potential investments and help guide decision making. However, there are several other aspects that are important to consider when looking at the economic value of One Health.

Economic evaluations of unintended consequences require a design that allows keeping track of what is happening and incorporating new consequences (both positive and negative) as they emerge in the system. These can then be embedded in retrospective (*ex-post*) economic evaluations. Alternatively, modelling approaches make use of dynamic modelling techniques that simulate complex interactions and feedback loops, aiding in predicting long-term economic implications, such as system dynamics or agent-based modelling. Another approach can be to use scenario analysis to consider wider potential effects.

The Network for the Evaluation of One Health (NEOH) proposed a framework to assess the level of One Health integration of an intervention or an institution operating in the One Health context (Rüegg *et al.*, 2017, 2018a, b). This framework could be helpful to investigate correlations between the economic value created by an intervention and its 'One Healthness' (i.e. the level of One Health). Currently, there are not many peer-reviewed studies available that are targeting this question explicitly. A systematic literature review (Auplish *et al.*, 2024) found only seven studies that looked at the added value of One Health coordination, collaboration, communication or capacities. However, the authors found a good body of evidence from studies that showed that the consideration of effects across sectors may generate a positive return on the investment. Some of these studies explicitly compared a uni-sectoral with a cross-sectoral intervention and thereby demonstrated the added value of One Health. It should be noted that One Health economic evaluations that do not show an added value are still useful because they allow understanding in which situations One Health may or may not generate an added value.

When expanding the scale and complexity, scenario analysis (see Chapters 10 and 11) can be useful to shed light on different options and their potential outcomes. They could refer to different scenarios as elaborated in the implementation cycle, or they could come up during the discussions on how to conduct the economic evaluations. In any case, they include the definition of differing scenarios or alternative futures that could affect the interventions. They could, for example, include different economic conditions, market trends, regulatory changes, technological advancements or environmental factors.

The challenges of dealing with complex systems and non-linear causality in economic analyses are multifaceted. While efficiency is a vital aspect of One Health initiatives, incorporating equity and sustainability aspects is challenging. Economic evaluations typically prioritize efficiency, aiming to maximize outcomes within resource constraints. However, this approach may not adequately address equity concerns or long-term sustainability, leading to potential inequities or unsustainable solutions. Efforts have been made to integrate equity considerations into health-oriented evaluations and incorporate sustainability goals into efficiency measures. Yet, these adaptations can sometimes conflict with the fundamental principles of economic evaluation, emphasizing the need for caution or alternative approaches as alluded to above. More information on this topic can be found in Häsler *et al.* (2021), for example.

Returning to our brucellosis example, the following expansions would be possible for a more comprehensive and in-depth economic analysis:

1. Assessing whether the effect of the One Health integration across sectors, **disciplines** or communities increases the added value of the intervention(s);
2. Conceptualizing the economic analysis at the systems level considering dynamic feedback loops and non-linear effects;
3. Including in the analysis a wide range of effects that span all One Health dimensions including social, economic, health and environment; and
4. Involving an explicit consideration of the value systems, rights and ethics of different groups affected by the intervention and incorporation of their priorities in a participatory way.

It is important to note, however, that these expansions may not be strictly necessary to inform decision making. An economic evaluation always needs to be structured with the decision maker in mind and what their needs are. The results of the economic analysis should be presented to them in an accessible way with clear guidance on how to interpret the results and what to do with them. This is particularly important when seeking to leverage investment in support of the One Health intervention.

13.9 Funding and Financing

There is a need for economic analyses providing information on the return on investment to orient financial resources towards One Health. While the One Health approach has the potential to generate efficiencies and positive outcomes, its implementation does require funding. To investors, it is relevant to understand the impacts and implications of One Health investments.

It is essential to clearly define the scope and objectives of the initiatives, whether focusing on zoonotic disease control, ecosystem health, antimicrobial resistance or food safety. Identifying potential stakeholders, partners and collaborators is an important step because it allows for collaborative funding efforts that leverage diverse resources and expertise from government agencies, NGOs, research institutions, private sector entities and international organizations.

For example, the global cost of emerging diseases has been shown to outweigh significantly the expenses of prevention at the source, highlighting the importance of proactive measures (Bernstein *et al.*, 2022). This has been recognized by the Pandemic Fund,[6] which is a financing mechanism aimed at prevention, response, containment efforts, healthcare infrastructure, research and development of vaccines or treatments, workforce development and other critical interventions. By pooling resources from various stakeholders and countries, the Pandemic Fund aims to enhance preparedness and response capabilities, minimize economic disruptions, and prevent the escalation of health crises into full-blown pandemics as seen during the COVID-19 pandemic.

Detailed budgeting and financial planning aligned with initiative objectives and timelines are essential. This involves developing short-term and long-term financial projections, conducting cost–benefit analyses, and assessing risks associated with funding uncertainties, budget overruns, economic fluctuations and political challenges. Strong grant applications and funding proposals tailored to different funding agencies' requirements are essential when aiming to secure financial support in line with the investor's interests. An awareness of different mechanisms can help you to think about how to prepare and present your investment case, as well as alignment with budget cycles.

Common funding and financing mechanisms include government grants, philanthropic donations, loans, private investments, private–public partnerships and crowdfunding. Another potential new mechanism is the proposed global subsidiary principle, akin to the Global Fund to Fight AIDS, Tuberculosis and Malaria, that could be beneficial for addressing emerging and endemic zoonoses, advocating for collective global support in funding initiatives. Additionally, newer funding instruments such as Development Impact Bonds, which share risk between donors and private investors, offer potential avenues for zoonosis control projects (Häsler *et al.*, 2021).

13.10 Conclusions

In this chapter, you have learned about how we can use economic evaluation to support decision making in the One Health implementation cycle. This information might help you to comprehend how evaluations can be conceptualized and the challenges of working across different sectors and scales. Further, you might have improved your understanding of the limits of economic evaluation and difficulties when trying to combine different paradigms and schools of economic thought in One Health. With this chapter, we have completed the One Health implementation cycle, and you are now equipped with information that helps you to support the different aspects of implementing a One Health initiative.

Acknowledgements

We thank Maria Garza for reviewing and fact-checking Box 13.1 on alternative schools of economic thought.

Notes

[1] A concept called discounting, which is explained later in the chapter.

[2] WTP is an economic concept that represents the maximum amount of money an individual or group is willing to spend to acquire a good or service, or to avoid something undesirable, such as a negative outcome or risk.

[3] https://ec.europa.eu/regional_policy/sources/studies/cba_guide.pdf

[4] A perspective in economic evaluation that focuses on maximizing overall wellbeing or welfare for society as a whole with the goal to assess interventions or policies based on their impact on the welfare of individuals within society.

[5] In One Health cross-sectoral evaluations, when the monetary benefits outweigh the monetary costs, the numerator in the ICER can become negative. The Roth *et al.* (2003) study estimated −373 US$ per DALY averted, which can be difficult to understand for decision makers. Therefore, different approaches have been developed to present these effects across sectors, such as the separable cost method (Roth *et al.*, 2003), the aggregate net cost, the zoonotic DALY (Torgerson *et al.*, 2018) or an integrative CBA. For a discussion of these approaches, see Häsler *et al.* (2021).

[6] https://www.thepandemicfund.org

[7] www.ipbes.net

References

Aenishaenslin, C., Hongoh, V., Cissé, H.D., Hoen, A.G., Samoura, K. *et al.* (2013) Multi-criteria decision analysis as an innovative approach to managing zoonoses: Results from a study on Lyme disease in Canada. *BMC Public Health* 13, 897. DOI: 10.1186/1471-2458-13-897.

Al Hamada, A., Bruce, M., Barnes, A., Habib, I. and Robertson, D.I. (2021) Cost–benefit analysis of a mass vaccination strategy to control brucellosis in sheep and goats in Northern Iraq. *Vaccines (Basel)* 9, 878. DOI: 10.3390/vaccines9080878.

Alonso, M.E., González-Montaña, J.R. and Lomillos, J.M. (2020) Consumers' concerns and perceptions of farm animal welfare. *Animals (Basel)* 10, 385. DOI: 10.3390/ani10030385.

Alumasa, L., Thomas, L.F., Amanya, F., Njoroge, S.M., Moriyón, I. *et al.* (2021) Hospital-based evidence on cost-effectiveness of brucellosis diagnostic tests and treatment in Kenyan hospitals. *PLoS Neglected Tropical Diseases* 15, e0008977. DOI : 10.1371/journal.pntd.0008977.

Antonopoulos, R. and Hirway, I. (2010) *Unpaid Work and the Economy: Gender, Time-Use and Poverty in Developing Countries*. Springer, Cham, Switzerland.

Anyanwu, U., Dimov, A., Zinsstag, J., Tediosi, F. and Markosyan, T. (2024) Profitability and cost-effectiveness analysis of brucellosis control in Armenia: A One Health approach. *CABI One Health* 3, 1. DOI: 10.1079/cabionehealth.2024.0010.

Aragrande, M., Romanelli, C. and Canali, M. (2020) *Valutazione dei costi di diverse strategie di sorveglianza della brucellosi bovina in allevamenti da latte*. Bologna.

Attfield, R. (1998) Existence value and intrinsic value. *Ecological Economics* 24(2–3), 163–168. DOI: 10.1016/S0921-8009(97)00140-7.

Auplish, A., Raj, E., Booijink, Y., de Balogh, K., Peyre, M. *et al.* (2024) Current evidence of the economic value of One Health initiatives: A systematic literature review. *One Health* 18, 100755. DOI: 10.1016/j.onehlt.2024.100755.

Bachelet, M. (2022) Transforming Global Governance for Social Justice: Feminist Economics and the Fight for Human Rights. International Association for Feminist Economics Annual Conference, 29 June–1 July, Graduate Institute, Geneva. Available at: https://www.ohchr.org/en/statements/2022/06/feminist-economics-and-fight-human-rights (accessed 8 August 2024).

Banke-Thomas, A.O., Madaj, B., Charles, A. and van den Broek, N. (2015) Social Return on Investment (SROI) methodology to account for value for money of public health interventions: A systematic review. *BMC Public Health* 15, 582. DOI: 10.1186/s12889-015-1935-7.

Baron, J. (2008) *Thinking and Deciding* (4th edn). Cambridge University Press, New York. DOI: 10.1017/9781009263672.

Basu, A. and Ganiats, T.G. (2016) Discounting in cost-effectiveness analysis. In: Neumann, P.J., Ganiats, T.G., Russell, L.B., Sanders, G.D. and Siegel, J.E. (eds) *Cost-Effectiveness in Health and Medicine*. Oxford

University Press, Oxford, pp. 277–288. DOI: 10.1093/acprof:oso/9780190492939.003.0010.

Batavia, C. and Nelson, M.P. (2017) For goodness sake! What is intrinsic value and why should we care? *Biological Conservation* 209, 366–376. DOI: 10.1016/j.biocon.2017.03.003.

Baumgärtner, S., Becker, C., Frank, K., Müller, B. and Quaas, M. (2008) Relating the philosophy and practice of ecological economics: The role of concepts, models, and case studies in inter- and transdisciplinary sustainability research. *Ecological Economics* 67, 384–393. DOI: 10.1016/J.ECOLECON.2008.07.018.

Benería, L., Berik, G. and Floro, M.S. (2015) *Gender, Development, and Globalization*. Routledge, Abingdon, UK. DOI: 10.4324/9780203107935.

Bentham, J. (1879) *An Introduction to the Principles of Morals and Legislation*. Clarendon Press, Oxford, UK.

Bernstein, A.S., Ando, A.W., Loch-Temzelides, T., Vale, M.M., Li, B.V. *et al.* (2022) The costs and benefits of primary prevention of zoonotic pandemics. *Science Advances* 8. DOI: 10.1126/sciadv.abl4183.

Bozzo, G., Barrasso, R., Grimaldi, C.A., Tantillo, G. and Roma, R. (2019) Consumer attitudes towards animal welfare and their willingness to pay. *Veterinaria Italiana* 55, 289–297. DOI: 10.12834/VetIt.1209.6739.4.

Braunstein, E. (2015) Economic growth and social reproduction: Gender inequality as cause and consequence (No. 5), UN Women. New York.

Briggs, A.H., Claxton, K. and Sculpher, M.J. (2006) *Decision Modelling for Health Economic Evaluation*. Oxford University Press, Oxford, UK.

Broome, J. (1992) *Counting the Cost of Global Warming*. White Horse Press, Cambridge, UK.

Brouwer, W.B.F., Culyer, A.J., van Exel, N.J.A. and Rutten, F.F.H. (2008) Welfarism vs. extra-welfarism. *Journal of Health Economics* 27, 325–338. DOI: 10.1016/J.JHEALECO.2007.07.003.

Buttigieg, S.C., Savić, S., Cauchi, D., Lautier, E., Canali, M. and Aragrande, M. (2018) Brucellosis control in Malta and Serbia: A One Health evaluation. *Frontiers in Veterinary Science* 5, 147. DOI: 10.3389/fvets.2018.00147.

Canali, M., Aragrande, M., Cuevas, S., Cornelsen, L., Bruce, M. *et al.* (2018) (eds) *Integrated Approaches to Health: A Handbook for the Evaluation of One Health*. Wageningen Academic Publishers, Wageningen, The Netherlands, pp. 170–226. DOI: 10.3920/978-90-8686-875-9.

Chawla, K. (1987) *Social Cost-benefit Analysis: An Introduction to Financial and Economic Appraisal of Projects*. Mittal Publications, New Delhi, India.

Coons, S.J. and Kaplan, R.M. (1996) Cost-utility analysis. In: Bootman, J.L., Townsend, R.J. and McGhan, W.F. (eds) *Principles of Pharmacoeconomics*. Harvey Whitney Books, Cincinnati, pp. 102–126.

Destoumieux-Garzón, D., Mavingui, P., Boetsch, G., Boissier, J., Darriet, F. *et al.* (2018) The One Health concept: 10 years old and a long road ahead. *Frontiers in Veterinary Science* 5, 306018. DOI: 10.3389/fvets.2018.00014.

Diamond, G.A. and Kaul, S. (2009) Cost, effectiveness, and cost-effectiveness. *Circulation: Cardiovascular Quality and Outcomes* 2, 49–54. DOI: 10.1161/CIRCOUTCOMES.108.793406.

Drummond, M.F., Sculpher, M.J., Claxton, K., Stoddart, G.L. and Torrance, G.W. (2015) *Methods for the Economic Evaluation of Health Care Programmes* (4th edn). Oxford University Press, Oxford, UK.

Esteves, A.M., Franks, D. and Vanclay, F. (2012) Social impact assessment: The state of the art. *Impact Assessment and Project Appraisal* 30, 34–42. DOI: 10.1080/14615517.2012.660356.

FAO, UNEP, WHO and WOAH (2022) One Health joint plan of action (2022–2026): Working together for the health of humans, animals, plants and the environment. Rome. DOI: 10.4060/cc2289en.

Franc, K.A., Krecek, R.C., Häsler, B.N. and Arenas-Gamboa, A.M. (2018) Brucellosis remains a neglected disease in the developing world: A call for interdisciplinary action. *BMC Public Health* 18, 125. DOI: 10.1186/s12889-017-5016-y.

Freudenburg, W.R. (1986) Social impact assessment. *Annual Review of Sociology* 12, 451–478. DOI: 10.1146/annurev.so.12.080186.002315.

Ghanbari, M.K., Gorji, H.A., Behzadifar, M., Sanee, N., Mehedi, N. and Bragazzi, N.L. (2020) One health approach to tackle brucellosis: A systematic review. *Tropical Medicine and Health* 48, 86. DOI: 10.1186/s41182-020-00272-1.

Glick, H. (2015a) Cost-Effectiveness Analysis. Lecture's Slide Presentation, Course Epidemiology (Epi 550), Penn Medicine, University of Pennsylvania, Philadelphia, Pennsylvania. Available at: http://www.uphs.upenn.edu/dgimhsr/documents/EPI550.ceatopics.sp15.pdf (accessed 26 August 2024).

Glick, H. (2015b) Welfare Economic Foundations of Cost-Benefit/Cost-Effectiveness Analysis. Health Services Research Unit, University of Pennsylvania Health System, Philadelphia, Pennsylvania. Available at: http://www.uphs.upenn.edu/dgimhsr/documents/welfareeconomics.fall2015.pdf (accessed 26 August 2024).

Guerriero, C. and Pacelli, A. (2020) Discounting benefits and costs. In: Guerriero, C. (ed.) *Cost-benefit Analysis of Environmental Health Interventions*. Elsevier, London, pp. 129–143. DOI: 10.1016/b978-0-12-812885-5.00007-x.

Haacker, M., Hallett, T.B. and Atun, R. (2020) On discount rates for economic evaluations in global health. *Health Policy Plan* 35, 107–114. DOI: 10.1093/heapol/czz127.

Hansen, A. Chr. (2006) Do declining discount rates lead to time inconsistent economic advice? *Ecological Economics* 60, 138–144. DOI: 10.1016/J.ECOLECON.2006.03.007.

Hansson, S.O. (2007) Philosophical problems in cost-benefit analysis. *Economics Philosophy* 23, 163–183. DOI: 10.1017/S0266267107001356.

Häsler, B., Cuevas, S., Canali, M., Aragrande, M., Shaw, A. and Zinsstag, J. (2021) One Health Economics. In: Zinsstag, J., Schelling, E., Crump, L., Whittaker, M., Tanner, M. and Stephen, C. (eds) *One Health: The Theory and Practice of Integrated Health Approaches*. CABI, Wallingford, UK, pp. 118–134. DOI: 10.1079/9781789242577.0118.

Hénaux, V. and Calavas, D. (2017) Evaluation of the cost-effectiveness of bovine brucellosis surveillance in a disease-free country using stochastic scenario tree modelling. *PLoS One* 12, e0183037. DOI: 10.1371/journal.pone.0183037.

Hitziger, M., Esposito, R., Canali, M., Aragrande, M., Häsler, B. and Rüegg, S.R. (2018) Knowledge integration in One Health policy formulation, implementation and evaluation. *Bulletin of the World Health Organization* 96, 211–218. DOI: 10.2471/BLT.17.202705.

Hurley, J. (2000) An overview of the normative economics of the health sector. In: *Handbook of Health Economics*. Elsevier, The Netherlands, pp. 55–118. DOI: 10.1016/S1574-0064(00)80161-4.

Kahneman, D. (2011) *Thinking, Fast and Slow*. Macmillan Publishers, New York.

Kahneman, D. and Tversky, A. (1979) Prospect theory: An analysis of decision under risk. *Econometrica* 47, 263. DOI: 10.2307/1914185.

Kelman, S. (1981) Cost-benefit analysis: An ethical critique. *AEI Journal on Government and Society Regulation* 5, 33–40.

Kumar, S. (2017) Does 'Participation' in common pool resource management help the poor? A social cost-benefit analysis of joint forest management in Jharkhand, India. In: *Development*. Routledge, Abingdon, UK, pp. 295–314. DOI: 10.4324/9781315258027-16.

Lefrançois, T., Malvy, D., Atlani-Duault, L., Benamouzig, D., Druais, P.-L. *et al.* (2023) After 2 years of the COVID-19 pandemic, translating One Health into action is urgent. *The Lancet* 401, 789–794. DOI: 10.1016/S0140-6736(22)01840-2.

Mair, S. (2020) Neoliberal economics, planetary health, and the COVID-19 pandemic: A Marxist ecofeminist analysis. *The Lancet Planetary Health* 4(12), e588–e596. DOI: 10.1016/S2542-5196(20)30252-7.

Manisalidis, I., Stavropoulou, E., Stavropoulos, A. and Bezirtzoglou, E. (2020) Environmental and health impacts of air pollution: A review. *Frontiers in Public Health* 8, 505570. DOI: 10.3389/fpubh.2020.00014.

Martinez-Alier, J. and Schlupmann, K. (1987) *Ecological Economics: Energy, Environment and Society*. Basil Blackwell, Oxford, UK.

Mill, J.S. (1863) *Utilitarianism* (1st ed.). Parker, Son & Bourn, West Strand, London.

Moriyón, I., Blasco, J.M., Letesson, J.J., De Massis, F. and Moreno, E. (2023) Brucellosis and One Health: Inherited and Future Challenges. *Microorganisms* 11, 2070. DOI: 10.3390/microorganisms11082070.

Nelson, J.A. (1995) Feminism and economics. *Journal of Economic Perspectives* 9(2), 131–148. DOI: 10.1257/jep.9.2.131.

Nordhaus, W.D. (2017) Revisiting the social cost of carbon. *Proceedings of the National Academy of Sciences of the United States of America* 114(7), 1518–1523. DOI: 10.1073/pnas.1609244114.

Nuijten, M.J.C. and Dubois, D.J. (2011) Cost-utility analysis: Current methodological issues and future perspectives. *Frontiers in Pharmacology* 2, 29. DOI: 10.3389/fphar.2011.00029.

Pal, M., Gizaw, F., Fekadu, G., Alemayehu, G. and Kandi, V. (2017) Public health and economic importance of bovine brucellosis: An overview. *American Journal of Epidemiology and Infectious Disease* 5, 27–34. DOI: 10.12691/ajeid-5-2-2.

Palmer, S. and Raftery, J. (1999) Economic notes: Opportunity cost. *BMJ* 318, 1551–1552. DOI: 10.1136/bmj.318.7197.1551.

Pansini, R. and Shi, L. (2022) COVID-19, air pollution and one health at the climate change turning point. In: *Air Quality and Health*. IntechOpen. DOI: 10.5772/intechopen.102943.

Pareto, V. (1923) *Manuale di Economia Politica, Con Una Introduzione Alla Scienza Sociale*. Società Editrice Libraria, Milan.

Pascual, U., Balvanera, P., Díaz, S., Pataki, G., Roth, E. *et al.* (2017) Valuing nature's contributions to people: The IPBES approach. *Current Opinion in Environmental Sustainability* 26–27, 7–16. DOI: 10.1016/J.COSUST.2016.12.006.

Pearce, D., Groom, B., Hepburn, C. and Koundouri, P. (2003) Valuing the future. *World Economics* 4, 121–141.

Pearce, D., Atkinson, G. and Mourato, S. (2006) *Cost-benefit Analysis and the Environment: Recent Developments*. OECD, Paris.

Pigou, A.C. (1920) *The Economics of Welfare*. Macmillan, London.

Pitt, S.J. and Gunn, A. (2024) The One Health concept. *British Journal of Biomedical Science* 81, 12366. DOI: 10.3389/bjbs.2024.12366.

Polasky, S. and Dampha, N.K. (2021) Discounting and global environmental change. *Annual Review of Environment and Resources* 46, 691–717. DOI: 10.1146/annurev-environ-020420-042100.

Rai, M. and Goyal, R. (2018) Pharmacoeconomics in Healthcare. In: Vohora, D. and Singh, G. (eds) *Pharmaceutical Medicine and Translational Clinical Research*. Academic Press, Elsevier, London, pp. 465–472. DOI: 10.1016/B978-0-12-802103-3.00034-1.

Raworth, K. (2017a) *Doughnut Economics: Seven Ways to Think Like a 21st Century Economist*. Chelsea Green Publishing, White River Junction, Vermont.

Raworth, K. (2017b) A Doughnut for the Anthropocene: Humanity's compass in the 21st century. *Lancet Planet Health* 1, e48–e49. DOI: 10.1016/S2542-5196(17)30028-1.

Razavi, S., Arza, C., Braunstein, E., Cook, S. and Goulding, K. (2012) Gendered impacts of globalization employment and social protection (No. 16), *Gender and Development*. Geneva.

Robinson, R. (1993) Cost-utility analysis. *The Bio-Medical Journal* 307, 859–862.

Roth, F., Zinsstag, J., Orkhon, D., Chimed-Ochir, G., Hutton, G. *et al.* (2003) Human health benefits from livestock vaccination for brucellosis: Case study. *Bulletin of the World Health Organization* 81(12), 867–876.

Rüegg, S.R., McMahon, B.J., Häsler, B., Esposito, R., Nielsen, L.R. *et al.* (2017) A blueprint to evaluate One Health. *Frontiers in Public Health* 5, 20. DOI: 10.3389/fpubh.2017.00020.

Rüegg, S.R., Häsler, B. and Zinsstag, J. (eds) (2018a) *Integrated Approaches to Health: A Handbook for the Evaluation of One Health.* Wageningen Academic Publishers, Wageningen, The Netherlands. DOI: 10.3920/978-90-8686-875-9.

Rüegg, S.R., Nielsen, L.R., Buttigieg, S.C., Santa, M., Aragrande, M. *et al.* (2018b) A systems approach to evaluate One Health initiatives. *Frontiers in Veterinary Science* 5, 23. DOI: 10.3389/fvets.2018.00023.

Sent, E.M. (2018) Rationality and bounded rationality: You can't have one without the other. *The European Journal of the History of Economic Thought* 25, 1370–1386. DOI: 10.1080/09672567.2018.1523206.

Simon, H.A. (1957) *Models of Man*. John Wiley and Sons, New York.

Stevano, S., Mezzadri, A., Lombardozzi, L. and Bargawi, H. (2021) Hidden Abodes in plain sight: The social reproduction of households and labor in the COVID-19 pandemic. *Feminist Economics* 27(1–2), 271–287. DOI: 10.1080/13545701.2020.1854478.

Sunstein, C.R. (2005) Cost-benefit analysis and the environment. *Ethics* 115, 351–385.

Tan-Torres Edejer, T., Baltussen, R., Adam, T., Hutubessy, R., Acharya, A., Evans, D.B. and Murray, C.J.L. (eds) (2003) *WHO Guide to Cost-Effectiveness Analysis.* World Health Organization, Geneva.

Teng, K.T.Y., Devleesschauwer, B., De Noordhout, C.M., Bennett, P., McGreevy, P.D. *et al.* (2018) Welfare-Adjusted Life Years (WALY): A novel metric of animal welfare that combines the impacts of impaired welfare and abbreviated lifespan. *PLoS One* 13, e0202580. DOI: 10.1371/JOURNAL.PONE.0202580.

The World Bank Group (2023) *Pandemic Fund Trust Fund Financial Report.* Washington, DC.

Torgerson, P.R., Rüegg, S., Devleesschauwer, B., Abela-Ridder, B., Havelaar, A.H. *et al.* (2018) zDALY: An adjusted indicator to estimate the burden of zoonotic diseases. *One Health* 5, 40–45. DOI: 10.1016/J.ONEHLT.2017.11.003.

Turner, R.A. and Wills, J. (2022) Downscaling doughnut economics for sustainability governance. *Current Opinion in Environmental Sustainability* 56, 101180. DOI: 10.1016/J.COSUST.2022.101180.

Van den Bergh, J.C.J.M. (2001) Ecological economics: Themes, approaches, and differences with environmental economics. *Regional Environmental Change* 2, 13–23. DOI: 10.1007/s101130000020.

Vanclay, F., Esteves, A.M., Aucamp, I. and Franks, D. (2015) *Social Impact Assessment: Guidance for Assessing and Managing the Social Impacts of Projects.* Fargo, North Dakota.

Von Neumann, J. and Morgenstern, O. (1953) *Theory of Games and Economic Behavior.* Princeton University Press, New Jersey.

Whitehead, J.C., Pattanayak, S.K., Van Houtven, G.L. and Gelso, B.R. (2008) Combining revealed and stated preference data to estimate the nonmarket value of ecological services: An assessment of the state of the science. *Journal of Economic Surveys* 22(5), 872–908, DOI: 10.1111/j.1467-6419.2008.00552.x.

Winders, J. and Smith, B.E. (2019) Social reproduction and capitalist production: A genealogy of dominant imaginaries. *Progress in Human Geography* 43(5), 871–889. DOI: 10.1177/0309132518791730.

Zhuang, J., Liang, Z., Lin, T. and De Guzman, F. (2007) *Theory and Practice in the Choice of Social Discount Rate for Cost-Benefit Analysis: A Survey*. ERD Working Paper. Manila.

14 Policy and Governance

Gabrielle Laing[1,2], Didier Wernli[1,3], Deborah J. Thomson[1,4], Massimo Canali[1,5], Patrícia Inácio[1,6], Manuela Vilhena[1,7], Hamisi Msagama[1,8], Sithar Dorjee[9] and Claire Lajaunie[1,10]

[1]NEOH (Network for Ecohealth and One Health); [2]Unlimit Health, London, UK; [3]Global Studies Institute, University of Geneva, Geneva, Switzerland; [4]One Health Lessons, Arlington, Virginia, USA; [5]Department of Agricultural and Food Sciences, University of Bologna, Bologna, Italy; [6]LEAF (Linking Landscape, Environment, Agriculture and Food Research Unit), School of Agriculture, University of Lisbon and National Institute for Agrarian and Veterinary Research, Oeiras, Portugal; [7]Mediterranean Institute for Agriculture, Environment and Development & CHANGE (MED), Global Change and Sustainability Institute, Department of Veterinary Medicine, University of Évora, Évora, Portugal; [8]One Health Society, Dar es salaam, Tanzania; [9]Khesar Gyalpo University of Medical Sciences of Bhutan, Thimphu, Bhutan; [10]Inserm, LPED (IRD-Aix-Marseille Université), Marseille, France and Strathclyde Centre for Environmental Law and Governance, Strathclyde University, Glasgow, Scotland, UK

Contents

DOI: 10.1079/9781800623002.0015

Chapter Overview

Elevator pitch

It's important for the application of the One Health approach that there is an enabling environment to facilitate its uptake and implementation. Policy and governance structure across sectors, groups and levels can be varied and have a large influence on the realization of the added value taking a One Health approach can deliver. It is therefore important for the One Health practitioner to understand different governance structures and mechanisms and how health policy is formed.

Book objectives the chapter relates to

- ☐ 1. Understand what One Health and Ecohealth mean
- ☑ 2. Think in a One Health and Ecohealth way
- ☑ 3. Apply One Health and Ecohealth in their professional and personal life
- ☐ 4. Know how to share One Health and Ecohealth knowledge
- ☐ 5. Integrate One Health and Ecohealth knowledge actively
- ☐ 6. Acquire or enhance core One Health competencies

Main One Health competencies covered

- ☑ 1. Effective communication
- ☑ 2. Collaborative and resilient working
- ☐ 3. Systems understanding
- ☐ 4. Transdisciplinarity
- ☑ 5. Social, cultural and gender equity and inclusiveness
- ☑ 6. Collective learning and reflective practice
- ☐ 7. One Health concepts
- ☐ 8. Theoretical and methodological pluralism
- ☑ 9. Harnessing uncertainty, paradox and limited knowledge

After having worked through this chapter, you will have an understanding of governance and policy as relevant to One Health.

Learning outcomes

1. Understand what is meant by governance and policy, and the policy-making process.
2. Be able to identify policy actors and governance structures in One Health.
3. Discuss use of evidence in policy and evidence in informed decision making.
4. Explain aspects of governance of particular relevance to the delivery of One Health.

Summary

This chapter discusses aspects of policy making and varying governance systems to equip the reader with a diverse understanding of policy systems, actors and the policy-making process. It discusses the use of evidence in decision making and how to interact across the science–policy interface. It is important for those looking to further the practice of One Health that they have an understanding of how policies and governance can both facilitate and challenge its implementation.

Note: The first half of the chapter can be read as a continuous section of prose so that the focus is on understanding the underlying concepts and not a case of memorizing facts. This first half of the chapter will explain policy-making processes and governance. The second part of this chapter will take a closer look at the specifics for One Health. Key concepts and terms are highlighted throughout. There are applied examples included to demonstrate the concepts described. Activities are deliberately thought provoking and complex with no right or wrong answer, but some suggested discussion points are included.

14.1 Why is it Important for a One Health Practitioner to Understand Policy and Governance?

One Health practitioners may be directly involved in **policy**, as decision makers or advisers or tasked with designing the governance for One Health institutions or groups. To embed the **One Health approach** into institutions, the principles or rules that are set, or how it will be organized, i.e. the **governance** structures, play a key role in its success. Similarly, when policies are being created, by a government, for example, a One Health practitioner may be needed to make sure there is consideration of all the One Health implications or to identify relevant people to be involved in the policy-making process.

We can group these roles into two sections: (i) the governance **of** One Health and (ii) governance **for** One Health. It is important for those looking to further the practice of One Health that they have an understanding of how policies and governance can both facilitate and challenge its use. The first half of this chapter will explain policy-making processes and governance. The second part of this chapter will take a closer look at the specifics for One Health. Key concepts are highlighted, and there are applied examples given and learning reflection points suggested.

What does Ebola have to do with fishing policy?

Ebola is a thankfully rare viral haemorrhagic disease with a 50% average fatality rate. It is passed human-to-human via direct contact. Outbreaks in humans are thought to re-emerge when people are in close contact with fruit bats, primates or other wildlife (or their bodily fluids) that are a natural host of the virus.

In 2013, the European Union (EU) made changes to the Common Fisheries Policy and arguably contributed to the largest outbreak of Ebola in history, some 5000 miles away in West Africa.

Policy: A 'sustainable fishing partnership agreement' gave European Union member countries fishing rights in third (i.e. non-EU) countries, including West Africa (Fig. 14.1).

The policy, in conjunction with illegal fishing, depleted fish stocks and endangered the marine **ecosystems** (Ifesinachi Okafor-Yarwood, 2020). This led to a reduction of fish available for local coastal villages where locally caught fish represented the primary source of protein for these communities (Khan, 2015).

Coastal communities were then forced to source alternative protein sources, entering the forests and jungles to hunt for wildlife (Fig. 14.2). This 'bushmeat' replacement was an essential source of protein but brought communities into closer contact with wild animal species that were potential vectors of Ebola virus.

In addition, there was increasing deforestation in these Western African countries (Fig. 14.3). Deforestation leads to widespread loss of **biodiversity** and reduces food sources such as fruit. This means animals of different species coming together around those remaining sources, alongside people (Rulli et al., 2017).

The first case of the most recent Ebola outbreak was identified in December 2014 in Guinea (Fig. 14.4). Weak surveillance systems and underfunded public health infrastructure hampered efforts to contain the outbreak and it quickly spread to Guinea's bordering countries, Liberia and Sierra Leone. Two and a half years after the first case was discovered, the outbreak ended with more than 28,600 cases and 11,325 deaths.

This tragically illustrates the complexity of the interactions between ecosystems, animals and humans. If we are going to prepare for and prevent infectious disease outbreaks with pandemic potential, we must consider **systems** more widely and how they are interconnected.

Governance **of** One Health is concerned with how we structure processes in One Health. Governance **for** One Health refers to how we incorporate One Health considerations into all relevant policies and sectors to achieve healthy societies, healthy animals and healthy ecosystems.

It can be difficult to define **governance** because there are various interpretations from different **disciplines** and **sectors**. The United Nations Commission on Global Governance (1995) defined it as 'the sum of the many ways individuals

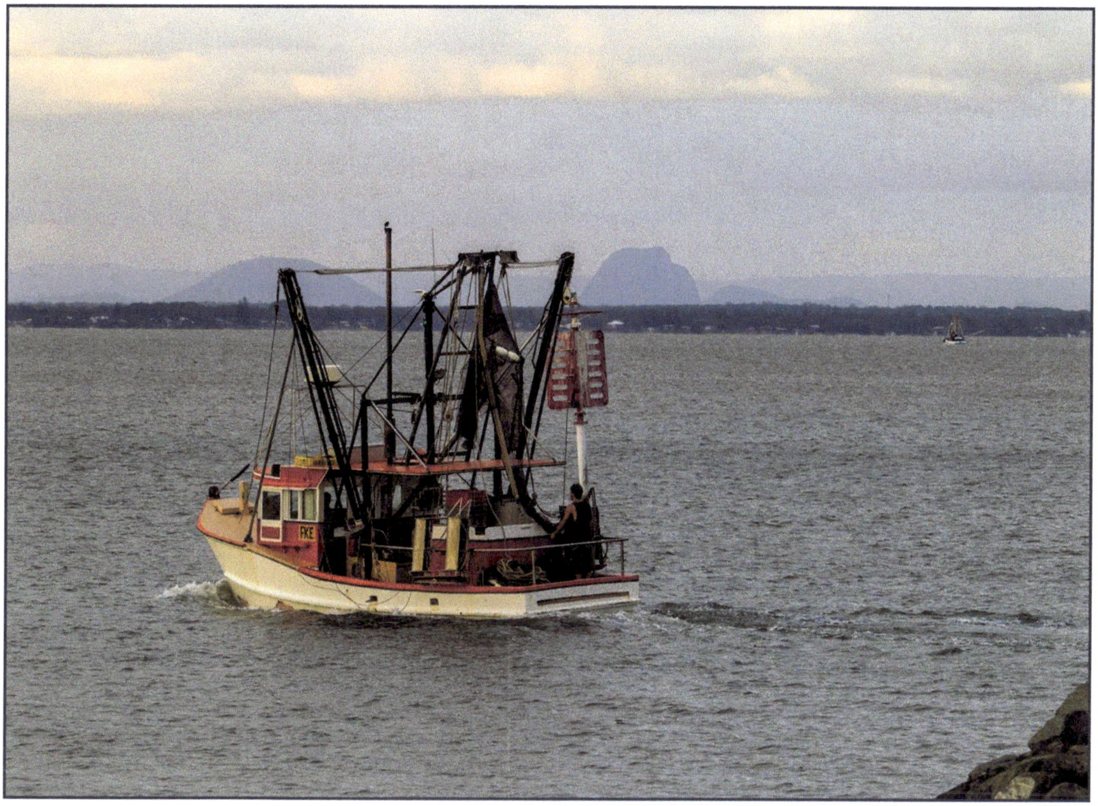

Fig. 14.1. EU policy changes to allow international fishing in 'third' countries including West Africa. Image: flickr.com, John.

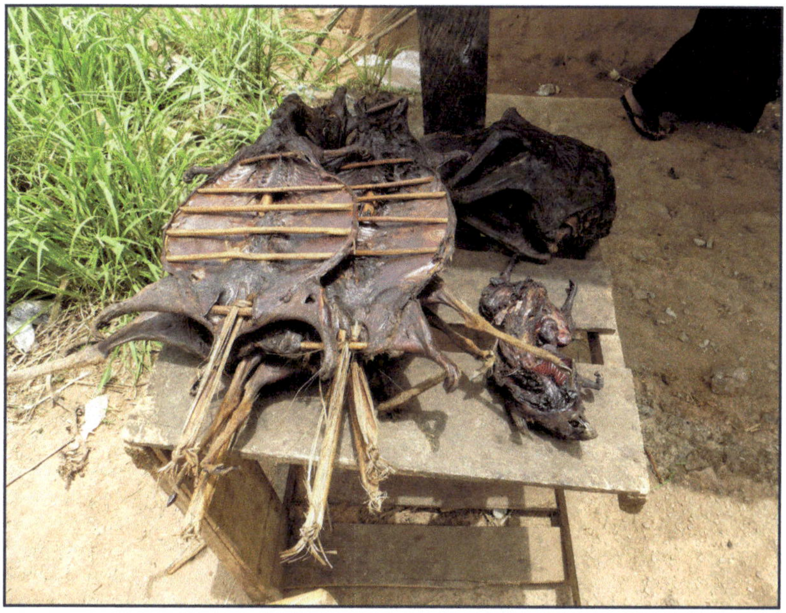

Fig. 14.2. Local communities unable to source fish protein turn to wildlife hunting. Image: Buschfleisch Ghana, Wikiseal.

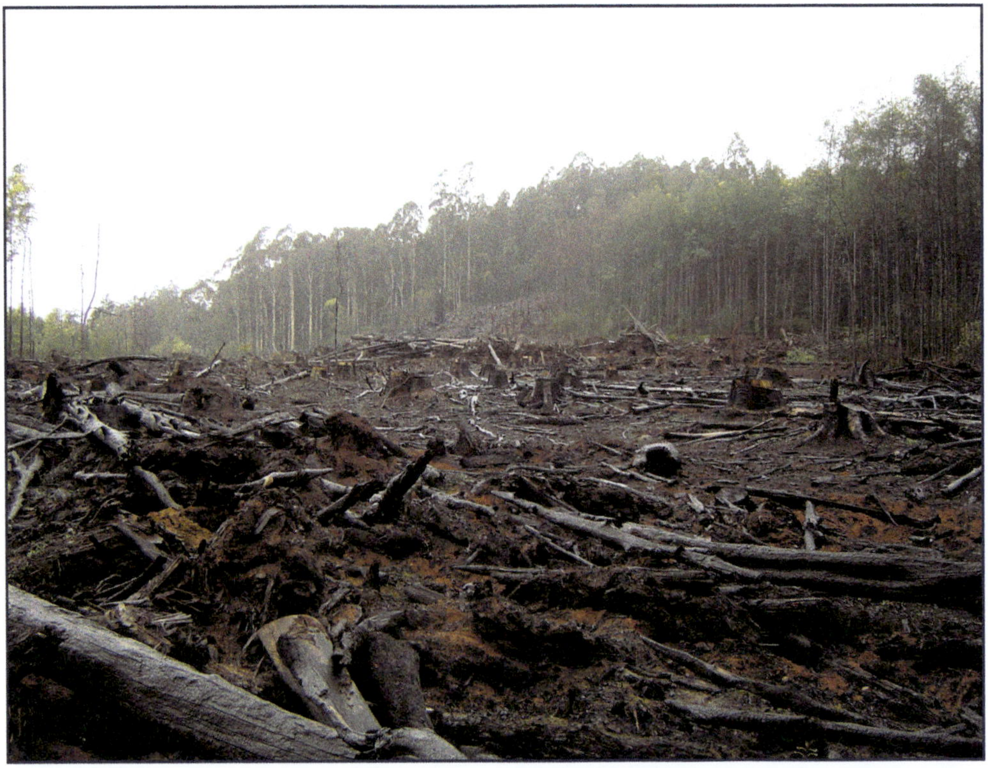

Fig. 14.3. Deforestation and climate change can reduce forest areas, concentrating animals and people into smaller areas. Image: flickr.com / Crustmania.

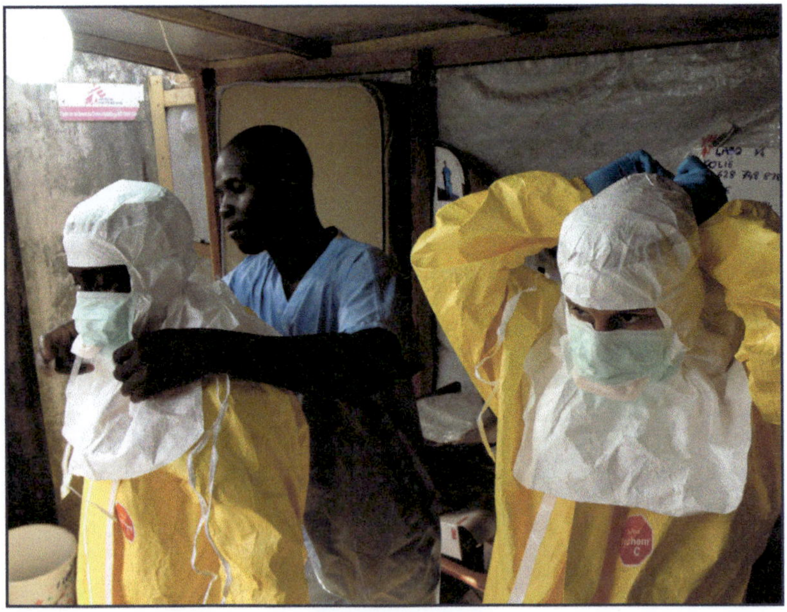

Fig. 14.4. Ebola killed over 11,000 people and left 22,000 orphaned. Image: flickr.com / Global Panorama.

and institutions, public and private, manage their common affairs'. In a review by Dodgson *et al.* (2002), the World Health Organization says it is 'the actions and means adopted by a society to promote collective action and deliver collective solutions in pursuit of common goals'. Another definition considers governance as 'a social function centred on steering societies toward collectively desirable outcomes and away from collectively undesirable outcomes' (Young, 2017).

Essentially, this means the various ways **stakeholder** groups (see Chapter 10 for details on stakeholders and their engagement) are organized and run, both formally and informally. These groups can range from democratically elected national governments to self-organized local community groups. Each group of people that come together may be influenced by social norms, customs or rules on how to interact or resolve conflicts, or they will need to agree on a common set of goals and rules for operating. These can range from legally binding laws (hard law) to simpler informal agreements and non-legally binding decisions (see the discussion on types of policies below).

Governance applies to both private and public groups, including commercial companies, charities and community groups. 'Governments' therefore are a particular example of a formally organized governance system.

The classic understanding of governance is a 'hierarchical governance' structure where leaders decide what needs to be done for everyone else.

In other words, this is a top-down model of decision making that is frequently used by national governments. Often this governance structure shares out these responsibilities between different sectors, such as government ministries or departments, who will have their own area of activity, each with separate lines of decision making. For example, human medicine is traditionally the responsibility of a Ministry of Health. This may be separate from other areas of One Health such as veterinary public health or **environment health**, which may be the shared responsibility of several departments such as a Ministry of Agriculture, Water, Wildlife, Forestry or Environment.

In today's world, there are many variations that have emerged from this hierarchical governance model, some that are more inclusive of other groups or ***actors*** than others. When governments are making decisions and developing policies to become law, the World Health Organization (2017) recommends that countries should be transparent in their decision making and allow public participation. This is to ensure that governments take responsibility for their actions, uphold principles of justice and ***equity*** and comply with the existing rule of law. The involvement or participation of the public or external experts in deliberation and decision making is usually considered a form of good governance.

'Good governance', therefore, can refer to the behaviour of a government or body in how it develops and implements policies and the way it exercises its power.

Policies set the rules that direct the behaviour and actions of a population, as agreed upon through the governance structure. For example, governments establish state laws (i.e. policies) that are the formal rules that a country sets for the relationship between citizens and institutions. In private business, companies may have a set of self-defined standard operating practices (i.e. policies) that incorporate external requirements such as regulations arising from government policy, e.g. meat inspection protocols, or industry standards like 'fair trade' or 'organic', alongside internal corporate values like 'good customer service', 'wearing a uniform' or 'high welfare animal handling'.

In crafting a solution to a problem, governments and other entities can consider a range of push-and-pull policy instruments: from enforced regulations, to offering incentives, or simply advisory information.

Laws are the legally binding rules that govern a population and national legislation (which sets out these laws for a country) comprises the main policies that governments set. The process by which these are made differs from country to country. If laws are the rules laid down, regulations are what are used to monitor or enforce them.

Regulations are adopted by governments and their ministries or authorities in the classic top-down, hierarchical governance approach mentioned above. Regulations can also develop outside governments. In some situations, stakeholders such as private industry can choose to adopt their own standards or self-regulation, for example as might be seen when companies commit to higher standards of animal welfare or lowered environmental impact (compared to government standards). Such standards often come in when there is a dearth of public regulation.

Similarly, there can be regulations agreed upon from the interactions between different non-governmental organizations (NGOs); in this case they can be called ***co-regulation***. An example of co-regulation might be where a house-building company agrees with a community group to protect a local woodland habitat that might exist on land they own and wish to develop, or where livestock farmers agree not to graze land adjoining wildlife reserves to reduce competition and risk of disease transmission.

Legally regulating as a means to guide a population's behaviour may be considered a **'push' mechanism**, but there is also the option to employ **'pull' mechanisms** to encourage a certain behaviour. This might include incentivization: for example, when governments want citizens to save for old age through a pension, they offer tax relief to working people if they add money to their pension fund, and nudging behaviour by making the enrolment onto a pension scheme the default position so that people have to opt out if they prefer (Thaler and Sunstein, 2009). Making the desired behaviour easier for people can be a powerful tool. For example, chlorine tablets added to water can help to prevent waterborne diseases such as cholera. Usage rates are low, however, because it can be inconvenient or easy to forget to do. Instead, researchers saw greater success when offering liquid chlorine at water points, which was an obvious reminder and convenient for those collecting water (Kremer *et al.*, 2010).

Alternatively, a body can try to influence behaviour in a solely advisory way, providing information on the preferred behaviour. An example would be health warnings on tobacco products, where you are still free to make an unhealthy choice and receive no compensation for making a 'good choice' but the government is interested in encouraging people to stop smoking. This advisory information can be communicated in different forms, such as through school education programmes and television advertising to increase awareness or warnings on packets.

Government policies are often developed by the relevant government ministry in response to an identified problem. In democratic systems, there are several stages where stakeholders can input on draft legislation before a policy is finalized and passed into law. In non-democratic or authoritarian regimes, the policy-making process may be more centralized and less inclusive, with decisions being made by a select group of individuals or ruling authorities without significant input from external stakeholders or the general public.

Classically in democratic societies, the process of making policy can be broken down into several steps, starting with **(i) problem identification** (Fig. 14.5). This might be a result of new research emerging or an event such as a natural disaster which demands new policy or an update to existing legislation. Once the problem has been identified, then the government needs to commit to give attention to this area by prioritizing it and **(ii) getting it on the agenda**.

Once the issue has been featured on the government's agenda, **(iii) a draft policy is formulated**. In general, policies are drafted by the relevant public sector departments following inputs from the government, sometimes in consultation with external stakeholders or the public. For stakeholder engagement, there needs to be a systematic identification of individuals and institutions who have a stake in the issue (see Chapter 10 on the process of how to include stakeholders). Their participation will help make sure that all aspects of the proposal are properly considered and the 'bigger picture' of a policy's impact can be understood. This should minimize unexpected negative impacts or loopholes that may arise. During stakeholder engagement there should be a mechanism to ensure equitable opportunity to participate no matter their sector or background. Not all stakeholders will have an equal interest in the issue so in any co-design process there may be some stakeholders more involved than others (see Chapter 10 for more details). This will be discussed in Section 14.2. At this stage it is also important to consider how the policy will interact with other existing policies both nationally and globally.

Following the initial development, draft policies are proposed to the wider group of policy makers, often elected members of a parliament or congress, for consideration. There may be debates held, specialist committee scrutiny and public consultation on the draft policy (as shown in the following applied example from

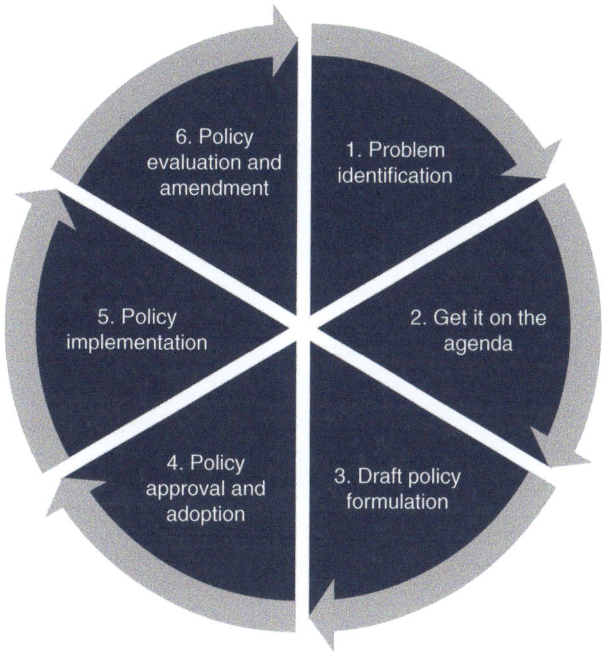

Fig. 14.5. Policy-making process. The six stages of policy making are often a continuous process of design, approval, implementation, evaluation and amendment. Developed by the authors.

Tanzania). Amendments might also be suggested and further debated during these stages. Once any amendments are agreed or rejected then **(iv) the policy is adopted** and passed into law.

Adoption of laws is often not sufficient to entirely change behaviour and thus **(v) policy implementation** will need to be decided upon, considering how best to achieve the law's goal. These different approaches or 'policy instruments' have been described above.

After a policy is implemented, it should be regularly **(vi) evaluated**, and the results used to review and **amend** the policy to improve its performance. See Chapter 12 for guidance on how to conduct ***evaluations*** of One Health initiatives.

Influencing policy: Youth-led organizations in Tanzania

In university, there are often student associations linked to various health-related professions. In Tanzania the student association of pharmacists led a campaign to join forces with others to tackle antimicrobial resistance (AMR) and neglected tropical diseases (NTDs). Different student bodies, such as those for medics, vets, environment science and laboratory technicians, came together to advocate for action, influence policy and promote ***sustainability***. This student task force had around 3000 members and petitioned government ministers to attend their meetings and to value a youth perspective on AMR and NTDs. After this, the Ministry invited youth representatives to participate in reviewing national policies on NTDs and their One Health Strategic Plan.

In 2019, the One Health Society (OHS) Tanzania was founded as a youth-led NGO (Fig. 14.6). The society acts as a platform for youth to engage, influence policy and impact their community through translating documents into local languages, running community engagement activities and advocating for continued youth representation in government policy making.

Once agreed upon, policies, e.g. laws, then need to be interpreted and upheld for them to function effectively.

Fig. 14.6. OHS Tanzania's logo.

The legal system plays a vital role in interpreting the meaning, intention and scope of the law, as well as judging when the law has been broken. Legislation (i.e. laws) and other policies should specify the authorities responsible for enforcing them, and grant the necessary powers to that authority to carry out this task.

Sometimes people adapt to laws in a way that can defeat or avoid their purpose. A common example is people finding new ways to evade taxes or failing to report environmental contamination or disease outbreaks. Sometimes, someone's interpretation of the law may be tested in the courts. If this unintended interpretation of the law is deemed allowable and it defeats the purpose of the law, then laws might need to be amended and evolve to be able to deliver on their original aims.

Are laws the best way to get things done?
Task: The process of passing legally binding rules for a governance system, as with national laws, is a powerful tool to influence behaviour but it can be very slow to establish and demand enforcement interventions to uphold. These can take a lot more resources than persuading a change in behaviour through a public advice campaign, for example.

Can you think of examples where there have been efforts to change behaviour through different mechanisms, such as laws, incentive schemes or public advice campaigns?

Discussion points and examples: Think about your own daily life:

- **How are you persuaded to brush your teeth in the morning or wash your hands after going to the toilet?** Public information campaigns provide information but are not regulated. This information might be delivered through school or through other media channels. Often the advice is targeted on children and families to build good hygiene habits from a young age to prevent dental disease or infection spread.
- **How do you choose a healthy meal?** You may receive information through advertising or education campaigns that teach people not to eat too much salt, fat or sugar, for example. The food you buy may be labelled and the companies must meet regulations around food safety or added ingredients such as allergens or sugar. Your choice is not mandated by law but there are several factors influencing your choice: for example, public health information warning against too much sugar in your diet versus the marketing campaigns attempting to persuade you to purchase the item.
- **How do you get to work or school?** If you travel in a car, in many countries it is a legal requirement to have a regular vehicle safety check and the driver is legally required to pass a driving test. There are legally imposed speed limits. What makes people comply with these rules? Public safety information and peer pressure can help to persuade good behaviour, but the rules need to be enforced for them to be upheld. These could be through traffic officers or automatic speed cameras that will catch people driving too fast and issue a fine. Multiple infringements of the rules often also incur a negative mark on your record. Commit multiple small offences and you could lose your licence to allow you to drive legally.

Policies should be based on evidence but evidence may take different forms and come from varying perspectives. Additionally, policies may need to be drafted before all the evidence is available or an issue is fully understood.

The interface between science, evidence and policy is a very important one but may not be a direct one. There are different ways that evidence, such as clinical trial data or environmental survey results, might be used to help inform a new policy or to update an existing one. Evidence can be presented to policy makers, for example, through government expert advisory groups or 'non-state actors' such as academics when they publish reports or give seminars. Policy makers may also hold consultations with the public or civil society organizations (such as charities) to invite their input at different stages of the process. An applied example of written policy briefs or evidence syntheses from the UK's Parliament is provided later in the chapter.

It is important to recognize that policy makers will also bring their own personal experience or professional ***knowledge*** into any work. This perspective may have been influenced through mainstream or social media or they may have lived experiences. It is important to understand the weight that different types of evidence hold and how to integrate quantitative and qualitative information as well as different forms of knowledge, and to consider where evidence gaps exist and how to handle conflicting evidence. See also Chapters 3–5 for more information on this.

There is increasing emphasis being placed on using evidence to inform policy decisions, but evidence is not the only influencing factor for policy makers. We must consider politics and the potential for conflicting views on what is the right way forward.

Taking a One Health approach involves different sectors working together and it is possible for there to be differences or conflict about the desired outcome or the best way to achieve it. Scientific evidence can help balance and guide the discussion, but it will not solve the problem by itself. There might need to be **trade-offs** or compromise between the aims and strategies of the different stakeholders. Deciding what to prioritize involves deciding why this issue is more important than another. In a democratic system, politicians are elected to deliberate between a number of options, but the ruling party will get ultimate power to make the final selection, e.g. through a vote where they can expect to win a majority. In a few countries with a 'direct democracy', the population can vote directly on issues. In Switzerland, for example, the citizens voted directly to phase out nuclear reactors and instead increase renewable energy sources for their electricity.

In business, decisions may be put to the company shareholders for a vote or the Board of Directors to decide upon. Other tools to resolve disagreements on contentious issues can include a citizen assembly or panel. This is where a group of the public are selected at random (similar to a jury in a court of law) to represent society in discussion sessions around the policy issue. The citizen's panel then make a final recommendation to the government.

At a local level, communities may form their own groups with a particular focus to take local action. For example, community-managed conservation areas, such as community forests, marine protected areas and Indigenous territories, could be established to maintain and safeguard local natural resources. These areas might be subject to certain rules agreed between the community members, with local residents actively participating in decision making, patrolling and enforcement to safeguard these habitats.

Because One Health issues often touch on fundamental issues, such as how we live, how we eat and how we care for our environment, it is often unavoidably a political issue. The challenge of deciding on a shared or common goal is made more complicated by the often broad diversity of stakeholders and countries involved, each with their own political agenda and cultural sensitivities. In achieving the common goal, there are likely to be some countries or stakeholders that stand to benefit more than others, or those who will have to work harder to achieve the goal, alongside differences in the financial contribution made. Here the roles of international organizations such as the United Nations (UN) agencies or regional organizations like the African Union are crucial to finding common solutions. The UN agencies most concerned with One Health issues have formed an alliance known as the Quadripartite alliance for One Health to support the mainstreaming of One Health.

UN Quadripartite alliance for One Health: To identify common goals between stakeholders and help address the potential conflicts that might arise when multiple partners work together for One Health issues, alliances can be formed. The Food and Agriculture Organization of the United Nations (FAO), the UN Environment Programme (UNEP), the World Health Organization (WHO) and the World Organisation for Animal Health (WOAH) have agreed to cooperate to combat health risks at the human–animal–ecosystems interface and sustainably balance and optimize the health of humans, animals, plants and the environment. This alliance is known as the Quadripartite and has a Chair position that rotates between each of the agencies.

The Quadripartite helps deliver 'global public goods', i.e. those goods that are available to everyone and do not diminish after use, such as clean air, by motivating each organization to work towards these common goals in a shared way. Successes of this alliance have been the setting of shared goals where each UN agency has a stake either in the delivery or outcome of the goal.

The Quadripartite agreed upon an initial framework for action with a set of activities that the four organizations can offer together to enable countries to mainstream and sustainably scale up One Health in managing health threats to humans, animals, plants and the environment. This is known as the One Health Joint Plan of Action (Quadripartite, 2022) and includes goals for curbing AMR, reducing the risk of emerging zoonotic pandemics, controlling and eliminating zoonotic neglected tropical disease and food safety amongst others (Fig. 14.7). Countries can then align their National Action Plans to this global Joint Plan of Action in what might be considered a form of top-down governance influence.

Collaboration can prove challenging, however, when each agency has its own responsibilities or objectives, and there may be differences in the size of budget or resources each must work with. There is also potential for inequity in agenda setting given the discrepancy between each participating agency's influence in the wider UN structure. There are also potential gains, however, with smaller bodies such as WOAH and UNEP joining the wider alliance, as they could benefit from improved advocacy or influencing power as part of a bigger stakeholder.

International agreements, such as a treaty, can be a way to unite countries to a common goal but allow each country to implement the policy as they see best.

A **TREATY** is a written agreement between two or more countries on an issue of global concern, such as antimicrobial resistance or climate change. There is agreement on the intent to act but the decision-making power is placed on the country

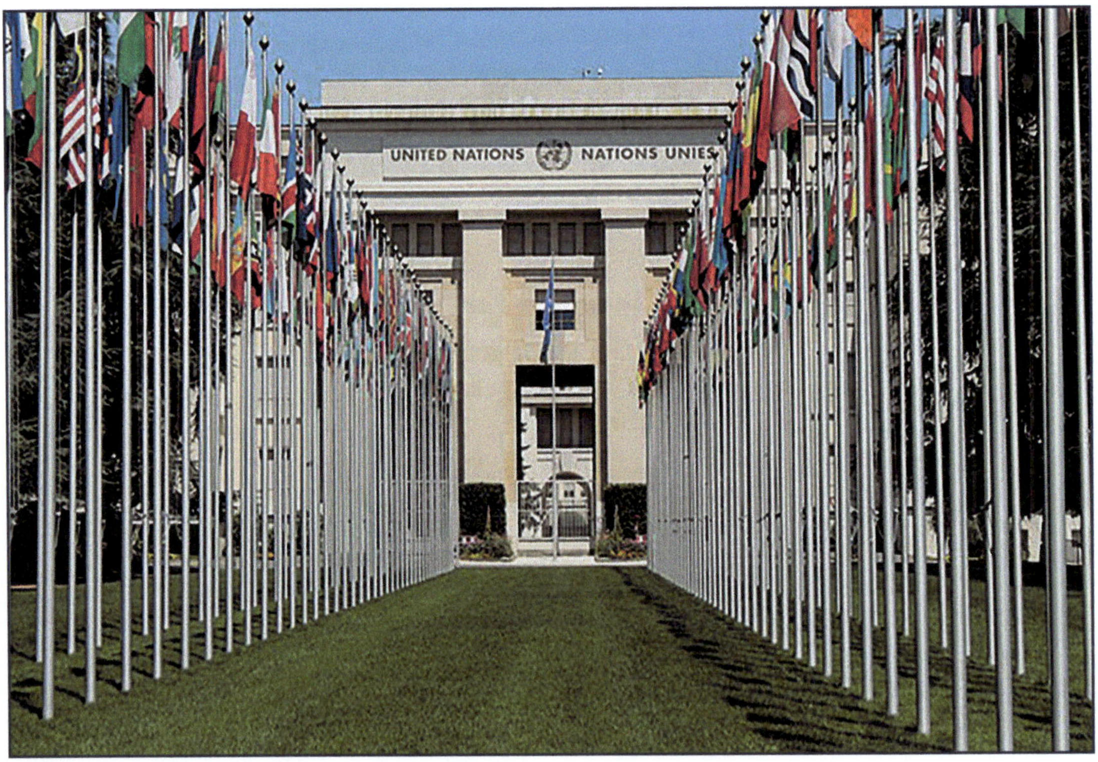

Fig. 14.7. United Nations, Geneva (CC BY-SA 4.0 DEED Attribution-ShareAlike 4.0 International).

to interpret the treaty or convention and select the best route for implementation. For example, the Convention on Biological Diversity (UNTS, 1992) is an international environmental agreement or framework that sets standards and requires countries to develop National Biodiversity Strategies and Action Plans (NBSAPs). It proposes legally binding obligations for each country that is party to the convention, but each member state has the flexibility to achieve these obligations in their own way, through their own national laws according to their own national or regional priorities. As part of those obligations, countries must report back on the actions taken to implement the Convention and their ***effectiveness***.

Once a policy has been developed, then it needs to be implemented. This often requires allocation of responsibilities and resources, including the financial means to pay for implementation and enforcement. It is also important to decide how to measure impact, success or value for money.

Any policy proposal should include an analysis of the (i) financial costs and (ii) economic consequences related to its implementation. This may be retrospective as part of an evaluation process or prospective, for example, when proposing a new policy to the Ministry of Finance or a national treasury for funding approval.

1. The financial aspect concerns the money and resources to be allocated to the public and private entities involved in policy implementation. These provisions must be sufficient to ensure that each collaborating entity is able to procure the material resources and the technical skills necessary to conduct the policy's commitments in the suggested timescale.
2. The economic aspect concerns the potential of the new policy to create a net social benefit, i.e. the policy outcomes should bring an overall benefit that society values more than the costs incurred for its implementation. Furthermore, the net social benefit must exceed the one created by alternative policies, including 'business-as-usual' solutions in which no change is initiated. One Health analysis across the whole system, incorporating the costs and benefits in human, animal, plant and environment sectors, should provide a more comprehensive analysis of a policy's costs and impact than traditional single-sector review. See Chapter 13 for more information on how to structure economic evaluations of One Health initiatives.

14.2 Why Do We Need One Health-Specific Governance?

One Health governance refers to the structures and organizations that play a role in or exert influence over the health of humans, animals and the environment, and is underpinned by several considerations and norms that stress their interconnectedness. From a One Health governance perspective, it is important that institutions, finance structures and policies function across sectors to support healthy humans, animals and ecosystems in a more joined-up way.

These cross-sector governance mechanisms may not always be labelled One Health but, importantly, will serve to strengthen the whole health system.

Traditional, narrow and sector-specific approaches in policy making may not only miss opportunities for more effective or efficient policy solutions but, when policy development has been inconsiderate of other disciplines, as well as social, economic and cultural contexts, it may result in unforeseen and detrimental consequences. Collaboration of individuals, communities and organizations within and between different sectors maximizes the benefits of shared knowledge and can increase acceptance and 'buy in' to new policies. A diversity of perspectives and evidence considered helps to avoid any unintended impacts from a policy and can help to get the best value for money.

Governance structures can be both a barrier and facilitating contributor to implementing the One Health approach and seeing it widely adopted. Many One Health success stories have relied on informal mechanisms, such as personal relationships between staff in different institutions or suitable individuals just being in the right place at the right time, but it would be preferable to formalize the structures to increase the likelihood of this being the case. More recently, some countries have established formal One Health multi-sector coordination governance mechanisms through an inter-ministerial body (One Health platforms or units), which sit independently beneath the prime minister or president's office rather than in any one ministry. An applied example of this from Bhutan follows.

Bhutan's One Health Secretariat: In Bhutan, the government have established a formal One Health governance structure through an Inter-Ministerial Committee for One Health (IMCOH) supported by a Bhutan One Health Secretariat. The Secretariat acts as a focal point for coordinating all national activities related to One Health, such as development and implementation of a One Health agenda, coordinated disease surveillance, field outbreak investigation and response, risk communication, advocacy and engagement of the community and environment sectors, and collaborative research. The secretariat sits within a central department at the Royal Center for Disease Control (RCDC) to create an equitable space for participation from the key ministries. To make sure that the secretariat's work remains closely linked to the existing ministries, they use a shared leadership approach, with a rotating chair known as secretaries (highest bureaucratic position) taken from each of the two key ministries, the Ministry of Health and the Ministry of Agriculture and Livestock. The Secretariat will support members to agree on a list of priority issues that require a One Health approach, e.g. **zoonotic disease** control. They also organize One Health conferences regularly and help to determine the financial contributions needed from each ministry and agencies for each area of work.

There are many demands of a governance structure to allow for cross-sector, multilevel and transdisciplinary relationships that can also adapt as our understanding of the human–animal–plant–environment interface continues to evolve. **Here we discuss aspects of governance systems to allow the One Health approach to be fully realized.**

14.2.1 Communication, coordination and collaboration across sectors

One of the main challenges associated with intersectoral governance is the difference in problem perception or what priorities are set. For example, those working in human health tend to judge a situation in terms of improvement of human health, while those in animal health or food production will be interested in goals related to animal ***wellbeing*** and/or productivity.

Rather than eliminate these differences, good One Health governance can help to resolve conflict and competition between organizations which can often arise when the responsibility for addressing certain issues is not clearly assigned. Despite favourable governance structures, it can still be difficult to balance the importance of outcomes across the sectors or stakeholders (see Chapter 15 on ***Sustainable Development Goals***).

Task: How to manage differing priorities: One Health approaches consider and engage a range of stakeholders to work towards issues that involve them in some way. However, stakeholders may not always have been motivated by the same thing. For example, in the control of zoonotic parasitic diseases that pass through livestock as an intermediate host before infecting humans, it would be preferable to prevent the infection of people by controlling the parasites (e.g. *Echinococcus granulosus*) in the animal stage (e.g. sheep). Despite presenting a serious public health risk for people, the condition in sheep is not perceived as important to the productivity of sheep by farmers. It is important to foresee and accept there may be differing priorities for each stakeholder rather than expecting all stakeholders to automatically accept human health priorities, as is often the case. If possible, finding common ground for collaboration can achieve the same, shared or similar outcomes but helps to engage stakeholders on their own terms.

Understanding objectives from the whole system is important to help identify common ground for different sectors to collaborate, but what happens when those outcomes are conflicting?

For example, should tackling malnutrition by producing more safe food for the world come at the cost of poor farm animal welfare or increased deforestation for livestock? Try to present the arguments for and against these dilemmas.

Discussion points and examples:

Farm animal welfare vs food security: Within European law, some animals are recognized as 'sentient beings' but otherwise non-human animals are treated as 'things' under law, unlike the human species that has fundamental rights. Others recognize that improved farm-animal welfare can contribute to increased productivity (i.e. any costs to improving welfare will be paid for by the increase in productivity), so there can be a shared objective between those advocating food security concerns and those advocating animal welfare (Farm Animal Welfare Council, n.d.).

But what happens when we need to cut down prime rainforest areas to produce meat or to build new houses or hospitals? There may be long-term benefits to humans of protecting forests, such as carbon sequestration from the atmosphere, but in the short term there are obvious benefits of building new hospitals.

Is providing more farmed animals for food, or hospitals or houses, equally beneficial to human health as protecting the forest would be? Should human health outcomes always be prioritized over those of wildlife or the ecosystem? The outcomes of interest might occur over different timescales – often the human health outcomes are short term, dealing with affected people to cure or prevent disease now. But when we talk about climate change and ecosystem health, we might be talking about much longer timescales, decades, maybe centuries. The duration of democratic cycles, i.e. the length of time before a leader must face elections again, could influence the timescale over which the benefits will be assessed and prioritized.

Consider how the method of evaluation might have an impact. For example, economic assessment of costs and benefits might be over a specific timescale or only look at impacts in one sector and not fully assess unintended impacts elsewhere. For example, pollution from manufacturing may not be calculated in the assessment to build a new factory or facility.

14.2.2 Communication, coordination and collaboration across groups

Healthy ecosystems often involve many different stakeholders and organizations working on any particular issue. So, One Health issues often demand different groups to work together in a multilateral collaboration, with multilateral meaning to have contributors from three or more groups. This could be when multiple countries come together or when public (i.e. government) and private organizations collaborate.

The different groups may have their own methodologies, knowledge, beliefs or languages so it is important in One Health governance that there are respectful partnerships between groups of people from different backgrounds and disciplines. See also Chapter 3 on ***transdisciplinarity*** and Chapter 4 on ***knowledge integration.***

Collaborations across governance scales and bodies are very common and have been formalized to varying extents, for example, public–private partnerships (PPPs) where NGOs may be asked to deliver a government public health programme. An example of this is private pharmaceutical companies donating anthelmintic (deworming) drugs to school public health programmes. These public health programmes are coordinated by the World Health Organization and national governments but sometimes delivered by NGOs and local health workers and schools.

Communicating science evidence to policy makers

Policy briefs and evidence syntheses: A policy brief or evidence synthesis is the process of bringing together and evaluating multiple sources of evidence and presenting it in a way that helps describe the big picture. Often these will be on particular areas that are topical to current policy debates. They are a useful tool to bridge the gap between primary scientific research and data publications, which may focus on a technical or specific area of interest, and the need to understand the situation at large. These syntheses help to piece together many of these more specific evidence sources into a bigger picture view that communicates essential context, describes limitations of the evidence base and provides examples or case studies.

Policy makers may specifically commission evidence syntheses as 'policy briefs'. An effective policy brief must be written in an accessible way for those from different professional backgrounds that may be stakeholders in policy development or decision making. Thus, a policy brief or evidence synthesis should be unbiased and accurate, but also concise so that stakeholders can become

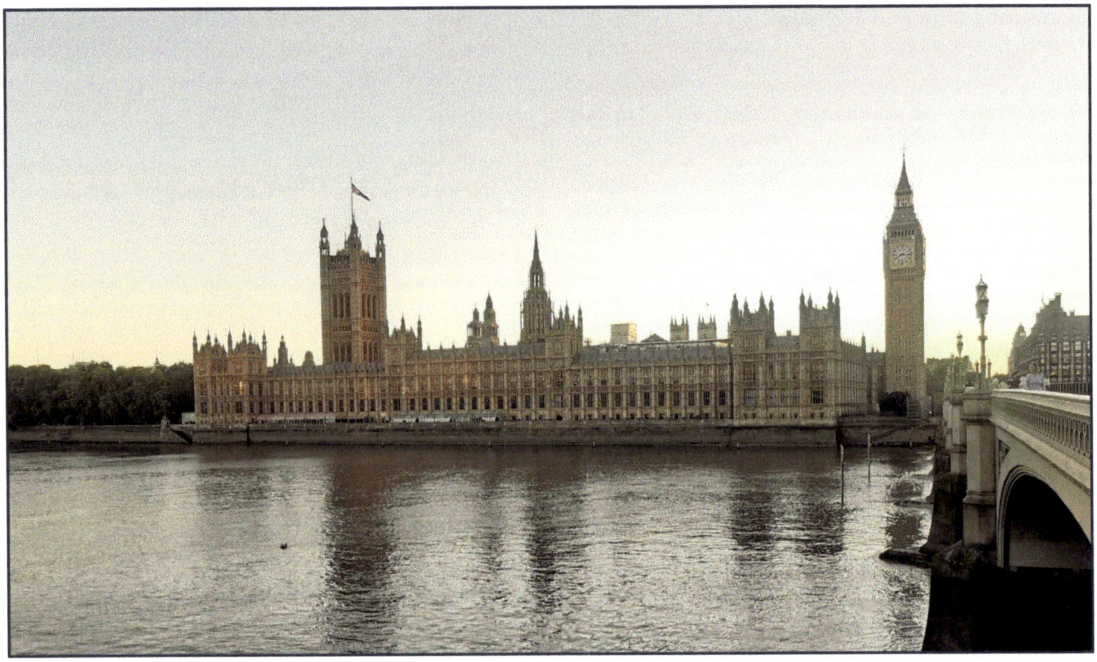

Fig. 14.8. In the UK, the Parliamentary Office of Science and Technology is one of the world's longest-standing legislative science advice networks. UK Parliament building. (Authors' own image.)

quickly informed on the overall situation while still understanding the limitations or complexity of the evidence relating to a particular subject.

In the UK, the Parliamentary Office of Science and Technology (POST, n.d.) is one of the world's longest standing legislative science advice networks. POST specializes in sourcing scientific evidence and making it accessible to all UK Parliamentarians, no matter their professional background (Fig. 14.8). Topics for these policy briefs are identified by horizon scanning for upcoming areas of interest or commissioned by government committees on topics they may be scrutinizing.

Rapid evidence assessments may be completed where there is an urgent need, e.g. in response to an unforeseen area for legislation or investigation by parliament. These will be done in partnerships with academic experts able to quickly review and synthesize the evidence. More routine briefings are mostly written by POST fellows, who are science and technology PhD students who specialize in the subject area and undertake a placement with supervision at POST in between their studies. This approach ensures the scientific rigour of these briefs and also helps to improve academia's understanding of the policy-making process and the needs of policy makers when these fellows return to their research institutions.

Examples include briefings on indoor air quality, environmentally sustainable diets or taking a One Health approach to public health and climate change. More information about speaking with policy makers can be found in Thomson (2021).

14.2.3 Communication, coordination and collaboration across levels

The distribution of responsibility and power will be different between sectors and countries for different issues. For some One Health issues, the focus might be national, such as for food safety policy, but some responsibility or power is also devolved to a more localized district authority. This can be helpful to allow the districts to tailor the national policy for their own local context, e.g. where a particular type of industry or crop occurs in one district but not in another.

One Health governance will need to be multi-level, i.e. function across levels, from the local to national or even international level. This demands coordinating several, potentially diverse, existing governance structures or groups. For example, trade of food products occurs across the world and a global policy might want to control disease spread. Multiple countries may agree to meet international trade regulations, but these policies may be quite general in order to be appropriate to lots of different country contexts. National or cross-border policies may therefore be developed with more detail to stop spread in or out of a country, with even more localized policies within countries to prevent spread into or out of individual districts or farms.

The extent to which decision-making power is devolved to national or district levels can vary a lot between countries and even between sectors within a country. For example, human health might be mostly governed at national level, where veterinary health services might be mostly devolved to district level. Good One Health governance and policies should be flexible enough to adapt to the idiosyncrasies of each local context, recognizing that a one-size-fits-all policy is often not appropriate for the many different political, social and economic realities that One Health issues involve.

As well as considering the flow of policy influence from top (international powers) to bottom (the local receiving population), there is also an influence running from bottom to top. With increased connectivity between people and goods in our modern world, what happens at the local level can have an impact anywhere in the world.

14.2.4 What governance may be most suitable for One Health?

The interconnected nature and ever-changing issues that are often found in a One Health system demand a suitable form of governance that can adapt to a changing situation when needed, can incorporate many perspectives and will consider different groups' needs. Given the interdependence of the various stakeholders within One Health, traditional top-down approaches may not be able to cope with the diverse challenges and opportunities presented. Instead, a more decentralized and collaborative approach may be better suited. Characteristics of such a form of governance should consider:

- **How to engage multiple stakeholders and be inclusive:** A suitable governance approach should allow for active participation and representation from diverse stakeholders. For example, in a food-related matter, this could mean farmers, producers, consumers, retailers, policy makers, scientists and civil society organizations. Engaging a broad range of stakeholders ensures that different perspectives, expertise and interests are considered in decision making. A limiting factor to stakeholder engagement could be: capacity, such as a time-pressed smallholder farmer; or where certain groups, e.g. women, might not be routinely involved in decisions about livestock health despite being the primary carers for their animals; or where a particular department or organization might be invited to many more meetings than they have staff available for. Having a governance system that can incorporate a diversity of power structures can also allow for locally led or bottom-up approaches.
- **Consider interactions across the whole system (systems thinking) and how sustainable any impact will be:** One Health systems are intricate webs of interactions and interdependencies. Governance should account for this by adopting a systems-thinking approach (see Chapter 10 for more information on ***systems thinking***). This will help to consider the interconnectedness of various components of any issue under consideration and the ripple effects of any policies and actions throughout the whole system. This also applies to how such policies or actions might be evaluated and which metrics are selected to indicate if it was good value-for-money or successful. Suitably considering and accounting for the impacts (desired and unintended) across the whole system, and over different timescales, will help to ensure that progress or behaviour change can be sustained.
- **How to adapt and respond to new information or changes in the system:** Health systems are subject to constant change: for example, environmental changes such as climate change; economic changes such as global oil prices; and social factors such as the different political views of ruling parties. A suitable governance approach therefore needs to be flexible, adaptive and capable of responding to any emerging challenges, such as infectious disease outbreaks. An adaptive and responsive approach can also capitalize on new opportunities in real time, such as those arising from a social movement.
- **Maximizing decision making informed by evidence and continuous learning:** Governance

decisions should be based on sound evidence and data where available. Rigorous research and analysis help policy makers understand the impacts of their decisions and inform effective strategies. It is important that this evidence and its limitations be presented to policy makers in an accessible way and that decisions be re-evaluated in the face of new evidence or any lessons learned during the implementation of a policy or action. (See the previous applied example of the UK Government on communicating science to policy makers.)

- **Cross-sector, multilevel and multilateral financing**: ***Financial governance*** for One Health needs to be able to work across levels, sectors and different stakeholder groups. It needs to recognize that responsibilities between stakeholders may not be equally distributed and that the costs and benefits may occur in different sectors. Similarly, any financial governance structure needs to account for the likely increased initial costs associated with establishing this new, integrated or collaborative way of working in health, where the benefits might be more difficult to measure or occur over a slower timescale (see Chapter 13 and the following applied example).

Economic aspects of One Health

1. Control of rabies demonstrates the issues that can arise when governance processes such as evaluation of costs and benefits do not support One Health working. Rabies is a viral infection that affects many species but preventing disease in humans is best achieved by preventing transmission from domestic dogs by controlling the disease in dogs rather than any interventions aimed directly at people. In fact, vaccinating dogs against rabies is about 50 times cheaper than providing post-exposure treatment to people and is the only way to sustainably prevent human rabies deaths (Hampson *et al.*, 2015). However, responsibility for dog-based interventions lies with the Ministry or district authority concerned with animal health and their priorities may lie elsewhere, for example, with food-producing animal health such as cattle or poultry.

Individual dog owners may listen to advisory information or act on incentives such as free dog vaccination to protect themselves and their animal; however, for those dogs without owners (stray), or where owners are unable or unwilling to vaccinate their dogs, there is an issue. Mobilizing funding from the human health sector to prevent human rabies deaths through dog vaccination can be problematic when the governance structures of funding institutions specify their responsibilities are to human health.

With a One Health governance structure, having the intervention (dog vaccination) sit in another sector to the benefit or funding institution (human health) could be less problematic. But this requires a suitable approach to evaluation of success, where this separation of costs and benefits between sectors is taken into account. In Latin America (Vigilato *et al.*, 2018), in order to overcome this mismatch of responsibilities, the liability for control of animal rabies now sits under the ministries responsible for human health.

2. Barriers to cross-sector working can relate to historic governance structures such as separation of those working with different samples in a diagnostics laboratory. In a laboratory processing samples from human, animal or environmental sources, the skills required from staff and the work they perform are similar. For example, laboratory technicians or the epidemiologists analysing data will perform similar work despite their training background or where their samples came from. They may, however, be offered different payment levels depending on the sector they belong to.

Here, having a One Health governance approach could allow for a more adaptive workforce structure. For example, in the global COVID-19 pandemic, laboratory staff trained in the animal health sector were able to help out in a time of increased surge demand on human health laboratories. However, there can be financial barriers to taking this approach when deciding where the responsibility for funding this work would sit. There may also be discrepancies between the pay offered to those from a human health background compared to those from animal or environmental health.

14.3 Conclusions: One Health Policy and Governance

- The modification of existing policy and governance structures, or the creation of new One Health governance structures, is required to create the 'enabling environment' that will allow the full benefits of taking a One Health approach to be realized.
- Those tasked with implementing a One Health approach need to be given enough decision-making responsibility and financial ability to effectively bring the sectors together, overcoming the inevitable challenges of establishing integrated working between normally segregated groups.
- Any new governance structure or policy will need to engage stakeholders on their own terms, such that common ground and shared objectives can motivate engagement from a wide range of partners (across levels, sectors and groups) with clear pathways for action.
- One Health practitioners must remain informed across a wide variety of evidence sources and types, representing fairly and respectfully a wide variety of disciplines and stakeholders outside their expertise and engaging their sector and policy makers with tailored communications.

14.4 Putting the Theory into Practice: Mapping One Health Systems, Implementing One Health Policy Making and Communicating to Decision Makers

This section of the chapter guides you through an activity that will help you to apply the learnings from the Policy and Governance chapter.

Task: You are invited to advise on a new Government policy

Scenario: The government have summoned a meeting of the scientific advisory group on which you sit. They tell you that they have ambitions to improve the economy, create jobs and reduce their carbon footprint by investing in renewable energy. They propose switching the national electricity generation away from coal-fired plants to a new hydroelectric dam (Fig. 14.9). To create this dam, they will need to increase the size of an existing lake by flooding a small rural valley. This may mean that some villages become separated on either side of the banks, and they will lose some agricultural land used to grow crops and graze cattle.

While this dam is being built, there will be downstream damage to the river ecosystem as water flow is drastically reduced. Additionally, the increase in standing water in the lake will increase the habitat for vectors of human and animal disease such as snails and insects.

Imagine this scenario as if you are scientists sitting on a government advisory group; you are tasked with advising on a solution that will best work for all stakeholders!

Identify the health system in your country or a selected country of choice: First, describe the governance structure of your selected country's One Health relevant institutions. Which government ministries or national institutions hold responsibility for human, animal, plant and ecosystem health? How do they communicate, coordinate or collaborate in their areas of shared interest?

Build your task team: Based on the scenario, who would you want to consult with? On what grounds would you approach these stakeholders to interest them in the issue?

Have a go at co-design: If you are able, form a small discussion group or, alternatively, imagine different stakeholders and their perspectives. Assume the roles of different stakeholders, e.g. national public health official, the village leader, veterinarian from World Organisation for Animal Health, government treasury representative, climate change scientist, or others. What would your main points for discussion be? How would you reach an agreement between your different priorities?

Developing policy solutions: Consider what policy solutions there might be to help achieve the best outcome for the government's hydroelectric dam proposal. How would you implement the policy ideas? What might the barriers be to implementation? Are there compromises that must be made to accommodate everyone's interests (Fig. 14.10)?

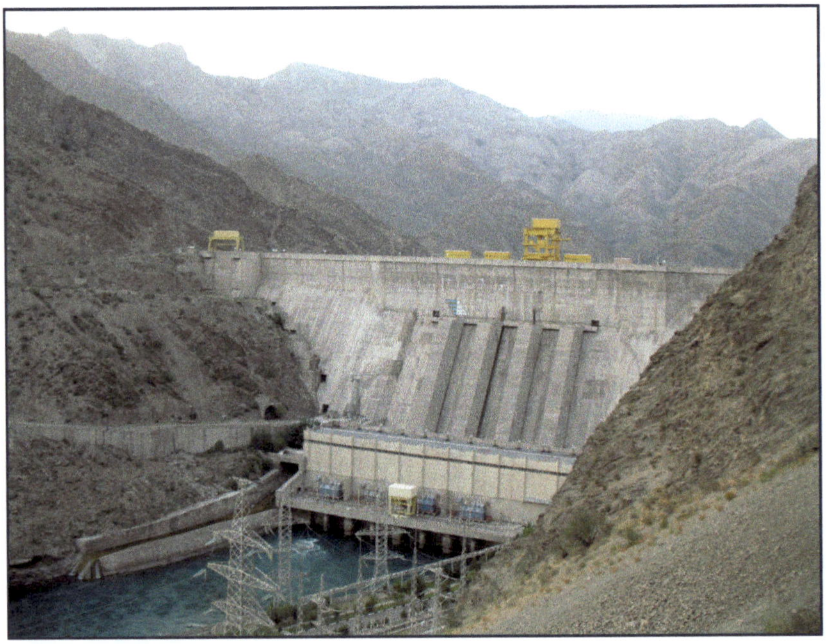

Fig. 14.9. Kürpsay hydroelectric dam in Kyrgyzstan. Image: Wikimedia/Firespeaker.

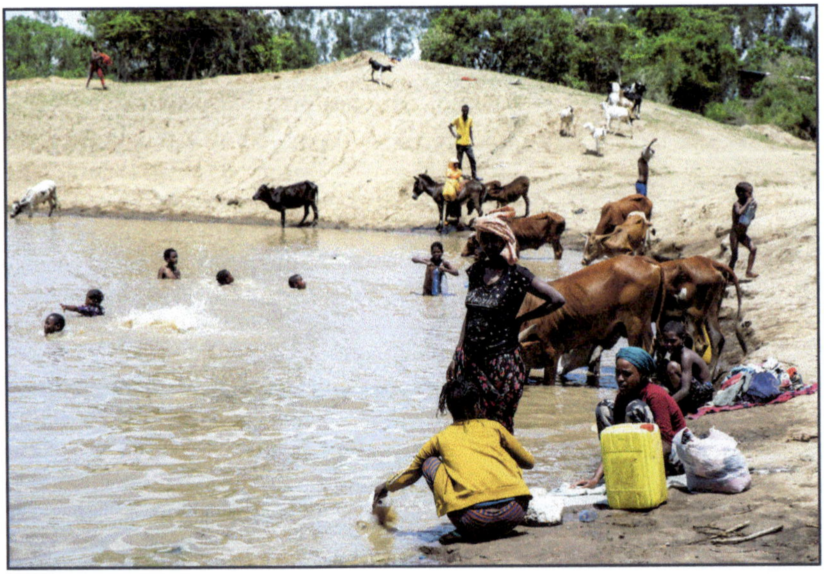

Fig. 14.10. The human-made dam in Keranso, Ethiopia traps water from the previous rainy season which the local community uses for washing clothes, bathing, swimming, taking home for household chores, as well as to provide water for their cattle. The pond is also home to freshwater snails that host schistosomiasis, otherwise known as bilharzia. Access to clean piped water, or even water from a clean protected source, is limited, and many people in the community rely on this and similarly unprotected pools, ponds, streams and rivers for bathing, washing clothes and other household chores. According to the villagers in Keranso, one 20-litre jerrycan of clean/safe drinking water costs 15 birr, and a 30-litre jerrycan costs 20 birr – a prohibitive amount for anything other than for drinking. Image: Indrias G. Kassaye, Unlimit Health.

Briefing the Minister: Write a policy brief or present a 3-minute pitch for your imagined Minister. You should set out the problem, need, current situation, political considerations and policy options with discussion of pros and cons of each. Think about how you will communicate your ideas and information to best inform the policy makers' (Minister's) decision. Ensure your briefing is suitable for someone from a non-science background and keep it brief – a maximum of two sides of A4 or a 3-minute presentation!

Activity discussion points:

1. Identify the health system in your country or a selected country of choice:

- Use government websites to identify the ministries or departments that might be relevant. What other public bodies exist (i.e. those tasked to deliver a public or government service but that do not have a Minister)? For example: technical advisory groups or non-executive government departments such as an office for statistics, meteorological data or a regulatory body such as those on health and safety or environmental inspection.
- The system map or list does not need to be exhaustive, but it is helpful to understand how governance systems can be arranged and separate out responsibilities differently. It is helpful to identify how some of the stakeholders communicate, influence or collaborate and where others may be excluded.
- Focus on the main ministries or bodies that are relevant to the scenario and what areas of the scenario might cross over between responsibilities of different ministries or bodies.
- Who are the non-state actors of relevance (e.g. NGOs or private companies)?

2. Build your task team and have a go at co-design:

- Refer to the list or systems map you created in step 1 to identify those public and non-state stakeholders that are of relevance to the scenario. Are there multiple people from some ministries? Are there particular job roles or advisory bodies that you would want to consult?
- Thinking about the example of snail vector increase as a risk factor for human and cattle schistosomiasis, the change of habitat from river to dam and increased water may provide more habitat for snails as a vector for schistosomiasis in both humans and cattle. Recognizing this risk early by involving the right stakeholders in the discussion can allow mitigation measures to be put in place. For more information see World Health Organization (2022, p. 1).
- Who are the non-state actors and what perspective are they coming from? NGOs also come from a diversity of backgrounds and could be interested in different things, e.g. preventing increased human or animal disease from vector habitat increase when the land is flooded, or they could be helping to represent small communities affected and ensure they are consulted. Private companies could be interested to win the contract to build the dam or to distribute the electricity it generates. Others may be concerned that local roads will be shut down, affecting transport of goods, or their agricultural land will be reduced.
- Stakeholders may be from different organizations but on what grounds are they engaging? For example, wildlife experts from government organizations or NGOs might share a similar interest in how ecosystems may be disrupted when the water flow is changed. Although coming from a different perspective, those from private water companies might also be interested in how water flow is disrupted but with their main concern for water supply, not ecosystem disruption.
- This does not need to be an exhaustive list but consider where the common issues or motivating factors might lie to persuade your team to engage with this issue and who they might find have similar aims despite coming from different backgrounds.

3. Developing policy solutions:

- Put yourselves in the shoes of different stakeholders around the table. What are the differing priorities for all those people who are linked to the scenario? Are there any areas of conflict and how could a compromise be reached? For example, creating dams may displace communities and businesses and affect how they interact with neighbouring villages. Some communities may feel unfairly disadvantaged despite recognizing that there may be a national benefit to the dam building. A compromise could be that the government or the construction contractor must include a boat pier and ferry service to ensure a way to travel across the area.

- Returning to the example of snail vector increase as a risk factor for human and cattle schistosomiasis, what policies could be put in place to mitigate public health risk? This could be a responsive action in the form of mass deworming treatment policy for local people or targeted at those who are at highest risk (e.g. in contact with the water or cattle). It could also take on a One Health approach by considering multisector control points such as environmental controls. These could include control of the snail vector through clearing vegetation from the water edges in occupied areas or introduction of natural predators (e.g. freshwater shrimp) if these are locally suitable for the ecosystem and community.
- Consider where resolution of conflicting priorities between stakeholders might be more difficult, e.g. there may be reduced carbon emissions from increasing renewable energy use, which would help mitigate climate change, and there may be economic benefits to increasing national reliance on a domestic and renewable energy source but this is at the cost of unavoidable ecosystem damage. Is reducing carbon emissions more important than preserving ecosystems in this scenario? What are the mitigation measures that could be put in place, e.g. creation of local protected habitats, documentation of species and relocation, protected wildlife corridors to aid migration.

4. **Briefing the Minister:**

- Find examples on the internet of briefs for other issues and decide on what sections your brief or presentation will have. Consider what a person new to the subject would need to know and explain it using non-technical language. Be careful to explain if there are limitations in the advice you are giving, e.g. there is no evidence in a certain area or the evidence is out of date. An absence of evidence is not evidence that there is no cause for concern!
- Search for existing systematic reviews, government reports or evidence syntheses that are related to your topic – these should give a good high-level overview in the abstract or introduction.
- Presenting the evidence in an unbiased way and noting the limitations is important but a policy brief will often go further and make recommendations based on the available evidence. Sometimes policies will need to be decided upon, even when there are gaps in the evidence, but part of the recommendations can be to gather more evidence and update the policy in the face of new information. Regular evaluations and adjustment of policies and a suggestion for a timeline over which this should occur can be helpful. For example, recommend that in parallel to the dam building (policy implementation) there should be ongoing monitoring and evaluation of the environmental impact or vector-borne disease incidence so that these impacts can be minimized or mitigated.
- In contrast to much science decision making, policy decision making will also need to consider public opinion or political consequences and thus becomes evidence-informed rather than fully evidence-based. Pointing out these influencing factors is helpful. For example, if the dam were to flood an area of national significance, then there might be public outcry and no Minister would want to sign off the project, even if this would be the best place to position the dam based on scientific factors such as topography.
- Keep your brief or your presentation short and clearly structured. Ministers are responsible for many different areas of work so require rapid information that does not require technical knowledge. You should always be clear and transparent about what the evidence says and where you have interpreted that evidence into a recommendation. As an expert you are there to offer your expert opinion so do not be scared to suggest solutions and your ideas – it is for the Minister to decide what the final decision will be!

References

Dodgson, R., Lee, K. and Drager, N. (2002) Global Health Governance: A Conceptual Review. World Health Organization. Available at: https://iris.who.int/bitstream/handle/10665/68934/a85727_eng.pdf;sequence=1 (accessed 8 August 2024).

Farm Animal Welfare Council (n.d.) *Report on Economics and Farm Animal Welfare*. London. Available at: https://assets.publishing.service.gov.uk/media/5a7d5b5840f0b60a7f1aa056/FAWC_report_on_economics_and_farm_animal_welfare.pdf (accessed 8 August 2024).

Hampson, K., Coudeville, L., Lembo, T., Sambo, M., Kieffer, A. *et al.* (2015) Estimating the global burden of endemic canine rabies. *PLoS Neglected Tropical Diseases* 9(5). DOI: 10.1371/journal.pntd.0003709.

Ifesinachi Okafor-Yarwood, D.B. (2020) The duplicity of the European Union Common Fisheries Policy in third countries: Evidence from the Gulf of Guinea. *Ocean and Coastal Management* 184. Available at: https://www.sciencedirect.com/science/article/abs/pii/S0964569119301620?via%3Dihub (accessed 8 August 2024).

Khan, A.S.S. (2015) Seafood insecurity, bush meat consumption, and public health emergency in West Africa: Did we miss the early warning signs of an Ebola epidemic? *Maritime Studies* 14(3). DOI: 10.1186/s40152-015-0020-2.

Kremer, M., Ahuja, A. and Zwane, A.P. (2010) Providing Safe Water: Evidence from Randomized Evaluations. Harvard Environmental Economics Program. Available at: https://heep.hks.harvard.edu/files/heep/files/dp23_kremer-ahuja-petersonzwane.pdf (accessed 8 August 2024).

Parliamentary Office of Science and Technology (POST) (n.d.). Available at: https://post.parliament.uk/ (accessed January 2024).

Quadripartite (2022) One Health Joint Plan of Action (2022–2026) Working Together for the Health of Humans, Animals, Plants and the Environment. Available at: https://www.who.int/publications/i/item/9789240059139 (accessed 8 August 2024).

Rulli, M.C., Santini, M., Hayman, D.T. and D'Odorico, P. (2017) The nexus between forest fragmentation in Africa and Ebola virus disease outbreaks. *Scientific Reports* 7, 41613. DOI: 10.1038/srep41613.

Thaler, R.H. and Sunstein, C.R. (2009) *Nudge: Improving Decisions about Health, Wealth, and Happiness*. Penguin, London.

The United Nations Commission on Global Governance (1995) *Our Global Neighborhood: The Report of the Commission on Global Governance*. Oxford University Press. Available at: https://apps.who.int/iris/bitstream/handle/10665/68934/a85727_eng.pdf;sequence=1 (accessed 8 August 2024).

Thomson, D.J. (2021) *The Art of Science Communication: Sharing Knowledge with Students, the Public, and Policymakers*. Thomson Publishing, Arlington, Virginia.

UNTS (1992) Convention on Biological Diversity. Available at: https://www.cbd.int/ (accessed 8 August 2024).

Vigilato, M.A.N., Molina-Flores, B., Del Rio Vilas, V.J., Pompei, J.C. and Cosivi, O. (2018) Canine rabies elimination: Governance principles. *Revue Scientifique et Technique* 37(2), 703–709.

World Health Organization (2017) *Advancing the Right to Health: The Vital Role of Law*. World Health Organization, Geneva. Available at: https://iris.who.int/handle/10665/252815 (accessed 8 August 2024).

World Health Organization (2022) Ending the neglect to attain the sustainable development goals. *One Health: Approach for Action Against Neglected Tropical Diseases 2021–2030*. Geneva. Available at: https://www.who.int/publications/i/item/9789240010352 (accessed 8 August 2024).

Young, O.R. (2017) *Governing Complex Systems: Social Capital for the Anthropocene (Earth System Governance)*. MIT Press, Cambridge, Massachusetts.

15 One Health and Sustainable Development Goals

Asta Tvarijonaviciute[1,2], Patrícia Inácio[2,3,4], Alberto Muñoz-Prieto[1,5], Dai Nakae[6] and Lorena Franco-Martínez[1,2,7]

[1]Interdisciplinary Laboratory of Clinical Pathology, Interlab-UMU, Campus of Excellence Mare Nostrum, University of Murcia, Murcia, Spain; [2]Network for Ecohealth and One Health (NEOH); [3]National Institute for Agrarian and Veterinary Research, IP, Portugal; [4]LEAF (Linking Landscape, Environment, Agriculture and Food Research Unit), ISA, University of Lisbon, Portugal; [5]Internal Diseases Clinic, Faculty of Veterinary Medicine, University of Zagreb, Zagreb, Croatia; [6]Department of Medical Sports, Faculty of Health Care and Medical Sports, Teikyo Heisei University, Chiba, Japan; [7]Moorepark Animal and Grassland Research Center, Teagasc, Irish Agriculture and Food Development Authority, Cork, Ireland

Contents

DOI: 10.1079/9781800623002.0016

Chapter Overview

Elevator pitch

One Health is a collaborative and interdisciplinary approach, cutting across boundaries of animal, human and environment health. One Health is increasingly gaining attention among scientists and the general population. In parallel, the United Nations have gathered 17 Sustainable Development Goals (SDGs) with the main aim to promote human prosperity while protecting the planet. The two perspectives (One Health and SDGs) seem to care about the health of humans, animals, plants and the environment, but are they really the same? This chapter will address the main similarities and unique differences of the two perspectives.

Book objectives the chapter relates to

☐ 1. Understand what One Health and Ecohealth mean
☑ 2. Think in a One Health and Ecohealth way
☑ 3. Apply One Health and Ecohealth in their professional and personal life
☐ 4. Know how to share One Health and Ecohealth knowledge
☑ 5. Integrate One Health and Ecohealth knowledge actively
☑ 6. Acquire or enhance core One Health competencies

One Health competencies covered

☐ 1. Effective communication
☐ 2. Collaborative and resilient working
☑ 3. Systems understanding
☑ 4. Transdisciplinarity
☐ 5. Social, cultural and gender equity and inclusiveness
☑ 6. Collective learning and reflective practice
☐ 7. One Health concepts
☐ 8. Theoretical and methodological pluralism
☐ 9. Harnessing uncertainty, paradox and limited knowledge

After having worked through this chapter, you will be familiar with the concept of the SDGs and how One Health links to them.

Learning outcomes

1. Enhance knowledge on SDGs.
2. Address the main benefits and limitations of SDGs regarding One Health.
3. Address agreements and disagreements of the two perspectives.
4. Develop (improve) personal skills such as critical and holistic thinking, ethical decision making and problem solving.

Summary

In this chapter, the 'what', 'why' and 'what for' of the SDGs will first be introduced. Subsequently, all SDGs are discussed, organized according to a framework in which each of the SDGs is assigned to one of three concentric layers: inner level, 'Wellbeing'; intermediate level, 'Infrastructure'; and outer level, 'Natural Environment'. In addition, each part is accompanied by a table in which the implicated SDGs are concisely described, presenting their aims, current situation and the importance of each SDG to achieve the change. In the chapter, you will find considerations on their benefits and interconnections, as well as a critical view on their limitations regarding One Health and even in relation to other SDGs.

15.1 Introduction

In the 19th century, the specialization and separation of **disciplines** gained momentum forced by the appearance of very large amounts of specific **knowledge** that required super-specialists[1] to better manage multifaceted problems (Kalra *et al.*, 2003). Even if in some cases this proved to be a useful approach, however, the super-specialization had some limitations and drawbacks. For example, in medicine, super-specialists became highly technology dependent and had a profound knowledge in their field, but very little understanding outside it. Thus, in many cases, super-specialization has led patients to move from one super-specialist to another, resulting in fragmentation of patient care, diffusion of responsibilities and increased costs, among other issues (Peter *et al.*, 1999). For this reason, the need for generalist trained doctors with knowledge about all body systems and their interactions has been claimed by different authors in the 20th and 21st centuries (Loefler and Turnberg, 2000; Kalra *et al.*, 2003; Weisz, 2003). Similarly, the separation of human and veterinary medicines and related professions and disciplines (e.g. ecology, sociology, economics) constituted a major obstacle to the holistic vision of public, animal and **ecosystem** health, and the resolution of related problems. This raised the need for the implementation of interdisciplinary and cross-sectoral initiatives to address and target the problems involving different **sectors** more effectively, and to ensure the **health** and **wellbeing** not only of humans but also of animals and the environment. Thus, One Health initiatives promote the integrative holistic approach to addressing human–animal–plant–environment health issues. However, the path back from super-specializations and the separation of disciplines to integrative thinking and working in science, politics and society in general is complex and hampered by siloed education, traditions, policies and personal beliefs.

In 2015, the United Nations General Assembly set 'Transforming our World: The 2030 Agenda for Sustainable Development' (https://sdgs.un.org/publications/transforming-our-world-2030-agenda-sustainable-development-17981). The agenda includes a pack of 17 'integrated and indivisible' **Sustainable Development Goals** (SDGs) and 169 targets that balance three dimensions of sustainable development – social, environmental and economic – by focusing on five main topics: people, planet, prosperity, peace and partnership. The SDGs were built on the basis of Millennium Development Goals (MDGs) and besides new aims also seek to finish and complete initiated tasks during MDGs. With these goals, it is intended to direct the actions from 2015 to 2030 towards improved lives for all and transform the world by strengthening universal peace and freedom, and moving towards a sustainable and resilient path.

The 17 SDGs have been clustered in different ways by different authors (Fig. 15.1). In the present chapter, however, the framework proposed by Waage *et al.* (2015) and represented in Fig. 15.2 will be used because of its common use by other scientists in the field. In this framework, each of the SDGs is assigned to one of three concentric layers:

1. **Inner layer: Wellbeing** includes six goals (SDGs 1, 3, 4, 5, 10, 16) directly related to human wealth – health, education and inequality.
2. **Middle layer: Infrastructure** includes seven goals (SDGs 2, 6, 7, 8, 9, 11, 12) related to different networks and mechanisms to achieve the essentials of modern society such as clean water, sanitation and waste management, among others.
3. **Outer layer: Natural Environment** includes three goals (SDGs 13, 14, 15) that address the management of ocean and terrestrial ecosystems to preserve **biodiversity** and actions to lessen **climate** change.

In this framework, SDG 17 was left out because it was considered a cross-cutting goal relating to goals at all levels (Waage *et al.*, 2015). Later on, the framework was extended by other authors to include SDG 17 for the global partnership for sustainable development because it was seen as a key goal with regards to One Health (Kock *et al.*, 2018). Overall, this framework and its graphic representation highlight the human-centred origin of the goals. Nevertheless, it was argued that the SDGs represent the first steps permitting to drive a shift in policy and daily practice towards a fully integrated approach of whole health and wellbeing (Zinsstag *et al.*, 2011; Kock *et al.*, 2018).

In the following paragraphs, the relationship between the different layers of the concentric circles of the framework and the SDGs that compose it in relation to the **One Health approach** will be addressed.

15.2 Inner Level: 'Wellbeing'

WELLBEING is a positive outcome that is meaningful for people and for many sectors of

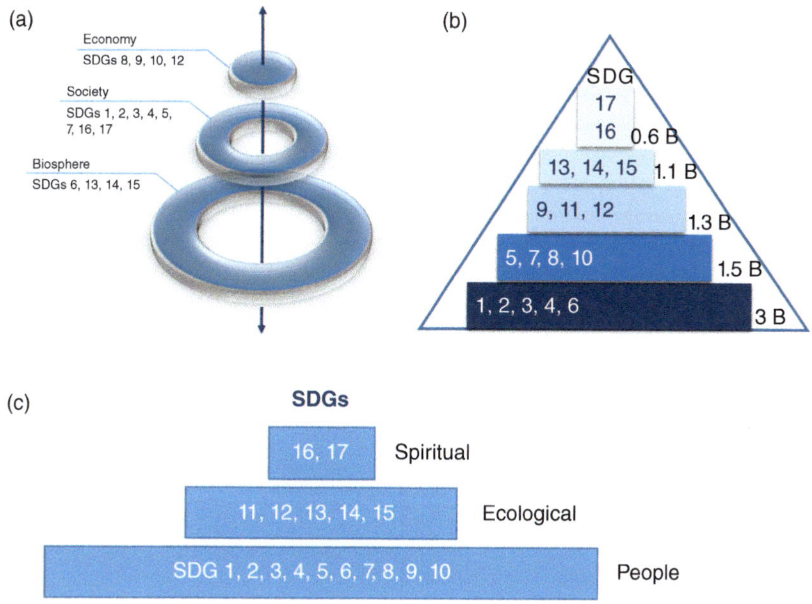

Fig. 15.1. Sustainable Development Goal (SDG) clusters proposed by different authors: (a) economies and societies are integral parts of the biosphere (Rockström and Sukhdev, 2017); (b) pyramid of SDGs based on affected number of people (B = billion) (Jaiswal, 2018); (c) SDGs presented in a three-level pyramid based on the Tri Hita Karana, a traditional Indonesian philosophy for life (https://sdgpyramid.org/).

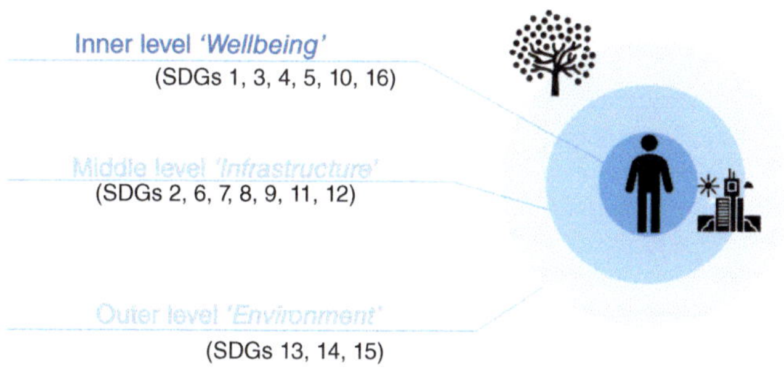

Fig. 15.2. Framework proposed by Waage *et al.* (2015).

society, because it tells us that people perceive that their lives are going well. Good living conditions (e.g. housing, employment, sanitation, food security) are fundamental to wellbeing. However, many **indicators** that measure living conditions fail to measure what people think and feel about their lives, such as the quality of their relationships, their positive emotions and resilience, the realization of their potential, or their overall satisfaction with life – i.e. their 'wellbeing'. Wellbeing generally includes global judgements of life satisfaction and feelings ranging from depression to joy (according to the Centers for Disease Control and Prevention (CDC)).

The inner level is composed of six interrelated SDGs that aim to deliver individual and collective outcomes, such as health, education and nutrition, equally between individuals and countries, which directly pertain to the **welfare** and wellbeing of **humans** (Waage *et al.*, 2015) (Figs 15.2 and 15.3, Table 15.1). An example of synergies that could be achieved can be seen by aligning the designs of health (SDG3), **gender equality** (SDG5) and education (SDG4) goals to

Table 15.1. SDGs belonging to inner 'Wellbeing' level.

Goal	Short description
1. No Poverty	**Aim:** To end poverty in all its forms everywhere (https://www.un.org/development/desa/disabilities/envision2030-goal1.html). **Current situation:** Globally, the number of people living in extreme poverty declined from 36% in 1990 to 10% in 2015. Progress towards Goal 1 had slowed and, even before COVID-19, baseline projections suggested that 7% of the global population would still be living in extreme poverty in 2030, missing the target of ending poverty (https://www.un.org/sustainabledevelopment/poverty/) **SDG1 to achieve the change:** Strong social protection systems are essential for mitigating the effects and preventing many people from falling into poverty. Nevertheless, 53.1% of the world's population did not benefit from any form of social protection in 2020, and behind this global average, there are significant inequalities across and within regions. Only 18.6% of unemployed workers were covered by unemployment benefits (https://www.ilo.org/global/publications/books/WCMS_817574/lang--en/index.htm). Active engagement in policy making can make a difference in addressing poverty: governments should create an enabling environment to generate productive employment and job opportunities, while the private sector should promote inclusive economic growth with opportunities for the poor.
3. Good Health and Wellbeing	**Aim:** To ensure healthy lives and promote wellbeing for all at all ages (https://www.un.org/development/desa/disabilities/envision2030-goal3.html). **Current situation:** In 2017, only around one-third to half of the global population was covered by essential health services. If current trends continue, only 39% to 63% of the global population will be covered by essential health services by 2030. Progress in many health areas, such as reduced maternal and child mortality, increased vaccination coverage and reduction of some infectious diseases, continues, but the rate of improvement has slowed down, especially during COVID-19. This pandemic crisis has disrupted essential health services around the world and, together with the decrease in food availability, the increase in child and maternal deaths could be devastating (https://www.un.org/sustainabledevelopment/wp-content/uploads/2017/03/3_Why-It-Matters-2020.pdf). **SDG3 to achieve the change:** All its targets focus on reducing mortality and morbidity rates by addressing the main health threats including infection, non-communicable and pollution-engendered diseases, road accidents and drug abuse by fostering access to quality health services, improved universal health coverage and education (Meurs *et al.*, 2019). To achieve the change, it is important to support the research on these areas, mainly on the development of vaccines and medicines, and providing affordable access to them. The pandemic crises have provided more evidence of the importance of strengthening the capacity of all countries for early warning, risk reduction and management of national and global health risks.
4. Quality Education	**Aim:** To ensure inclusive and equitable quality education and promote lifelong learning opportunities for all (https://www.un.org/development/desa/disabilities/envision2030-goal4.html). **Current situation:** Although in 2000–2009 major progress was made regarding access to education, this trend was stalled in recent years with, in 2018, more than 258 million (one in five) of primary- and secondary-age children, adolescents and youth out of school (UN, 2020). Girls still face more barriers than boys at the primary level. During the COVID-19 pandemic, many schools offered remote learning to students through virtual classrooms to mitigate the impact of school closures, but at least 500 million children and youth were excluded from these options, increasing inequalities (https://unstats.un.org/sdgs/report/2020/goal-04/). **SDG4 to achieve the change:** Education is a pillar of personal and social development and progression, contributing to practically all SDGs in one or another way. SDG4 stands up for equitable, gender-impartial and quality primary, secondary, technical, vocational and tertiary education. Furthermore, SDG4 addresses the need for and supply of qualified teachers and the implementation of information and communication technologies (ICT) to create effective learning environments to deal with the learning crisis. There is currently a large gap between what is taught and what is sought in the labour market (https://www.unicef.org/media/59856/file/UNICEF-education-strategy-2019-2030.pdf).

Continued

Table 15.1. Continued.

Goal	Short description
5. Gender Equality	**Aim:** To achieve gender equality and empower all women and girls (https://www.un.org/development/desa/disabilities/envision2030-goal5.html). **Current situation:** Besides 15,000 reforms performed worldwide in the last 50 years, women are still disadvantaged in terms of schooling, rates of unpaid care and domestic work, earnings, and still have only three-quarters of the legal rights of men (https://www.worldbank.org/en/topic/gender/overview#1). The pandemic crises of COVID-19 intensified the risk of violence against women and girls. Moreover, women were likely to take on most additional care work owing to the closure of schools and day-care centres. They were also on the front lines in fighting the coronavirus because women account for nearly 70% of health and social workers globally (https://www.oecd.org/coronavirus/policy-responses/women-at-the-core-of-the-fight-against-covid-19-crisis-553a8269/). **SDG5 to achieve the change:** SDG5 goals are focused on women's rights and gender equality and are supported by at least another 11 SDGs that contain targets addressing gender equality issues. SDG5 seeks to end all types of discrimination, violence and exploitation of women and girls, foster equal rights to economic resources and access and use of technology through the adoption of new policies and legislation (https://www.un.org/sustainabledevelopment/gender-equality/).
10. Reduced Inequality	**Aim:** To reduce income inequality within and among countries (https://www.un.org/development/desa/disabilities/envision2030-goal10.html). **Current situation:** During the period 2012–2017, the incomes grew of the bottom 40% of the population living in 90 countries. Yet even so, the poorest 40% of the population received less than 25% of the income or general consumption, while the richest 10% received at least 20% of the income (secretary-general-sdg-report-2020--EN.pdf (un.org)). Moreover, women are more likely to be victims of discrimination than men. Among those with disabilities, 3 in 10 personally experienced discrimination, with higher levels still among women with disabilities (https://www.un.org/development/desa/disabilities/wp-content/uploads/sites/15/2019/10/Making-SDGs-count-for-women-with-disabilities.pdf). **SDG10 to achieve the change:** SDG10 calls to reduce inequality irrespective of age, sex, disability, race, ethnicity, religion and economic status, among others, and to foster income growth of the bottom 40% of the population and enhance representation and the voice of the developing countries via adoption and adjustment of policies (https://www.un.org/sustainabledevelopment/inequality/). Moreover, establishing adequate migration policies is needed to promote cooperation and partnerships and to facilitate safe, orderly and regular migration to protect the vulnerable population and leave no one behind.
16. Peace, Justice and Strong Institutions	**Aim:** To promote peaceful and inclusive societies for sustainable development, provide access to justice for all and build effective, accountable and inclusive institutions at all levels (https://www.un.org/development/desa/disabilities/envision2030-goal16.html). **Current situation:** Conflict, insecurity, weak institutions and limited access to justice remain threats to sustainable development. In 2019, the number of people fleeing war, persecution and conflict exceeded 79.5 million, the highest level recorded (https://unstats.un.org/sdgs/report/2020/goal-16/). The implication of the institutions in the development of an egalitarian and fair society is essential, but judicial and police institutions are the most affected by corruption. Corruption has a significant economic impact, limiting the resource distribution between the different social classes. Furthermore, inequality in society seriously affects children, being regularly exposed to multiple forms of violence, many of which are unrecognized and unreported (https://unstats.un.org/sdgs/report/2020/goal-16/). **SDG16 to achieve the change:** Governments, civil society and communities must work together to implement lasting solutions to reduce violence, deliver justice, combat corruption and always ensure inclusive participation. Promote inclusion and respect towards people of different ethnic origins, religions, gender, sexual orientations or different opinions.

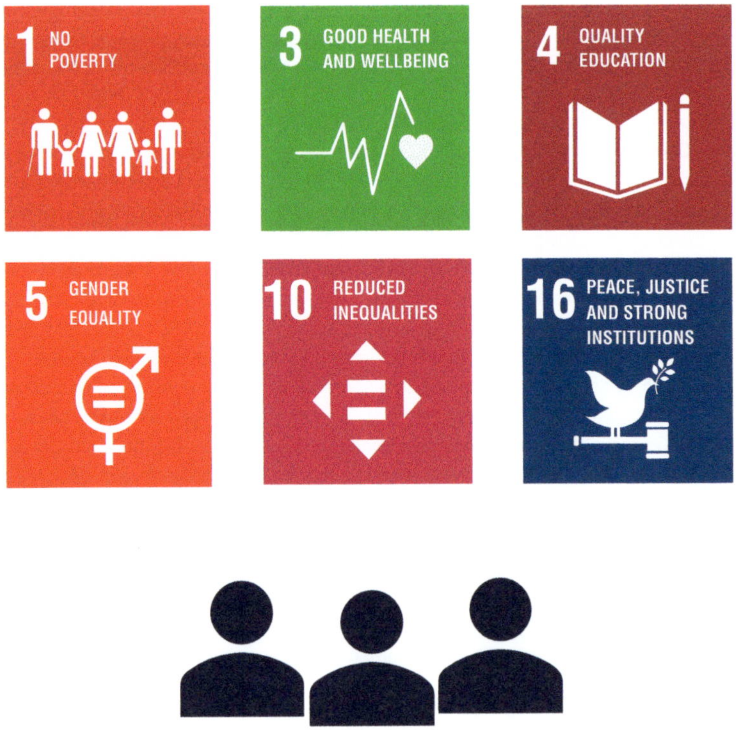

Fig. 15.3. The 'wellbeing' people-centred goals: SDGs 1, 3, 4, 5, 10, 16 (https://www.un.org/sustainabledevelopment/). The content of this publication has not been approved by the United Nations and does not reflect the views of the United Nations or its officials or Member States.

improve sexual and reproductive health, as well as the **empowerment** of women and girls (Waage *et al.*, 2015).

15.2.1 How is human wellbeing measured?

Measurement of wellbeing can be performed using:

- **objective** wellbeing indicators (OWI), e.g. observable health status, economic incomes, material outcomes, biological markers, etc.
- **subjective** wellbeing measures (SWM) that are based on respondents' self-evaluations of their own life.

Based on scientific evidence, the use of mixed evaluation is recommended because the **OWIs** have a limited capacity to assess and solve global health problems and define success, as such, whereas **SWMs** do play an important role in defining success and, therefore, are gaining increasing significance in policy making, but are imperfect due to their subjective origin (Adams, 2016; Benjamin *et al.*, 2019).

15.2.2 Wellbeing measures and SDGs

The current version of the SDGs only includes objective indicators. For example, the monitoring of achievements of SDG3 (Health and wellbeing) targets are mainly based on objective quantitative metrics, such as mortality rates. Furthermore, although the title of SDG3 includes the term 'wellbeing', which according to WHO refers to 'a state of complete physical, mental and social well-being and not merely the absence of disease or infirmity' (https://apps.who.int/gb/bd/PDF/bd47/EN/constitution-en.pdf?ua=1), none of the 13 targets refers to ways to assess, improve or achieve it. In addition, different authors claimed that, besides focusing on incomes or other material indicators, one of the essential ways toward reducing inequality (SDG10) is promoting advancements of healthcare systems worldwide with special emphasis in low- and middle-income countries (Tangcharoensathien *et al.*, 2015; Hone *et al.*, 2017). In the same way, SDG1 (no poverty) only includes economic and material metrics (https://read.dukeupress.edu/books/book/78/MetricsWhat-Counts-in-Global-Health). Nevertheless, there is a strong correlation between achieving sustainable development and self-reported measures of wellbeing. Moreover, the analyses indicate that there are increasing marginal returns to sustainable development in terms of wellbeing (De Neve and Sachs, 2020a, b).

Learning questions:

- Reflect on how the achievement of inner-level SDGs could affect animals and the environment.
- Could you list at least three positive and/or negative aspects of how the achievement of these goals could affect the wellbeing of animals and nature?

Consider that:

- Animal wellbeing is conceptualized as the overall state of an animal's physical, mental and emotional health and its ability to experience positive welfare. It encompasses the animal's ability to thrive and adapt to its environment, avoid suffering and have positive experiences. Animal wellbeing is a multidimensional concept that considers various factors influencing an animal's quality of life.
- The concept of the wellbeing of nature refers to the overall health, functioning and resilience of ecosystems, biodiversity and natural habitats. It extends the idea of wellbeing beyond individual organisms to encompass the health and **sustainability** of the entire natural world. The wellbeing of nature is a holistic concept that emphasizes the interconnectedness and interdependence of all living organisms and their environment. From the 'One Health Joint Plan of Action' glossary (FAO *et al.*, 2022):
  - Health of the environment: The extent to which the environment is able to function, maintain biological and chemical processes, adapt to change or cope with the impacts of human activity.
  - Ecosystem health: The extent to which an ecosystem (or group of ecosystems) is able to function, maintain ecological and evolutionary processes, adapt to change and cope with the impacts of human activity.

This is not to be confused with **environmental health** – the branch of public health concerned with studying and regulating factors in the environment that affect human health and disease and those with alleviating detrimental effects; often attributive; (also) the general condition of the natural environment.

Example answer:

The goals included in the inner level are people-centred and include little to nothing on the health and wellbeing of animals and the environment. Nevertheless, the achievement of these inner-level goals could affect or are dependent on animal and/or environment health. For example, SDG1, to end poverty in all its forms, aims to fight against poor housing, lack of food and animal feed, unsafe water supplies and sanitation, and lack of human, animal and plant healthcare. The most marginalized rural populations are characteristically dependent on livestock and also carry the heaviest burden from diseases that infect both humans and animals (Queenan *et al.*, 2017). The eradication of **zoonotic diseases**, however, is addressed in Goal 3 (good health and wellbeing), although its success largely depends on the management of risk at the human–animal interface and the intact health of the ecosystems. Lastly, the expected economic growth compiled in SDG10 (reduced inequality) could have a negative effect on the environment, animal health and overall sustainability, unless they are based on green actions.

Following on SDG1, no poverty, as an example, three positive aspects of the achievement of this goal could be related to: (i) the protection of the natural habitats of wild animals, biodiversity and conservation of ecosystems by rising awareness on their wellbeing because impoverished societies were shown to rely on illegal activities such as poaching, logging for fuelwood, and abuse of land, air and water bodies for survival (Harper, 2023; Isibor *et al.*, 2023); (ii) the poverty was related to increased antimicrobial resistance (AMR) (Alvarez-Uria *et al.*, 2016) so the reduction of poverty would help to reduce AMR, leading to increased health and welfare of animals and ecosystems;

(iii) persons living in higher-income countries were more sensitized to animal health and wellbeing (Morris, 2013; Muñoz-Prieto *et al.*, 2018), thus, reducing/ eliminating poverty would lead to a more generalized awareness and sensitization.

> Education is the most powerful weapon which you can use to change the world.
>
> Nelson Mandela

Education is a central pillar of society: it provides opportunities and is a basis for development and progression at an individual and societal level. Furthermore, education is crucial for decent living and the creation of conflict-free cultures. Because of the importance education has, it is regulated by policies to preserve and equalize it for all (or at least this should be an aim in general). Therefore, SDG4 (quality education) promotes 'free, equitable and quality' gender-non-specific education at all levels (primary, secondary, tertiary, technical, etc.) around the world. In regard to sustainability, target 4.7 is explicitly intended to highlight the importance of the acquisition of knowledge and skills needed to promote sustainability in all sectors. In this sense, a WHO/UNICEF/Lancet commission called childhood the ideal time to intervene and thus accelerate progress in previously neglected areas, such as environmental issues (Clark *et al.*, 2020). Therefore, the incorporation of sustainability and One Health concepts in the curricula from very early ages could help promote critical thinking skills and understanding of linkages between human, animal and environmental health, among others.

Conflict, insecurity, weak institutions and limited access to justice remain a great threat to sustainable development because it depends on promoting peace, justice and strong institutions (SDG16). The targets 16.5, 16.6, 16.10 and 16.12 can contribute to promote the protection of animals (health and welfare) and the environment (e.g. rules against water, air and land pollution, biodiversity maintenance). Tracking these conditions is important for public policy; they represent well-established terrain for governments and are a key component of accountability (the social contract between the state and society) and state legitimation strategies. The institutional structures for delivering wellbeing goals stem from the historical role of states in providing health, education and welfare. Synergistic opportunities for implementation are associated with the alignment of goals that link education, health and gender equality. The intersectoral cooperation needed to achieve these synergies in wellbeing goals is challenging, but there are institutional forms to realize this (Waage *et al.*, 2015).

15.3 Middle Level: 'Infrastructure'

The principal function of the SDGs allocated in the 'Infrastructure' layer is to support and provide a platform for the 'Wellbeing' layer by addressing essential functions of modern societies (Waage *et al.*, 2015). These include food production, water availability and sanitation, access to energy and decent work while reducing the use of natural resources, improved waste management and promotion of sustainable industrialization (Table 15.2). Therefore, the achievement of the goals from the middle level would result in an improvement of human wellbeing, helping directly to attain the goals of the inner level, and vice versa, resulting in a close positive interaction between the two levels. For example, the achievement of SDG2 (Zero Hunger – End hunger, achieve food security and improved nutrition and promote sustainable agriculture) (Fig. 15.4) would help to tackle:

- **SDG1:** End poverty in all its forms everywhere through achievement of targets 2.1 and 2.2.
- **SDG5:** Achieve gender equality and empower all women and girls – mainly through fulfilment of target SDG 2.2 and 2.3.
- **SDG10:** Reduce income inequality within and among countries through achievement of targets 2.5, 2.6 and 2.7.
- **SDG16:** Promote peaceful and inclusive societies for sustainable development, provide access to justice for all and build effective, accountable and inclusive institutions at all levels – through achievement of targets 2.5, 2.6 and 2.7.

The **achievement of some targets could have contradictory effects on outer-level goals**, however. For example, if target 2.3 of SDG2 which seeks to 'double the agricultural productivity and incomes of small-scale

Table 15.2. SDGs belonging to middle 'Infrastructure' level.

Goal	Short description
2 Zero Hunger	**Aim:** To end hunger, achieve food security and improved nutrition and promote sustainable agriculture (https://www.un.org/development/desa/disabilities/envision2030-goal2.html). **Current situation:** Up to 462 million adults and 205 million children under 5 years suffer undernutrition, while an estimated 1.9 billion adults and 41 million children are overweight or obese worldwide. Furthermore, almost half of deaths among children under 5 years of age are linked to undernutrition (https://www.who.int/news-room/q-a-detail/malnutrition). These data indicate the urgency and importance of malnutrition in all its forms (undernutrition, overweight, obesity, inadequate minerals or vitamins) being addressed in this Agenda. **SDG2 to achieve the change:** Five out of seven targets of SDG2 aim to improve sustainable agriculture and overall food production systems by implementing 'resilient agricultural practices that increase productivity and production, that help maintain ecosystems, that strengthen capacity for adaptation to climate change' (Target 4). Passing sustainable food systems (from production to consumption), supporting small-scale producers and nutrition-sensitive healthcare, and adopting adequate policies, among other elements, were highlighted to be the main drivers to end hunger and elimination of all forms of malnutrition while respecting ecosystems and overcoming climate change-related devastating effects (https://unglobalcompact.org/take-action/action/sdg2).
6 Clean Water and Sanitation	**Aim:** To ensure the availability and sustainable management of water and sanitation for all (https://www.un.org/development/desa/disabilities/envision2030-goal6.html). **Current situation:** Water and sanitation are the very core of sustainable development, critical for the planet's survival. Despite the progress made, in 2017 only 71% of the global population used safely managed-to-drink water and just 45% used safely managed sanitation services, one in four healthcare facilities throughout the world lacked basic water services, and one in five had no sanitation services. Integrated management of water resources is needed, and the success of the programmes depend also on the stakeholder's engagement, including local communities. Nevertheless, countries face growing challenges linked to water scarcity, aquatic pollution, degraded water-related ecosystems, and cooperation over transboundary water basins. Holistic management of the water cycle means taking into account the level of 'water stress', which affects more than 2 billion people around the world. It is important to establish key interventions to improve water-use efficiency (e.g. industry and agriculture) (https://unstats.un.org/sdgs/report/2020/The-Sustainable-Development-Goals-Report-2020.pdf). **SDG6 to achieve the change:** Goal 6 addresses not only the issues relating to drinking water, sanitation and hygiene, but also the quality and sustainability of water resources worldwide.
7 Affordable and Clean Energy	**Aim:** To ensure access to affordable, reliable, sustainable and modern energy for all (https://www.un.org/development/desa/disabilities/envision2030-goal7.html). **Current situation:** Energy is crucial for achieving most of the SDGs, from its role in the eradication of poverty through advancements in health, education, water supply and industrialization, to combating climate change. The world is making good progress in increasing access to electricity and improving energy efficiency. However, millions of people throughout the world still lack such access, and progress in facilitating access to clean cooking fuels and technologies is too slow. Access to affordable and reliable energy is needed and urgent (e.g. hospitals and health facilities to treat patients, communities to pump clean water, access vital information and maintain the food supply chain). The share of renewable energy (derived from hydropower, solid and liquid biofuels, wind, the sun, biogas, geothermal and marine sources, and waste) in the world's total final energy consumption has increased slowly. Improving energy efficiency is crucial to reaching the global climate goal of reducing greenhouse gas emissions, but during the last few years the progress was slow and the improvements are below what is necessary to achieve the target (https://unstats.un.org/sdgs/report/2020/The-Sustainable-Development-Goals-Report-2020.pdf). **SDG7 to achieve the change:** First, SDG7 acknowledges the importance that everybody would have access 'to affordable, reliable and modern energy services' (Target 1) and highlights the necessity of international cooperation to advance in green-energy research, technology and accessibility, as well as improve energy efficiency.

Continued

Table 15.2. Continued.

Goal	Short description
8 Decent Work and Economic Growth	**Aim:** To promote inclusive and sustainable economic growth, full and productive employment and decent work for all (https://www.un.org/development/desa/disabilities/envision2030-goal8.html). **Current situation:** Sustained and inclusive economic growth is necessary for achieving sustainable development. During the past 10 years, the world witnessed rising labour productivity and improved unemployment rates, but after 2018 it started to decrease, with an adverse impact on the labour markets. After 2020, workers in informal employment, the self-employed, daily wage earners, and workers in sectors at the highest risk of disruption are the most negatively affected. This crisis poses a serious threat to the occupational safety and health of workers and may increase the risk of child labour. Although the number of children engaged in child labour has declined globally, more than half were engaged in hazardous forms of work. In 2019, 22% of the world's young people were not in employment, education or training, a figure that has hardly changed since 2005. While economic growth and employment are important for economic security, access to financial services is an essential component of inclusive growth. Financial exclusion disproportionately affected women and the poor (https://unstats.un.org/sdgs/report/2020/The-Sustainable-Development-Goals-Report-2020.pdf). **SDG8 to achieve the change:** This SDG, through its 12 targets, calls for the improvement of economic productivity and new development-oriented policies to assure decent work creation for all men and women, support of micro-, small and medium enterprises, and to eradicate forced labour among others. However, this SDG also included the most disputed target among the scientific community, namely, Target 1, which calls to 'Sustain per capita economic growth in accordance with national circumstances and, in particular, at least 7 per cent gross domestic product growth per annum in the least developed countries' because of being incompatible with sustainability (Shirin *et al.*, 2019; Kreinin and Aigner, 2022).
9 Industry, Innovation and Infrastructure	**Aim:** To build resilient infrastructure, promote inclusive and sustainable industrialization and foster innovation (https://www.un.org/development/desa/disabilities/envision2030-goal9.html). **Current situation:** Promoting inclusive and sustainable industries and continuing to invest in physical infrastructure, innovation and research are vital to long-term economic development. Investment in research and development (R&D) increased globally, as well as the financing for economic infrastructure in developing countries. But global manufacturing growth decelerated in 2018 and continued to decline due to tariffs and trade tensions between the world's most dominant economies. The slowdown affected all regions and country groups, with serious impacts on the global economy. The intensity of global CO_2 emissions has declined, by nearly one quarter since 2000, showing a general decoupling of CO_2 emissions from GDP growth. Impressive progress has been made in mobile connectivity. It is estimated that, in 2019, 96.5% of the global population thereof was covered by at least a 2G network, with 81.8% covered by at least a long-term evolution network. However, just 54% of the global population actually uses the internet. Most of the offline population live in the least developed countries, where only 19% use the internet, compared with 87% in developed countries. Key reasons for this large gap are the cost of using the internet and the lack of necessary skills (https://unstats.un.org/sdgs/report/2020/The-Sustainable-Development-Goals-Report-2020.pdf). **SDG9 to achieve the change:** Goal 9 encompasses three important aspects of sustainable development: infrastructure, industrialization and innovation.
11 Sustainable Cities and Communities	**Aim:** To make cities and human settlements inclusive, safe, resilient and sustainable (https://www.un.org/development/desa/disabilities/envision2030-goal11.html). **Current situation:** Globally, more than half of people (54% in 2014) live in urban areas with this trend being on the rise, and it is expected that the percentage of the population living in urban areas will reach 66% in 2050 (https://population.un.org/wup/Publications/Files/WUP2014-Highlights.pdf). These population movements result in the rapid expansion of cities and urbanization development, leading to high consumption of suburban green spaces, environmental degradation, increased air pollution, large volumes of solid waste, an increasing number of slum dwellers, insufficient or unaffordable basic services and infrastructure, among many other problems, which are bringing social tensions and challenges (Cai, 2020). **SDG11 to achieve the change:** SDG11 addresses these challenges by promoting the adoption of policies to provide access to safe, affordable and sustainable housing, basic services and transport systems. Special attention is put on air quality, waste management and green and public spaces planning, among others. Furthermore, using local materials for sustainable and resilient buildings is encouraged.

Continued

Table 15.2. Continued.

Goal	Short description
12 Responsible Consumption and Production	**Aim:** To ensure sustainable consumption and production patterns (https://www.un.org/development/desa/disabilities/envision2030-goal12.html). **Current situation:** Consumption and production drive the world economy, but they also damage environmental health through the unsustainable use of natural resources and increasing waste accumulation, resulting in pollution and greenhouse gas emissions (https://unstats.un.org/sdgs/report/2020/The-Sustainable-Development-Goals-Report-2020.pdf). Furthermore, a vast number of studies have shown the direct negative effect of pollution on human, animal and environmental health (Igbedioh, 1991; Almetwally *et al.*, 2020). **SDG12 to achieve the change:** SDG12 calls for sustainable consumption and production, sustainable use of natural resources, ubiquitous environmentally friendly types of waste management and overall waste reduction, and a decrease in fossil fuel subsidies, among others. In this sense, passing from a 'linear economy' (take, make and dispose of) to a 'circular economy' (prevent, reduce, recycle and reuse) has been proposed. Implementation of a circular economy would help to reduce the use of natural resources, material footprint (amount of primary materials required to meet basic needs) and waste generation.

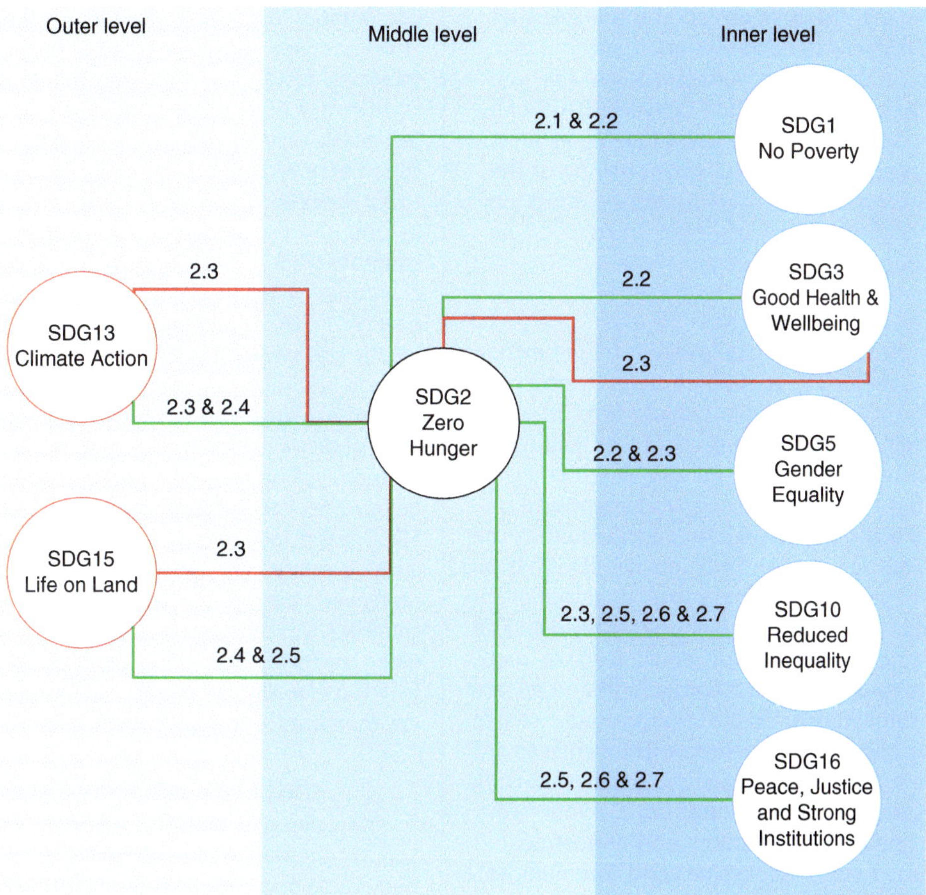

Fig. 15.4. Simplified relationship between SDG2 and other SDGs. Green line: positive effect; red line: negative effect; numbers above lines: most implicated SDG2 targets.

food producers (...)' is achieved, it could have a detrimental effect on terrestrial and sweet water ecosystems and the climate (SDG13, SDG15), leading to zoonosis overflow by interfering with target 3.3 (end zoonotic diseases, among others). Overall, although SDG2 is a people-centred goal, it also envisions the importance of reshaping the current model of agriculture and overall food system to more sustainable and climate-compatible practices. By this, although indirectly, the importance of environment health is addressed. Nevertheless, this goal could be further improved regarding One Health by also addressing animal health. Special focus should be placed on farm animals[2] because they constitute a big part of food systems, thus, their health and welfare should be assured.

Learning questions: Based on the example above of SDG2, analyse and assess the relationship and the role that SDG6 (clean water and sanitation) plays in relation to other SDGs at different levels. Can you identify a positive relation between SDG6 and other SDGs? If so, which SDG6 targets are most implicated? Could the fulfilment of any of the SDG6 targets have a contradictory effect on other SDG achievements? How could SDG6 be improved?

Although the middle layer's main function seems to be to support and provide a platform for 'Wellbeing', the achievement of some goals from the middle level could also lead to the improvement not only of human health and wellbeing but also that of the environment and animals (the three main sectors represented in the One Health approach). For example, SDG12 is almost entirely focused on a sustainable way of living and the ways it could be achieved. The achievement of this goal would lead to great benefits to all – environment, human and animal health through reduced pollution, natural resource wasting and waste generation. The achievement of others, however, especially SDG8 (decent work and economic growth) and, on a minor scale, SDG9 (industry, innovation and infrastructure) and SDG11 (sustainable cities and communities), would not be compatible with or are even antagonistic to health spreading beyond the human being (Hickel, 2019).

SDG8 calls for decent work and economic growth, assuming that economic growth is necessary for the eradication of poverty and human development. According to existing data and empirical models, however, the 7 % economic growth per capita (target 8.1) and achievement of 'higher levels of economic productivity' (target 8.2) together with target 9.2, which indicates that this growth should be primarily industrial, are opposed to the majority of the sustainability objectives. This is due to the fact that even economic growth at 3 % makes it impossible to reduce the use of natural resources and carbon emissions enough to stay within the 2°C warming limits (Hickel, 2019). Therefore, the achievement of SDG8 would not be feasible, in particular with the reduction of natural resources use (contemplated in SDG12, responsible consumption and production) and greenhouse gas emissions (key target of SDG13, climate action), thus also failing to reach One Health objectives. Furthermore, the primary rationale for including 'economic growth' within the agenda – the eradication of poverty and human development – seems to not have enough weight as to overcome sustainability and is not justifiable unless in very low-income countries (Hickel, 2019; Carr, 2021). This is because a number of other goals, such as SDG1 (ending poverty), SDG2 (ending hunger), SDG3 (good health and wellbeing) and SDG4 (education), are directly committed to achieving these objectives. Moreover, Carr (2021) claims that poverty should not just be measured by access to materials as well as money, but also by people's subjective wellbeing. The modification or even elimination of SDG8 (especially target 8.1) was proposed to generate a more resilient economy (Hickel, 2019). Moreover, 'sustainable de-growth' in high-income countries was suggested as a possible solution to meet sustainability goals leading to improved health and wellbeing of all – humans, animals and environment (Schneider *et al.*, 2010; Hickel, 2019).

SDG11 is specific for sustainable urban development. It is primarily focused on human wellbeing and the creation of equitable and socially inclusive cities. However, environmental sustainability is also addressed to guide policy makers and planners (https://

unstats.un.org/sdgs/metadata). Nevertheless, any new constructions leading to the interruption of suburban spaces and expansion of cities could have a devastating effect on the surrounding environment and wild animal wellbeing and even survival. Some studies point out that rapid urban land growth exceeds by more than three times the growth of the urban population (Horn and Grugel, 2018). This rapid urbanization, besides leading to encroachment and alteration of natural ecosystems, also increases pollution. Therefore, ideally, the existing urban areas should be transformed into more resilient cities, while new buildings and encroachment on green spaces (within and outside the city) should be avoided to meet the overall sustainability objectives and align with the One Health approach. SDG11 is very closely related to SDG7 (affordable and clean energy), which focuses exclusively on the material domain (physical infrastructure) of the current socio-technological energy system but remains mainly silent on the social (user practices and meanings, lifestyles, business models, markets, power, etc.) aspect (Menton *et al.*, 2020). The call for green energy could, however, reduce the use of natural resources, allowing conservation of natural ecosystems. Ideally, the technology for the production of green energy, e.g. solar panels, would have to be incorporated locally where this energy is used (individual houses, etc.), instead of building solar panel fields. These panel fields, although helpful to reduce the use of fossil fuel, disrupt ecosystems and would mainly contribute to increasing profits of large companies instead of the individual final users, contributing to deepening inequality (Hu, 2023). The expenses for the acquisition of these technologies are, however, usually very high and many people cannot afford them. Therefore, governments have the main role to promote aids via new policy adoption to make these changes feasible.

In this sense, Sovacool (2021), after reviewing 20 years of geography and political ecology literature on the energy justice implications of climate change mitigation, calls for reflection in his final article lines:

> As climate mitigation actions become more integral in future resource planning discussions, attract more investment, and become more instrumental to economies, we must collectively ensure its rise in prominence is not accompanied by an inexcusable tragedy of equally compelling problems.

Learning questions: Think about the solar panel fields [or wind farms]:

- Identify positive and negative effects on the health and wellbeing of humans, animals, biodiversity and ecosystems.
- Identify implicated/affected sectors and the multiple connections among them.
- Identify implicated SDGs.
- Reflect on how passing from solar panel fields [or wind farms] to the *in-situ* generation of green energy would affect the health and wellbeing of humans, animals and nature.
- Could you suggest any alternative?
- How is this topic addressed in the place/region/country where you live? Have you noticed any changes in the society's approach to solar panel fields in recent years?

Example answer: Fuente Librilla is a small village in the south-east of Spain. For years, it was surrounded by agricultural plantations of trees of great tradition and importance in the Mediterranean area, such as olive and almond trees. In addition, some citizens owned small extensive farms of goats and sheep. In 2019, a huge solar panel field was built in the nearby lands by the promoters and executors of the private international company and the local policy makers. In addition, the landowners contributed by renting their lands. The trees and small farms were replaced by the grey metal structures (Fig. 15.5). The energy produced in this field travels kilometres through cables hooked on newly installed electricity towers without contributing to the use of this green energy by the citizens of the nearby villages. The village lost its charm and nice landscape. Furthermore, the possible long-term consequences on the health of the people, animals, biodiversity and ecosystems are still unknown. It is clear, however, that the elimination of trees that grow and provide food have contributed to the desertification of the area, further impacting life in the area.

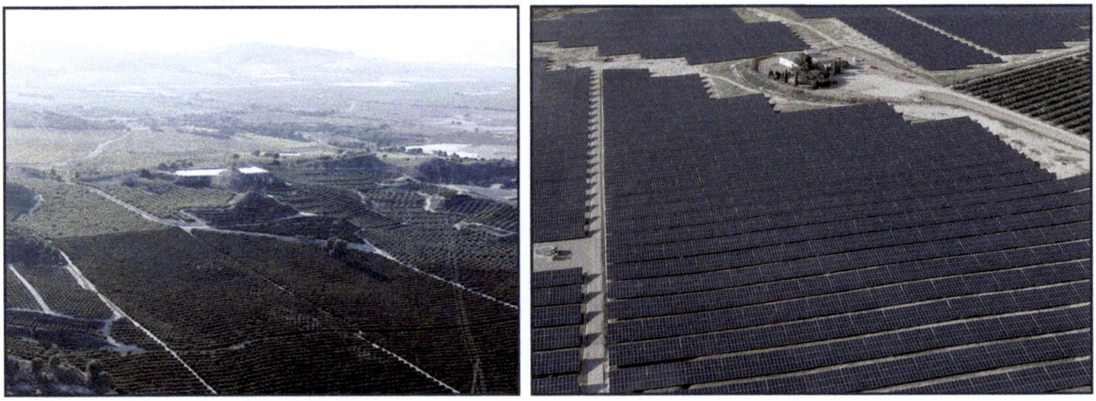

Fig. 15.5. Photo of the Mula Photovoltaic Power Plant in Murcia, Spain (right) that replaced fields of almond and olive trees (left) by solar panels, disrupting ecosystems and contributing to visual pollution. Photos courtesy of Maria Ceron Madrigal.

Similar problems were detected in other parts of Spain and, in 2023, protests against wind farms have been organized claiming that 'renewable energy yes, but not in this way' (in Spanish, '*Energía renovable si, pero no así*'). As a possible alternative to the panel fields, a pilot study was initiated in 2023 in Germany. In it, a roof was assembled made of photovoltaic modules fixed to a steel structure that rises 5.5 m above the asphalt of the highway. If successful, the solar panels could be installed along kilometres of existing highways and roads, without the need to break into new green spaces and thus preserve nature. In addition, it will provide shade to vehicles.

15.4 Outer Level: 'Natural Environment'

The outer level of the framework proposed by Waage *et al.* (2015) includes three goals (SDGs 13, 14 and 15) that encompass objectives related to global resources management including land, sea, air and biodiversity (Table 15.3). The three goals are closely and inseparably interconnected and link to the goals belonging to the 'Wellbeing' and 'Infrastructure' levels (Fig. 15.6).

SDG13 (Climate Action) stresses the need to take immediate action to curb climate change. The global average surface air temperature increased by 0.85°C between 1880 and 2012, while the rate of increase has been much higher since 1971 (~0.2°C/decade). For decades, protection actions against climate change have been oriented toward human health (Wheeler and Watts, 2018). However, as seen in Fig. 15.6, global warming is a central gear between the results of anthropogenic activities and the cause of decreased health and wellbeing of all – humans, animals and the environment. Importantly, while human wellbeing is highly protected by SDGs forming inner (six goals) and intermediate (seven goals) levels, only two (SDG14, Life Below Water, and SDG15, Life on Land) seek to protect the aquatic and terrestrial environments and promote animal and plant biodiversity. Preserving species and conserving biodiversity has value not only for the natural ecosystem but also for human health and wellbeing (Nielsen *et al.*, 2021). This constitutes the cornerstone for the sustainability of the ecosystem. Therefore, SDGs should be further improved to give importance and equal recognition to animals and the environment as it gives to humans.

The Intergovernmental Panel on Climate Change (IPCC) pointed out that population and economic growth are the primary drivers of growing climate-altering emissions (IPCC, 2014). In this sense, the three outer-level SDGs call for the adoption of policies essential for mitigating climate change, pollution of all kinds and protection of ecosystems. For instance, economic investment in sustainable agriculture and environmental sanitation can help meet the goal of alleviating hunger without decisively affecting climate change (Zinsstag *et al.*, 2018; Sulser *et al.*, 2021). Furthermore, improving sexual education could help to balance population

Table 15.3. SDGs belonging to outer 'Natural environment' level.

Goal	Short description
13 Climate Action	**Aim**: To take urgent action to combat climate change and its impacts (https://www.un.org/development/desa/disabilities/envision2030-goal13.html). **Current situation**: Global warming and its related climate disasters across the continents – wildfires, hurricanes, floods, etc. – continue to worsen while the global community shuns engagement. The global temperature is expected to rise by up to 3.2°C by the end of the century, while ocean acidity has increased by 26% since pre-industrial times and is expected to rapidly increase by 100–150% in the next century owing to carbon dioxide emissions. **SDG13 to achieve the change:** SDG13 encourages the adoption or modification of national policies, strategies and planning to strengthen resilience and adaptive capacity to climate-related hazards and natural disasters in all countries, improving education, awareness and mitigation of climate change.
14 Life Below Water	**Aim:** To conserve and sustainably use the oceans, seas and marine resources for sustainable development (https://www.un.org/development/desa/disabilities/envision2030-goal14.html). **Current situation:** Oceans impact people's lives on several levels. They are indispensable for the sustainability of populations and commerce since over 3 billion people depend on marine and coastal resources. The over-pollution of marine environments as a result of the incorrect disposal of waste (it is estimated that 4.8 to 12.7 million metric tons of plastic waste enter the oceans from coastal countries per year), as well as the extensive use of the oceans for transportation, are degenerating the marine natural environments. **SDG14 to achieve the change:** This goal promotes the protection of the oceans, marine and coastal ecosystems through more effective regulation of fisheries, aquaculture and tourism among others by adopting appropriate scientific information-based legal frameworks that would guarantee its execution.
15 Life on Land	**Aim:** To protect, restore and promote sustainable use of terrestrial ecosystems, sustainably manage forests, combat desertification, and halt and reverse land degradation and halt biodiversity loss (https://www.un.org/development/desa/disabilities/envision2030-goal15.html). **Current situation:** The forested areas are diminished every year due to the adaptation of the land to settlements, agriculture, mining and infrastructures (road, railway, etc.). As a result, life on land is extensively modified to facilitate human-made activities that might provide short-term benefits, while posing long-term threats to biodiversity. The endangered species are increasing every year owing to the loss of natural habitat, poaching and the presence of invasive species. **SDG15 to achieve the change:** This SDG aims to preserve biodiversity and sustainability through economic reinforcement that allows forest conservation and avoids desertification. With the intention of maintaining the biodiversity of the species, the Nagoya protocol was ratified among 123 countries and the European Union to guarantee access to genetic resources and the dissemination of information from the Convention on Biological Diversity and the United Nations launched a Decade on Ecosystem Restoration (2021–2030) (https://www.decadeonrestoration.org/) to pursue this objective.

growth (United Nations Population Fund, 2020; Dodson *et al*., 2020). However, these policies should be adopted not just nationally; international co-operation is essential to reduce climate change and preserve our ecosystems. Chapter 7 provides further insight into ecosystems, biodiversity and their conservation. It presents a great difficulty owing to the need for high interoperability between different countries. Therefore, different actions, such as the Paris Agreement, adopted in 2015, were taken to encourage international collaboration to fight global warming and other major environment-related issues. In this way, the application of SDG17 ('Partnerships for the Goals') is considered essential for optimal inclusion of the different stakeholders in achieving the common goals.

15.5 Sustainable Development Goal 17

Goal SDG17 is considered as a cornerstone of the SDGs and of One Health (Queenan *et al.*, 2017; Kock *et al.*, 2018). It seeks to 'strengthen the means of implementation and revitalize the global partnership for

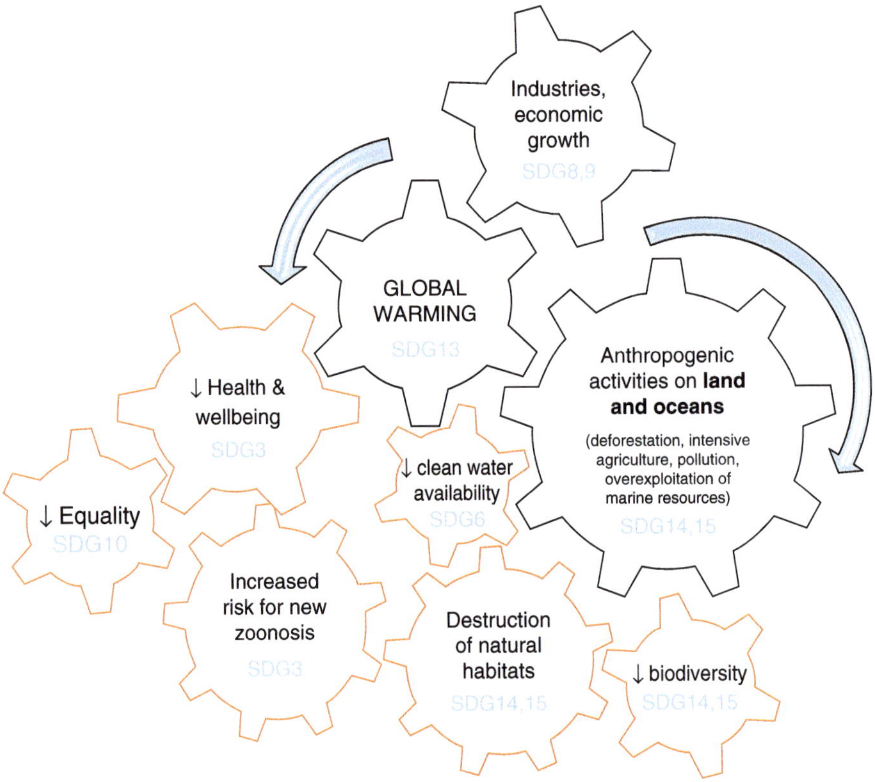

Fig. 15.6. A schematic representation of negative consequences related to economic growth (grey gears) resulting in negative effects on different sustainability targets (orange gears). Involved SDGs are also included.

sustainable development' (https://www.un.org/development/desa/disabilities/envision2030-goal17.html). To ensure the success of the different SDGs, productive international cooperation between all stakeholders is necessary. This cooperation is especially important in the context of the pandemic-induced recessions. While developed economies were able to roll out large fiscal stimulus packages to support their recoveries, many developing countries were faced with protracted scarring to potential output, amid larger cumulative investment and output losses (World Bank, 2021). In general, donor countries have been failing to achieve the objective of increasing funding to be destined for developing countries. This has brought many difficulties in the implementation and execution of the SDGs. Thus, to achieve the objective, SDG17 establishes a joint action at several levels, namely: 'financial, technological, capacity building, trade, systemic issues, multistakeholder partnership, and data, monitoring and accountability' (https://sdgs.un.org/goals/goal17). Only a close collaboration of governments, civil society, scientists, academia and the private sector constitutes the framework to rebuild better and succeed in the change. Therefore, a fully integrated approach including both policy and daily practice has to be implemented to ensure the health and wellbeing of humans, animals and the environment (Zinsstag *et al.*, 2011; Gostin and Friedman, 2015; Kock *et al.*, 2018). Overall, SDG17 summarized the need for a global partnership to achieve the goals and is also a fundamental pillar for One Health.

15.6 Conclusions

Key issue: Although most SDGs are focused on a human-centred strategy and some may be considered negative to One Health, in general, the achievement of these goals can trigger the recognition of the existence of the connection between the health of people, animals and the environment, potentially resulting in better health and wellbeing of all if the trade-offs can be managed successfully.

- The SDGs provide a unique opportunity to move towards a more integrated approach as encouraged by One Health.
- It is crucial to recognize that humans are only one component of the ecosystem, on which they depend and which they must support rather than undermine.
- Education is the basis for development and progress in all aspects, having a key role in successfully achieving the 2030 Agenda Goals and One Health.
- Achievements of some SDGs (8, 9, 11) could have a detrimental effect on animal and environment health unless they are approached carefully, taking these aspects into account.
- The climate crisis must be addressed urgently to mitigate the negative effects it already produces on the health of humans, animals and the environment.
- SDG17 emphasizes the need for global collaboration to reach the objectives of the 2030 Sustainable Agenda. As stated by One Health, this collaboration is crucial to preserve health and wellbeing and has to be performed for all (institutional, industry and personal) from international to local levels.

Notes

[1] As an example, most human medical doctors have extra expertise in one or another area and, therefore, they are considered specialists, e.g. cardiologist, endocrinologist or gynaecologist. A super-specialist, however, is considered to be a medical doctor who has special training in and knowledge of a very particular area of medicine, e.g. a specific disorder.

[2] The importance of focusing on livestock is also due to its extent and thus the effect it has on the ecology: the biomass of livestock (~0.1 Gt C, dominated by cattle and pigs) surpasses that of wild mammals (~0.007 Gt C). Similarly, the biomass of domesticated poultry (~0.005 Gt C, dominated by chickens) is about threefold higher than that of wild birds (~0.002 Gt C) (Bar-Ona *et al.*, 2018).

References

Adams, V. (ed.) (2016) *Metrics: What Counts in Global Health.* Duke University Press, Durham, North Carolina. DOI: 10.2307/j.ctv1168c3w.

Almetwally, A.A., Bin-Jumah, M. and Allam, A.A. (2020) Ambient air pollution and its influence on human health and welfare: An overview. *Environmental Science and Pollution Research* 27, 24815–24830. DOI: 10.1007/s11356-020-09042-2.

Alvarez-Uria, G., Gandra, S. and Laxminarayan, R. (2016) Poverty and prevalence of antimicrobial resistance in invasive isolates. *International Journal of Infectious Diseases* 52, 59–61. DOI: 10.1016/j.ijid.2016.09.026.

Bar-Ona, Y.M., Phillips, R. and Milo, R. (2018) The biomass distribution on Earth. *Proceedings of the National Academy of Sciences of the United States of America* 115(25), 6506–6511. DOI: 10.1073/pnas.1711842115.

Benjamin, D.J., Cooper, K.B., Hefetz, O. and Kimball, M.S. (2019) Self-reported wellbeing indicators are a valuable complement to traditional economic indicators but aren't yet ready to compete with them. *Behavioural Public Policy.* DOI: 10.2139/ssrn.3463478.

Cai, Y. (2020) Opportunities for all: Inclusive and equitable sustainable development. In: Leal Filho, W., Marisa Azul, A., Brandli, L., Gökçin Özuyar, P. and Wall, T. (eds) *Sustainable Cities and Communities: Encyclopedia of the UN Sustainable Development Goals.* Springer, Cham.

Carr, S.C. (2021) Setting 'poverty thresholds': Whose experience counts? *Sustainability Science* 16, 31–36. DOI: 10.1007/s11625-020-00859-x.

Clark, H., Coll-Seck, A.M., Banerjee, A., Peterson, S., Dalglish, S.L. *et al.* (2020) A future for the world's children? A WHO-UNICEF-Lancet commission. *Lancet* 395(10224), 605–658. DOI: 10.1016/S0140-6736(19)32540-1.

De Neve, J.-E. and Sachs, J.D. (2020a) Sustainable Development and Human Well-Being. World Happiness Report, 2020.

De Neve, J.-E. and Sachs, J.D. (2020b) The SDGs and human well-being: A global analysis of synergies, trade-offs, and regional differences. *Nature Scientific Reports.* DOI: 10.1038/s41598-020-71916-9.

Dodson, J.C., Dérer, P., Cafaro, P. and Götmark, F. (2020) Population growth and climate change: Addressing the overlooked threat multiplier. *Science of the Total Environment* 748, 141346. DOI: 10.1016/j.scitotenv.2020.141346.

FAO, UNEP, WHO and WOAH (2022) One Health Joint Plan of Action (2022–2026). Working Together for the Health of Humans, Animals, Plants and the Environment. Rome. DOI: 10.4060/cc2289en.

Gostin, L.O. and Friedman, E.A. (2015) The sustainable development goals One-Health in the world's development agenda. *JAMA* 314(24), 2621–2622. DOI:10.1001/jama.2015.16281.

Harper, C.K. (2023) Poaching forensics: Animal victims in the courtroom. *Annual Review of Animal Biosciences* 11, 269–286. DOI:10.1146/annurev-animal-070722-084803.

Hickel, J. (2019) The contradiction of the sustainable development goals: Growth versus ecology on a finite planet. *Sustainable Development* 27(5), 873–884.

Hone, T., Rasella, D., Barreto, M.L., Majeed, A. and Millett, C. (2017) Association between expansion of primary healthcare and racial inequalities in mortality amenable to primary care in Brazil: A national longitudinal analysis.

PLoS Medicine 14(5), e1002306. DOI: 10.1371/journal.pmed.1002306.

Horn, P. and Grugel, J. (2018) The SDGs in middle-income countries: Setting or serving domestic development agendas? Evidence from Ecuador. *World Development* 109, 73–84. DOI: 10.1016/j.worlddev.2018.04.005.

Hu, Z. (2023) Towards solar extractivism? A political ecology understanding of the solar energy and agriculture boom in rural China. *Energy Research and Social Science* 98, 102988. DOI: 10.1016/j.erss.2023.102988.

Igbedioh, S.O. (1991) Effects of agricultural pesticides on humans, animals, and higher plants in developing countries. *Archives of Environmental Health: An International Journal* 46(4), 218–224. DOI: 10.1080/00039896.1991.9937452.

IPCC (2014) Climate Change 2014: Mitigation of Climate Change. Contribution of Working Group III to the Fifth Assessment Report of the Intergovernmental Panel on Climate Change. Cambridge. DOI: 10.1017/CBO9781107415416.

Isibor, P.O., Onwaeze, O.O., Kayode-Edwards, I.I., Agbontaen, D.O., Ifebem-Ezima, I.M. *et al.* (2023) Investigating and combatting the key drivers of viral zoonoses in Africa: An analysis of eight epidemics. *Brazilian Journal of Biology* 84, e270857. DOI: 10.1590/1519-6984.270857.

Jaiswal, B.K. (2018) E-Commerce of Handicraft. Bachelor's Thesis. Available at: https://www.researchgate.net/publication/331742924_E-commerce_of_Handicraft_Degree_Programme_in_Logistics_Engineering_E-commerce_of_Handicraft_Case_South_Asian_Handicraft/figures?lo=1 (accessed 9 August 2024).

Kalra, S.P., Anand, A.C. and Shah, B.N. (2003) The relevance of general medicine today: Role of super-specialists vis-à-vis internists. *Journal Indian Academy of Clinical Medicine* 4(1), 14–17.

Kock, R., Queenan, K., Garnier, J., Rosenbaum Nielsen, L., Buttigieg, S. *et al.* (2018) Chapter 2 Health solutions: Theoretical foundations of the shift from sectoral to integrated systems. In: Rüegg, S.R., Häsler, B. and Zinsstag, J. (eds) *Integrated Approaches to Health: A Handbook for the Evaluation of One Health.* Wageningen Academic Publishers, pp. 22–37.

Kreinin, H. and Aigner, E. (2022) From 'Decent work and economic growth' to 'Sustainable work and economic degrowth': A new framework for SDG 8. *Empirica* 49, 281–311. DOI: 10.1007/s10663-021-09526-5.

Loefler, I.J.P. and Turnberg, L. (2000) Are generalists still needed in a specialised world? *British Medical Journal* 320, 436–440.

Menton, M., Larrea, C., Latorre, S., Martinze-Alier, J., Peck, M. *et al.* (2020) Environmental justice and the SDGs: From synergies to gaps and contradictions. *Sustainability Science* 15, 1621–1636. DOI: 10.1007/s11625-020-00789-8.

Meurs, M., Seidelmann, L. and Koutsoumpa, M. (2019) How healthy is a 'healthy economy'? Incompatibility between current pathways towards SDG3 and SDG8. *Global Health* 15, 83. DOI: 10.1186/s12992-019-0532-4.

Morris, M.C. (2013) Improved nonhuman animal welfare is related more to income equality than it is to income. *Journal of Applied Animal Welfare Science.* 16(3), 272–293. DOI: 10.1080/10888705.2013.768921.

Muñoz-Prieto, A., Nielsen, L.R., Dąbrowski, R., Bjørnvad, C.R., Söder, J. *et al.* (2018) European dog owner perceptions of obesity and factors associated with human and canine obesity. *Scientific Reports* 8(1), 13353. DOI: 10.1038/s41598-018-31532-0.

Nielsen, K.S., Marteau, T.M., Bauer, J.M., Bradbury, R.B., Broad, S. *et al.* (2021) Biodiversity conservation as a promising frontier for behavioural science. *Nature Human Behaviour* 5, 550–556. DOI: 10.1038/s41562-021-01109-5.

Peter, R.F., Reed, M.C., Kemper, P. and Blumenthal, D. (1999) Changes in the scope of care provided by primary care physicians. *The New England Journal of Medicine* 341, 1980–1985.

Queenan, K., Garnier, J., Nielsen, L.R., Buttigieg, S., Meneghi, D.D. *et al.* (2017) Roadmap to a One Health agenda 2030. *CABI Reviews* 12, 14.

Rockström, J. and Sukhdev, P. (2017) Stockholm Resilience Centre's (SRC) Contribution to the 2016 Swedish 2030 Agenda HLPF report. Stockholm. Available at: https://www.stockholmresilience.org/download/18.2561f5bf15a1a341a523695/1488272270868/SRCs%202016%20Swedish%202030%20Agenda%20HLPF%20report%20Final.pdf (accessed 9 August 2024).

Schneider, F., Kallis, G. and Martinez-Alier, J. (2010) Crisis or opportunity? Economic degrowth for social equity and ecological sustainability. Introduction to this special issue. *Journal of Cleaner Production* 18(6), 511–518. DOI: 10.1016/j.jclepro.2010.01.014.

Shirin, M.R., Benjamin, D.B. and Kanchana, N.R. (2019) SDG 8: Decent work and economic growth – A gendered analysis. *World Development* 113, 368–380. DOI: 10.1016/j.worlddev.2018.09.006.

Sovacool, B.K. (2021) Who are the victims of low-carbon transitions? Towards a political ecology of climate change mitigation. *Energy Research and Social Science* 73, 101916. DOI: 10.1016/j.erss.2021.101916.

Sulser, T., Wiebe, K.D., Dunston, S., Cenacchi, N., Nin-Pratt, A. *et al.* (2021) Climate Change and Hunger: Estimating Costs of Adaptation in the Agrifood System. Food policy reports 9780896294165, International Food Policy Research Institute (IFPRI).

Tangcharoensathien, V., Mills, A. and Palu, P. (2015) Accelerating health equity: The key role of universal health coverage in the sustainable development goals. *BMC Medicine* 13, 101. DOI: 10.1186/s12916-015-0342-3.

United Nations Population Fund (2020) Comprehensive Sexuality Education. Available at: https://www.unfpa.org/comprehensive-sexuality-education (accessed 22 October 2022).

Waage, J., Yap, C., Bell, S., Levy, C., Mace, G. *et al.* (2015) Governing sustainable development goals: Interactions, infrastructures, and institutions. In: Waage, J. and Yap, C. (eds) *Thinking beyond Sectors for Sustainable Development*. Ubiquity Press, London, UK.

Weisz, G. (2003) The Emergence of Medical Specialization in the Nineteenth Century. *Bulletin of the History of Medicine* 77(3), 536–575.

Wheeler, N. and Watts, N. (2018) Climate change: From science to practice. *Current Environmental Health Reports* 5, 170–178. DOI: 10.1007/s40572-018-0187-y.

World Bank (2021) Global Economic Prospects, 2021. Available at: https://www.worldbank.org/en/news/press-release/2021/06/08/world-bank-global-economic-prospects-2021 (accessed 9 August 2024).

Zinsstag, J., Crump, L., Schelling, E., Hattendorf, J., Maidane, Y.O. *et al.* (2018) Climate change and One Health. *FEMS Microbiology Letters* 365(11), fny085. DOI: 10.1093/femsle/fny085.

Zinsstag, J., Schelling, E., Waltner-Toews, D. and Tanner, M. (2011) From 'One Medicine' to 'One Health' and systemic approaches to health and well-being. *Preventive Veterinary Medicine* 101, 148–156.

16 Bringing 'One Health' Home

Deborah J. Thomson[1,2]

[1]One Health Lessons, Arlington, Virginia, USA; [2]Network for Ecohealth and One Health (NEOH)

Contents

DOI: 10.1079/9781800623002.0017

Chapter Overview

Elevator pitch

Knowledge of One Health is good but application of One Health is better. This chapter applies knowledge learned in previous chapters through several activities that simulate realistic situations. You are challenged to apply your new knowledge in different ways and with different novice audiences throughout the chapter and then to apply your knowledge in your community.

Book objectives the chapter relates to

☐ 1. Understand what One Health and Ecohealth mean
☑ 2. Think in a One Health and Ecohealth way
☑ 3. Apply One Health and Ecohealth in their professional and personal life
☑ 4. Know how to share One Health and Ecohealth knowledge
☑ 5. Integrate One Health and Ecohealth knowledge actively
☑ 6. Acquire or enhance core One Health competencies

Main One Health competencies covered

☑ 1. Effective communication
☐ 2. Collaborative and resilient working
☐ 3. Systems understanding
☐ 4. Transdisciplinarity
☑ 5. Social, cultural and gender equity and inclusiveness
☑ 6. Collective learning and reflective practice
☑ 7. One Health concepts
☐ 8. Theoretical and methodological pluralism
☐ 9. Harnessing uncertainty, paradox and limited knowledge

Learning outcomes

Be able to:

1. Explain One Health in under 15 seconds.
2. Navigate provocative conversations in relation to One Health.
3. Apply knowledge from other chapters to real-life situations.
4. Effectively and strategically use infographics to demonstrate One Health.
5. Converse with novice audiences about One Health.

Summary

This chapter challenges you to apply your One Health knowledge to real-world scenarios. It focuses on methods and techniques needed to communicate with audiences that are new to the idea and terminology of One Health. It teaches you effective communication skills through sharing true stories and working on practical activities that have been designed to improve your word choice, your messaging strategy, and stretch your creativity to overcome unexpected obstacles. After finishing this chapter, you should be better equipped to communicate with new audiences today about One Health.

16.1 Introduction

This chapter is written in a tone different from all other chapters. This was done on purpose. You will be reading short sentences. You will be reading direct sentences. Some sentences may even be light-hearted. Sometimes there are stories written in the first person. But they are constructed to clearly deliver the message of how to introduce One Health topics into a variety of communities.

After engaging with the content of this textbook, you have expanded your vocabulary. **Did you notice?** Perhaps at the start of your readings you did but, over time, you became accustomed to encountering new words. Perhaps you have even started using them in everyday speech – that is, while you speak with colleagues and classmates!

Like it or not, you may sound somewhat foreign to your neighbours back home when you use words like 'stakeholders' and 'One Health'. Or worse, you may be misinterpreted when using these terms. After all, when somebody hears '**stakeholders**' for the first time, they may envision somebody holding onto a stake in the ground or somebody holding a piece of beef steak (Fig. 16.1).

Now, can you only imagine what they would think of hearing 'One Health'? Some may think it's the name of a health insurance company or something else similarly far off!

In this chapter, you will be challenged to detangle definitions and interpret, and then translate, excerpts of dense One Health text. In addition, you will learn from real-life examples of successful implementation and delivery of the One Health message to stimulate community engagement and buy-in. This chapter may remind you of having growing pains as an adolescent. It may hurt but it will bring you to the next level. After all, you now have substantial knowledge that needs to be shared with others who are new to hearing the words 'One Health'. In order to make a lasting impact at the community level, **you** need to be relatable and your message needs to be relatable but you first need to understand your audience (Thomson, 2021). As described in *The Art of Science Communication: Sharing Knowledge with Students, the Public, and Policymakers*, the first action of a good communicator is to actively listen. Listen with your ears. Listen with your eyes. Listen without an agenda. When speaking with a new group, find the answers to: What are their backgrounds? What are their priorities? Why are they here speaking with you? Who is the thought leader in the group? Who inspires action in the group? What are the dynamics and relationships within the group? Do not rush this step. It is crucial to understand and appreciate each other's backgrounds, strengths and priorities. You should then share your story. You can reflect on points mentioned previously and be sure to include phrases that build a relationship like 'similar to you, I also have brothers' or 'your story made me smile because I also met a person just like that'. After building trust, the next step is to ensure your audience: (i) cares about One Health (especially if they did not previously care about it); then (ii) takes action to protect their community's health and wellbeing;

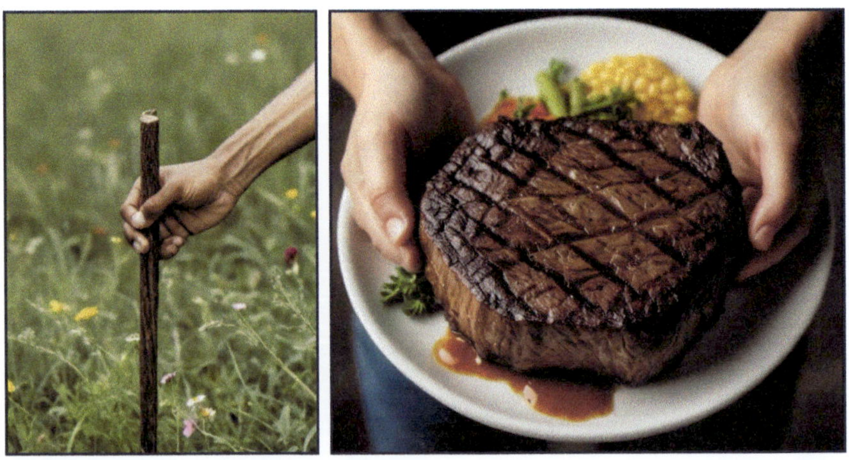

Fig. 16.1. Artificial Intelligence-generated images from Freepik.com demonstrating two possible misinterpretations when people first hear the word 'stakeholder'. Personal collection of the author.

and (iii) maintains an open mind that encourages respectful dialogue and knowledge exchange (Thomson, 2021; Searight and Sheehan, 2023) (Fig. 16.2).

16.2 Breaking Down the Definition of 'One Health'

Can you explain One Health in 15 seconds or less? This challenge is important because you must immediately capture the attention and interest of anybody who is new to hearing about 'One Health'. Attention spans are short. You need to beat the clock. If you can already explain One Health in 15 seconds or less, please skip to the next section entitled 'Word Choice Matters'. If not, please read on.

This challenging question of concisely defining One Health arose during a conference when I was having a one-on-one conversation with a highly esteemed professional in his field. I had explained that I was starting a new position in the United States Congress and I was hoping to work on One Health legislation. (For more information about One Health **policy** and **governance**, please see Chapter 14.) He said that my wish would be impossible because One Health is too complicated a topic to harness in policy. I said that it is worth trying and his immediate response was: 'Oh yeah? Can you explain One Health in 15 seconds? To that, I responded that it is possible. He took off his wristwatch and put it on the table sitting between us and then he said 'go'.

I stated that 'One Health can be explained as both a concept and an approach. The One Health concept is the **interconnection** between public health and the health of the environment, animals, and plants.' I then explained these sentences are the opener to use to start the conversation. It is not worth sharing the 'One Health approach' definition (explained later) if the 'One Health concept' is not initially understood.

The United Nations' Quadripartite (FAO *et al.*, 2022) welcomed the following definition of One Health from the One Health High-Level Expert Panel (OHHLEP *et al.*, 2022):

> One Health is an integrated, unifying approach that aims to sustainably balance and optimize the health of people, animals, and ecosystems. It recognizes the health of humans, domestic and wild animals, plants, and the wider environment (including ecosystems) are closely linked and interdependent.
>
> The approach mobilizes multiple sectors, disciplines, and communities at varying levels of society to work together to foster well-being and tackle threats to health and ecosystems, while addressing the collective need for healthy food, water, energy, and air, taking action on climate change and contributing to sustainable development.

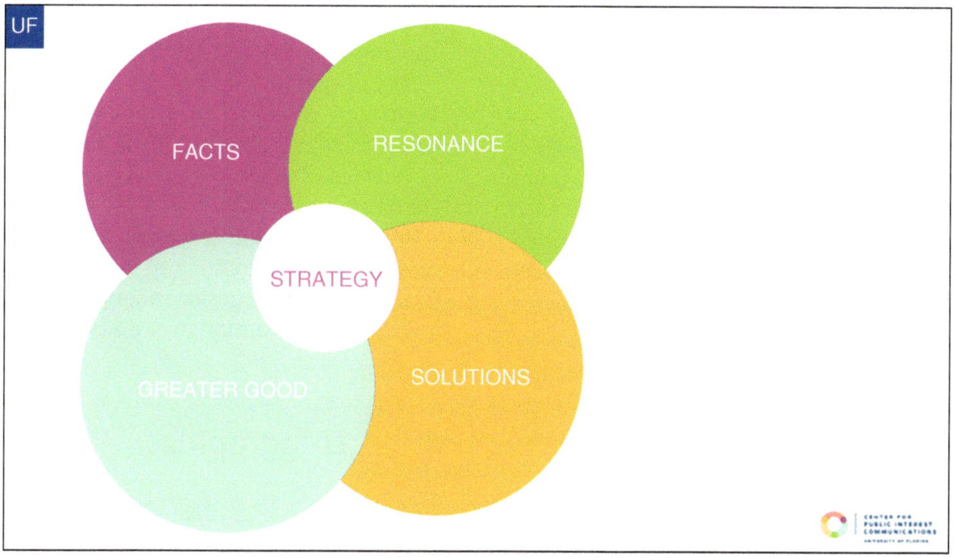

Fig. 16.2. The essential elements of public interest communication. Credit: Searight and Sheehan (2023).

Learning questions: After reading this 88-word definition, who do you think this definition is designed for? What parts of this definition are necessary to include when introducing One Health to a novice audience? Which words can be better clarified? Can you circle the words that are appropriate for scientists and health professionals?

Recently, I ran an impromptu survey in a local coffee shop and asked several strangers without a science background to read and interpret this 88-word definition of One Health. I then asked them to explain One Health back to me to see if they understood the full breadth of One Health. I also asked them for an explanation of certain words in the aforementioned definition. The words with the highest incidence of misinterpretations were: ecosystems, domestic (animals), interdependent, sectors and disciplines.

Can you run a similar survey at your school with non-health and non-science students? Did you find similar or different points of confusion or opportunity for misinterpretation that could possibly lead to misinformation? More on this later.

16.3 Word Choice Matters

Do you think the general public (particularly people who have not recently taken a biology class or claim to be a biologist) will readily explain the difference between '**ecosystems**' and '**environment**'? Do you think all final-year secondary school students will understand the difference between '**sectors**' and '**disciplines**'?

Recently, I was teaching about One Health in a classroom full of 17- and 18-year-old students at a secondary school. English was the first language of all students in the classroom. I explained the '**One Health approach**' as 'teamwork between people of different backgrounds, disciplines and strengths to prevent and solve health problems'. I then asked the students what type of disciplines could be engaged to prevent a disease outbreak. There was silence. I realized that they were stuck on the word 'discipline'. I asked what 'discipline' means to them and was told by the students that they were thinking of the definition that is related to punishment. No wonder there was silence! I agreed with them that this is one definition but there is another meaning to the word as well – one that has to do with the study area a person dedicates their life to and gave examples like a veterinarian, a nurse, etc. The conversation continued seamlessly after that explanation, but it was a reminder that, despite having taught thousands of students about One Health, not all audiences are the same. Choose your words carefully and do frequent subtle check-ins to ensure there is no confusion, or worse, misinformation.

16.4 Misinformation vs Disinformation

After the COVID-19 pandemic, the general public has become accustomed to hearing the powerful terms of '**misinformation**' and '**disinformation**'. These words have been heard on the radio and seen in print and are thrown around to such a degree that it is generally assumed that people know the difference. Unfortunately, this is not the case as described in the World Health Organization's Infodemic Management Course (WHO, 2021). Both terms relate to wrong information but let's be clear on the distinct difference: misinformation is an honest mistake and disinformation is purposefully feeding wrong information in order to manipulate a population's views.

Learning questions: Can you think of examples in your life when you encountered (or spread) misinformation? Can you think of examples in your life when you encountered (or spread) disinformation?

Let's now think through your adolescent years. What type of gossip went through your school or social group? Where did you hear the news? Social media? Radio? Television? Friends? News? Healthcare experts?

Similarly, have you seen examples of misinformation or disinformation in films? If so, which films and do you consider your examples to be related to misinformation or disinformation?

16.5 Infographics

Images can be powerful. They can tell stories. They can also cause confusion. They also limit the audience by excluding visually impaired people, unless additional alternative texts are made available with technology.

Does the image translate equally as well to people who have colour blindness? Be aware of where and when to utilize any type of image. Is it accessible to everybody in the audience? When choosing an infographic to describe One Health, or anything else, a tip is to select one that accompanies a concise explanation. Can you try to explain the infographic in Fig. 16.3 concisely?

Would you explain the entire infographic at once or would you try to break it up into sections? If sections, then which part would you choose to tackle first? Honestly, the answer should be 'it depends on the audience'.

When speaking with university professors and other academics, starting on the far left 'sectors and disciplines' would be the most relatable because universities are divided into categories – College of Engineering, Ecology Department, etc.

However, where would you start if you are speaking with children? The most logical answer is the lower central circle where there is the merging of healthy animals, healthy ecosystems and healthy humans. Out of these three sections, which do you think should be spoken first – humans, ecosystems or animals? Typically, children gravitate toward animals so you will probably be able to capture your young audience's attention more easily if you first mention 'healthy animals'. Keep in mind, however, that words matter and you will need to ensure that the young audience understands the word 'ecosystems' before moving beyond this circle to any other place in the infographic.

What type of audience would care the most about the far-right circle with the 'society' heading? Do you think children would care very much? Depending on the age, some children may (and some may not) know what the word 'society' means. The answer to the initial question here is government workers, including legislators and other policy makers. Similarly, non-government workers at the international level would also probably value the 'society' circle the most, if forced to choose.

The next section of the infographic to dissect is the central area with gears and the words: Communication, Coordination, Collaboration and Capacity Building. Who would pay particular attention to these words? The answer could be everybody who works within a One Health team unit, as well as those who sponsor such units. It is important, however, to ensure that your audience understands these words because one in particular can be fraught with vague definitions. Can you guess which term is the vaguest? It is '**Capacity Building**'. How would you define it? How would your classmate define it?

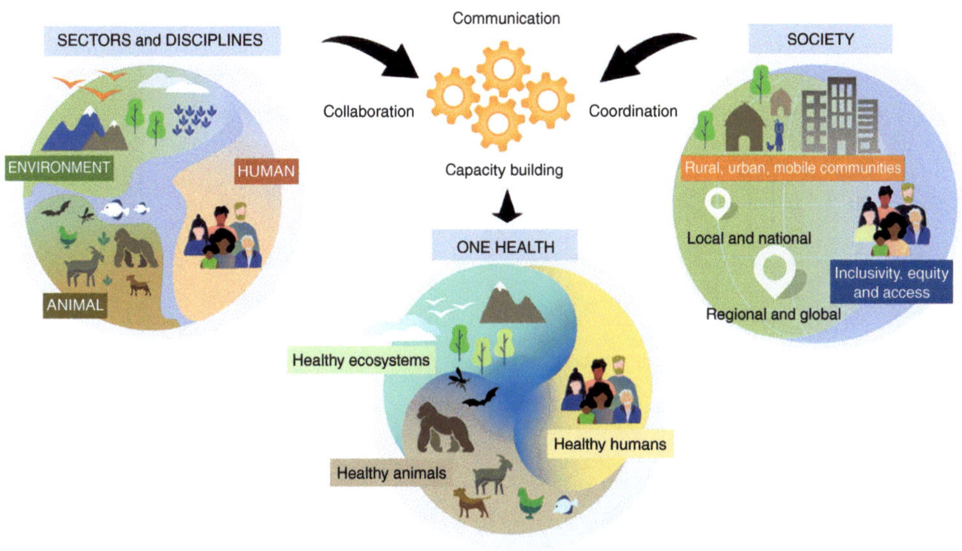

Fig. 16.3. Infographic describing how the sectors, disciplines and society come together in a process of communication, collaboration, coordination and capacity building to achieve healthy ecosystems, humans and animals through One Health (OHHLEP *et al.*, 2022). (From Mettenleiter *et al.*, 2023, unmodified, CC BY 4.0 DEED: https://creativecommons.org/licenses/by/4.0/.)

Learning questions: I recommend to pause here and write your definition of Capacity Building down and have a classmate do the same. Now compare your answers. Are the two definitions identical? 'Capacity Building' is considered to be jargon and can be open to interpretation, based on where you first learned the term.

To illustrate the variety of interpretations of 'Capacity Building', I asked the Artificial Intelligence program Freepik for an image expressing 'Capacity Building', and two of the search results included the images in Fig. 16.4. Can you create a story out of these two images? Do the two stories have much overlap?

Similar to 'misinformation' and 'disinformation', 'Capacity Building' may be recognized as familiar by an audience but it may not be clearly understood. The United Nations defines Capacity Building as 'the process of developing and strengthening the skills, instincts, abilities, processes and resources that organizations and communities need to survive, adapt, and thrive in a fast-changing world' (United Nations, 2024). How can you explain Capacity Building using fewer words? A suggested answer may be 'training to make others self-sufficient'. What other abbreviated definitions can you create to ensure your audience understands the general concept of Capacity Building?

16.6 Practise Translating One Health

I am trusting that you have engaged with various chapters of the textbook and can remember (or at least go back and review) certain figures from different chapters. Here, we will work toward translating specific figures and create a message that is palatable and digestible to a diverse audience.

Let's start with a topic that has been referenced in several chapters but was truly the focus of Chapter 15. You may have guessed it; it is the United Nations' **Sustainable Development Goals** as seen in Fig. 16.5 here.

Learning questions: Now pretend that you are standing in front of an audience and there is a large printed version of these Sustainable Development Goals (SDGs) on a poster situated behind you. You need to explain the SDGs to people who are hearing about them for the first time. How would you present the SDGs to different audiences?

1. Describe the SDGs to a group of children between 3 and 12 years old. Would you use words alone or would you create activities? Write down your presentation and thought process behind it.

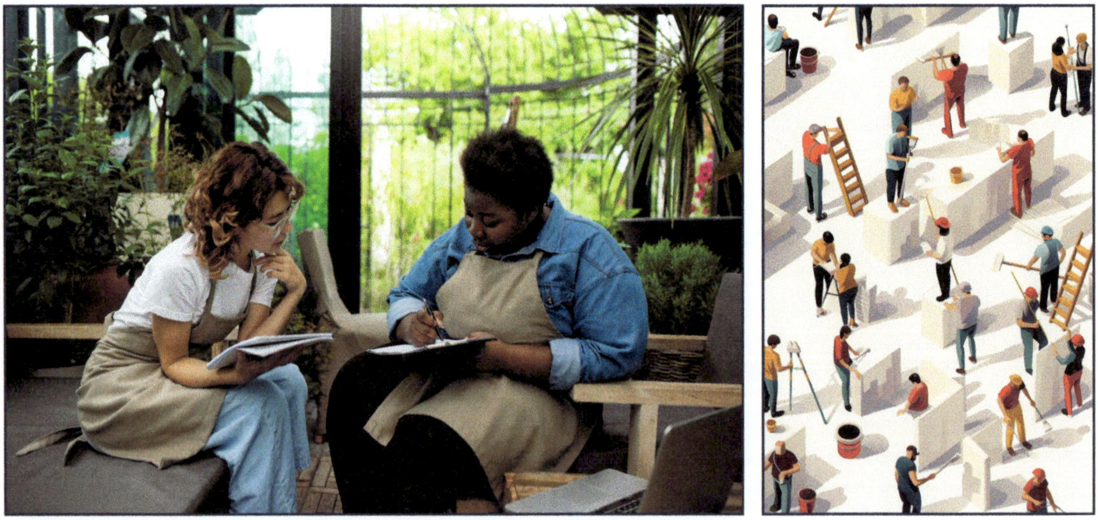

Fig. 16.4. Artificial Intelligence-generated images from Freepik.com demonstrating two possible interpretations when people first hear the words 'Capacity Building'. Personal collection of the author.

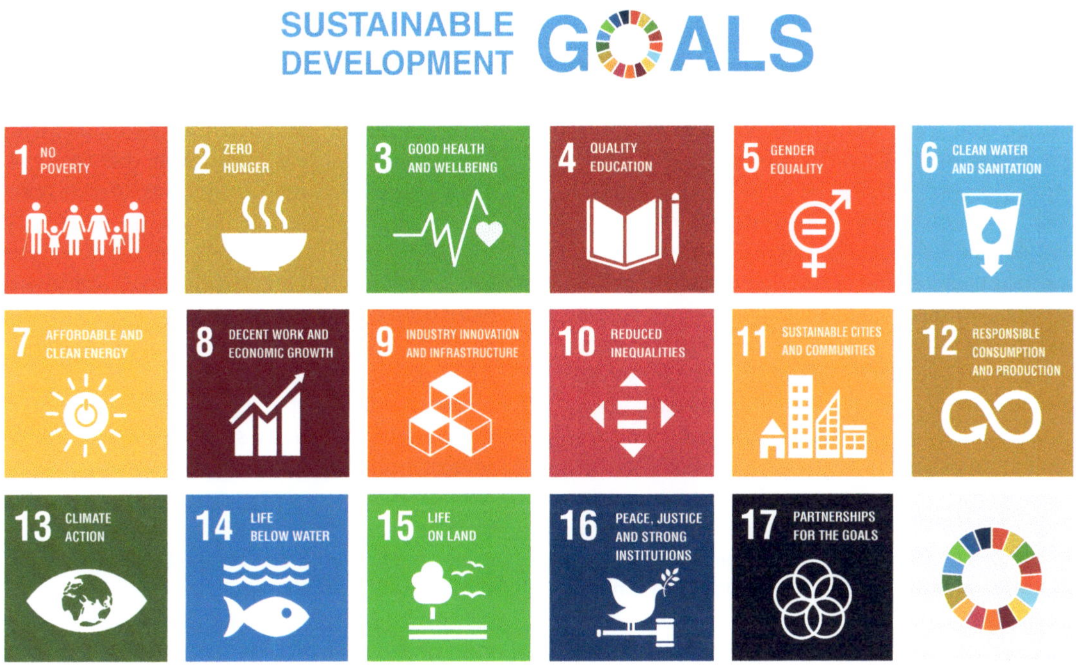
SUSTAINABLE DEVELOPMENT GOALS
1 NO POVERTY
2 ZERO HUNGER
3 GOOD HEALTH AND WELLBEING
4 QUALITY EDUCATION
5 GENDER EQUALITY
6 CLEAN WATER AND SANITATION
7 AFFORDABLE AND CLEAN ENERGY
8 DECENT WORK AND ECONOMIC GROWTH
9 INDUSTRY INNOVATION AND INFRASTRUCTURE
10 REDUCED INEQUALITIES
11 SUSTAINABLE CITIES AND COMMUNITIES
12 RESPONSIBLE CONSUMPTION AND PRODUCTION
13 CLIMATE ACTION
14 LIFE BELOW WATER
15 LIFE ON LAND
16 PEACE, JUSTICE AND STRONG INSTITUTIONS
17 PARTNERSHIPS FOR THE GOALS

Fig. 16.5. The United Nations' Sustainable Development Goals (United Nations, 2019). From https://www.un.org/sustainabledevelopment/. The content of this publication has not been approved by the United Nations and does not reflect the views of the United Nations or its officials or Member States.

2. Describe the SDGs to a group of students between 13 and 22 years old. Would you use words alone or would you create activities? Write down your presentation and thought process behind it.
3. Describe the SDGs to a group of people older than 23 years old who are university-educated adults. Would you use words alone or would you create activities? Write down your presentation and thought process behind it.
4. Describe the SDGs to a group of people older than 23 years old who are adults without a university background. Would you use words alone or would you create activities? Write down your presentation and thought process behind it.
5. Describe the SDGs to a group of people older than 23 years old who are adults without a secondary school background. Would you use words alone or would you create activities? Write down your presentation and thought process behind it.
6. Describe the SDGs to a group of people older than 23 years old who are adults who do not speak the language you are using. Would you use words alone or would you create activities? Write down your presentation and thought process behind it.
7. Describe the SDGs to a group of people older than 23 years old who are adults who have various physical or cognitive challenges. Would you use words alone or would you create activities? Write down your presentation and thought process behind it

Example answers or key points to inspire consideration and discussion:

1. At One Health Lessons, a global educational charity that teaches communities about One Health (One Health Lessons, 2024), I have taught children between the ages of 2 and 12 about the Sustainable Development Goals (SDGs). Young children do not consider much, if anything, beyond themselves but they can identify different colours and sometimes numbers. Older children can understand various relationships within a community and beyond, depending on the age of the child. However, most children between 2 and 12 can identify differences between objects. Therefore, you need to use the large colourful visual aid positioned behind you to capture their interest. Briefly speak about some key words found in the image that they may not understand like 'wellbeing', 'sanitation' or 'community' (the keywords of choice would change depending on the particular age of the children). Then create an engaging activity that encourages the children to move based on the numbers or the colours seen in the infographic. For instance, when SDG programmes are taught to young children at One Health Lessons, the colour 'blue' is called out and the young students are encouraged to rush to the poster and put a hand on any blue box. Immediately afterward, the young students are asked questions about the box they approached. From there, they are asked questions related to similar boxes like 'how does box 6 relate to box 14?' or 'does the cleanliness of the water affect the health of fish?' or 'what happens if a person eats an unhealthy fish?' or 'what can make a fish unhealthy?' and so forth. More communication and educational material for communities can be found on the One Health Lessons' website (https://onehealthlessons.org/).

2. This age range would be able to understand most of the SDGs but may need help with some choice keywords. Which keywords do you think a 13-year-old may struggle with? Once all students understand the point of the SDGs, they can enter into competitions in relation to different boxes as seen on the infographic. You could pose trivia questions or have them solve problems where the problems and solutions can be found in all areas of the world, regardless of the community's resources.

3. This group will have been exposed to disciplinary silos. Leverage their expertise to various problems that may not 'naturally fit into' their field of study. For instance, ask a veterinarian 'how can veterinarians work toward building "peace, justice, and strong institutions" (SDG16) with their skillset?' and follow up with 'who else would be ideal to work with in order to accomplish SDG16?'. This last question focuses on the One Health approach.

4. It is important to remember that everybody has something to offer and there are countless reasons for somebody to not attend or graduate from university – it could be due to financial hardship, it could be because of disinterest, it could be due to family obligations, the list goes on and on. Regardless of the reason, remember that they have much to offer and acknowledge their intelligence. It is crucial to stay humble and learn from them as much as they learn from you when discussing the SDGs. With that in mind, speak about a relatable One Health story. An example could be that you kept seeing litter being thrown into the nearby stream and that posed several problems because: (i) the litter attracted animals that could bring diseases to your community; (ii) the litter smelled bad and attracted insects; (iii) the litter blocked the downflow stream and led to flooding, increased the mosquito burden, and affected your backyard animals and your family, etc.

5. See answer to number 4.

6. With this group, you must rely heavily on the visual aid (infographic) behind you. You also must be familiar with common basic words that are familiar to the audience in their language such as 'eat', 'drink', 'breathe', 'education', 'health' and 'clean'. It is also important to have somebody with you from the community who you trust and can accurately translate your message into the other language. Messaging is always better received when delivered in a language comfortable to one's upbringing.

7. You first need to understand the goal and abilities of your audience. Why and what do they want to learn from you about the SDGs? How much information can they understand in one sitting? Again, it depends on the audience. You must tailor your message to meet the needs of the audience. If you are speaking with people who have visual impairments, then describing scenarios that the SDG infographic would represent would lead to a fulfilling conversation. If you are speaking with a group of people who cannot speak much or have cognitive challenges, then you will need to speak with this group's organizer and learn what communication techniques work the best with this particular group.

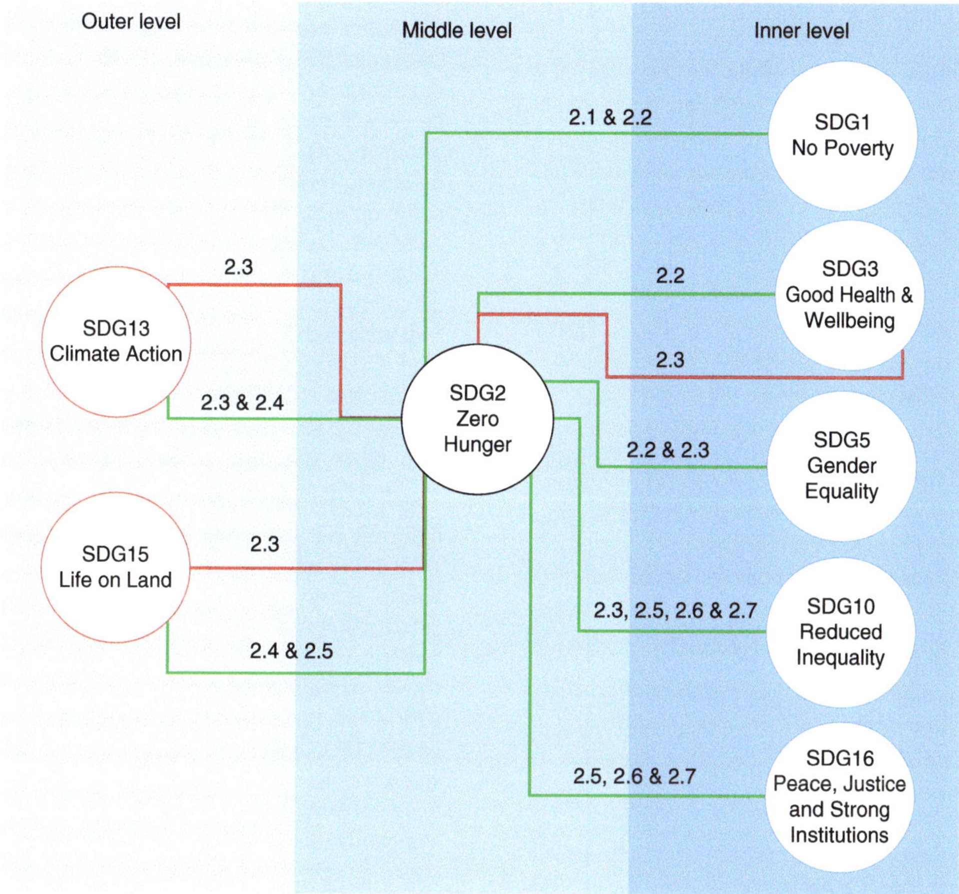

Fig. 16.6. Simplified relation between SDG2 and other SDGs. Green line, positive effect; red line, negative effect; numbers over lines, most implicated SDG2 targets.

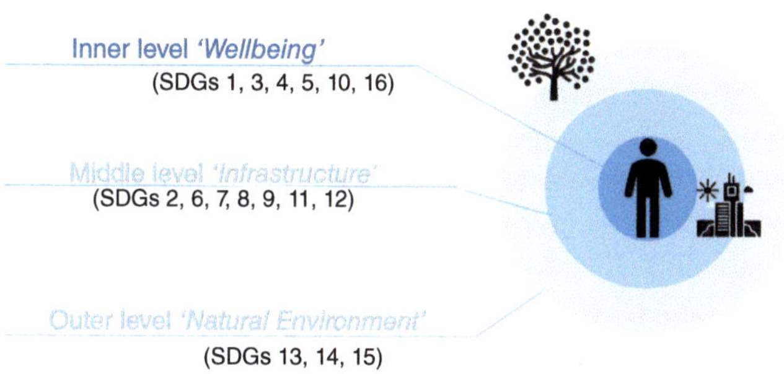

Fig. 16.7. Framework proposed by Waage *et al.* (2015).

Now let's apply what you have learned about communication and translation of complex images to something that you have seen before in this textbook. Specifically, we are focusing on Fig. 15.4 of Chapter 15 as seen here (as Fig. 16.6).

Do you remember what the authors were explaining about 'outer level', 'middle level' and 'inner level'? If not, the infographic in Fig. 16.7 was also provided in Chapter 15 (as Fig. 15.2), and it would be worth a review of this section before proceeding here.

Task:

1. Translate the message associated with Figs 16.6 and 16.7 to an audience that already understands SDG2. There is no limit to your number of words or sentences.
2. Translate the message associated with Figs 16.6 and 16.7 to an audience that already understands SDG2. Limit your explanation to 2 minutes.
3. Translate the message associated with Figs 16.6 and 16.7 to an audience that already understands SDG2. Limit your explanation to 1 minute.

Let's now leave Chapter 15 and move on to Chapter 9 that focused on **gender equality** in the context of One Health.

After reading Chapter 9, you understand that a person's '**gender**' encompasses much more than a person's '**sex**'. Instead of the usual paradox of gender being seen as only a difference of sex, you now know that 'gender' also encompasses a person's culture, ethnicity and more.

Task: Imagine that you are sitting and eating at a lunch table while at an international One Health conference. You are the youngest person at the table by at least ten years. At that table, there are men and women from different areas of the world and they are having a discussion in English. You observe that there is one person wearing a hijab, another person wearing a dastar, and you learn that there are at least three different countries represented at this one table. You hear somebody mention that they are interested in attending a lecture later that day on Gender in One Health. In response, another person expresses an opinion that this lecture would likely be very short because there is not much to say about it. You hear the second person continue by saying 'equity, equality, give everybody the same opportunity and skills and that is all they need to succeed'.

You want to add to the conversation. What do you say and how would you say it? Remember that you are the youngest at the table. Remember that English may not be their first language. Remember that respect needs to be paid to different cultures in your response. Remember that there are often many different cultures within a single country.

Example answers or key points to inspire consideration and discussion:
Your primary goal here is to approach this delicate topic strategically, avoid embarrassing anybody at the table, open others' minds to what the word 'gender' encompasses, and choose your words carefully. Given that there is a large variety of cultures represented at the table, a safe place to start is to bring everybody together in agreement; you need to start with a topic that everybody can relate to. In this example, the most obvious topic is to speak about the conference that you are all attending. From there, you may want to lightly reflect on the variety of conference speakers (keynote speakers, panellists, moderators) in relation to their impressive qualifications and backgrounds, their disciplines, their gender, their sex, their country of origin, etc.; from there, you could encourage discussion at the table by inquiring if anybody knows about the culture (and not just the country) where the speakers are found. Stay objective in your comments. Ask questions that you sincerely want to know the answers to or, at least, the opinions of others at your table. From there, you ask stimulating questions like 'I wonder if boys and girls are traditionally educated, or treated, the same way in that culture. Do you know?' or 'If a disease killed many village chickens in that community, who would be the first person in a family to be affected by it?' and then proceed to stay quiet and listen to the responses and following discussion. If the discussion does not naturally follow, you

can proceed to answer your own questions in relation to your culture but then ask others at the table how their experiences compare.

Task: Similar to the previous activity, you find yourself sitting at a lunch table but the others at your table are your friends and classmates who have the same sex as you. You hear a friend complaining that there is a newly required lecture that is focused on gender that afternoon. Your friend says 'equity, equality, give everybody the same opportunity and skills and that is all they need to succeed'. Your friend wants to skip the lecture and asks you to sign their name on the attendance sheet to hide their absence.

All your friends at the table are watching you both closely. What do you say in response and how would you say it?

Bringing Your Knowledge to Your Capital

Let's now jump from the lunch table with your peers to your country's capital city where you are preparing to speak with a government official about One Health. This official represents your area of the country and is creating a law that will ultimately permit the building of local dams that will negatively impact several homes, farms and forests. You are bringing reading material for the official and their staff to reference after you finish your meeting with them. Using your knowledge gained from Chapter 4 (**knowledge integration**), Chapter 5 (**data–information–knowledge–wisdom**), Chapter 7 (**biodiversity** and **ecosystems**), Chapter 13 (One Health economics) and Chapter 14 (**policy** and **governance**), complete the following activity.

Task: Create a one-page document that you plan to leave with the official's office after your meeting. This is often known as a policy brief. This document should include:

- The proposed law's name.
- The law's consequences on people, animals, plants and the environment in the lawmaker's territory.
- The financial implications of the law (both good and bad).
- The types of people affected by the proposed law.
- The people and organizations that oppose the proposed law.
- Your recommendations about supporting, modifying or objecting to the law's development.

Remember three important points while creating this document:

- You must avoid jargon.
- There needs to be 'more white on the page than ink' (Thomson, 2021).
- You need to understand why the official is proposing this law.

Possible helpful points to inspire consideration and discussion:

In the book entitled *The Art of Science Communication: Sharing Knowledge with Students, the Public, and Policymakers* (Thomson, 2021), a policy brief has been described as follows:

> This single page has the science policy's objective, how it affects the [area's voters], how it looks good, how it can look bad (politicians need to know both sides of a policy idea before making a decision), who already supports the policy idea, and how much the policy change would cost the country [or area]. Don't just note the problem. List at least three realistic solutions! Remember that every policy idea revolves around feasibility, timing, and money.

16.7 Conclusions

Throughout this book, you have acquired an outstanding amount of new knowledge. With this chapter, you have experienced activities that challenged you to apply that knowledge in different ways and with different audiences. Now, it is time for you to go out into your community, engage your networks, and speak about One Health in an efficient, relatable and digestible way to create positive change in the world.

References

FAO, UNEP, WHO and WOAH (2022) One Health joint plan of action (2022–2026). *Working Together for the Health of Humans, Animals, Plants and the Environment*. FAO, Rome. DOI: 10.4060/cc2289en.

Mettenleiter, T.C., Markotter, W., Charron, D.F., Adisasmito, W.B., Almuhairi, S. *et al.* (2023) The One Health High-Level Expert Panel (OHHLEP). *One Health Outlook* 5, 18.

OHHLEP, Adisasmito, W.B., Almuhairi, S., Behravesh, C.B., Bilivogui, P., Bukachi, S.A. *et al.* (2022) One Health: A new definition for a sustainable and healthy future. *PLoS Pathogens* 18(6), e1010537. DOI: 10.1371/journal.ppat.1010537.

One Health Lessons (2024) One Health Lessons [online]. Available at: https://onehealthlessons.org (accessed 11 January 2024).

Searight, A. and Sheehan, M. (2023) Just Because It's True Doesn't Mean People Care – The Science of What Makes People Care [online]. Center for Public Interest Communications. University of Florida.

Thomson, D.J. (2021) *The Art of Science Communication: Sharing Knowledge with Students, the Public, and Policymakers*. Thomson Publishing, Arlington, Virginia.

United Nations (2019) Sustainable Development Goals. Available at: https://www.un.org/sustainabledevelopment/news/communications-material/ (accessed 11 January 2024).

United Nations (2024) United Nations Academic Impact. Available at: https://www.un.org/en/academic-impact/capacity-building (accessed 5 January 2024).

Waage, J., Yap, C., Bell, S., Levy, C., Mace, G. *et al.* (2015) Governing sustainable development goals: Interactions, infrastructures, and institutions. In: Waage, J. and Yap, C. (eds) *Thinking beyond Sectors for Sustainable Development*. Ubiquity Press, London.

World Health Organization (2021) World Health Organization's Infodemic Management Course. Available at: https://openwho.org/courses/infodemic-management-101 (accessed 20 November 2023).

Glossary

We recognize that definitions are culturally constructed and can therefore have multiple meanings and that this means some terms have several alternative definitions.

Actors – includes the various individuals, groups, organizations or entities that play a role in or are affected by the functioning of a system or sub-system or network. They exert influence, perform actions, make decisions and have roles within the system or network.

Agroecology is an approach to farming that applies ecological principles to agricultural systems, aiming to create sustainable, resilient and socially just food systems. It integrates traditional knowledge, scientific research and social values.

Anthropocene refers to the current geological era, characterized by significant human impact on Earth's geology and ecosystems, including climate change, biodiversity loss and altered disease dynamics.

Anthropocentric – a world view characterized by an assumption that humans are at the centre of importance and are apart from nature and the cosmos.

Assumptions can be ontological and epistemological and will determine the methodological approach taken in research inquiry. In the One Health implementation cycle, assumptions are underlying beliefs about necessary conditions for achieving outcomes that need to be identified, evaluated and tested during implementation.

Beyond One Ocean Health or Oceans Health highlights transdisciplinary actions emphasizing aquatic ecosystems and all interconnected integrated systems and health through sustainable development, linking a healthy ocean with health and equity.

Biocentric – values all living beings, including animals, and considers their intrinsic worth and rights; recognizes the importance of non-human life forms and ecosystems, recognizing the interconnectedness of life.

Biodiversity – the variety of life in the world on earth, everything from genes to landscapes. An anthropocentric view of biodiversity assigns it value because it is crucial for ecosystem resilience and agricultural production and supports human wellbeing by enhancing species richness and diversity.

Capacity building is the process of developing and strengthening the skills, instincts, abilities, processes and resources that organizations and communities need to survive, adapt and thrive in a fast-changing world.

Chaotic system – system without obvious structure or patterns.

Citizen science – involves public participation in scientific research, where non-professional scientists contribute to data collection, analysis and problem solving.

Climate – long-term average of weather conditions in a specific region over extended periods, typically decades to centuries, encompassing temperature, precipitation, humidity, wind patterns and atmospheric pressure.

Coherence – can be a synonym for integration or the quality of building a unified whole, and means a form of oneness with significance for One Health.

Comparative medicine – an interdisciplinary and translational approach to biomedical research benefiting animal and human medicine. In an anthropocentric perspective, it is related to translational science when using animal models of disease for human medicine evolution.

Complex adaptive systems – systems, such as businesses, ecosystems, social systems or other organizations, that consist of many interconnected parts and should change as conditions evolve in order to succeed. They are open and dynamic, continually adapting to new developments.

Complex system – system having multiple pathways leading to multiple different interactive possibilities

DOI: 10.1079/9781800623002.0018

and therefore outcomes. Complex systems show emerging properties that are not predictable from the sum of their components and links (distinction to complicated systems), among other special characteristics.

Complicated system – system having multiple paths leading to an outcome. Can be (dis-)assembled and understood as the sum of its parts.

Conceptual pathway – a theoretical construct that describes the sequence of steps or events leading to a particular outcome often including visual representations of relationships between concepts.

Conservation medicine – an interdisciplinary field of study that examines the interrelationships between animal and human health within the context of ecosystems. It draws upon a diverse range of disciplines, including veterinary medicine, public health, ecology and environmental arts, humanities and sciences, to elucidate the effects of environmental change, biodiversity loss and human activities on the health of all species. This approach fosters an interdisciplinary or transdisciplinary approach to research.

Constructivism – an epistemological viewpoint that posits that the representation of reality (knowledge and understanding) emerges from the interactions of the mind(s) with the environment to construct a worldview. Thus, everyone's worldview is conditional on their personal history (*see also* objectivism and subjectivism). As a research methodology, constructivism recognises that our perception of reality is constructed and therefore available to transformation. Constructivism is also used to describe a learning theory that says people actively create their own understanding and knowledge by building on their experiences and interactions with the world around them in a cognitive or social process that starts from subjective thoughts, perceptions and individual pieces of evidence.

Core competencies – a set of skills needed in order to be proficient at a job, or other activity.

Data – symbolic representations of the real world such as numbers, letters of the alphabet, words and text, created by human observation or measurement and/or recording by machines.

Disciplines – segments of knowledge and practices that are grounded in specific intellectual traditions or paradigms. Over time, they often solidify their boundaries to maintain coherence and legitimacy and may adopt ways to ensure adherence to established norms and protect the domain.

Discounting determines the present value of future costs or benefits by applying a discount rate that reflects the time preference of people.

Disinformation is the deliberated release of false or misleading information.

Ecocentrism is a perspective that values ecosystems as a whole, independent of their utility to humans. It emphasizes the wellbeing of all species and ecological integrity. Some interpretations suggest it can involve a shift in consciousness where the ego dissolves and gives way to a sense of relational connectedness and interbeing.

Ecohealth / eco (systems) approach to health – emphasizes the intertwined connections between health and sustainable development. The central tenet of Ecohealth is the premise that human and animal health and wellbeing is dependent on that of the environment and cannot be sustained in a resource-depleted, contaminated and socially unstable planet. A wider interpretation recognizes that the relational system of processes that sustain life has health that we can choose to align and work with.

Ecosystem – biological community of interacting organisms and their physical environment. An ecosystem can also be used as a way of referring to a wider system and the processes that sustain it at individual, organizational and collective levels. An ecosystem recognizes that the thoughts, emotions, and awareness of individuals and communities are part of its overall functioning. More holistic definitions of ecosystems understand that the quality of relationships, interactions, and shared experiences within the ecosystem directly contributes to its health and effectiveness.

Ecosystem resilience – the ability of an ecosystem to absorb disturbances and still maintain or evolve its basic structure and functions. These functions can, however, be threatened by rapid climate, biodiversity loss, and other changes.

Ecosystem services are gains or benefits to humankind derived from surrounding ecosystems, including provisioning (e.g. food, water), regulating (e.g. disease control, climate regulation), supporting (e.g. nutrient cycling) and cultural services (e.g. recreation, spiritual benefits).

Effectiveness – a degree to which an initiative achieves its intended objectives and desired outcomes.

Efficiency – an extent to which an initiative uses resources effectively to achieve its outcomes, maximizing impact for input.

Emergent properties are the new characteristics or behaviours that arise from interactions within a system, often unexpected and unpredictable.

Empowerment – an ability to control one's life through actions that promote change in the factors limiting the individual's ability to take charge of his or her own life.

Environment – the surroundings or conditions in which a person, animal or plant lives or operates and the natural world, as a whole or in a particular geographical area, especially as affected by human activity.

Environmental health – anthropocentric approach of how the environment affects human health.

Epistemic practices – socially organized activities and ways through which knowledge can be and is generated, validated, interpreted and communicated. These practices vary depending on the context and underlying values, beliefs, and assumptions pertaining to the social group that determine how knowledge is generated, understood and applied. A post-humanist approach will recognize that knowledge (epistemic) practices are about how we know and recognize that there are many ways of knowing, including multispecies ways of knowing. Thus, epistemic practices can go beyond socially organized activities and respect wider ways of interpreting, validating and sharing energy, data, information and therefore knowledge.

Epistemology – branch of philosophy that tackles questions around acquiring knowledge, its nature, origins, possibilities and limits.

Equity – the fair treatment of individuals or groups, regardless of their gender, health status, species, knowledge system or worldview and just access to opportunities realized through making adjustments and taking action to account for different circumstances, needs, and disadvantages (*see also* gender equity, interspecies equity, health equity, and knowledge systems).

Evaluation is the systematic process of determining the value, quality, effectiveness or performance of a programme, project, policy or other initiative.

Externalities – the consequences of an economic activity that affects third parties who are not directly involved in the activity; they can be positive or negative.

Feasibility – the practicality and possibility of implementing an initiative or evaluation plan given the available resources and constraints.

Financial governance – the way an organization manages its financial information. It includes data collection and analysis along with monitoring usage and wastage.

Gender – socially constructed roles and characteristics associated commonly with being male or female, which can influence the impacts of health programmes owing to differing needs, access to services and societal roles. Gender is a primary way of signifying relationships of power.

Gender analysis – identifies, analyses and informs action to address inequalities that arise from the different roles of women and men, the distribution of resources, opportunities and power between them, and the consequences of these inequalities on their lives.

Gender aware – taking into consideration the set of economic, social and political roles, responsibilities, rights, entitlements, obligations and power relations associated commonly with being female and male and the dynamics between and among gender, and also taking into consideration how these factors intersect with other factors.

Gender blind – without prior analysis of the culturally defined set of economic, social and political roles, responsibilities, rights, entitlements, obligations and power relations associated with different genders and the dynamics between and among them.

Gender equality refers to women, men and people who identify differently having equal and equally respected rights, and equal access to resources and opportunities.

Gender equity refers to the process of ensuring fairness for women, men and people who identify differently as part of a gender transformative approach creating a level playing field for them.

Gender mainstreaming refers to the process of assessing the implications for women and men of any planned action, including legislation, policies or development programmes, in all areas and at all levels.

Gender norms – ability to control one's life through actions that promote change in the factors limiting the individual's ability to take charge of his or her own life.

Gender perspective – focuses particularly on gender-based differences in status and power, and considers how such discrimination shapes the immediate needs, as well as the long-term interests, of women and men.

Gender planning – planning that recognizes that because women and men play different roles in society, they often have different needs.

Gender roles – in most societies low-income women have a triple role: women undertake reproductive, productive and community managing activities, while primarily men undertake productive and community politics activities.

Governance – structures and processes to steer a particular issue. Governance occurs at different levels of a social system, often simultaneously, for example in companies, organizations, countries, or communities. Self-governance refers to the ability of individuals or groups to regulate their own behaviour, make decisions, and take responsibility without external guidance. At individual level, self-governance entails the behaviours mobilized to warrant personal wellbeing.

Habitat fragmentation – describes the process by which large and continuous habitats are divided into smaller, isolated sections, disrupting natural wildlife movement and exchange patterns.

Health – the overall wellbeing and harmonic functioning of an individual's (whether that of human or other-than-human organisms) physical, mental and behavioural states, and the degree to which they can lead a fulfilling life within their species-specific context. Health goes beyond the absence of disease or illness and includes the presence of positive factors that contribute to quality of life, equity and wellbeing. More holistic definitions take into account an individual's relations with the whole and recognize relational and spiritual health. Ultimately, health is a construct that depends on many personal, cultural and environmental aspects and may be interpreted differently in different contexts.

Health equity refers to the fair and just opportunity for everyone to attain their highest level of health. It means that no one is disadvantaged from achieving their potential due to social, economic, demographic or geographic differences.

Impact refers to the effect or influence of an initiative on its intended outcomes and the broader system or population.

Implementation research seeks to bridge the gap between research and practical application, improving how innovations are integrated into everyday systems and services.

Inclusiveness refers to the practice of ensuring that all individuals, regardless of their background, identity or abilities, are welcomed, valued and given equal opportunities to participate and contribute.

Indicator – a specific, measurable piece of data that reflects the status, progress, or change of a particular aspect of an initiative.

Indigenous Peoples – self-identification, cultural difference from other groups in a state, a special relationship with their traditional territory, and an experience of subjugation and discrimination under a dominant cultural model.

Indigenous and traditional belief systems – the health of the environment is inherently linked and inseparable from the physical and spiritual health of humans, animals and plants (*see also* knowledge systems).

Information is created when data are processed, organized, structured, analysed and interpreted, and has meaning and value.

Intangible costs and **intangible benefits** – those that cannot be easily quantified or measured in monetary terms but still have value.

Integrated approaches to health – holistic approaches that consider the interconnected aspects of health including social, economic, environmental, biological and spiritual factors. They involve collaboration among diverse people, including Indigenous knowledge holders, medical professionals, veterinarians, ecologists and policy makers in collaboration with communities, to address complex health challenges.

Integration – the action or process of integrating, successfully joining or mixing with a different group.

Interdisciplinarity – process of integration of knowledge between two or more disciplines to tackle a common problem. It entails a shared and mutual learning between disciplines, with co-adaptation of their methodologies. Interdisciplinarity has to contend and engage with the dissolution of disciplinary boundaries to allow the free exchange of insights and the development of new insights.

Interspecies equity – the consideration of non-human animals based upon their inherent self-interests.

Knowledge – the application of data and information through analysis and interpretation referring to the understanding of a subject based on experiences, insights and organized information. Knowledge can also encompass energy and be pre-informational and intuited via a right hemisphere approach.

Knowledge integration – a cognitive process of critically evaluating multiple knowledge models (or representations) and creating common ground among divergent perspectives to construct a more comprehensive understanding through integration into a common model (representation).

Knowledge systems are networks of linked actors, organizations and objects that facilitate communication and translation across diverse perspectives and between actors. They link knowledge, expertise, and practical know-how with action. They exist in various traditions that have different ways of acquiring, conserving and conveying knowledge, such as scientific knowledge, traditional ecological knowledge, or indigenous knowledge systems. In One Health and transdisciplinary processes, all forms of knowledge should be respected and utilized in decision making and action.

Land-use change refers to the alteration of land from one use to another, such as from forest to cropland, often driven by agricultural intensification.

Meta-analysis – a statistical analysis that combines results from multiple independent studies to determine patterns, relationships or effects on a particular research question.

Misinformation is incorrect or misleading information resulting from honest mistake.

Multidisciplinarity – collaborations that use knowledge and practices from different disciplines but stay within the boundaries of each field.

Nature-based solutions centre on utilizing nature to address societal challenges.

Nature contributions to people encompasses the multifaceted ways in which nature enriches human lives beyond material benefits.

Neo-classical economics – a school of economic thought that emphasizes the role of individual rational behaviour, market mechanisms and the efficient allocation of resources to maximize societal welfare.

Objectivism – an epistemic viewpoint that emphasizes the existence of an objective reality (valid and true for everyone) and holds that knowledge about reality is based on factual observation. It implies that knowledge held by a party is valid for everyone. If parties disagree, either they need to adopt the same epistemic foundation or they cannot reach consensus. This leads inevitably to epistemic inequity and disfavours all worldviews except the dominant one. Therefore, in the context of One Health, where equity is an underlying principle, objectivism is limited as a practical foundation (*see also* constructivism and subjectivism).

One Health implementation cycle – based on the concept of the policy life cycle or project life cycle, the One Health implementation cycle contains all steps through which a project or policy will exist when it is put into practice. The terms can thus be used interchangeably. The particularity about this cycle in the context of One Health is that emphasis is put on participation, co-creation and equity.

One Medicine – recognizes the similarities between human and veterinary medicine and that they can mutually benefit from each other for their development.

One Welfare – recognizes the interconnections and interdependencies between animal welfare, human wellbeing and their physical and social environment. This initiative promotes the awareness of the consequences of human activities with animals (direct and indirect use), which have profound impacts on the environment, law making, commerce and finance development, and ultimately conditioning humans' and animals' health.

Ontology – the (commonly) philosophical study of reality or being, exploring what exists in the world and relating this to epistemic practices and how we acquire knowledge about reality. It helps us better understand the concepts and categories within a subject area or domain that are used to classify and relate things.

Open awareness is an energy state (or state of receptivity) where people are connected to the field of possibility.

Opportunity cost – the value of the next best alternative that is forgone when a decision is made, reflecting the trade-offs between different choices.

Outcomes – the specific changes or effects (both intended and unintended) that result from the implementation of an initiative.

Outputs – the direct measurable and tangible products, services or activities that result from the implementation of an initiative.

Pathogen – an organism, such as a virus, bacterium, or parasite, that causes disease in its host.

Pathological states or disease – a deviation from normal physiological functioning in an individual, leading to a disturbance in its health and wellbeing.

Planetary Health focuses on the intricate connections between the health of human populations, the health of ecosystems, and the health of the planet as a whole.

Policies set the rules that direct the behaviour and actions of a population, as agreed upon through the governance structure.

Private good – excludable and rivalrous in consumption and includes most consumer products.

Problem statement – explains what the problem is in a way that covers as many perspectives as possible.

Public good – non-excludable and non-rivalrous in consumption, i.e. consumption is open to all and if one individual consumes it, there is still availability or benefits for others.

Reflective practice – a way of exploring honestly and deeply an experience to identify what happened, what one's role in the action was, to learn from this reviewing and apply insights to future situations.

Reflexivity – the practice of uncritically befriending one's being and inner purpose. This can then inform the critical examination of one's beliefs, values, attitudes, impulses and actions. The development of such awareness focuses on nurturing consciousness. The ability to enter into relational experience with awareness is described as mentalization.

Satisficing refers to the decision-making strategy of choosing an option that meets acceptable criteria rather than seeking the optimal solution (which is non-existent in open systems).

Sector – set of agencies, institutions, professions and actors operating throughout society around one domain of concern.

Sensitivity analysis assesses how the variation in the output of a model can be attributed to different variations in its input parameters.

Sex refers to biological aspects (chromosomes, genitalia, hormones, reproductive functions). These are the strictly biological, anatomical and physiological characteristics that differentiate individuals.

Simple system – a single path leads to a single output and causalities are clear.

Sixth mass extinction refers to the unprecedented rate of species extinction currently occurring, often called the 'biodiversity crisis', largely driven by human activities.

Social Determinants of Health (SDH) are the conditions in which people are born, grow, live, work and age that influence their overall health and wellbeing. These factors are shaped by the distribution of money, power and resources at global, national and local levels.

Social justice involves ensuring that the needs of marginalized communities, vulnerable populations and underserved areas are considered. (See Equity and social justice.)

Social norms – shared standards of acceptable behaviour by groups.

Social organization – the arrangement and structure of society, including social groups and institutions, which varies across cultures and time and interacts with economic and political organization.

Socio-ecological system – an integrated and dynamic system that includes both social components (socially/collectively constructed or established) and those of the ecological system, as well as their interactions, highlighting how social and ecological components co-evolve and impact each other, influencing sustainability and resilience.

Soil degradation – the decline in soil quality caused by factors such as overgrazing, deforestation, insufficient crop rotation and conventional tilling methods, reducing the capacity of the land to support plant life.

Stakeholders – all the people, groups and interested parties affecting and affected by the system. At a social level this can include customers, employees, suppliers and regulators each playing a role in different stages of the system's life. At a multispecies level in One Health, animals, plants, ecosystems and the environment can be recognized as stakeholders with interests and rights.

Subjectivism – an epistemic viewpoint that emphasizes the role of individual perception and subjective experience in the construction of knowledge. Reality is shaped by an individual's personal experiences, feelings, and biases. Subjectivism thus assumes multiple realities. In the context of One Health, it allows for the integration of diverse, often marginalized perspectives, acknowledging that each community's experiences and cultural understandings of health may differ (*see also* constructivism and objectivism). A possible challenge for subjectivism is that there is no assumed common truth and that in the context of One Health or transdisciplinary approaches it may be difficult to find a common way forward based on a common reference.

Sustainability – the ability to maintain or support a process continuously over time and avoidance of the depletion of natural resources in order to maintain an ecological balance.

Sustainable Development Goals (SDGs) – collection of 17 global objectives set by the United Nations in 2015 as part of the 2030 Agenda for Sustainable Development.

Sustainable intensification – an approach to agriculture that aims to increase food production while simultaneously protecting the environment without depleting its resources (see sustainability).

System – an interacting or interdependent group of items that work together to form a unified whole. Alternatively, a system can be seen as a set of processes in relationship that give rise to items provisionally (i.e. they are evolving and in flux).

Systems thinking – a holistic approach to investigate factors and interactions that could contribute to a possible outcome using interdisciplinary and transdisciplinary knowledge to understand complex systems, including the variety of relationships, feedback loops and dynamics within the system.

Tacit knowledge – typically gained through personal experience and practice and including insights, skills and intuitions that people acquire over time. It is often not easily described or documented.

Tangible costs and **tangible benefits** – those that are easily quantified or measured in monetary terms.

Theory of change (ToC) – a comprehensive and systematic approach that outlines the causal pathways between inputs, activities, outputs, outcomes and impacts, including causal linkages, assumptions and barriers, of an intervention or programme representing visually how and why desired changes are expected to occur.

Tipping points – critical thresholds, where small changes can lead to significant and potentially irreversible impacts, such as the collapse of the Greenland ice sheet or dieback of the Amazon rainforest.

Trade-offs – in the context of One Health interventions, trade-offs refer to the need to balance competing needs or goals across sectors.

Transdisciplinarity – the integration of academic and social knowledge through collaboration among various disciplines and stakeholders to address complex problems and challenges.

Treaty – a written agreement between two or more countries on an issue of global concern, such as antimicrobial resistance or climate change. There is agreement on the intent to act but the decision-making power is placed on the country to interpret the treaty or convention and select the best route for implementation.

Uncertainty – involves situations where the probabilities of outcomes are unknown or not well defined (probable, but not certain, situations). Working with uncertainty involves working with possibilities and addressing our desire for certainty and control. Recognizing this is particularly important when traditional science engages with philosophy, theology, social science, art and the humanities to explore co-creative methodologies and sympoietic becomings, where we embrace emergence and evolve together.

Utility – the satisfaction, happiness or benefit that a person derives from consuming goods or services based on personal and subjective preference over a set of choices.

Valuation – process of assigning a quantifiable monetary value to various entities, outcomes or impacts.

Value – worth or importance assigned to something based on its benefits, usefulness or significance that it has to people in society as well as its inherent value, which reflects the intrinsic qualities and significance it holds regardless of human perception or use.

Welfare – state of doing well, efforts to provide a basic level of wellbeing through different services.

Wellbeing – broad concept that refers to the overall quality of an individual's life, encompassing physical, mental, emotional and social health.

Wholeness – the state of forming a complete and harmonious whole; unity, the state of being unbroken or undamaged. It also refers to the state of being undivided by human dualistic thought.

Wicked problem – a complex, multifaceted issue that is difficult to define, has no clear boundaries or solution, and involves many interconnected factors, often leading to conflicting goals among stakeholders.

Wisdom – viewed through an analytical lens, wisdom extends beyond accumulated data, information and knowledge to involve the application of knowledge and experience with judgement to make sound decisions. Viewed through a process lens, wisdom involves the transcendence of paradox and duality.

Zoocentric – focus on animals and their welfare, including ethics.

Zoonotic diseases – infectious diseases shared between humans and animals, often through direct contact, vectors, or environmental exposure, with the risk of transmission increasing due to changes in climate and proximity to water sources during droughts.

Editors' Afterword

The journey we have taken through the chapters of this book has been nothing short of enlightening for us. It is the result of many years of dialogue, reflection, learning, and opening our minds and hearts to the possibilities that come when being willing to be taken into new (and sometimes uncomfortable) realms of knowledge. We hope that you have found pleasure in this book and that it has given you inspiration and useful competencies that you can apply in your professional and personal life, and that it helps you to look at and do things differently and thereby promote better health and sustainability – for us all.

The chapters in this book serve as a foundation, but the real work begins with each of us applying the One Health competencies locally, regionally and globally. Maybe you find empowerment and motivation through a better understanding of what One Health is and how we can use One Health in practice. Or you have new ideas of how you could bring certain principles or methods into your work. You might feel stimulated by deeper connections or moved by emotions that came up while engaging with the content. Maybe your curiosity is piqued, and you want to know, learn and connect more. Whatever it is, we hope that you continue the One Health learning journey, share it with others, and use your newly acquired or deepened competencies to make a positive contribution.

You might already have ideas of how you could help others to learn about One Health – whether that is in a classroom or elsewhere. It was important for us to make this book available as open access so that it can be a resource for anybody who would like to learn on their own or support others in gaining One Health competencies. As we said at the beginning of this book, it is an entry-level textbook for people who have already (or are obtaining) a tertiary education or other relevant experience and possess foundational relevant knowledge but are not yet very familiar with One Health and would like to understand what One Health is about. This of course leaves out other audiences that would also benefit greatly from One Health competencies and the empowerment they can provide. Unfortunately, it was not possible for us to create a book that would speak to all audiences, and we therefore had to decide on who to focus on as target learners for this book.

This does not mean, however, that we restrict our efforts only to the target audience. While many of the authors work in higher education and with health and other professionals, there are also several colleagues who care deeply and passionately about bringing One Health into all levels of education. By introducing One Health concepts at primary and secondary school levels, we can lay the groundwork for a generation that not only understands the interconnectedness of human, animal, plant and environment health, but also develops a mindset of collaboration, dealing with different perspectives and systems thinking from a young age. This early exposure can shape future citizens, leaders, policy makers and professionals who are equipped to tackle complex global challenges with a holistic approach. Moreover, fostering One Health awareness among younger generations can lead to sustainable behaviour changes and responsible decision making regarding environmental conservation, health practices and community wellbeing.

We often observe that children naturally demonstrate aspects of systems thinking owing to their innate curiosity, exploration and ability to make connections. At a young age, they observe, experiment and learn through interactions with their environment. They learn playfully how different elements interact within a system, explore how patterns develop, and what action may cause different expected and unexpected effects. We think that as educators, caregivers and parents we

DOI: 10.1079/9781800623002.0019

can nurture and enhance children's innate abilities through experiential learning, problem-solving activities and exposure to interdisciplinary concepts. Thus, we can extend our efforts to help children become One Health knowledgeable, skilled and capable individuals who can contribute positively to society and the planet. Given the multiple crises that we are faced with each day, this is more important than ever.

Therefore, while this book targets individuals with tertiary education or relevant experience, the overarching goal is to contribute to a broader movement that supports comprehensive One Health learning at all levels, empowering individuals of all ages to become stewards of multiple healths for those who cannot speak for themselves. We encourage you to join us on this journey. If you are interested in doing this via a particular initiative, you might look at and engage with the International One Health For One Planet Education Initiative (1HOPE) with regional groups to enhance One Health education at multiple levels (primary/secondary; tertiary/college/universities; governance/policy/advocacy/international organizations) or its spin-off activity 1HOPE-transdisciplinary research (1HOPE-TDR). Similarly, the One Health Lessons mentioned in this book provide an excellent entry point for teaching One Health concepts to children and adults. If you are interested in teaching resources, the One Health Commission website has a rich repository of useful resources. You are of course most welcome also to join our Network for Ecohealth and One Health!

At this point, you are aware that we no longer can afford to view any type of health in isolation and that we must consider the broader ecological, economic and social determinants that shape wellbeing, welfare and sustainability. Whatever path you choose for the application of your knowledge, we hope that it leverages change for a healthier, more sustainable future.

Barbara Häsler, Asta Tvarijonaviciute, Sara Savić

Index

Note: page numbers in **bold** type refer to **figures**; page numbers in *italic* type refer to *tables*.